ENDOCRINE
PHYSIOLOGY

Notice

ENDOCRINE PHYSIOLOGY

BALINT KACSOH, M.D., Ph.D.

Associate Professor of Anatomy, Physiology, and Pediatrics
Mercer University School of Medicine
Division of Basic Medical Sciences and Department of Pediatrics
Macon, Georgia

McGraw-Hill

HEALTH PROFESSIONS DIVISION

New York St. Louis San Francisco Auckland Bogotá Caracas Lisbon London
Madrid Mexico City Milan Montreal New Delhi San Juan
Singapore Sydney Tokyo Toronto

McGraw-Hill

A Division of The McGraw·Hill Companies

Endocrine Physiology

1234567890 DOCDOC 09876543210

ISBN 0-07-034432-9

This book was set in Times Roman by The PRD Group, Inc.
The editor was John Dolan.
The production supervisor was Richard Ruzycka.
Project supervision was performed by The PRD Group, Inc.
The cover was designed by Marsha Cohen.
The index was prepared by Joann Woy.

This book is printed on acid-free paper.

Cataloging-in-Publication Data is on file for this title at the Library of Congress.

To my mentors, colleagues and students with humility and respect. To my wife Gabriella, to our children Balint and Dorottya, and to our parents with love.

CONTENTS

PREFACE

Endocrine Physiology is intended to provide the physiologic foundation of clinical endocrinology: It explains humoral regulatory mechanisms, demonstrates how these processes operate in health and disease, and provides the physiologic basis for the diagnosis and therapy of endocrine diseases. The text emphasizes the molecular and cellular mechanisms of endocrine regulation in context with whole-body processes during the human life span. The mechanisms are explained in sufficient detail to support independent learning by first-year medical students. At the same time, the text intends to satisfy the needs of graduate medical education by incorporating the recent advances of basic and clinical endocrine research. The text aids both the development of skills for laboratory diagnosis of endocrine diseases and relating laboratory findings to clinical manifestations. Although the book is not case based, it facilitates the discussion of a typical case lineup used in problem-based curricula.

Endocrine Physiology is primarily intended as a core text for medical students, and as an up-to-date review of endocrinology for residents, fellows, and practicing physicians in the fields of internal medicine, pediatrics, obstetrics/gynecology, family medicine, dermatology, and psychiatry. Students and professionals of allied health sciences (e.g., physician's assistants and endocrine nurses), and graduate students enrolled in Ph.D. programs may also find it useful. The book is structured to meet the needs of these target audiences.

Part 1 covers the general concepts of endocrinology, including homeostasis, the feedback relationship between the regulator hormone and its regulated physiologic parameter, the chemical nature of hormones, the cellular aspects of hormone synthesis, secretion, and action, the general characteristics of hormone receptors and signaling mechanisms, the transport of hormones from their site of synthesis to their site of action, and the elimination of hormonal signals. The endocrine glands and their most important hormones are introduced in general terms. The last chapter of Part 1 is dedicated to clinical laboratory measurements with the intent of preparing the reader through general concepts and concrete examples to associate and interpret laboratory tests.

Part 2 covers system-based endocrinology. It is assumed that the reader will already be familiar with the material presented in Part 1 before engaging in the study of system-based endocrinology. The sequence of the chapters in Part 2 proceeds from relatively simple to more complicated systems. For this reason, calcium homeostasis and the endocrine pancreas are discussed before the hypothalamohypophyseal system and its target glands. Understanding reproductive endocrinology requires proficiency in all preceding chapters. A principal feature of endocrine regulation is the interaction between hormones. The discussion of these interactions often involves hormones that are covered in detail only in subsequent chapters. In these cases, whenever possible, sufficient information is provided to make the interactions meaningful without extensive cross-referencing.

Each chapter begins with learning objectives that help readers to identify the general scope of the presentation and to determine the emphasis of independent study. Course directors may provide a more detailed set of learning objectives tailored to specific programs. The text box format is utilized throughout the book as an extended footnote: Logic requires the material to be introduced at that point, but it breaks the main thrust of the presentation. Thus, the reader is recommended to refer to the corresponding text box, then return to the line of reasoning that preceded the text box. The content of the text boxes is heterogenous: They contain basic concepts, pathophysiologic, clinical, and other topics.

There are certain areas of endocrinology that are traditionally covered in chapters or volumes of general physiology texts that discuss the systems regulated by these hormones, most notably the hormones of the gut. In line with this tradition, this book provides only minimal coverage of gut hormones. Renal function is extensively covered from an endocrine point of view; the kidney is discussed as a target and source of hormones, as a regulator of homeostasis, and as a determinant of the elimination of hormones. However, this book does not cover every aspect of the urinary system and renal function, and its organization is different from renal physiology texts.

Both basic and clinical endocrinology are very dynamically developing fields. Today the use of database searches (such as Medline) via the Internet is within the reach of most students. Therefore, the bibliography portion of this book is very limited, and the reader is encouraged to perform on-line searches using the terms found in this book as keywords. The omission of references is by no means meant to be disrespectful to the scientists who made the discoveries; it is merely in consideration of the main target audience of this book because medical students will not benefit from extensive references and bibliographies.

I am indebted to my colleagues, who have unselfishly dedicated their time and expertise to peer-reviewing this text: Ferenc Obál, Jr, M.D., Ph.D., D.Sci. (Professor of Physiology at the Albert Szent-Györgyi Medical University, Szeged, Hungary), and my colleagues at Mercer University School of Medicine in Macon, Georgia, USA: Colleen M. Smith, Ph.D. (Professor of Biochemistry), Tarek Bisat, M.D. (Associate Professor of Pediatrics/Clinical Endocrinology), and Ananda Weerasuriya, Ph.D. (Professor of Physiology and Neuroscience). My alma mater, the Semmelweis University of Medicine (Budapest, Hungary) and Mercer University School of Medicine have always viewed medical education as a top priority. I am grateful for the institutional environment that has made this work possible. Special thanks are due to Mr. John J. Dolan, the editor at McGraw-Hill. Finally I would like to thank the support, help, and sacrifice of my family: my wife, Gabriella, our parents, and our children Balint and Dorottya.

Balint Kacsoh, M.D., Ph.D.

P.S.: In case you have been wondering, my name is pronounced as Baalint Kacho, similar to *macho* only with a *K*.

LIST OF ABBREVIATIONS

1α-OHase	25-hydroxy-vitamin D 1α-hydroxylase
24-OHase	vitamin D 24-hydroxylase
5-HIAA	5-hydroxy-indoleacetic acid
13-HODE	13-hydroxyoctadecadienoic acid
5HT	5-hydroxy tryptamine (=serotonin)
5HTP	5-hydroxy-L-tryptophan
25OH-VitD	25-hydroxy-vitamin D
1,25(OH)₂-VitD	1,25-dihydroxy-vitamin D, calcitriol
A-II	angiotensin II
AA-NAT	arylalkylamine N-acetyltransferase
ABP	androgen-binding protein
ACh	acetylcholine
ACE	angiotensin converting enzyme
ACTH	adrenocorticotroph hormone
ActR	activin receptor
ADD1	adipocyte determination and differentiation factor-1
ADH	antidiuretic hormone (=AVP)
ADP	adenosine 5′ diphosphate
AFP	α-fetoprotein
AGE	advanced glycosylation end product
AGP	α₁-acid glycoprotein, orosomucoid
AGRP	agouti-related peptide (=ART)
AHO	Albright's hereditary osteodystrophy
AhR	arylhydrocarbon receptor (dioxin receptor)
ALB	albumin
ALS	acid-labile subunit
AM	adrenomedullin
AME	apparent mineralocorticoid excess
AMH	anti-Müllerian hormone (=MIH)
AMP	adenosine 5′ monophosphate
AMPA	α-amino-3-hydroxy-5methyl-4-isoxazole propionic acid
ANP	atrial natriuretic peptide
apo	apolipoprotein
apobec-1	apoB mRNA-editing catalytic polypeptide-1
APUD	amine precursor uptake and decarboxylation
AQP	aquaporin
AR	androgen receptor

ARC	arcuate nucleus of the hypothalamus
ARNT	AhR nuclear translocator
ART	agouti-related transcript (=AGRP)
ATM	ataxia telangiectasia mutated
ATP	adenosine 5′ triphosphate
AV3V	a brain region anteroventral to the 3rd ventricle
AVP	arginine vasopressin (=ADH)
AZF	azoospermia factor
B	corticosterone
B_0	binding at zero concentration of the cold antigen in RIA (=TB)
βARK	β-adrenergic receptor kinase
BAT	brown adipose tissue
BBB	blood-brain barrier
bFGF	basic fibroblast growth factor
BGP	osteocalcin (=bone Gla protein)
bHLH	basic-helix-loop-helix (a family of transcription factors named after their conformation)
BMAL1	brain/muscle ARNT-like protein 1
BMD	bone mineral density
BMI	body mass index
BMP	bone morphogenetic protein
BMR	basal metabolic rate
BMU	basic multicellular unit (=bone remodeling unit)
BRCA	breast cancer genes and their products
BUN	blood urea nitrogen
CAH	congenital adrenal hyperplasia
CaM-kinases	calmodulin-dependent protein kinases
CAM	cell-cell adhesion molecule
cAMP	cyclic 3′,5′-adenosine monophosphate
CaR	calcium-sensing receptor
CART	cocaine and amphetamine regulated transcript
CASH	cortical androgen-stimulating hormone (uncharacterized entity)
CBC	complete blood count
CBG	cortisol-binding globulin, transcortin
CBP	CREB-binding protein
CCD	cortical collecting duct
CCK	cholecystokinin
CDK	cyclin-dependent kinase
cDNA	complementary DNA
C/EBP	CCAAT/enhancer binding protein
CFTR	cystic fibrosis transmembrane regulator
CFU-GM	granulocyte-macrophage colony forming units
cGMP	cyclic 3′,5′-guanosine monophosphate

CGRP	calcitonin gene-related peptide
CHIP	channel-forming integral protein
CIRP	cold-inducible RNA-binding protein
CLIP	corticotropin-like intermediate lobe peptide
CLOCK	circadian locomotor output cycles kaput (Zeitgeber gene)
CMO	corticosterone methyl-oxidase
CNS	central nervous system
CNTF	ciliary neurotrophic factor
CoA	coenzyme A
COMT	catechol-O-methyltransferase
COX	cyclooxygenase (=PGHS)
cPDE	cyclic phosphodiesterase
CPHD	combined pituitary hormone deficiency
CRE	cAMP response element
CREB	cAMP response element-binding [protein/transcription factor]
CRF	corticotrophin-releasing factor (=CRH)
CRH	corticotrophin-releasing hormone (=CRF)
CRH-BP	CRH-binding protein
CSF	cerebrospinal fluid
CT	1. calcitonin; 2. computed tomography
CYP	cytochrome pigment/protein
DAG	diacylglycerol
DAO	diamine oxidase
DAZ	deleted in azoospermia
DAZH	DAZ-homologue (=DAZLA)
DAZLA	DAZ-like autosomal (=DAZH)
DBD	DNA-binding domain
DBH	dopamine β-hydroxylase
DBP	vitamin D-binding globulin (= Gc)
DCT	distal convoluted tubule
DES	diethylstylbestrol
DHEA	dehydroepiandrosterone
DHEAS	dehydroepiandrosterone sulfate
DHT	dihydrotestosterone
DIC	disseminated intravascular coagulation
DIDS	4,4'-di-isothiocyanatostilbene-2,2'-disulfonic acid
DIT	3,5-diiodotyrosine
DKA	diabetic ketoacidosis
DMN	dorsomedial nucleus of the hypothalamus
DNA	deoxyribonucleic acid
DOC	11-deoxycorticosterone
DOMA	dihydroxymandelic acid
DOPA	dihydroxyphenylalanine

DSS	dosage-sensitive sex reversal gene
E_1	estrone
E_2	estradiol
E_3	estriol
ECF	extracellular fluid
ECG	electrocardiogram (=EKG)
EDTA	ethylenediaminetetraacetic acid
EGF	epidermal growth factor
EKG	electrocardiogram (=ECG)
EPAS1	endothelial PAS-domain protein-1
EPO	erythropoietin
ER	1. estrogen receptor; 2. endoplasmic reticulum
ERE	estrogen-response element
ERK	extracellular-signal-regulated kinase (=MAPK)
ET	endothelin
F	cortisol
FA-1	fertilization antigen-1
$FABP_{pm}$	plasma membrane fatty acid binding protein
FAT	fatty acid translocase (=CD36)
FATP	fatty acid transport protein
FBP	fructose-bisphosphatase
FFA	free fatty acid
FHH	familial hypocalciuric hypercalcemia (=familial benign hypercalcemia)
FHHI	familial hyperinsulinemic hypoglycemia of infancy
FKBP12	FK-binding protein 12 (FK506 is the code name of a drug)
FLAP	5-lipoxygenase activating protein
FMTC	familial medullary thyroid cancer
FRAP	FKBP-rapamycin associated protein
FSH	follicle stimulating hormone
FTI	free thyroxine index
G6PDH	glucose-6-phosphate dehydrogenase
GABA	gamma amino butyric acid
GAD	glutamic acid decarboxylase
GAG	glycosaminoglycans
GAPs	GTPase-activating proteins
Gc	group-specific component = DBP
GDF	growth and differentiation factor
GDM	gestational diabetes mellitus
GDNF	glial cell-line-derived neurotrophic factor
GDP	guanosine 5′ diphosphate
GFR	glomerular filtration rate
GH	growth hormone (=STH)
GHBP	growth hormone-binding protein

GHRH	GH-releasing hormone (often used as GRF)
GHRP	GH-releasing peptide (a type of GH secretagogue)
GHS	GH secretagogue
GHSR	GHS receptor
GHT	geniculohypothalamic tract
GI	gastrointestinal
GIP	gastric inhibitory peptide
GK	glucokinase
GLP	glucagon-like peptide
GLUT	glucose transporter
GnRH	gonadotropin-releasing hormone (=LHRH)
GR	glucocorticoid receptor (Type II glucocorticoid receptor)
GRA	glucocorticoid-remediable (hyper)aldosteronism
GRE	glucocorticoid response element
GRF	GH-releasing factor (often = GHRH)
GRP	glycine-rich RNA-binding protein (a family of proteins)
GRPP	glicentin-related pancreatic polypeptide
GSH	reduced glutathione
GTH	gonadotroph hormone(s) = gonadotropin(s)
GTP	guanosine 5′ triphosphate
Hb	hemoglobin
HBD	hormone-binding domain
HBP	helix-bundle peptide
hCG	human chorionic gonadotropin
hCS	human chorionic somatomammotropin (=hPL)
HDL	high density lipoprotein
HGO	hepatic glucose output
HHM	humoral hypercalcemia of malignancy
HIF-1α	hypoxia-inducible factor-1α
HIOMT	hydroxyindole-O-methyltransferase
HIV	human immunodeficiency virus
HLA	histocompatibility locus (or human leukocyte) antigen
HMG	1. human menopausal gonadotropin (menotropin; mainly FSH-like activity); 2. high mobility group box
HMG-CoA	3-hydroxy-3-methyglutaryl-coenzyme A
HNF-4α	hepatocyte nuclear factor-4α
HNP-4	human neutrophil peptide-4 (corticostatin)
hPL	human placental lactogen (=hCS)
HRE	hormone response element
HSD	hydroxysteroid dehydrogenase
Hsp	heat shock protein
HVA	homovanillic acid
IAPP	islet amyloid polypeptide (=amylin)
ICA	islet cell antigen

ICF	intracellular fluid
IDDM	insulin-dependent diabetes mellitus (=Type I diabetes mellitus)
IDL	intermediate density lipoprotein
IDO	indoleamine 2,3-dioxygenase
IFN-γ	interferon-γ
IGF-1	insulin-like growth factor-1 (=Sm-C)
IGF-2	insulin-like growth factor-2 (=Sm-A)
IGFBP	IGF-binding protein
IgG	immunoglobulin G
IGT	impaired glucose tolerance
IL-1β	interleukin-1β
IP	intervening peptide
IP$_3$	inositol triphosphate
IPF-1	insulin promoter factor-1 (=IDX-1)
IR	insulin receptor
IRKO	insulin receptor knockout
IRMA	immunoradiometric assay
IRS	insulin receptor substrate
ISR	insulin secretory response
IU	international unit
IVGTT	intravenous glucose tolerance test
Jak	Janus kinase
JGA	juxtaglomerular apparatus
K$_{ir}$6.2	inward rectifying (ATP-sensitive) K$^+$-channel 6.2
LAP	liver-enriched activating protein
LATS	long-acting thyroid stimulator (= TSAb = TSI)
LCAT	lecithin cholesterol acyltransferase
LDL	low density lipoprotein
LH	luteinizing hormone
LHRH	LH-releasing hormone (=GnRH)
LIF	leukemia inhibiting factor
LIP	liver-enriched inhibiting protein
LMP	last menstrual period
LPH	lipotropin
LPL	lipoprotein lipase
LPS	lipopolysaccharide (=endotoxin)
LRP	LDL receptor-related protein
M6P/IGF-2R	mannose-6-phosphate/IGF-2 receptor
MAO	monoamine oxidase
MAPK	mitogen-activated protein kinase (MAP kinase = ERK)
MCD	medullary collecting duct
MCH	melanin-concentrating hormone
MC4R	melanocortin 4 receptor
MCP	membrane cofactor protein (= TLX = CD46)

M-CSF	macrophage colony stimulating factor
MDR	multidrug resistance protein
MEK	MAP/ERK kinase
MEKK	MEK kinase
MELAS syndrome	myopathy, encephalopathy, lactic acidosis, strokelike episodes
MEN	multiple endocrine neoplasia
MGDI	mammary-derived growth inhibitor (heart-type FABP)
MGP	matrix Gla protein
MHC	1. major histocompatibility complex; 2. myosin heavy chain
MIBG	^{131}metaiodobenzylguanidine
MIH	Müllerian inhibiting hormone (=AMH)
MIP	membrane integral protein
MIT	3-monoiodotyrosine
MIX	methylisobutylxanthine
MMP	matrix metalloproteinase
MODY	maturity-onset diabetes of the young
MPF	major proglucagon fragment
MPO	myeloperoxidase
MR	mineralocorticoid receptor (Type I glucocorticoid receptor)
MRI	magnetic resonance imaging
mRNA	messenger RNA
α-MSH	α-melanocyte-stimulating hormone
MTC	medullary thyroid cancer
mtDNA	mitochondrial DNA
NADPH	nicotine adenine dinucleotide phosphate, reduced form
N-CAM	neural cell adhesion molecule
NE	norepinephrine
NEM	N-ethylmaleimide
NF-κB	nuclear factor-κB
NICTH	non-islet-cell tumor-induced hypoglycemia
NIDDM	non-insulin-dependent diabetes mellitus (=Type II diabetes mellitus)
NIS	sodium iodide (Na^+/I^-) symporter
NK	natural killer (a type of lymphocytes)
NLS	nuclear localization signal motif
NMDA	N-methyl-D-aspartate
NO	nitric oxide
NOS	NO synthase
NPR	natriuretic peptide receptor
NPY	neuropeptide Y
NRBA	neutrophil respiratory burst activity
NREM	non-REM (a stage of sleep)

NSAIDs	nonsteroidal anti-inflammatory drugs
NSB	nonspecific binding
NSILA	nonsuppressible insulinlike activity (=IGFs)
NTS	nucleus tractus solitarii
OCIF	osteoclastogenesis-inhibitory factor (=OPG)
ODC	ornithine decarboxylase
ODF	osteoclast differentiation factor (= TRANCE = RANKL = SOFA)
OGTT	oral glucose tolerance test
OHase	hydroxylase
OPG	osteoprotegerin (=OCIF)
ORF	open reading frame
OT	oxytocin
OVLT	organum vasculosum laminae terminalis
P	progesterone
p70S6k	protein 70 kDa S6 ribosomal subunit kinase
PACAP	pituitary adenylyl cyclase activating peptide
PAI-1	plasminogen activator inhibitor-1
PAS	1. protein domain having homology with Period, ARNT, and Sim (single-minded); 2. periodic acid Schiff (cytochemical staining)
PAMP	proadrenomedullin N-20 terminal peptide
PBM	peripheral blood monocytes
PBR	peripheral-type benzodiazepine receptor
PC	proprotein convertase
PCT	proximal convoluted tubule
PCOS	polycystic ovary syndrome
PDGF	platelet-derived growth factor
PDH	pyruvate dehydrogenase
PDK	3-phosphoinositide-dependent protein kinase
PEPCK	phosphoenolpyruvate carboxykinase
PER	"period" gene
PEX	*phosphate-regulating gene with homologies to endopeptidases found at the HYP locus on the X chromosome*
PFK	1. phosphofructokinase; 2. periodically fluctuating protein kinase
PGHS	prostaglandin H synthase (=COX)
PGI_2	prostacyclin
PGE_2	prostaglandin E_2
$PGF_{2\alpha}$	prostaglandin $F_{2\alpha}$
Pgp	P-glycoprotein
PH	pleckstrin homology domain
PHM-27	peptide hystidyl-methionine-27
PHP	pseudohypoparathyroidism
P_i	inorganic (ortho)phosphate

PIF	prolactin-inhibiting factor (mainly dopamine)
PIH	prolactin-inhibiting hormone (dopamine)
PI3-K	phosphatidylinositol 3'-kinase
PIP_2	phosphatidylinositol 4,5-bisphosphate
PKA	protein kinase A (A-kinase, cAMP-dependent protein kinase)
PKB	protein kinase B (=AKT)
PKC	protein kinase C (calcium-dependent protein kinase)
PKG	protein kinase G (cGMP-dependent protein kinase)
PLA_2	phospholipase A_2
PLC	phospholipase C
PMS	premenstrual syndrome
PNMT	phenylethanolamine N-methyl transferase
POA	preoptic area of the hypothalamus
Pol II	RNA polymerase II
POMC	proopiomelanocortin
PP	1. pancreatic polypeptide; 2. pyrophosphate (usually as PP_i)
PPAR	peroxisome proliferator-actived receptor
PPHP	pseudo-pseudohypoparathyroidism
PR	progesterone receptor
Pref-1	preadipocyte factor-1 (= ZOG)
PRF	prolactin-releasing factor
PRL	prolactin
PROP-1	prophet of Pit-1 (a transcription factor)
PSA	prostate-specific antigen
PTB	phosphotyrosine-binding domain
PTH	parathyroid hormone
PTHrP	parathyroid hormone-related protein
PTU	propylthiouracil
PVN	paraventricular nucleus of the hypothalamus
RAIU	radioactive iodine uptake
RANK	receptor activator of NF-κB
RANKL	RANK-ligand (= ODF = TRANCE = SOFA)
RAR	retinoic acid receptor
RBC	red blood cell
RBG	retinol-binding globulin
RBM	RNA-binding motif
RDA	recommended daily (dietary) allowance
REM	rapid eye movement (a stage of sleep)
rER	rough endoplasmic reticulum (=ergastoplasm; in neurons: Nissl substance)
RET	"rearranged during transformation" (a specific oncogene)
Rh	rhesus factor (blood group antigen)

RHT	retinohypothalamic tract
RIA	radioimmunoassay
RNA	ribonucleic acid
ROR	retinoic acid-related orphan receptor
rT_3	reverse T_3 (3,3′,5′-triiodothyronine)
RTK	receptor tyrosine kinase
RXR	retinoid X receptor
RZR	retinoid Z receptor
S	11-deoxycortisol (compound S)
SAD	seasonal affective disorder
SAM	S-adenosyl-L-methionine
SCN	suprachiasmatic nucleus of the hypothalamus
sER	smooth endoplasmic reticulum
SERCA	sarcoplasmic/endoplasmic reticulum calcium ATPase
serpin	serine-protease inhibitor (a family of proteins)
SF-1	steroidogenic factor-1
SFO	subfornical organ
SGP	stress-generated potential
SGLT	sodium glucose (co-)transporter
SH2	Src (Rous sarcoma viral oncogenic protein) homology 2 domain
SHBG	sex hormone-binding globulin = TeBG
SIADH	syndrome of inappropriate ADH secretion
Sm-A	somatomedin A (=IGF-2)
Sm-C	somatomedin C (=IGF-1)
snRNA	small nuclear RNA
SOCS-3	suppressor of cytokine signaling 3 (=ODF=RANKL= TRANCE)
SOFA	stromal osteoclast-forming activity
SON	supraoptic nucleus of the hypothalamus
SOS	"son of sevenless"
SREBP	sterol regulatory element binding protein
SRIF	somatostatin
SRY	[male] sex determining region of the Y chromosome
StAR	steroidogenic acute regulatory protein
STAT	signal transducer and activator of transcription
STH	somatotroph hormone (=GH)
SUR	sulfonylurea receptor
T	testosterone
T_3	triiodothyronine
T_3RU	T_3 resin uptake [test]
T_4	thyroxine (tetraiodothyronine)
TAF	transactivation factor/domain
TAL	thick ascending limb
TB	total bound (=B_0)

TBG	thyroxine-binding globulin
TBPA	thyroxine-binding prealbumin (=TTR)
TCA	tricarboxylic acid
TDF	testis determining factor
TeBG	testosterone binding globulin = SHBG
Tg	thyroglobulin
TGF-β	transforming growth factor-β
THBR	thyroid hormone-binding ratio
THDA	tuberohypophyseal dopaminergic neurons
TIDA	tuberoinfundibular dopaminergic neurons
TIM	"timeless" gene
TIMP-1	tissue inhibitor of metalloproteinases-1
TLX	trophoblast-lymphocyte cross-reactive alloantigen system (= MCP = CD46)
T_m	tubular transport maximum
TNF-α	tumor necrosis factor-α
tPA	tissue plasminogen activator
TPO	thyroid peroxidase
TR	thyroid hormone receptor
TRAF	tumor necrosis factor receptor-associated factor (a signal transducer)
TRANCE	tumor necrosis factor-related activation-induced cytokine (= ODF = RANKL = SOFA)
TRAP	tartrate-resistant acid phosphatase
TRE	thyroid hormone-response element
TRH	thyrotropin-releasing hormone (thyroliberin)
TRH-DE	TRH-degrading ectoenzyme (pyroglutamyl peptidase II)
TRIAC	3,5,3'-triiodothyroacetic acid
tRNA	transfer ribonucleic acid
TSAb	thyroid-stimulating antibody (=TSI)
TSBAb	thyroid stimulation-blocking antibody
TSH	thyroid stimulating hormone (thyrotropin)
TSH-R	thyroid stimulating hormone receptor
TSI	thyroid stimulating immunoglobulin (=TSAb)
TTF-1	thyroid transcription factor 1
TTR	transthyretin (= TBPA)
UCP	uncoupling protein (thermogenin)
USP	uterine-stimulating potency (units of oxytocin-like activity)
UT	urea transporter
UTR	untranslated region
UV	ultraviolet
VDAC	voltage-dependent anion channel (mitochondrial porin)
VDR	vitamin D receptor

VDRE	vitamin D response element
VEGF	vascular endothelial growth factor
VHL	von Hippel-Lindau (a tumor suppressor gene)
VIP	vasoactive intestinal polypeptide
VLDL	very low density lipoprotein
VMA	vanillylmandelic acid
VMAT	vesicular monoamine transporter
VMN	ventromedial nucleus of the hypothalamus
WAT	white adipose tissue
WBC	white blood cells
WDHA	syndrome of watery diarrhea, hypokalemia, and achlorhydria
WHR	waist-to-hip ratio
WT1	Wilms' tumor 1 (a transcription factor)
XLH	X-linked hypophosphatemic rickets
XRE	xenobiotic response element
ZOG	zona glomerulosa protein (=Pref-1)
ZP3	zona pellucida receptor glycoprotein 3

ENDOCRINE PHYSIOLOGY

Part 1

General Principles of Endocrinology

1

HOMEOSTASIS: STEADY-STATE AND ADAPTIVE RESPONSES

OBJECTIVES

1. Define the major fluid compartments of the body.
2. Compare and contrast the composition of the intracellular and extracellular fluids.
3. Discuss the causes of the resting membrane potential. Identify the unique features of "excitable tissues."
4. Define osmolality and be familiar with the quantitative aspects and consequences of osmotic changes.
5. Identify the relationship between cytosolic osmolality and the resting membrane potential.
6. Discuss the concept of pH and be familiar with the quantitative aspects and consequences of pH-changes in bodily fluids.
7. Define the terms acidosis and alkalosis, and identify their respiratory and metabolic components.
8. Identify the most important biologic buffers in the main fluid compartments of the body.

METABOLIC ENERGY MAINTAINS THE COMPOSITION OF THE INTRACELLULAR ENVIRONMENT AGAINST A DIFFERENT COMPOSITION OF THE EXTRACELLULAR ENVIRONMENT

The smallest unit capable of independent life is the cell. In a thermodynamic sense, life is a highly organized state of matter. To maintain spatial and temporal organization (to prevent an increase in entropy), cells require energy. Energy is used to (1) maintain the organization of the cell and (2) reproduce the cell. To generate chemical energy and obtain structural components, the cell must take up materials from its environment. The cell also must eliminate the byproducts of its chemical reactions. Thus, the cell must meet the challenge of exchanging materials with the environment while maintaining its organization and structure. The phenotype of the cell (the structure and function displayed by a cell) ultimately relies on the expression of specific portions of its genotype. Two aspects of the phenotype play crucial roles in the maintenance of life:

    1.   Compartmentalization—membranes that separate, for example, the extracellular and the intracellular fluid compartments; and
    2.   Function of proteins—enzymes, ion channels, and so on.

The enzymes (mainly proteins and sometimes RNA molecules) are biologic catalysts that reduce the activation energy of specific chemical reactions. These chemical reactions occur in an aqueous solution. Enzymes function well only within a narrow range of environmental parameters, which are necessary to maintain their active conformation. These parameters include temperature, ionic strength, and pH of the solution. The compartmentalization by membranes necessitates that osmotic concentration of fluids be kept within a narrow range; otherwise, dehydration or swelling/rupture would inflict osmotic injury on the cells. At the expense of energy, single-cell organisms maintain their intracellular environment in a remarkably steady state, in spite of facing an everchanging extracellular (external) environment. Single-cell organisms thus maintain the active conformation of their enzymes and the integrity of their genome. In multicellular organisms, *homeostasis* is the maintenance of the volume and composition of the extracellular environment. The maintenance of the intracellular environment is in essence *intracellular homeostasis,* which is interrelated with the extracellular environment.

THE DEVELOPMENT OF THE MULTICELLULAR ORGANISM LEADS TO THE DEVELOPMENT OF AN INTERNAL EXTRACELLULAR FLUID COMPARTMENT

During ontogeny, the development of the multicellular organism from the fertilized egg presents the cells with a new set of challenges. Even a small cluster of cells will have some cells that are directly exposed to the external environment (in the case of an embryo, the mother's bodily fluids), whereas others are enclosed by a fluid compartment surrounding the cells, and are therefore not in direct contact with the external environment. The fluid compartment surrounding the enclosed cells is an internal, yet extracellular, fluid compartment. This internal fluid known as the *extracellular fluid* (ECF) compartment is shared by the enclosed and the surface cells of the multicellular organism. As will be discussed in detail, the ECF is further compartmentalized. As a first approximation, it consists of the *intravascular compartment* (the space occupied by blood) and the *interstitial fluid compartment* (the extravascular space that immediately surrounds the cells in tissues). Advanced multicellular organisms maintain the composition of the ECF within relatively narrow limits known as the *physiological range*. The central dogma of classical endocrinology is that this "milieu intérieur" (a term coined by Claude Bernard) is steady; this is also known as *homeostasis* (a term coined by W.B. Cannon). The composition of the interstitial fluid supposedly reflects the composition of the primordial sea that served as the extracellular environment of the early cellular life forms during evolution. The composition of the *intracellular fluid* (ICF) and ECF compartments is shown in Table 1-1.

Although homeostasis is a useful initial concept in the understanding of the regulation of metabolism, this dogma is an oversimplification. *The physiological range may normally vary* with the time of the day (it may follow a circadian rhythm) and other conditions (e.g., fasting versus postprandial levels of blood plasma glucose). The conditions that require an *adaptational response* from the organism to maintain the composition of bodily fluids within the physiological range are known as *stress* (a term coined by Selye).

The surface cells of a multicellular organism are more exposed to sudden and potentially deleterious changes in the external environment than the enclosed cells. On the other hand, they are potentially better positioned to obtain nutrients (e.g., the epithelial lining of the gut). The enclosed cells (e.g., muscle or brain) enjoy protection against changes in

Table 1-1   Composition of Extracellular and Intracellular Fluids

	Extracellular (blood plasma*) concentration	Intracellular (cytoplasmic) concentration
Cations		
Na^+ (mM or mEq/L)	136–145	5–15
K^+ (mM or mEq/L)	3.5–5.1	140
Total Ca^{2+} (mM)	2.15–2.50	1–2
Free Ca^{2+}	1.16–1.32 mM	≤0.1 μM (resting)
		≤6 μM (stimulated)
Total Mg^{2+} (mM)	0.66–1.07	20
Free Mg^{2+} (mM)	0.43–0.75	0.5
pH (negative logarithm of H^+ concentration in mEq/L)	7.35–7.45 (arterial) 7.32–7.43 (venous)	7.2
Anions		
Cl^- (mM or mEq/L)	98–107	5–15
HCO_3^- (mM or mEq/L)	21–28 (arterial) 22–29 (venous)	9–18
HPO_4^{2-} (mM)	0.87–1.45	60
Proteins (mM)	About 2 mM	About 6 mM
(g/dL)	6.4–8.3 (serum)	
Osmolality (mOsm/kg H_2O)	275–295	275–295

* Extracellular fluid is exemplified by its most often tested compartment, blood plasma.

the external environment but must rely on nutrients provided to them by the surface cells through the interstitial fluid compartment. During evolution, the position of the cells therefore led to differences in their function: this specialization is the first type of *cellular differentiation.*

Having a set of protected enclosed cells offers a *survival advantage* to multicellular organisms over single-cell organisms; the protected inner cells may replenish lost surface cells with genetically identical and appropriately differentiated cells. Thus, the survival advantage manifests not at the level of any given cell of a multicellular organism, but for the multicellular organism as a whole.

HIGH INTRACELLULAR PROTEIN CONCENTRATION, THE NA⁺-K⁺ ATPase, AND THE RELATIVE IMPERMEABILITY OF THE LIPID BILAYER OF THE CELL MEMBRANE FOR IONS CONTRIBUTE TO THE MAINTENANCE OF THE RESTING MEMBRANE POTENTIAL, ISOTONICITY OF THE CYTOPLASM, AND CELLULAR VOLUME

The different composition of the intracellular and extracellular fluids, together with the characteristics of the cell membrane yield an electrical potential, known as the *resting membrane potential.* Compared to the cell surface, the inside of the cell is negatively charged; the resting membrane potential is about -90 mV. This membrane potential is in part generated by the *Donnan effect* of proteins: the higher intracellular concentration of negatively charged protein anions, which cannot penetrate the cell membrane, results in a force that favors movement of positively charged ions into the cell. (Note that cells, other than blood and endothelial cells, are not in direct contact with plasma but with the interstitial fluid, which has an even lower protein concentration than plasma, < 1 mM.)

The *electrical gradient* (or voltage gradient) of an ion is defined by the charge difference between the intracellular and extracellular compartments; the flux of any ion is driven by this gradient toward the opposite charge. The difference in concentration of an ion is known as the *chemical gradient:* this drives the flux from high toward low concentration. The vectorial sum of the two gradients is known as the *electrochemical gradient.* If the vectorial sum of the two gradients is zero for a given ion, there is no net flux between the intracellular and extracellular compartments. This state, which is known as *equilibrium,* can be calculated from the *Nernst equation* (Box 1-1).

The actual (measured) electrical potential is different from the values calculated from the concentrations of ions such as Na⁺ or K⁺; in other words, the concentrations of Na⁺ and K⁺ ions are different from equilibrium conditions. In the case of potassium, the electrical gradient favors K⁺ flux toward the intracellular compartment, but the chemical gradient points in

BOX 1-1 The Nernst Equation

The Nernst equation describes the relationship between the electrical potential and the concentration gradient of a given ion under equilibrium conditions:

$$E = \frac{RT}{zF} \ln \frac{C_e}{C_i}$$

where E is the electrical potential in volts; C_e and C_i are the molar concentrations of the ion in the extracellular and intracellular fluid, respectively; R is the universal gas constant (2 cal/mol/°K); T is absolute temperature (in °K, or °C + 273); F is Faraday's constant (2.3×10^4 cal/V/mol); z is the valence of the ion; and ln is the natural logarithm.

Although the Nernst equation is undoubtedly very useful for research and the development of a conceptual understanding, it is not routinely used in clinical practice. Thus, for a medical student it is more important to understand the implications of the equation than the ability to perform the calculations.

the opposite direction. The net electrochemical gradient favors K^+ flux toward the extracellular fluid compartment. However, owing to the opposing forces, K^+ is close to its equilibrium concentration. In contrast, both the electrical and the chemical gradients of sodium favor Na^+ flux toward the intracellular compartment leading to a high electrochemical gradient.

The difference between the actual and the equilibrium concentrations is generated by the ouabain-sensitive Na^+-K^+ ATPase, which pumps out 3 Na^+ for every 2 K^+ pumped in at the expense of the energy of one ATP molecule. Because there is a change in the net intracellular charge during this active transport, the process is *electrogenic* (approximately 5 to 10 mV).

Of the total number of ions present in the cell, only a very small quantity is actually involved in the development of the membrane potential. The lipid bilayer functions as an electrical insulation, and the ions generating the electrical potential form a layer on either side of the membrane. This arrangement is similar to that in condensers/capacitors. However, away from the membrane (i.e., in solution), electroneutrality must exist. This means that the amount of positive charge must equal that of the negative charge. As discussed below, this has a major impact on cellular osmolality.

Compared to the extracellular (especially the interstitial) fluid, the cytoplasm has high concentrations of negatively charged proteins. Although the protein concentration is high when expressed as g/dL, these high concentrations are due to the large molecular weight of proteins and translate into low molar concentrations. Because each mole of a *particle* (either undissociated molecule or dissociated ion) counts as one mole towards osmolality, the proteins themselves contribute little to osmolality. However, each protein molecule carries several negative charges, which suggests the presence of positively charged *counterions.* The presence of high (g/dL) pro-tein concentrations through this indirect mechanism means that the intra-cellular fluid would have a higher osmolality than the interstitial fluid (i.e., *hyperosmotic* or *hypertonic*). Because the membrane is permeable to water, this would lead to swelling and eventually rupture of the cells. The action of Na^+-K^+ ATPase is important not only in generating the resting potential but also in attaining *isotonicity:* it lowers intracellular osmolality by keep-ing the intracellular concentration of sodium low. Approximately 30% of the energy expenditure of an average cell is used by Na^+-Ka^+ ATPase.

Even with this energy expenditure, the physiologic distribution of ex-tracellular and intracellular ions could not be maintained if it were not for the relative impermeability of the membrane to ions, particularly Na^+. The presence of *potassium leak channels* in the membrane means that the membrane's permeability to K^+ is far greater than to Na^+. This Na^+ impermeability is the most important factor in maintaining the electrochem-ical gradient of Na^+ and the resting potential. The membrane, however, is not absolutely impermeable to Na^+; if the Na^+-K^+ ATPase is inhibited, the resting potential is gradually dissipated, with a concomitant increase in cellular volume.

Nerve and muscle are *electrically excitable cells* because their mem-branes contain *voltage-gated Na^+- and K^+-channels,* which are sequentially activated during the generation of *action potentials.* The electrically excit-able property of cells can also be conferred by *voltage-gated Ca^{2+}-channels;* this mechanism is utilized by certain endocrine cells.

HYPEROSMOLAR COMA DEVELOPS WHEN PLASMA OSMOLALITY EXCEEDS 340 mOsm/kg, AND CEREBRAL EDEMA DEVELOPS WHEN PLASMA OSMOLALITY DROPS ACUTELY BELOW 250 mOsm/kg

The quantity (not the concentration!) of osmotically active particles is expressed as *osmoles.* The moles of a substance multiplied by the number of particles into which the substance dissociates in solution determines the number of osmoles. For example, 0.15 moles of NaCl dissociates into 0.15 moles of Na^+ ions plus 0.15 moles of Cl^- ions, and therefore 0.15 moles of NaCl equals 0.3 osmoles. The *concentration* of osmotically active substances can be expressed either as osmolarity or as osmolality, which usually leads to lots of confusion. Let us first define these terms.

- *Osmolarity*—the number of osmoles per liter of plasma (i.e., total volume of solution); its unit is Osm/L.
- *Osmolality*—the number of osmoles per kilogram solvent (weight of *water* in plasma); its unit is Osm/kg. However, because the density of water is approximately 1 kg/L (it is by definition 1 kg/L at 4°C), osmolality

is often expressed as Osm/L. Note that this means per liter water (volume of *water* in plasma) and not per liter plasma.

The volume of various solutes in plasma affects only osmolarity. The density of water is affected by temperature; if osmolality is expressed as Osm/kg, it is independent of temperature. Osmolality in practice is measured by the freezing point of the solution: the freezing point of distilled water (0°C) is depressed by 1.86°C by every Osm/kg water. *The normal laboratory value of plasma osmolality by direct measurement is 275 to 295 mOsm/kg water.* A solution that has an osmolality within the normal range of plasma is termed *isotonic* (or *isosmotic*); those having higher and lower osmolalities are called *hypertonic* and *hypotonic* solutions, respectively.

In clinical practice, the effective plasma osmolality can be estimated as

$$\text{Osmolality} = 2\,[Na^+] + 2\,[K^+] + \frac{[\text{glucose}]}{18}$$

The osmolality is obtained in mOsm/kg if the concentrations of Na and K are expressed as mEq/L (or mM), and plasma glucose is expressed as mg/dL. (The division of glucose concentration by 18 is the conversion factor for glucose between mg/dL and mM.) Note that the doubling of the cation concentrations is needed for estimating the counterions (such as Cl^-), which are also osmotically active. Some texts add the molar concentration of urea (*blood urea nitrogen,* or BUN) to the formula for estimating plasma osmolality, and some neglect potassium. This is legitimate in the sense that (1) extracellular potassium concentration is normally a relatively minor component of the total osmolality; and (2) urea has an impact on osmolality measured by freezing point; however, urea in most places of the body does not contribute to osmotic forces, because depending on the presence of water channels (aquaporins) and urea transporters the cell membrane is permeable to this small, uncharged, polar molecule (in this regard, urea, water, and glycerol are similar). This difference in the calculations is reflected by the terms *osmolality* and *effective osmolality.* Note that the above calculation uses concentrations of solutes obtained in units similar to osmolarity (i.e., weight per total volume), yet in clinical practice the formula is used for *estimating* osmolality.

Plasma osmolality is strictly regulated by several factors, most notably by antidiuretic hormone (ADH; see Chap. 10). The most important determinant of plasma osmolality is the concentration of sodium, but under pathological conditions, e.g., diabetes mellitus, the contribution of glucose becomes clinically important.

Hyperosmotic and hyposmotic conditions exert a profound effect on cell volume. Depending on the membrane's permeability for the solute and the dynamics of water movement between fluid compartments, hyperosmolality may result either in cellular dehydration or cell swelling. Plasma hyperosmolality exceeding 340 mOsm/L interferes with brain function and results in *hyperosmolar coma.* Similarly, an *acute drop* of osmolality below 250 mOsm/kg, which usually happens when plasma sodium drops below 120 meq/L (known as *water intoxication*), causes cerebral edema and a high rate of mortality.

THE OSMOLALITY OF URINE IS OFTEN ESTIMATED BY MEASURING ITS SPECIFIC GRAVITY

As mentioned above, plasma osmolality is kept within a narrow range by regulatory mechanisms. The most prominent effector organ regulating plasma osmolality is the kidney. When the osmolality of plasma is high, the kidney attempts to retain more water than solute, and produces a urine with a very high osmolality (up to 1200 mOsm/kg). In contrast, when plasma osmolality is low, the kidney attempts to retain the solutes and minimize the retention of water. Under these circumstances, the osmolality of urine becomes extremely low (down to about 50 mOsm/kg). Thus, to maintain a tight control of plasma, urinary osmolality varies markedly, and the ratio of plasma and urinary osmolality may normally range between about 0.2 and 4.7.

For the assessment of urinary osmolality, an inexpensive and rapid alternative to the measurement of freezing-point depression is the measurement of *specific gravity* with a urinometer. In spite of its limitations, specific gravity is widely utilized in clinical practice.

Although proteins contribute to osmolality only to a negligible degree, the specific gravity of a bodily fluid is significantly increased by its protein concentration: for each 0.4 g/dL of protein, the specific gravity increases by 0.001 units. Thus, specific gravity is not practical for the assessment of plasma osmolality. In addition, in case of proteinuria (the presence of significant amounts of protein in urine, a pathologic condition) specific gravity values can be misleading.

The specific gravity of distilled water is by definition 1.000. The specific gravity of 1.012 approximately equals 300 mOsm/kg water; this is the specific gravity of *protein-free* plasma. In urine, the osmotic peak (1200 mOsm/kg) equals an approximate specific gravity of 1.040. Maximally diluted urine (50 mOsm/kg) equals an approximate specific gravity of 1.002.

LIFE IS COMPATIBLE WITH A PLASMA pH RANGING BETWEEN 6.80 AND 7.80

The pH of bodily fluids is tightly regulated and normally ranges in arterial plasma between 7.35 and 7.45. If pH is higher than 7.45, it is described as *alkalosis;* if it is below 7.35, it is described as *acidosis.* Thus, in a physiologic sense, a pH of 7.1 is a severe acidosis, whereas in a chemical sense a solution with a pH of 7.1 would be considered mildly alkaline.

Metabolism generates H^+ ions, which are first buffered (see below) but ultimately must be eliminated for the maintenance of intracellular pH. Although the concentration gradient of H^+ would favor diffusion towards the extracellular compartment, the net electrochemical gradient would drive the flux of H^+ towards the intracellular space. There are two major mechanisms to expell H^+ from the cells:

1. *H^+-ATPase* (proton-pump), an electrogenic transport mechanism that can be inhibited by *N-ethylmaleimide* (NEM) or *bafilomycin A* (note that this is a reversible pump, a characteristic that is exploited by mitochondrial ATP synthesis).

2. The family of *Na^+/H^+-ion exchangers* (*antiporters*), an electroneutral transport mechanism that can be inhibited by *amiloride* (a potassium-sparing diuretic drug). The transport of H^+ out of the cell utilizes the Na^+-gradient generated by the Na^+-K^+ ATPase; thus, Na^+/H^+-ion exchanger is an indirect active transport mechanism.

The secretion of H^+ by active transport mechanisms acidifies the interstitial fluid and in turn venous blood so that the arteriovenous pH difference is normally 0.01 to 0.03; that is, venous blood has a higher H^+ concentration and a lower pH. The H^+ expelled from within the cells, however, is still within the ECF, where it is buffered. The eventual elimination of H^+ from the body involves two major mechanisms:

1. Excretion, mainly in urine, by the kidneys (involves filtration and active tubular H^+ secretion processes).

2. Respiration, which blows off carbonic acid as CO_2.

The First Line of Defense against Acidic pH Is Buffering the H+ Generated by Metabolism

Buffer systems are formed by

- Weak acids plus the salt of the weak acid formed with a strong base.
- Weak base plus the salt of the weak base formed with a strong acid.

In a buffer system, the relationship between pH and the ratio of acid anion/nondissociated acid is described by the *Henderson-Hasselbalch equation:*

$$pH = pK + \log \frac{[A^-]}{[HA]} \text{ or } pH = pK + \log \frac{[salt]}{[acid]}$$

Table 1-2   Principal Buffers in the Main
Fluid Compartments

Compartment	Buffer(s)
Intravascular fluid	Bicarbonate/carbonic acid
	Prot⁻/HProt (mainly albumin)
	Within RBCs: Hb⁻/HHb
Interstitial fluid	Bicarbonate/carbonic acid
Intracellular fluid	Bicarbonate/carbonic acid
	Prot⁻/HProt
	$HPO_4^{2-}/H_2PO_4^-$

where pK is the negative logarithm of K_d (K_d is the equilibrium dissociation constant of the electrolyte). Table 1-2 displays the most important in vivo buffers and their compartmentalization.

The bicarbonate buffer system is one of the most important in vivo buffers. The chemically dissolved CO_2 (bicarbonate anion) keeps a dynamic equilibrium with the CO_2 gas, which is physically dissolved in water at the site of production of CO_2 (i.e., at the site of the citric acid cycle in tissues). The physically dissolved CO_2 is in a dynamic equilibrium with the CO_2 present in the alveolar air in the lungs. The following chemical reaction proceeds from left to right in tissues and from right to left in the lungs:

$$CO_2 + H_2O \rightleftarrows H_2CO_3 \rightleftarrows H^+ + HCO_3^-$$

An important property of this buffer system is that CO_2 as a gas readily penetrates lipid bilayers (cell membranes), but bicarbonate can penentrate the membrane only by protein-mediated transport mechanisms. The main regulator of physically dissolved CO_2 in plasma is the lung. In contrast, bicarbonate is mainly regulated by the kidneys. Thus, the Henderson-Hasselbalch equation for the bicarbonate buffer system is:

$$pH = 6.10 + \log \frac{[HCO_3^-]}{0.0301\ P_{CO_2}} \text{ or } pH = 6.10 + \log \frac{\text{kidney}}{\text{lung}} \text{ or}$$

$$pH = 6.10 + \log \frac{\text{metabolism}}{\text{ventilation}}$$

where 6.10 is the pK of the bicarbonate/carbonic acid buffer, and 0.0301 is the solubility factor of CO_2 in water used for the conversion of partial pressure of CO_2 in mmHg (P_{CO_2}) into H_2CO_3 in mM.

When the protons generated by metabolism are not precisely balanced by renal bicarbonate generation, plasma bicarbonate and pH levels decrease. This condition is referred to as *metabolic acidosis*. Causes of metabolic acidosis include

- Overproduction of acids.
- Intestinal loss of bicarbonate.
- Failure of the kidney to excrete protons, which is equivalent with failure to regenerate bicarbonate.

An important cause of metabolic acidosis is the overproduction of metabolic acids (e.g., lactic acidosis, diabetic and starvation ketoacidoses; see Chap. 9). These forms of metabolic acidoses belong to the group of *anion-gap acidoses* (Box 1-2). Lactic acidosis is an example of anion-gap acidosis where lactate anion plus Na^+ are filtered by the kidney. The Na^+ is exchanged for H^+, which is actively secreted by the kidney; the H^+ is derived from H_2CO_3 generated by carbonic anhydrase enzyme in the renal tubular cells. Thus, while the kidney secretes H^+ and eliminates lactate, it secretes bicarbonate into the circulation.

When metabolic acidosis occurs, hyperventilation can reduce the carbonic acid concentration (P_{CO_2}) of plasma; this is known as *respiratory compensation*. It is easily deduced from the equation that if acids are generated by metabolism, carbonic acid needs to be reduced to maintain

BOX 1-2   Anion-Gap Acidosis

Anion gap is defined as the difference between the concentration of the major cations and anions in serum or heparinized plasma. There are two formulae used for the calculation that yield different normal values:

- $Na^+ - (Cl^- + HCO_3^-)$: 7 to 16 mEq/L
- $(Na^+ + K^+) - (Cl^- + HCO_3^-)$: 10 to 20 mEq/L

Of course, if all cations and anions were accounted for, the difference would be zero. By using sodium (and potassium) in the formulae, most cations of the ECF are accounted for. However, a significant proportion of anions typically remains unmeasured. The anion gap is an approximation of the unmeasured anions. These anions may include proteins (mainly albumin), lactate, ketone bodies (β-hydroxybutyrate and acetoacetate), negatively charged amino acids, phosphate, sulfate, and others. If the concentration of ketone bodies increases, for example, $Cl^- + HCO_3^-$ must decrease to maintain the net zero charge in plasma. This means that the anion gap increases. Even if the ketone bodies were not directly measured, one can estimate their concentration by the anion gap. The anion gap is not increased in every form of acidosis: for example, *hyperchloremic acidosis* due to intestinal loss of bicarbonate during diarrhea and *aldosterone-deficient hyperkalemic acidosis* are associated with a normal anion gap. The reason for a normal anion gap is that the sum of $(Cl^- + HCO_3^-)$ is normal because the decreased bicarbonate is compensated by an increase in chloride.

the normal ratio and hence pH. Respiratory compensation may be sufficient to normalize pH; however, if it is insufficient, and the pH decreases, it is described as *uncompensated metabolic acidosis*. The rapid, deep breathing usually observed in diabetic ketoacidosis is referred to as *Kussmaul respiration*.

Proteins Are Large Capacity Biological Buffers

Proteins are amphoteric molecules: they contain residues that are negatively (dicarboxylic acids) or positively (lysine, arginine) charged at physiologic pH. On the average, proteins are negatively charged at physiologic pH. Due to the pK of the imidazole group of histidine (6.4 to 7.0), histidine residues perform most of the buffering function of proteins in vivo.

Intracellular proteins contribute more to the maintenance of both cytosolic and extracellular pH than extracellular proteins. This greater buffering capacity is related to the higher intracellular than extracellular concentration of proteins and an ICF fluid volume that is about twice the ECF volume. Hemoglobin, which is found in the red blood cell (RBC), has a buffering capacity about six times larger than that of plasma proteins. This is due to both its high concentration and its high histidine content. For example, during diabetic ketoacidosis, most of the H^+ (generated by the liver and dumped into the circulation as organic acid) is buffered by intracellular proteins; the extracellular H^+ enters the cell and is exchanged for K^+, which leaves the cell.

2

PRINCIPLES OF SIGNALING

OBJECTIVES

1. Compare and contrast cell signaling by nutrients and specialized molecules.
2. Compare and contrast the signaling mechanisms utilized by the nervous, endocrine, and immune systems.
3. Discuss the quantitative aspects of fluid compartments. Define the terms plasma, serum, and hematocrit.
4. Describe the transport of dissolved substances between fluid compartments through barriers. Identify mechanisms that limit accessibility of a fluid compartment for signaling molecules. Identify the types of cell signaling in which the signaling molecule reaches its target only by diffusion without entering the bloodstream. Contrast these types of signaling with those that exceed the limits of diffusion.
5. Define, compare, and contrast the terms *hormone, growth factor, cytokine, neurotransmitter, neurohormone,* and *neuromodulator.*
6. Identify the sources of hormones, and define ectopic hormone secretion and paraneoplastic syndrome.
7. Define and contrast the terminology used for describing the quantitative aspects of hormone secretion, such as in the terms *euthyroidism, hypothyroidism,* and *hyperthyroidism.* Discuss the concept of negative feedback regulation. Explain the normal range of hormones and their regulated substances in the context of negative feedback and homeostasis.
8. Discuss the mechanisms of growth and its relationship with differentiation. Describe the action of growth factors. Explain the relationship between the growth of tissues and their vascular supply. Identify cytokines as growth factors of the immune system and understand their role in the interaction between the immune and endocrine systems.

THE SIGNALING PROCESS LEADING TO COORDINATED CELLULAR FUNCTION INVOLVES NUTRIENTS, METABOLITES, AND SPECIFIC SIGNALING MOLECULES

The multicellular organism is a community of cells. As such, it must distinguish between self and nonself, and eliminate any foreign cells and macromolecules that may invade the organism. This need is met by the immune system, which maintains the antigenic integrity of the organism. The differentiation/specialization of cellular function also necessitates that the *cells coordinate their metabolic functions.* The maintenance of antigenic integrity and the coordination of metabolic function is achieved by *cell signaling.*

In its simplest form, cell signaling involves changing the composition of the extracellular fluid by taking up nutrients from, and by discharging metabolites (the products and byproducts of metabolism) into, the extracellular fluid (ECF) compartment (e.g., acidifying the ECF during the fermentation of glucose into lactic acid). This change may have an impact on the function of all cells that are reached by sufficiently high concentrations of these "signaling molecules" diffusing through the interstitial fluid. Signaling by nutrients and metabolites in the extracellular (interstitial and intravascular) fluid is an important means of coordinating metabolic function, even in higher organisms.

However, advanced multicellular organisms developed molecules specialized for signaling. These molecules are involved in the regulatory processes that help the organism as a whole to maintain its internal environment and to adapt to acute challenges. Unlike nutrients and metabolites, which act at high concentrations (mM range), most of the signaling molecules act at very low concentrations (pM to μM) and exert their effects on specialized cellular targets known as the *receptors,* which act as signal transducers. These low effective concentrations reflect high-affinity interactions between the ligand and its receptor. This high affinity contributes to the high specificity of the ligand-receptor interaction. At any given moment, the extracellular fluid contains a mixture of signaling molecules. The specificity of the ligand-receptor interaction assures that of all cells exposed to a given signaling molecule in the mixture, only those cells that have the appropriate receptor will respond to it. Thus, the availability of nutrients or an acidic environment affects the function of all cells. In contrast, any given specialized signaling molecule affects the function of only those cells that express a specific receptor.

It is important to note that low concentrations of signaling molecules have an impact on metabolites that are present in over 1000-fold concentrations. This implies that these signaling mechanisms always include *signal amplification.* For example, minute quantities of hypothalamic releasing factors evoke the secretion of far larger quantities of anterior pituitary hormones; binding of glucagon to its receptor induces adenylyl cyclase activity, which in turn activates protein kinase A (another enzyme); each enzyme acts on multiple copies of its substrate. Thus, the signal amplification cascade involves extracellular and intracellular pathways and regulation of enzyme activities.

Cell Signaling at Distances Exceeding the Limits of Diffusion Is Achieved by Nerve Fibers, Hormones, and Mobile Cells

Diffusion is suitable for transporting signaling molecules (as well as nutrients, oxygen, metabolic byproducts) only at very short distances (μm to mm range). The development of larger multicellular organisms required an effective means of distributing these substances throughout the body at distances exceeding the limitations of diffusion. Signaling at distances exceeding the limitations of diffusion is achieved by three different means, nerve fibers, hormones, and mobile cells, exemplified by the nervous, endocrine, and immune systems, respectively.

The nervous and the endocrine systems typically consist of immobile cellular components, whereas the immune system extensively uses mobile cells. Nerve cells most often form synapses with each other or with their target cells, and the transport of their signaling molecules is achieved by diffusion in the narrow synaptic cleft between the presynaptic nerve terminal (source) and the postsynaptic membrane (target). However, the nerve fiber (the axon with myelin and/or Schwann envelope), which carries the signal from the perikaryon (cell body of the neuron) to the terminal, utilizes the spread of an electrical signal known as the *action potential* along its surface. The propagated action potential is by far the fastest signaling modality used by cells.

The extracellular fluid compartment, mainly blood circulation, provides the means of delivering hormones and mobile immune cells rapidly to the target sites in effective concentrations or numbers. The main difference in cell signaling between the nervous and endocrine systems stems from the mode of delivering their signaling molecules. A given nerve cell targets only a very specific subset of potentially responsive cells, namely the ones they have a synaptic contact with. For example, all skeletal muscle fibers respond to acetylcholine (ACh), but the release of ACh at the neuromuscular junctions (a type of synapse) of the gluteus maximus muscle will not result in a generalized muscle contraction of the body. In contrast, hormones may exert a biologic effect on any potentially responsive target cell that is in a fluid compartment accessible to the hormone. For this reason, *hormonal signaling* is also referred to as *humoral signaling* (*humor* means fluid, liquid, or juice). For example, adrenaline released by the adrenal medulla into the circulation will have an effect on all vascular smooth muscle cells expressing adrenergic receptors. Hence, endocrine signaling tends to be more diffuse, more generalized throughout the body, and relatively slow (taking at least several seconds), whereas nerve signaling tends to be spatially more restricted (nerve projection-specific) and relatively fast (on the order of milliseconds).

The signaling molecules of the nervous, endocrine, and immune systems are often the same. This enables these three major regulatory systems to interact with each other and maintain homeostasis in a cooperative, integrated fashion. For the same reason, pathologic conditions affecting any of these systems may have a significant impact on the other systems.

The Development of the Circulatory System Resulted in the Partitioning of the Extracellular Fluid Compartment into Intravascular and Extravascular-Interstitial Fluid Compartments

In clinical practice, the biologic fluid samples utilized most often are systemic blood (whole blood, plasma, or serum), urine, and cerebrospinal fluid (CSF). Interpretation of the composition of these samples requires a thorough understanding of the relationship among the fluid compartments of the body.

Approximately 60% of the body weight is water. Figure 2-1 displays the distribution of water in the fluid compartments of the body. In many respects, water in the transcellular fluid and in dense connective tissue behaves as if it were in the intracellular fluid (ICF) compartment. Thus, for quick approximation, it is useful to remember that about two-thirds of this volume (40% body weight) is in the ICF compartment and one-third (20% body weight) is in the ECF compartment. Of the ECF, 75% (15% body weight) is in the form of interstitial fluid, and 25% (5% body weight) is blood plasma. (Note that the volume of blood cells is intracellular fluid.) It is important to understand that, because of the relative volumes of these fluid compartments, relatively small but generalized changes in cellular metabolic activities may lead to major changes in the composition and/or volume of the extracellular fluid.

The intravascular fluid compartment is filled with blood. Blood is a specialized connective tissue that has a liquid-phase extracellular matrix known as the *plasma. Serum* is the liquid fraction of coagulated plasma. The bulk of the cellular elements in blood belongs to the red blood cells. *Hematocrit* is the volume of packed red blood cells (RBCs) expressed as a percentage of total blood volume. Because the volume of white blood cells (WBCs) is normally negligible, the relative plasma volume can be

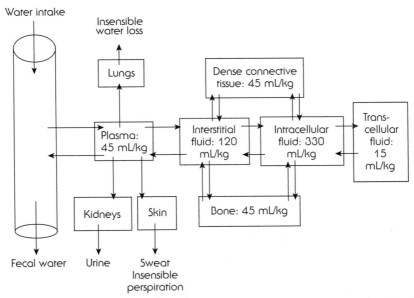

Figure 2-1. Distribution of water in the fluid compartments of the body. The total body water is approximately 600 mL/kg (60%).

expressed as $100 -$ hematocrit. The normal value of hematocrit in adults is 39 to 50% in males and 35 to 47% in females.

Specialized portions of the ECF compartment of the body (CSF; endolymph and perilymph in the inner ear; aqueous humor of the eye, etc.) are sometimes referred to as *transcellular fluid compartments*. The transcellular fluid is separated from other compartments by specialized epithelia, for example, the ependymal lining of the choroid plexus and the capillary endothelium together form a double barrier, which separates plasma from CSF.

Communication between the Intravascular and Interstitial Fluid Compartments Is Influenced by the Structure of Exchange Vessels

The vascular system has two main components: conducting vessels and exchange vessels. Significant communication between the intravascular and the interstitial fluid compartments occurs only at the exchange vessels (the capillaries, sinusoids, and pericytic postcapillary venules). All blood vessels are lined by a single layer of endothelial cells. The *capillary endothelium* may belong to one of three types: *continuous, fenestrated,* or *discontinuous.*

The continuous endothelial lining provides the tightest barrier against nonselective diffusion. *Tight junctions* (*zonulae occludentes*) limit the paracellular route of transport (i.e., through the space between adjacent endothelial cells), and cellular mechanisms limit *transcytosis* (vesicular transport involving endocytosis on one side of the endothelium and exocytosis on the other; see in more detail in Chaps. 4 and 5). Continuous capillaries are found in muscle, adipose, and connective tissues. A very tight continuous endothelial lining is found in brain capillaries and is a major constituent of the *blood-brain barrier.*

Such a tight barrier would limit the delivery of water-soluble secretory products of endocrine glands into blood and/or limit the delivery of water-soluble hormones from blood regulating the function of the endocrine gland. Most endocrine glands achieve rapid diffusion between their interstitial and intravascular fluid compartments by having a fenestrated endothelium, which has pores through the endothelial cells (Fig. 2-2). In the intestines, delivery of gut hormones into plasma is also facilitated by the presence of fenestrated capillaries.

A discontinuous endothelium associated with a discontinuous basal lamina is found in the liver. This type of endothelial lining does not represent a barrier for solutes, but prevents extravasation of RBCs. Albumin, which is the main determinant of oncotic pressure (see below) and cannot readily penetrate any other type of capillary barrier, is solely produced by the liver. In addition, the liver needs to take up and secrete high-molecular-weight lipoproteins. Thus, the discontinuous endothelium is a must for hepatic function.

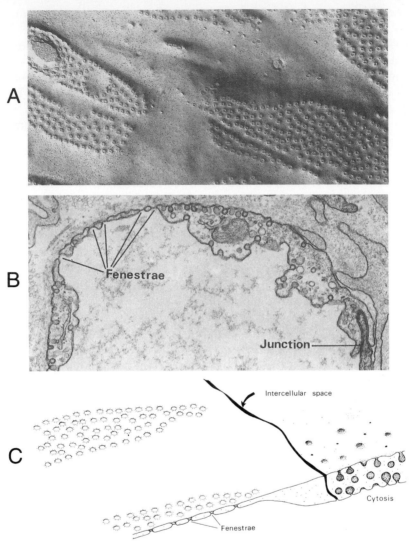

A

B Fenestrae Junction

C Intercellular space

Cytosis

Fenestrae

Figure 2-2. Fenestrated endothelial lining of capillaries. *A.* Scanning electron micrograph of the endothelial surface. The smooth areas are the thick parts of the endothelial cells, which contain the nucleus and other organelles. The small round openings arranged in clusters are the *fenestrae* (windows), which facilitate diffusion between blood plasma and the interstitial fluid. *B.* Transmission electron micrograph of a fenestrated capillary in cross section. Note the thin areas with fenestrae and thick areas with organelles and signs of vesicular transport. The fenestrae are "closed" by an electron-dense material called the *diaphragm.* The basal surface of the endothelium (i.e., away from the lumen) has a continuous basal lamina. *C.* The schematic diagram illustrates that the fenestrations are openings through the cells and not gaping spaces between adjacent endothelial cells. The cells are joined by tight junctions, which block passage of materials through the narrow intercellular space. (Source: B and C: Fig. 57, p. 90; A: Fig. 60, p. 93 in Hopkins CR: *Structure and Function of Cells,* London, Philadelphia, Toronto, Saunders, 1978.)

Transport between the Intravascular and Interstitial Compartments Is Determined by Diffusion of Solutes and Filtration of Solutions   Movement of the extracellular *fluid* between the intravascular and interstitial compartments is determined by filtration forces (Fig. 2-3). The filtration forces (also known as *Starling forces*) depend on hydrostatic pressure and colloid osmotic (oncotic) pressure. Movement of blood along the vasculature is maintained by the *hydrostatic pressure gradient* that exists between the aorta and the right atrium (or, for the pulmonary circulation, between the pulmonary trunk and the left atrium).

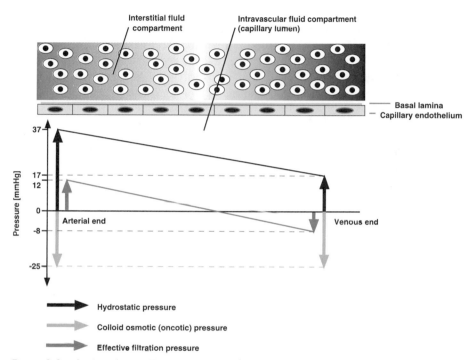

Figure 2-3.   Starling forces. The top portion of the figure symbolizes the interstitial fluid compartment, which contains metabolically active cells, and is separated from blood by the capillary endothelium and its basal lamina. The bottom portion of the figure illustrates the changes of pressure along the length of the capillary from its arterial to the venous end. The drop of hydrostatic force from 37 to 17 mmHg propels blood in the capillary lumen toward the venous end. The colloid osmotic pressure, a force opposing the hydrostatic pressure, remains practically unchanged at −25 mmHg because of the relative impermeability of the capillary to albumin. The vectorial sum of the opposing forces is the effective filtration pressure. This is positive at the arterial end, meaning that fluid moves toward the interstitial compartment, and negative at the venous end, implying resorption of fluid. Thus, the direction of the fluid movement in the interstitium parallels that in the capillary. The composition of the fluid, however, changes due to the metabolic activity of the cells, which is indicated by the color gradient in the upper part of the figure. The albumin that escaped from the intravascular compartment cannot re-enter blood at the venous end because it would have to move against the concentration gradient. The escaped albumin is taken up by lymphatic capillaries present in most tissues and eventually returns to blood with lymph (not shown).

The *oncotic pressure* is generated by the concentration gradient of nonfilterable components of the fluids found on either side of the capillary wall. What is nonfilterable is mainly determined by the pore size of the basal lamina of the capillary endothelium. The pore size of the basal lamina in the tissues is in general somewhat smaller than the pore size of the renal glomerular basement membrane (see Chap. 6). Quantitatively, the most important contributor to oncotic pressure is albumin.

The transport of *solutes,* however, is also determined by diffusion. Transport between plasma and the interstitial fluid is influenced by the solute's ability to equilibrate between the two compartments. Small molecules may rapidly cross the capillary wall in either direction, which often results in a diffusion equilibrium near the arteriolar end of the capillary. Consequently, an increase in blood flow will increase total diffusion, which means that the amount of molecules exchanged between plasma and the interstitial fluid is *flow limited.* The transport of solutes that do not reach diffusion equilibrium in the exchange vessel is *diffusion limited.*

The Concept of Hormonal Signaling Is Best Understood from the Evolving Definition of Hormones

Hormones (from the Greek word *hormao,* to stimulate) were originally defined as stimulatory chemical signals, which were secreted by endocrine glands and reached their site of action via the blood stream.

The *exocrine glands,* usually by means of ducts, secrete their products into the external environment (e.g., skin or mucosal surfaces, such as the conjunctiva, or the lumen of the gastrointestinal, respiratory, urinary, or genital tracts). In contrast, the *endocrine glands* are ductless, and secrete their products (hormones) into the interstitial fluid compartment, from which the products may enter the blood stream through the capillary wall. A list of the classical major endocrine glands and their main secretory products is shown in Table 2-1. The above definition of hormones has been revised extensively.

- Not all hormones stimulate cellular function. The discovery of inhibitory hormones (such as the general turn-off signal molecule somatostatin) led to the conclusion that hormones are regulators of cellular function.
- Not all hormones are produced by the classical endocrine (ductless) glands. Important examples include
    - Active vitamin D_3, a product of the coordinated function of the skin, liver, and kidney.
    - Oxytocin and antidiuretic hormone, produced by neurons in the hypothalamus.
    - Erythropoietin, secreted by peritubular endothelial cells of the renal cortex.
    - Atrial natriuretic peptide, secreted by cardiomyocytes.

Table 2-1   Major Endocrine Glands and Their Main Secretory Products

Endocrine gland	Subdivision	Main secretory products
Pineal gland (epiphysis)	—	Melatonin
Pituitary gland (hypophysis)	Adenohypophysis	Growth hormone (GH); prolactin (PRL); adrenocorticotroph hormone (ACTH); gonadotropins (follicle-stimulating hormone [FSH]; luteinizing hormone [LH]); thyroid-stimulating hormone (TSH).
	Neurohypophysis	Oxytocin (OT); arginine vasopressin (AVP or antidiuretic hormone [ADH]).
Adrenal gland	Cortex	Aldosterone; cortisol (F); androstenedione; dehydroepiandrosterone (DHEA); DHEA-sulfate (DHEAS).
	Medulla	Adrenaline (epinephrine); noradrenaline (norepinephrine).
Testis	Leydig cells	Testosterone (T); Estradiol (E_2).
	Sertoli cells	Inhibin, Müllerian inhibitory hormone. (MIH or anti-Müllerian hormone [AMH])
Ovary	Hilar cells	Testosterone
	Follicles	Estradiol (E_2); androstenedione; testosterone; inhibin.
	Corpus luteum	Progesterone, Estradiol (E_2); inhibin.
Thyroid gland	Follicles	Thyroxine (T_4); triiodothyronine (T_3).
	Parafollicular cells	Calcitonin (CT)
Parathyroid gland	—	Parathyroid hormone (PTH)
Pancreatic islets	—	Insulin; glucagon; somatostatin (SRIF); pancreatic polypeptide.

- Several hormones are produced by cells scattered along the bronchial tree and the gastrointestinal tract, belonging to the *diffuse endocrine system.*

Certain substances act like hormones, yet either the hormone-like substance or its precursor is derived from the diet; this is exemplified by vitamin D and retinoids. When hormones are produced by neurons, they are often called *neurohormones,* and the secretory process is referred to as neurosecretion or neuroendocrine secretion.

- Hormones do not necessarily reach their site of action via the blood stream. When a hormone is secreted into the interstitial fluid compartment, it may bind to its specific receptor on the surface of the very cell which secreted it. This mode of action is known as *autocrine secretion.* When the target cell of the hormone is reached by diffusion within the interstitial fluid compartment without entering the blood stream, it is called *paracrine secretion.*

A single cell may produce several different hormones, and a given hormone may have more than one site of production or cellular origin. For example, the pituitary gonadotroph cells secrete luteinizing hormone (LH), follicle-stimulating hormone (FSH), and angiotensin II; pancreatic β cells secrete insulin, amyloid peptide, and GABA. In females, androgens are secreted by the adrenal cortex and the ovaries.

If the hormone is derived from its normal cellular source, it is described as *eutopic* hormone secretion. In contrast, if the hormone is derived from a distinct site, it is described as *ectopic* hormone secretion. Antidiuretic hormone (ADH) or ACTH produced by small-cell bronchial cancer and growth hormone-releasing hormone (GHRH) produced by pancreatic tumor are examples of ectopic hormone secretion. Ectopic hormone production is often a feature of tumors; the hormone secretion results in an endocrine dysfunction described as a *paraneoplastic syndrome*. The progression of the tumor can be monitored by measuring its hormone product.

THE ORIGINAL PARADIGM OF ENDOCRINOLOGY WAS STUDYING THE EFFECTS OF THE ABSENCE, REPLACEMENT, AND EXCESS OF HORMONES

Hormones were originally discovered by removing endocrine glands from experimental animals and studying the symptoms of the absence of their products. Cell-free extracts of the same endocrine glands were then administered to these animals, and the reversal of the symptoms was evaluated. Further fractionation and purification of the extracts led to the isolation and chemical identification of the hormones. Another experimental approach called for the administration of endocrine gland extracts to intact animals, thereby generating an excess of certain hormones. These experiments provided the foundation of the physiologic roles of the endocrine glands and their hormones.

The experimental paradigms described above are especially important from a clinical standpoint; many patients present with symptoms of diminished production, and others present with symptoms of overproduction of a certain hormone or hormones. The terminology used for describing these states includes prefixes followed by the name of either a hormone or an endocrine gland:

- *eu-* for normal hormone secretion, such as euthyroidism, eucortisolemia
- *hypo-* for subnormal hormone secretion, such as hypothyroidism, hypocortisolemia
- *hyper-* for supranormal hormone secretion, such as hyperthyroidism, hypercortisolemia

Similar to the experimental setting, hypofunction is treated with the administration of exogenous hormones. Hyperfunction may call for removal or pharmacologic inhibition of an endocrine gland. Note that the normal hormone concentration (e.g., euthyroid state) cannot be described with a single number but as a range. Patients who present with clinical symptoms of hypo- or hyperthyroidism typically have blood thyroid hormone concentrations below or above the normal range, respectively. As will be discussed later, this original paradigm is still useful, but in itself is insufficient for understanding numerous disease states.

KEEPING THE CONCENTRATION OF HORMONES WITHIN THE NORMAL RANGE IS ACHIEVED BY NEGATIVE FEEDBACK REGULATION

To achieve homeostasis, the organism attempts to keep the concentrations of regulated substances (metabolytes, electrolytes, nutrients, etc.) within the relatively narrow range of normal values. Any impact that sways these concentrations outside the normal range provokes an effort from the organism to restore the initial values. Keeping the concentration of the hormones (regulator substances) within the normal range follows the same concept of homeostasis as described for the regulated substances.

A major mechanism involved in the maintenance of the homeostasis of hormones is *negative feedback* regulation. The concept of negative feedback is that if the value of the regulated parameter is altered (falls outside the preset normal range), it serves as a signal that modulates the regulator in such a manner that the regulated parameter returns to the preset normal range. In other words, the regulated parameter is an important regulator of the regulator, which implies that the regulation is organized as a *loop* (Fig. 2-4).

This arrangement can be compared to the regulation of temperature in a house by a thermostat. If the thermostat is set to 20° to 22°C (normal range), temperatures rising above 22°C turn on the cooling system, which reduces the temperature to 20°C. At that point the thermostat turns further cooling off. Alternatively, temperatures falling below 20°C turn on the heating system, which increases the temperature to 22°C, when the thermostat turns further heating off (see Chap. 7).

The Same Signaling Molecule May Serve as a Hormone or as a Neurotransmitter

Hormones have usually been discovered as "biologic activities." This is followed by their purification and chemical identification (Box 2-1). The names of the hormones are typically related to the circumstances under which they were discovered. For example, growth hormone (GH) was discovered as a pituitary hormone that is an important regulator of somatic

A **B**

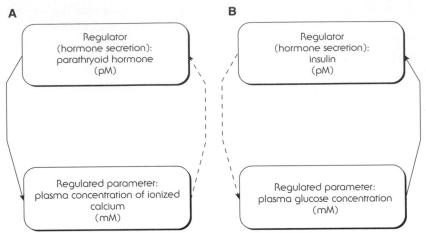

Figure 2-4. The principle of the negative feedback loop. *A.* The regulator hormone increases the regulated parameter. The increase in the regulated parameter inhibits further secretion of the hormone. In this case, a decrease in the regulated parameter serves as the activator of hormone secretion. *B.* The regulator hormone decreases the regulated parameter. Because an increase in the regulated parameter serves as the stimulus of hormone secretion, the decrease in the regulated parameter is perceived as the absence of the stimulus. Thus, a decrease in the regulated parameter inhibits further secretion of the hormone, thereby preventing its own further decrease. In both cases, the hormone-secreting cells respond to changes in regulated parameter, and the effect modulates both the hormone and the regulated parameter so as to hover around their respective normal values. The degree of normally allowed deviation from this value is the normal range, which reflects the tightness of the regulation. In these examples, the hormones and the regulated parameters are present in picomolar and millimolar concentrations, respectively. The hormones regulate the concentration of solutes that are present in 10^9-fold higher concentrations, indicating a high degree of signal amplification.

growth. The name GH, however, means neither that GH would be the only regulator of somatic growth, nor that promoting somatic growth would be the only biologic effect of GH. In fact, most hormones exert a number of different biologic actions, and most biologic processes are regulated by several hormones.

Several signaling molecules carried by the blood stream as hormones may also serve as neurotransmitters, either in the peripheral or in the central nervous system. Adrenaline, for example, is a hormone of the adrenal medulla that is also a neurotransmitter in the brain. Several peptide hormones (such as cholecystokinin and vasoactive intestinal peptide), which were originally discovered in the gut, are also neurotransmitters in the brain. These signaling molecules belong to the group of brain-gut peptides or to the *brain-gut axis.*

Neurotransmitters reach their receptors by diffusion in the confined space of the synaptic cleft. The receptors of neurotransmitters are restricted to the postsynaptic membrane. In contrast, membrane receptors of hormones may be found more or less evenly distributed on the surface of nonepithelial cells. In the autonomic (sympathetic and parasympathetic)

BOX 2-1   Orphan Receptors

The advent of recombinant DNA technology has dramatically changed the way hormones and their receptors are discovered. Quite often these molecules are cloned based on sequence homologies with previously identified hormones or receptors. This approach has resulted in the discovery of a number of molecules without known physiologic functions. The receptors discovered through this technology are usually called orphan receptors until their physiologic ligands are identified. It has been suggested that some of the intracellular orphan receptors might function as transcription factors either in a ligand-independent fashion, or that they are regulated by nonsecreted products of the same cell.

nervous system the postganglionic nerve fibers release the contents of their synaptic vesicles into the general extracellular fluid compartment; there is no synaptic cleft or defined postsynaptic membrane. The targeted smooth muscle cells carry receptors all over their surfaces; the targeted epithelial cells (usually glandular epithelium) display receptors on their basolateral membranes.

Surface-lining epithelial cells are asymmetric in nature (epithelial polarity). Their apical and basolateral surfaces are separated from each other by tight junctions that prevent lateral diffusion of membrane proteins. Membrane receptors of hormones are often distributed asymmetrically in epithelial cells.

In certain cases a hormone or a neurotransmitter has no detectable impact on cellular function when acting alone but will modulate (either enhance or inhibit) the action of another hormone or neurotransmitter. These signaling molecules are called *(neuro)modulators*. The same hormone/neurotransmitter may function as an effective stimulus for one cell type and only as a modulator for another cell type. A similar concept is covered by the term: *permissive action* of hormones/neurotransmitters (see Chap. 5).

Growth and Growth Factors

Growth factors are hormones that regulate cell growth and survival. Growth is an increase in size of the organism. Growth in a multicellular organism may include an increase of cellular size (*hypertrophy*), an increase in cell numbers achieved through proliferation (*hyperplasia*), or a combination of both. A common feature of both mechanisms is the synthesis of proteins. Hyperplasia invariably involves DNA synthesis; hypertrophy may or may not involve DNA synthesis, depending on the cell type. If hypertrophy involves DNA synthesis, it is not followed by cell division: the condition may result either in multinucleated or polyploidic cells. Deposition of fat in adipocytes and fluid retention increase the size and weight of the body, but they do not qualify as growth.

Growth of the organism from the zygote into an adult individual is a highly regulated process. Growth processes continue in the adult human body; examples include wound healing, continuous production of blood cells, and replacement of shed epithelial cells in skin and its appendages or intestinal lining. Derangement of the regulatory mechanisms results either in cell death or uncontrolled growth (tumors).

In a broad sense, growth factors are hormones or hormone-like signaling molecules that stimulate growth. This definition, however, requires the following refinements:

• Certain cell populations require the presence of a growth factor for survival. In the presence of the growth factor, the cells function normally but do not grow. Withdrawal of the growth factor causes the cells to undergo *apoptosis* (programmed cell death) or *atrophy* (reduced cellular size and diminished function).

• Certain growth factors may actually inhibit cell growth/proliferation. The antiproliferative activity of these growth factors is often associated with an ability to induce the differentiation of the target cell.

• Growth factors that induce hyperplasia must get their target cells past the G_1 checkpoint of the cell cycle.

These features display a high degree of plasticity; the same growth factor may stimulate proliferation and also be capable of inducing differentiation, depending on other factors present at the time of exposure. For example, a classic bioassay for prolactin (PRL) is the pigeon crop sac-stimulation assay. To produce crop milk, PRL exerts two different actions: It stimulates proliferation of the stem cells that are resting on the basal lamina of the stratified squamous epithelium of the crop, but it does not induce differentiation of these stem cells. PRL also induces differentiation of those crop epithelial cells that are no longer in contact with the basal lamina but does not stimulate their proliferation any longer. This example demonstrates that the extracellular matrix (e.g., basal lamina) also serves as a signaling molecule; the binding of the cells to the extracellular matrix via special membrane receptors called *integrins* results in an intracellular signaling cascade. In fact, several cell types depend on this signal for survival (*anchorage-dependence*).

A similar signaling mechanism arises from attachment of cells to each other via receptors called *cell-cell adhesion molecules* (CAMs), which are single-pass transmembrane proteins. There are two classes of CAMs: Ca^{2+}-dependent and Ca^{2+}-independent adhesion molecules. *Cadherins, selectins,* and certain *integrins* mediate Ca^{2+}-dependent adhesion. Ca^{2+}-independent adhesion is mediated by proteins that are structurally similar to immunoglobulins. The best characterized member of this class is the *neural cell adhesion molecule* (N-CAM).

Most hormones of the anterior pituitary gland are referred to as *tropic hormones* (e.g., corticotrope, thyrotrope). They are also referred to as *trophic hormones* (e.g., corticotroph, thyrotroph). Although the terms sound similar and are often used interchangeably, their meanings are quite different. Tropic (from the Greek *tropos,* direction) refers to the fact that these hormones direct hormone production by other endocrine glands, or they are targeting a specific tissue. For example, adrenocorticotrope hormone (ACTH) targets the adrenal cortex. Trophic (from the Greek *trophein,* feed, nurture) refers to the growth factor-like action of the hormone. ACTH is in fact trophic (i.e., a growth factor) for the adrenal cortex; thus the term adrenocorticotroph hormone is correct (see Chap. 12).

Many classical hormones fulfill growth factor functions in various target tissues: estrogens, for example, promote the growth of the endometrial lining, the ductal growth in the mammary epithelium, and the growth of estrogen-receptor positive breast cancer cells. However, many growth factors were discovered because of their abilities to maintain the growth of specific types of cells in culture. Later, growth factors were cloned and characterized based on their complementary DNA (cDNA) homology with already known growth factors. Sometimes the unveiling of these homologies led to the renaming of already known entities. For example, *somatomedin C,* which mediates the growth-promoting effects of growth hormone (GH), was renamed *insulin-like growth factor-1* (IGF-1) based on its homology with the amino acid sequence of insulin.

The cellular specificity of growth factors depends on the distribution of their receptors. Some growth factors, such as *epidermal growth factor* (EGF), *basic fibroblast growth factor* (bFGF) and IGF-1, display broad cellular specificity; they stimulate growth in various types of cells that express the appropriate receptor. Others display a narrow specificity and target only one type or very few types of cells. The sole targets of FSH are the granulosa cells in the ovary and the Sertoli cells in the testis. Most cells, however, require simultaneous exposure to a blend of growth factors.

In a narrow sense, *growth factor* is used for those signaling molecules that typically meet the following criteria:

- They act either on receptor tyrosine kinases or tyrosine kinase-associated receptors (see Chap. 5).
- They act in a paracrine/autocrine fashion at very low concentrations, in the range of 0.01 to 1 nM.

The transforming growth factor-β (TGF-β) family is an apparent exception because its members activate receptor serine/threonine kinases and usually induce cell differentiation and growth arrest.

Gain-of-function mutations of tyrosine kinase-activating growth factor receptors may result in tumor development. Certain *protooncogenes* and *oncogenes* have turned out to be growth factor receptors and gain-of-function mutations thereof, respectively. For example, gain-of-function mutations of RET, the receptor of *glial cell line–derived neurotrophic factor* (GDNF), may result in tumors of various cells derived from the neural crest. They present either as familial medullary thyroid cancer, type IIa or IIb *multiple endocrine neoplasia* (MEN) syndrome (see Chap. 12). Because growth factors are sometimes inhibitors of cellular growth, the gain-of-function mutation of their receptors may also lead to attenuated growth; this mechanism is seen in the development of *achondroplasia* (Chap. 8).

Angiogenesis-Regulating Growth Factors   Capillary beds are embedded within all tissues except cartilage and stratified epithelia. The growth of tissues implies that the vascular bed of the tissue grows proportionately, thereby providing appropriate nutrition and oxygen supply. The process is known as *neovascularization* or *angiogenesis*. Tumor angiogenesis is critical for the growth of primary cancers above 1 to 2 mm in diameter; above this size, the center of the solid cluster of epithelial cells does not obtain sufficient nutrition and dies (*necrosis*). The process of angiogenesis involves proliferation of mesenchymal stem cells and their differentiation into all components of the vascular wall, including endothelium. Angiogenesis is activated by turning on proto-oncogenes and upregulating the cellular hypoxia-sensing pathway (see Chap. 12). Angiogenesis is regulated by a balance of stimulating and inhibiting growth factors. Stimulators of angiogenesis include *vascular endothelial growth factor* (VEGF) and bFGF. The most potent and specific inhibitors of angiogenesis identified to date are endostatin and angiostatin, which might become useful in the treatment of certain tumors.

- *Endostatin* is a 20-kDa C-terminal fragment of type XVIII collagen. Endostatin inhibits angiogenesis and also induces apoptosis of endothelial cells.
- *Angiostatin* is a fragment of plasminogen that contains the first four *kringle domains* (triple-disulfide bridged regions of internal homology) of plasmin. Macrophage *elastase* (*matrix metalloproteinase-12* [MMP-12]) is an efficient angiostatin-producing enzyme. Angiostatin can inhibit matrix-enhanced plasminogen activation, resulting in reduced invasive activity of tumors, and thus may antagonize the progress of metastasis.

Cytokines Are the Hormones of the Immune System

The immune system guards the integrity of the organism against invasion by foreign (antigenically different, "nonself") organisms. The regulation of cellular responses in the immune system is achieved by hormones known as *cytokines*. The cytokines produced by mononuclear phagocytic cells are often called *monokines;* those produced by lymphocytes are called *lymphokines*. Because the cells involved in the signaling relationships are all leukocytes (i.e., WBCs), the cytokines communicating between them are also called *interleukins* (ILs). For many target cells, cytokines act as growth factors. Quite understandably, growth factor receptors and cytokine receptors share significant structural homology. Cytokines exert profound effects on both the nervous system (e.g., IL-1β induces sleep and fever; tumor necrosis factor alpha [TNFα] induces anorexia) and the endocrine system (e.g., IL-1β activates the CRH-ACTH-adrenal cortex axis). In return, many classical hormones modulate immune function (e.g., prolactin stimulates lymphocyte proliferation; glucocorticoids are immunosuppressive). The interactions between the immune and the neuroendocrine systems achieve an integrated adaptational response at a whole-body level.

3

THE CHEMICAL NATURE AND PRODUCTION OF HORMONES

OBJECTIVES

1. Discuss the chemical nature of hormones; be familiar with the groups and subgroups of signaling molecules based on their chemical structure.
2. Compare and contrast the typical characteristics of hydrophilic and lipophilic hormones.
3. Discuss the biosynthesis of polypeptide hormones. Discuss transcription, translation, and posttranslational modifications.
4. Discuss the action of lipophilic hormones on the transcription of polypeptide hormones.
5. Discuss transcriptional regulation and the significance of alternative promoters.
6. Discuss the impact of alternative splicing of the mRNA and of the prohormone polypeptide on the biosynthesis of hormones.
7. Discuss the difference in the regulation of synthesis and release of hormones.
8. Compare and contrast the biosynthesis, storage, and release of polypeptide, steroid, and thyroid hormones.
9. Distinguish the processes of secretion and excretion.

THE CHEMICAL NATURE OF HORMONES

Hormones may be grouped based on their chemical structure. It is useful to categorize the hormones in terms of their solubility in water and lipids as either *hydrophilic* or *lipophilic* (hydrophobic) *hormones* because their lipid/water solubility determines some of their major characteristics (Table 3-1).

Of course, there are exceptions to the guidelines presented in Table 3-1. Examples of these exceptions include the following:

• Certain polypeptide hormones, in spite of being water-soluble, circulate in plasma bound to carrier proteins. The most important example is insulin-like growth factor-1 (IGF-1); binding to its carrier proteins pro-

Table 3-1 Comparison of the Typical Characteristics of Hydrophilic and Lipophilic Hormones

Hydrophilic hormones	Lipophilic hormones
After biosynthesis, they are often stored in membrane-bounded secretory granules	Typically not stored but released as soon as synthesized
Circulate mainly in an unbound (free) form	Require binding proteins for transport in blood plasma
Short half-life in plasma	Long half-life in plasma
Cannot penetrate compartmental boundaries (e.g., blood-brain barrier) without receptor-mediated transport	Readily penetrate barriers due to their solubility in membrane lipids
Act upon plasma membrane receptors and activate second messenger systems; nongenomic action may be prominent, genomic action is indirect	Act upon intracellular receptors (ligand-regulated transcription factors): prominent direct genomic action
Most responses evoked are relatively fast and short-lived	Most responses evoked are relatively slow in onset but have a long duration
Often inactive if administered orally	Often active if administered orally
Often may be administered intravenously	Without special formulation, they must not be administered intravenously because they would cause life-threatening lipid embolism

longs its half-life to about 24 h. In comparison, insulin, which circulates in an unbound form, has a half-life of about 3 to 5 min.

• Certain lipophilic hormones transmit most of their actions via membrane receptors, e.g., melatonin and the hormonal metabolites of arachidonic acid (such as prostaglandins, leukotrienes, and anandamide).

• Steroid hormones are lipophilic, and as such circulate in a protein-bound form, but aldosterone (the main mineralocorticoid) circulates mainly in an unbound form.

• A nongenomic action of steroid and thyroid hormones has been demonstrated (see Chaps. 8, 11, and 12).

The rapid responses to hormones acting on membrane receptors are due to regulation of preexisting enzymes usually by means of phosphorylation by kinase enzymes and dephosphorylation by phosphatases.

Note that hormones acting on membrane receptors (such as the growth factors) may also regulate transcription. These responses are similar in their kinetics to those evoked by lipophilic hormones. The major groups of hydrophilic and lipophilic hormones are displayed in Table 3-2.

THE SYNTHESIS OF POLYPEPTIDE HORMONES

The biosynthesis of hormones can be classified into two major groups: (1) peptide/protein hormones, and (2) all other hormones. However, the

Table 3-2   Classification of Hormones Based on Their Chemical Composition

Hydrophilic hormones	Lipophilic hormones

Proteins/peptides (groups of peptides often have similar amino acid sequences and belong to *homology groups*)
• Simple proteins
• Glycoproteins
	Steroid hormones
	• Corticosteroids
	  —Glucocorticoids: cortisol (F)
	  —Mineralocorticoids: aldosterone, 11-deoxycorticosterone (DOC)
	• Sexual steroids
	  —Androgens: dehydroepiandrosterone (DHEA), DHEA-sulfate (DHEAS), androstenedione, testosterone (T), dihydrotestosterone (DHT)
	  —Estrogens: estrone (E$_1$), estradiol (E$_2$), estriol (E$_3$)
	  —Progestins: progesterone (P)
	• Vitamin D derivatives: 25(OH)D; 1,25(OH)$_2$D; 24,25(OH)$_2$D

Amino acid derivatives
Monoamines:
• Catecholamines
  —Dopamine
  —Noradrenaline (norepinephrine)
  —Adrenaline (epinephrine)
• Serotonin
• Histamine
Others (e.g., GABA)
	Amino acid derivatives:
	• thyroid hormones: thyroxine (T$_4$), triiodothyronine (T$_3$)
	• melatonin

	Retinoids (Vitamin A derivatives)
	Derivatives of arachidonic acid
	• Cyclooxygenase pathway
	  —Prostaglandins
	  —Prostacyclin
	  —Thromboxanes
	• Lipoxygenase pathway
	  —12-Lipoxygenase (12-HPETE, 12-HETE)
	  —5-Lipoxygenase (5-HPETE and Leukotrienes)

synthesis of all hormones requires the biosynthesis of proteins. The protein may be

• a secreted peptide hormone or its precursor (e.g., insulin, angiotensinogen);
• a nonsecreted enzyme involved in the intracellular biosynthetic process of the hormone (e.g., tyrosine hydroxylase);
• a secreted enzyme, which contributes to the hormone production in the extracellular fluid (e.g., renin, kallikreins).

The enzyme reactions are very specific for each non-peptide hormone and are best described separately. A common theme in these biosynthetic pathways is that the enzymes are usually regulated by extracellular as well as intracellular signals. The regulated enzymes are typically catalysts of the rate limiting step(s) of the pathway, and these are strategically positioned either as early steps or immediately follow branchpoints of the pathway. Here we discuss the generic scheme of the biosynthesis of polypeptide hormones.

The Biosynthesis of All Polypeptide Hormones Starts with Transcription

Biosynthesis starts with gene expression, i.e., transcription of mRNA from nuclear DNA found in accessible regions of the DNA known as the readily accessible *euchromatin* and the conditionally accessible *facultative heterochromatin*. The densely packed (supercoiled) nuclear DNA known as *constitutive heterochromatin* is by definition never accessible for transcription in a given type of cell. If more than one X chromosome is present in a cell, only one X chromosome will be active, while the other copy(ies) of the X chromosome is (are) inactivated, except for the *pseudoautosomal region*, and their constitutive heterochromatin is observed as the *Barr body*(ies) or *sex chromatin* (see Chap. 13).

Availability of DNA for transcription is also regulated by *methylation* of the DNA, which occurs as a part of cellular differentiation during ontogeny. In certain cases, this process leads to *genomic imprinting*, in which methylation restricts expression of a gene either only from the maternal or only from the paternal chromosome in a diploid cell.

Although certain mitochondrial proteins are encoded by *mitochondrial DNA* (*mtDNA*), none of these proteins are known secretory products of the cell.

Transcription is a regulated process. There are certain genes whose expression is always maximal and appears to be unaffected by physiologic changes. Such genes are needed for the unconditional survival of the cell and are known as *housekeeping genes*. On the other hand, the transcription of genes encoding hormones is usually regulated by other hormones and/or metabolic signals. The *intracellular (nuclear) hormone receptors* are in effect ligand-regulated transcription factors (see Chap. 5). Note that the initial steps of protein hormone synthesis described here coincide with the *actions* of other hormones described in subsequent chapters (see Chap. 5). This is due to the fact that hormones either directly or indirectly modulate the activity of transcription factors (genomic action).

Transcription is usually performed by *RNA polymerase II* (Pol II). However, Pol II requires a number of other *gene regulatory proteins* to initiate RNA synthesis (Fig. 3-1). The assembly of Pol II and *general* or *core* (i.e., not gene-specific) *transcription factors* occurs at the regulatory region of the gene known as the *core promoter*, which usually has the *TATA box* at its 5' end. Transcription starts approximately 25 base pairs

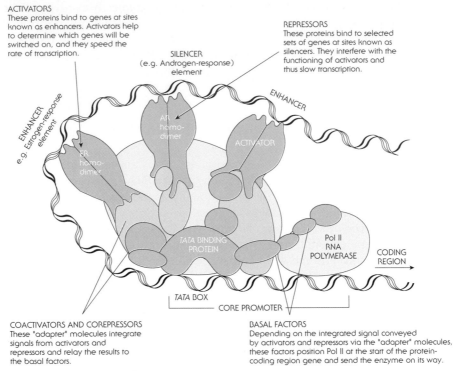

ACTIVATORS
These proteins bind to genes at sites
known as enhancers. Activators help
to determine which genes will be
switched on, and they speed the
rate of transcription.

SILENCER
(e.g. Androgen-response)
element

REPRESSORS
These proteins bind to selected
sets of genes at sites known as
silencers. They interfere with the
functioning of activators and
thus slow transcription.

ENHANCER
e.g. Estrogen-response
element

ENHANCER

AR
homo-
dimer

ACTIVATOR

ER
homo-
dimer

TATA BINDING
PROTEIN

Pol II
RNA
POLYMERASE

CODING
REGION

TATA BOX

CORE PROMOTER

COACTIVATORS AND COREPRESSORS
These "adapter" molecules integrate
signals from activators and
repressors and relay the results to
the basal factors.

BASAL FACTORS
Depending on the integrated signal conveyed
by activators and repressors via the "adapter" molecules,
these factors position Pol II at the start of the protein-
coding region gene and send the enzyme on its way.

Figure 3-1. Regulation of transcription.

(bp) downstream of the TATA box: this is the start of the *coding region* of the gene.

The general transcription factor assembly requires additional regulatory elements for its function. These are *DNA-sequence-specific transcription factors* and *adapter proteins*. Although there are many other sequence-specific transcription factors in the nucleus, we shall use the intracellular hormone receptors as an example. These ligand-regulated transcription factors bind to specific sequences of the DNA known as *hormone response elements (HREs)* found in the promoter region upstream from the TATA box. Due to folding of the double-stranded DNA, they also bind to the assembly of general transcription factors via adapter proteins. The specific transcription factors may either activate or repress transcription; in general, they are referred to as *trans-acting factors*. The trans-acting factors maybe either *activators* or *repressors*. Activators bind to *enhancer;* repressors bind to *silencer* DNA segments. HREs therefore may function either as enhancers or as silencers. The *DNA sequences* that are involved in the regulation of transcriptional activity are referred to as *cis-acting elements;* enhancers, silencers, and hormone response elements (HREs) are all *cis-*acting elements. The adapter proteins of the intracellular receptors are also known as *co-activators* and *co-repressors*.

The transcription of a given gene may be regulated by several enhancers and silencers. The transcriptional activity will be determined by the combined effect of the gene regulatory proteins binding to these DNA segments. Hormones may synergize with each other either to induce (activate) or to suppress (repress) gene expression; at other times the same hormones may antagonize each other's action. These interactions will be influenced by both the absolute and the relative concentrations of the hormones involved. A well-known example of this is the antagonism between estrogens and androgens; the current model of transcriptional regulation provides the molecular basis for the clinical considerations of *estrogen to androgen ratio*.

The set of available gene regulatory proteins depends on the differentiation and/or physiologic state of the cell. Therefore, the same hormone, depending on the cell type and/or conditions of the cell, may mediate an increase or decrease of transcription of the same gene. For example, consider that androgens cause hair growth in most regions of the body, yet they result in hair loss at the scalp (male pattern baldness).

The same gene may have several different promoter regions, all of which are located upstream of the coding region (i.e., closer to the 5' end than the 3' end of the gene). The use of different promoters is often cell-type specific, and is regulated by different signals. For example, the placenta is actively synthesizing most known hormones, and often utilizes alternative promoters in the process.

The Transcript Is Processed in the Nucleus: Splicing at Alternative Sites May Yield Different Mature mRNA Populations Derived from a Single Gene

Before leaving the nucleus, the *primary RNA transcript (pre-mRNA)* undergoes a maturation process, which (among other modifications) includes splicing of the pre-mRNA by complexes of small nuclear RNAs (snRNAs) and proteins called *spliceosomes* (Fig. 3-2). The splicing removes portions of the RNA known as *introns,* and joins the remainder of the RNA known as the *exons.* The mature RNA is exported through the nuclear pores into the cytoplasm, where it binds to ribosomes.

- The mRNA of *secreted* proteins binds to ribosomes, which are attached to the membrane of the endoplasmic reticulum (ER). This type of ER is called the *rough ER* (rER) in contrast with the smooth ER (sER), which is devoid of ribosomes.
- The mRNAs of proteins destined for the cytoplasmic and nuclear compartments, mitochondria and peroxisomes, are synthesized by free (non–membrane-attached) ribosomes.

The protein synthesis governed by the nucleotide sequence of the mRNA is called *translation.* Translation always starts at an *AUG* (or

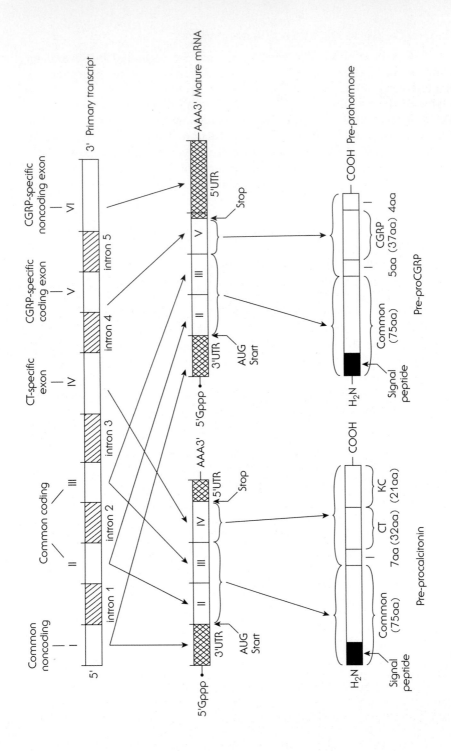

START) codon usually found within *Kozak's consensus translation initiation sequence*. The AUG codon also serves as the code for methionine. This would suggest that every protein should have a methionine at its N-terminal. (As we shall see, this is not the case.) It is important to remember that the entire nucleotide sequence of the mature mRNA will not be translated, only the *open reading frame (ORF)* found between the *START* and *STOP* codons. The mature mRNA contains a *5' and a 3' untranslated region (UTR)*.

As mentioned above, gene expression may utilize different promoters. The different promoters are associated with different first exons of the same gene. The first exon may in part, or as a whole, reside in the 5' UTR of the mature mRNA. Thus, *the use of different promoters may result in different regulation of gene expression and partially different mRNAs, but still yield the same protein*. As a consequence, mutations of the gene in this regulatory region may result in loss of function in some tissues, whereas others that rely on a different promoter will function normally.

In various cell types, the spliceosomes may differ in their sequence-specificity. These differences may result in *alternative splicing* of the same primary transcript. Alternative splicing may yield peptide products that are vastly different, yet encoded by the same gene. These peptides are usually referred to as *gene-related products. Calcitonin* (CT) and *calcitonin gene-related peptide* (CGRP) are two peptides generated by alternative splicing of the same primary transcript.

Families of Hormones and Receptors Arise during Evolution Mainly by Repeated Duplication of Genes Followed by Divergence

Many polypeptide hormones belong to so-called homology groups, which constitute "hormone families." The homology groups are identified by the amino acid sequence similarities of the peptides, and the nucleotide similarities of their mRNAs (Box 3-1). The shared genomic background can be verified by conserved intron-exon arrangements of the homologous protein genes. If a gene is accidentally duplicated during cell division, and both copies are present in germ cells, the next generation will carry an

---

Figure 3-2. Removal of introns during the posttranscriptional modification of the primary transcript and the coding of the pre-prohormone. The example shows the biosynthesis of calcitonin (CT), CT-gene related peptide (CGRP) and katacalcin (KC). The exons are shown by roman numerals. The 5' and 3' untranslated regions (UTRs) of the mature mRNA fall outside the open reading frame. Whereas in the C cells of the thyroid gland the preferred product is CT, CGRP is the main product in nerve tissue. The alternative splicing of the primary transcript is due to different specificity of the spliceosomes expressed in these tissues. (*Source:* Modified from Fig. 58-2, MacIntyre I: Calcitonin: Physiology, biosynthesis, secretion, metabolism and mode of action. Chapter 58, p. 979 in DeGroot LJ (ed): *Endocrinology*, 3rd ed., Philadelphia, Saunders 1995)

BOX 3-1   Messenger RNA *vs.* Complementary DNA

The mRNA sequence is usually referred to as the complementary DNA [cDNA] because the sequence is identified from the DNA obtained by reverse transcription of the mRNA template. The nucleotide sequence of the *sense* DNA strand is the same as in the mRNA, except that uridine is replaced by thymidine, and deoxyribonucleotides rather than ribonucleotides form the nucleotide chain.

extra copy of the gene. The second copy (mainly by point mutations) has a potential to diverge from the original copy as long as the first copy continues to perform its normal function. To establish the second copy as a separate hormone, it must have an appropriate receptor. The hormone receptors may also undergo duplication-divergence processes. The process may be repeated several times over millions of years leading to the development of hormone and hormone receptor families. This has two important medical applications:

• Hormones of a given family have the highest probability to cross-react on each other's receptors.
• Hormones of a given family tend to utilize similar second messenger systems, which maybe of importance in drug therapy.

An important example is the cross-reactivity of human growth hormone (GH) on the prolactin (PRL) receptor: GH-producing pituitary adenomas may lead to galactorrhea (milky discharge from the breasts) and amenorrhea (suspension of the menstrual cycle), which are also features of PRL-producing pituitary adenomas (prolactinomas). The receptors of GH and PRL belong to the superfamily of cytokine receptors. Accordingly, certain immunosuppressive drugs that have a postreceptor site of action (cyclosporin A), also interfere with some of the biologic effects of GH and PRL.

Thinking in terms of homology groups helps to memorize the various hormones, their biologic actions, receptor types, and second messenger systems.

Polypeptide Hormones Are Synthesized as Prehormones or Pre-prohormones: Alternative Proteolytic Processing of the Same Prohormone May Yield Different Final Products

Translation is a process whereby the nucleotide sequence of the mRNA is translated into an amino acid sequence (i.e., mRNA-directed protein synthesis). Translation consists of three phases: initiation, elongation, and termination, which will not be discussed here in detail.

Translation is a regulated process. Certain hormones, especially insulin and structurally related insulin-like growth factors stimulate translation in general, i.e., translation of practically any mRNA present in the hormone-responsive cell. This action is a major contributor to the anabolic effects of these hormones. Insulin stimulates translation via multiple pathways, affecting mainly initiation, and in part elongation, by altering the phosphorylation state of specific regulatory and ribosomal proteins involved in translation (see Chap. 9).

Secreted proteins and membrane proteins, such as membrane receptors, enter the cisternae (the lumen) of the rER during their translation. This process requires the protein to penetrate the membrane of the rER. This process is made possible by the N-terminal portion of the nascent protein known as the *leader sequence* or *signal peptide*. As the protein enters the cisterna of the rER, the leader sequence is cleaved by a proteolytic enzyme *(signal peptidase)* even before the translation of the peptide is completed. (Note that membrane proteins remain anchored to the lipid bilayer by specific transmembrane domains.) The cleaved signal peptide contains the N-terminal methionine of the nascent protein. Because all peptide hormones and peptide neurotransmitters are secretory products, they all have a signal peptide as nascent proteins. The peptide still containing the leader sequence is termed the *prehormone*.

The removal of the signal peptide may be followed by further proteolytic processing of the hormone that happens during the secretory process in the *trans Golgi network* and in the secretory vesicles (see below). If this is the case, the hormone precursor peptides *before* and *after* the removal of the signal peptide are called the *pre-prohormone* and *prohormone*, respectively. The prohormone is cleaved by *proprotein convertases (PCs)*, which are related to bacterial *subtilisins*. PC3 (identical with the independently discovered PC1) and PC2 are expressed only in neuroendocrine tissues, and their activities are calcium-dependent. Several other PCs have been discovered with different expression sites: e.g., PC4 in the testis, PC6/PC5 in the intestines and brain, and *furin*, which is almost ubiquitously expressed. PCs cut at recognition motifs which usually contain two adjacent positively charged amino acid residues, such as lysine and arginine.

Those prohormones that contain multiple copies of the same peptide hormone are sometimes called *polyproteins;* for example, there are six copies of *thyrotropin releasing hormone* (TRH) tripeptide in the single polypeptide of human proTRH. A single prohormone may yield several different peptide hormones. A good example for this is *pro-opiomelanocortin* (POMC), which may yield adrenocorticotrophic hormone (ACTH), α-melanocyte-stimulating hormone (α-MSH), β-endorphin, and other peptides (see Chap. 12). Depending on the PCs expressed by the cell, the same prohormone may be processed differently in a cell-type specific manner.

The Secretory Process of Polypeptides May Involve Posttranslational Modifications, Packaging, Storage, and Release

The prohormone released into the lumen of the rER is transported to the Golgi complex by means of vesicles budding off the rER and merging with the *cis-* face of the Golgi. While still in the lumen of the rER, the prohormone is often subject to *N-glycosylation*. This process is catalyzed by the *oligosaccharide transferase* enzyme, which requires the presence of a *glycosylation consensus motif* in the peptide. (This glycosylation is distinct from the *nonenzymatic* glycosylation of proteins, which is a major factor leading to complications of diabetes mellitus; see Chap. 9). The enzymatic glycosylation typically appends a preassembled oligosaccharide to an asparagine residue. This oligosaccharide is then modified in the Golgi and maybe processed into either a *complex* or a *high-mannose* oligosaccharide. Finally, secretory vesicles leave the *trans-* face of the Golgi. Note that glycosylation and proteolytic processing can occur simultaneously. These (and some other chemical modifications of the peptide chain, such as appending fatty acid chains as in the case of membrane-anchored proteins) are known as *posttranslational modifications*. The posttranslational modification does not necessarily affect every copy of the polypeptide molecule; this may lead to microheterogeneity of the hormone, which in turn may impact its biologic activity and immunoreactivity (see RIA, Chap. 7).

Usually peptide hormones are stored in secretory vesicles. The secretory vesicle may *concentrate* its hormone content; the concentration may involve crystallization of the peptide, which renders it osmotically inactive. If the appropriate stimulus reaches the cell, the vesicles move to the cell membrane by the aid of microtubules, and release their content into the extracellular fluid by means of exocytosis. This is known as *regulated secretion*. Note that in this context, the term secretion refers to the *release* of the hormone. The exocytosis of the secretory vesicles is often caused by a transient increase of Ca^{2+} in the ICF, which is triggered either by depolarization (voltage-gated Ca^{2+}-channels) or by postreceptor signaling mechanisms leading to activation of IP_3-gated Ca^{2+}-channels (see Chap. 5). In the absence of a secretory stimulus, some of the older stored vesicles will merge with primary lysosomes, and their content is degraded by proteases. However, some of the newly produced vesicles will be released even in the absence of a stimulus: this is known as *constitutive secretion*. The relative contribution of constitutive and regulated secretion varies with the cell types and the hormones.

The Synthesis and Release of Hormones Can Be Differentially Regulated if the Hormone Can Be Stored before Release

In general, the hormones that are packaged as mature hormones into secretory vesicles (peptides, biogenic amines) can be stored before release.

This also means that *the release process (exocytosis) is not directly coupled with the biosynthesis of these hormones.* Certain signals to these cells may stimulate both synthesis and release of their hormone(s), whereas others will affect only one or the other of these processes. For example, *growth hormone-releasing hormone* (GHRH) stimulates both the biosynthesis and the release of GH. The high levels of cortisol that reach the adrenal medulla due to the specialized circulation of the adrenal gland are important for inducing the enzyme PNMT *(phenylethanolamine N-methyl transferase),* which is required for the conversion of noradrenaline into adrenaline. Thus, cortisol is important for adrenaline synthesis. However, cortisol does not lead to the release of adrenaline from the adrenal medulla; the release is regulated by preganglionic cholinergic nerve fibers.

Lipid hormones (steroids, eicosanoids) are released as soon as they are synthesized because they cannot be retained by membrane barriers. In these cases the regulation of biosynthesis is directly coupled with that of release. For example, ACTH stimulates both the synthesis and the release of cortisol. Cortisol can be produced in large quantities upon stimulation by ACTH, but there is no "cortisol reserve" in the gland. Due to the trophic nature of ACTH, chronic exposure to ACTH will increase the cellular mass of the adrenal cortex: the increased mass is capable of synthesizing and secreting larger quantities of cortisol. Thus, hypertrophy may be used in lieu of storage of hormones.

Thyroid hormones are unique in the sense that they are stored as

Table 3-3 Differences in the Biosynthesis and Secretion of Peptide, Steroid and Thyroid Hormones

Peptides	Steroids	Thyroid hormones
Synthesized and processed sequentially in the rough ER and the Golgi complex	Synthesized in smooth ER and mitochondrial inner membrane	The precursor is synthesized and processed sequentially in the rough ER and the Golgi complex as a glycoprotein
Stored in significant quantities after synthesis in intracellular vesicles; the precursor amino acids are not stored	Not stored in significant quantities after synthesis, but the precursor cholesterol may be stored in cytoplasmic lipid droplets	The precursor (thyroglobulin) is secreted into the follicular lumen and thus stored in a transcellular fluid compartment
Either degraded within the cell or released upon appropriate stimulus	Released as soon as synthesized; no significant intracellular degradation occurs	The precursor is taken up from storage by endocytosis, and the hormone is liberated by lysosomal proteolytic cleavage
Secretion involves exocytosis of vesicles	Secretion of the lipophilic hormone occurs by diffusion through the cell membrane	Secretion of the lipophilic hormone occurs by diffusion through the lysosomal and the cell membranes

prohormones (thyroglobulin) in the transcellular fluid compartment (follicular fluid). While the thyroid hormones are highly lipophilic, and could not
be retained by cell membrane barriers, their precursor is a glycoprotein, and
thus hydrophilic. Table 3-3 contrasts the secretory process of polypeptide
hormones with that of steroid and thyroid hormones.

The term *secretion* is sometimes used interchangeably with "release"
of secretory vesicles. However, secretion implies that the same cell also
synthesized the hormone being released. In some cases, a hormone is not
synthesized by an epithelial cell, but is passing through it by transcytosis
(see Chap. 5). This involves receptor-mediated endocytosis, passing through
the endosomal compartment, and finally being released on the other side
of the cell by exocytosis. *Transcytosis* occurs, for example, in the choroid
plexus, where *leptin* (an appetite-suppressing hormone) may enter from
plasma into the cerebrospinal fluid (CSF) (see Chap. 15). Hormones under-
going transcytosis may be subject to posttranslational modifications. The
kidneys, salivary glands, sweat glands, and the mammary glands may contain
several components (including hormones) in their *exocrine* secretory products that were not synthesized by these glands, but entered the fluid by
means of filtration and/or transcytosis. This mechanism is distinct from
secretion and is called *excretion*.

4

TRANSPORT OF HORMONES TO THE SITE OF ACTION

OBJECTIVES

1. Discuss transport of hormones in blood, carrier proteins, and the concept of bound versus free hormones.
2. Compare the hormone-specificity, affinity, and binding capacity of carrier proteins. Identify factors that have significant impact on binding protein concentrations and may influence the distribution of circulating hormones between the free and the various protein-bound forms.
3. Discuss the relationship between the location of hormone release into the circulation and the effect/fate of the hormone.
4. Discuss how hormones may leave the circulation, crossing endothelial and epithelial barriers.
5. Discuss "protected" transcellular spaces and the characteristics of the blood-brain barrier (BBB). Be familiar with areas of the central nervous system (CNS) that are *not* protected by the BBB.

TRANSPORT IN BLOOD: CARRIER PROTEINS AND THE CONCEPT OF FREE HORMONE

Transport of hormones in blood is mainly determined by their solubilities in the aqueous fraction of blood. Most hydrophilic hormones circulate in plasma unbound to a carrier protein. However, lipophilic hormones, due to their physicochemical characteristics, require *carrier proteins* for transport in blood plasma. In addition, lipophilic hormones may penetrate the membrane of red blood cells (RBCs), and maybe transported partly in the cytoplasm of RBCs. Tables 4-1 and 4-2 summarize the most important proteins involved in the blood plasma transport of lipophilic hormones (these tables will be often referred to in subsequent chapters). Most carrier proteins are:

- synthesized in significant quantities by the liver and in certain cases by the yolk sac;
- retained by basement membranes, including the glomerular filter.

Table 4-1 The Main Hormone Carrier Proteins in Plasma

	MW	Plasma concentration	Half-life	% Binding sites normally occupied by the specific hormone	Ligand binding
RBG	21,000	1.4–2.9 μM (3–6 mg/dL)	Free: 3.5 hours; TBPA-bound: 12 hours	75	Vitamin A, TBPA
TBPA	55,000	2–8 μM (10–40 mg/dL)	1–2 days	?	T_4, RBG, (T_3)
TBG	54,000	0.28–0.56 μM	3 days (desialy-lated TBG: 15 min)	50	T_4, T_3, free fatty acids, drugs
CBG	58,200	323–433 nM (18.8–25.2 mg/dL) (male); 256–393 nM (14.9–22.9 mg/dL) (nonpregnant female); 541–1031 nM (31.5–60.0 mg/dL) (pregnancy)	5 days	50	Cortisol, DOC, pro-gesterone, aldo-sterone, (andro-gens, estrogens)
SHBG	95,000	10–80 nM (59–472 μg/dL) (male); 20–130 nM (118–767 μg/dL) (non-pregnant female); 321–456 nM (1.9–2.69 mg/dL) (35–40 wk of pregnancy)	2–8 h (initial) 33 h–4 days (depending on sialylation)	50	Androgens, estro-gens, (DOC, pro-gesterone, cortisol, aldosterone)
DBP	58,000	6 μM (35 mg/dL)	2.5 days	2	Vitamin-D and deriv-atives, actin, fatty acids, C5a and C5a des-Arg
AGP	41,000	13.4–34.1 μM (55–140 mg/dL)	5 days	?	Melatonin, proges-terone
Albumin	66,500	0.5–0.83 mM (3.2–5.4 g/dL)	18–20 days		Fatty acids, bilirubin, metals (e.g., Ca^{2+}), drugs, dyes, folate, steroids, Vitamin D deriva-tives, T_4, T_3, mela-tonin
AFP	70,000	Fetal peak (1st trimester) 28–57 μM (200–400 mg/dL); Maternal se-rum (screening time: 15th to 17th gestational week): 4.27–5.8 pM (29.9–40.6 ng/mL)	3–5 days		Fatty acids, bilirubin, metals, drugs, dyes, retinoids, di-ethylstylbestrol (DES)

ABBREVIATIONS: RBG, retinol-binding globulin; TBPA, thyroxine-binding prealbumin (also known as transthyretin [TTR]); TBG, thyroxine-binding globulin; CBG, cortisol-binding globulin, transcortin; SHBG, sex hormone-binding globulin (also known as TeBG, testosterone-binding globulin); DBP, vitamin D-binding protein (also known as G_c, group-specific component); AGP, α_1-acid glycoprotein, orosomucoid; ALB, albumin; AFP, α fetoprotein.

Although lipophilic hormones are mainly bound to carrier proteins, they are somewhat soluble in water. Thus, they exist in an unbound form known as the *free hormone* that is in equilibrium with the *bound hormone* fraction. The concentration of the free plus the bound hormone is known as the *total hormone* concentration. Traditionally the free hormone is con-sidered to be the biologically active fraction, because it is available for binding to its intracellular receptor after diffusing through the wall of

Table 4-2   Proportions of Lipophilic Hormones Carried in Plasma Free and Bound to Various Carrier Proteins (Basal Conditions)

Hormone	Half-life in plasma	Free hormone (%)	Albumin (%)	TBPA (%)	TBG (%)	CBG (%)	SHBG (%)	DBP (%)
T4	7 days	0.04	21.0	11	68	—	—	—
T3	1 day	0.4	16.6	1	80	—	—	—
Cortisol	70–90 min	4.0	6.5	—	—	89.3	0.2	—
Progesterone	5 min (initial), 38 min	2.4	79.3 (55.0, pregnancy)	—	—	17.7 (38.0, pregnancy)	0.6	—
Aldosterone	15–20 min	37.0	41.9 (25.0, pregnancy)	—	—	21.0 (42.0, pregnancy)	0.1 (1.8, pregnancy)	—
11-Deoxycorticosterone (DOC)	72 ± 31 min	2.7	59–60 (30.0, pregnancy)	—	—	36.3 (57.0, pregnancy)	0.8–1.9 (12.0, pregnancy)	—
DHEA	44 min	4.0	88–92 (46.0, pregnancy)	—	—	<0.1	3.4–7.9 (51.0, pregnancy)	—
Androstenedione		7.5	84–88 (47.0, pregnancy)	—	—	1.3	2.8–6.6 (45.0, pregnancy)	—
Testosterone	5 (initial) and 35 min	2.0 (0.2, pregnancy)	30–50 (4.0, pregnancy)	—	—	2.2–3.3 (0.8, pregnancy)	44–66 (95.0, pregnancy)	—
DHT		0.5 (F) 0.07% (pregnancy) 0.9 (M)	21.0 (F) 2.0 (pregnancy) 39.0 (M)	—	—	0.1–0.2	78 (F) 98 (pregnancy) 60 (M)	—
Estradiol	20–22 min (initial) and 7 hrs	1.8 (F; 0.5, pregnancy) 2.3 (M)	60.8 (F; 11.0, pregnancy) 78.0 (M)	—	—	<0.1	37.3 (F; 88.0, pregnancy) 19.6 (M)	—
Estrone		3.6 (1.3, pregnancy)	80.1 (F; 28.0, pregnancy) 88.6 (M)	—	—	<0.1	16.3 (F; 70, pregnancy) 7.4 (M)	—
Estriol		8.1 (9.8, pregnancy)	91.0 (79.0, pregnancy)	—	—	<0.5	1.0 (F; 11.0, pregnancy) 0.4 (M)	—
Vitamin D3		>0.4	10.0	—	—	—	—	—
25OHVitamin D3	12 days	0.04	10.0	—	—	—	—	—
1.25(OH)2Vitamin D3		0.4	10.0	—	—	—	—	88.0

ABBREVIATIONS: TBPA, thyroxine-binding prealbumin; TBG, thyroxine-binding globulin; CBG, cortisol-binding globulin; SHBG, sex hormone-binding globulin; DBP, vitamin D-binding protein; DOC, 11-deoxycorticosterone; DHEA, dehydroepiandrosterone; DHT, dihydrotestosterone; F, female; M, male.

continuous capillaries and through the lipid bilayer of the target cell's membrane. According to the traditional concept, the functions of carrier proteins are:

- to provide a circulating pool of the hormone that will replenish the free hormone as the free hormone is removed from the circulation by cellular uptake or excretion;
  - to limit the availability of the hormone to the target tissues
    - by keeping the concentration of the free hormone low (prevention of overexposure), and
    - by limiting the passage of bound hormones through continuous capillaries into the interstitial space;
- to prolong the half-life of the hormone by preventing filtration through the renal glomerulus.

Recent evidence has led to refinements of the traditional concept:

- certain carrier proteins have cell surface receptors that aid the delivery of the bound hormone to accessible cell populations;
  - the cell surface receptors that bind *carrier protein-ligand complexes* and ligand-free carrier proteins may transmit signals to the cells via second messengers (e.g., nongenomic action of steroid hormones);
  - *the biologically available hormone may also include the albumin-bound hormone fraction* of blood samples, because in the capillary bed the interaction of albumin (ALB) with the glycocalyx of the endothelium may liberate the hormone from ALB (but not from the more specific, high-affinity carrier proteins);
  - carrier proteins may be multifunctional proteins, and may have binding affinity for certain other carrier proteins.

The secretion of lipophilic hormones is usually regulated by polypeptide hormones (e.g., ACTH stimulates cortisol secretion). Most polypeptide hormones are secreted in a pulsatile fashion because the secretory granules exocytose in waves. The secretory profiles of steroid hormones regulated by these polypeptide hormones are also pulsatile. However, plasma levels of free steroid hormones show attenuated fluctuations because the carrier proteins "buffer" the changes in their secretion rates.

When lipophilic hormone precursors are ingested, they may become dissolved in the intestinal lipoproteins called *chylomicrons*. This mechanism is important in the transport of retinoids as *retinyl fatty acid esters*. Otherwise lipoproteins normally play a minor role in the plasma transport of lipophilic hormones.

A few peptide hormones have carrier proteins in plasma, most notably the insulin-like growth factor-binding proteins (IGFBPs), and growth hormone-binding protein (GHBP), and corticotrophin-releasing hormone-binding protein (CRH-BP). These binding proteins will be discussed later. The carrier proteins will be discussed in more detail in relationship with the hormone systems. Here we discuss some of the comparative aspects of carrier proteins.

The proportion of a lipophilic hormone bound to each of the various transport proteins is determined by its affinity for the carrier protein, and the concentration of the hormone and transport proteins present. The concentrations of carrier proteins vary markedly, and are regulated by several hormones (Table 4-3). In general, estrogens tend to increase the concentration of transport proteins. This is mainly achieved by prolonging their half-lives via increased sialylation, rather than by increasing the rate of protein synthesis. Glucocorticoids and androgens tend to decrease the concentration of transport proteins. Thyroid hormones increase plasma levels of binding proteins, but decrease the concentration of thyroxine-binding globulin (TBG), the specific binding protein of thyroid hormones.

As a rule of thumb, sex hormone-binding globulin (SHBG) has a higher affinity for androgens than for estrogens; for this reason, SHBG is also called testosterone-binding globulin (TeBG). Within the group of androgens or estrogens, the more biologically potent the sex steroid, the higher its affinity is for SHBG. Thus, for androgens, the binding preference is dihydrotestosterone (DHT) > testosterone (T) > androstenedione > dehydroepiandrosterone (DHEA) > DHEA sulfate (DHEAS); for estrogens, the binding preference is estradiol (E_2) > estrone (E_1) > estriol (E_3). In contrast, vitamin D-binding protein (DBP) has a much higher affinity for 25OHVitD (which has minimal biologic activity) than for the potent $1,25(OH)_2$VitD.

Pregnancy is associated with markedly altered hormone levels. An important feature is the increased production of estrogens and progesterone. Estrogens increase the concentration of most binding proteins, including SHBG. This increase results in a shift from albumin-binding toward increased SHBG binding of sex steroids, especially androgens. The tight binding of androgens contributes to the protection of the developing female fetus against the masculinizing effects of androgens.

Although progesterone is a sex steroid, it binds minimally to SHBG, and more to cortisol-binding globulin (CBG). Indeed, CBG has significant binding affinity for mineralocorticoids and progesterone in addition to its

Table 4-3   Factors Influencing Plasma Levels of Selected Hormone-Binding Globulins

	TBG	CBG	SHBG
Thyroid hormones	Decrease	Increase	Increase
Glucocorticoids	Decrease	Decrease	Decrease
Estrogens	Increase	Increase	Increase
Androgens	Decrease	Decrease	Decrease

ABBREVIATIONS: TBG, thyroid-binding globulin; CBG, cortisol-binding globulin; SHBG, sex hormone-binding globulin.

high affinity for cortisol. This feature is similar to the binding of these hormones by the glucocorticoid receptor, although the structure of CBG is distinct from the steroid hormone receptors.

Of all carrier proteins in plasma, ALB has the largest binding capacity. It has multiple binding sites; there are three separate binding sites for polyunsaturated fatty acids (e.g., arachidonic acid). ALB is the prototype of a family of *albuminoid proteins*, which also includes α fetoprotein (AFP), vitamin D-binding protein (DBP, also known as group-specific component or Gc globulin) and the recently discovered α-albumin. All these proteins are arranged in a tandem fashion on human chromosome 4. The expression of these carrier proteins is developmentally regulated.

•   AFP is often considered to be the equivalent of ALB during intra-uterine life. During embryonic life AFP expression is high and peaks in the first trimester. It is first expressed in the yolk sac, and then in the liver. Lower expression of AFP has been observed in some other organs (gut, pancreas, spleen, kidney, lung, and heart). Small quantities of AFP penetrate the placenta and enter the maternal circulation, where AFP concentration increases throughout pregnancy. After birth, both in the newborn and in the mother, AFP disappear from blood. Supranormal levels of AFP accompany twin pregnancies and neural tube defects of the fetus (such as *spina bifida* and *anencephaly*); subnormal levels of AFP are often associated with *Down syndrome* (trisomy of chromosome 21) and *hydatidiform mole* (see Box 13-10). *AFP in nonpregnant adults indicates tumor: liver tumors or yolk sac tumors of the gonads.*

•   *ALB is expressed by the same tissues as AFP, but its developmental pattern is the opposite: its production markedly increases after birth,* and it is mainly of hepatic and minimally of yolk-sac origin. In adults, there is no condition that would result in true hyperalbuminemia, but several conditions, such as nephrotic syndrome or hepatitis, may result in hypoalbuminemia that is associated with a decrease in other carrier proteins as well. ALB binds most lipophilic hormones with relatively low affinity. Therefore, *hormones are easily mobilized from the ALB-bound fraction, and typically have a shorter half-life than hormone molecules associated with their specific carrier proteins.* Note that ALB has a high-affinity binding site and several weak binding sites for thyroid hormones. ALB binds DHEAS tightly thereby prolonging its half-life, but binds DHEA with low affinity.

•   DBP expression commences between the 10th and 13th weeks of gestation in the fetal liver. ALB and DBP increase in a parallel fashion after birth. DBP/Gc displays polymorphism: it is encoded by three common codominant alleles leading to a combination of six phenotypes. The Gc system has been used as an adjunct for paternity testing. *Unlike the other specific ligand carrier proteins, DBP circulates in amounts far in excess of normal vitamin D metabolite concentrations in blood.* Estrogens increase plasma levels of DBP.

Binding of free fatty acids (FFAs) is not restricted to the albuminoid family: FFAs may compete for the thyroxine-binding site of TBG.

Thyroid hormones and retinoids are functionally related to each other (see Chap. 11). This relationship is demonstrated by the binding between transthyretin (TTR or thyroid hormone-binding prealbumin [TBPA]) and retinol binding globulin (RBG). The association aids the simultaneous delivery of retinol and thyroid hormones to the target tissues. Note that RBG is a small protein that is readily cleared from plasma by the kidney unless RBG is bound to TBPA.

RBG and α_1-acid glycoprotein (AGP) belong to the *lipocalin* protein family. Lipocalins are structurally diverse peptides that share characteristic sequence motifs enabling them to bind small lipophilic molecules. Lipocalins may bind to specific cell-surface receptors and also may form macromolecular complexes with other plasma proteins. In addition to their transport function, they may be involved in diverse functions such as olfaction, prostaglandin synthesis, regulation of cellular homeostasis/permeability, and modulation of immune response. AGP exemplifies these characteristics: it is an acute phase protein that, in addition to the liver, is synthesized by activated macrophages. It serves as a natural anti-inflammatory agent displaying antineutrophil, immunosuppressive, and anti-complement activities. The inflammatory process generates free radicals. By delivering melatonin (a potent free-radical scavenger) to the site of inflammation, AGP may be involved in the protection against cellular damage caused by free radicals.

LOCAL AND SYSTEMIC CIRCULATION

Blood circulation in mammals is maintained by a four-chamber heart, which functions as two, serially connected pumps. The *major circulation* originates in the left ventricle and leads to the right atrium; the *lesser (or pulmonary) circulation* originates in the right ventricle and leads to the left atrium. Most circulating hormones enter the bloodstream at the venous portion of the capillary beds of the major circulation.

However, hormones of the gut, pancreas, and spleen enter the bloodstream at sites collected by the *hepatic portal vein*. In the liver, the portal vein branches into the sinusoids of the liver, which in essence is a second capillarization. In the sinusoids, portal vein blood is mixed with the arterial blood of the hepatic artery. Hormones collected from the drainage area of the hepatic portal vein are effectively delivered to the hepatocytes, which clear a significant portion of these hormones *before* they can reach the inferior vena cava via the efferent hepatic veins. This fast and effective hepatic clearance is known as the *first-passage phenomenon*. The first-passage phenomenon explains why natural gonadal steroid hormones are ineffective when administered orally (their intestinal absorption takes them to the portal circulation) whereas the endogenously produced hormone is delivered to the inferior vena cava. Quite often the first-passage phenomenon is not simply a hormone degradation process: the liver is a target organ for several hormones. For example, the liver is the most important target organ of glucagon, which is produced by the pancreatic islets (see Chap. 9).

The lesser circulation and the lungs also play an important role in endocrine regulation. The bronchial tree contains an endocrine cell population (*Kulchitsky's cells*), which is part of the diffuse endocrine system. The normal function of the Kulchitsky's cells is not well understood, but under pathologic conditions, such as their tumors (carcinoids and small cell bronchial cancer), their secretory products can present in paraneoplastic syndromes.

The lungs are very important in the normal function of the renin-angiotensin-aldosterone axis: they contain the proteolytic enzyme which converts angiotensin I into angiotensin II (*angiotensin converting enzyme* [ACE]; see also Chap. 12). Most of ACE functions as an *ectoenzyme;* it is anchored to the membrane of the lung (and other tissues') capillary endothelium by a C-terminal hydrophobic tail, and the rest of the enzyme is in contact with circulating plasma. Due to enzymatic cleavage of tissue-bound ACE, minor quantities of ACE are also found in plasma as a circulat-

BOX 4-1   Autacoids and the Extracellular Activation of Prohormones

Autacoids (from the Greek *autos* [self] and *akos* [remedy]) are in essence locally acting hormones, which have a very brief half-life in the circulation. Thus, they typically act in a paracrine and/or autocrine manner, and they are often involved in the signaling process of the inflammatory reaction. They include mast cell-derived histamine, prostaglandins, the kinins and adenosine. The *kinins* (the nonapeptide *bradykinin* and the decapeptide *kallidin*) are generated from the *kininogens* (larger protein precursors) by proteolytic cleavage in the ECF by *kallikreins. Plasma kallikrein* is a proteolytic enzyme that is found in plasma as its inactive precursors (prekallikrein) that is activated by factor XIIa (activated Hageman factor) of the clotting cascade. *Tissue kallikrein* is an isoenzyme found in several tissues, mainly in the pancreas (in Greek: *kallikreas,* hence the name of the enzymes); its expression is regulated by hormones and nerves. Bradykinin and kallidin (lysyl-bradykinin) induce pain, vasodilation, increased vascular permeability, and prostaglandin synthesis. The kallikrein-kininogen-kinin system is a good example for the functional integration of clotting and the hormone systems. Note that angiotensin-converting enzyme (ACE) is important in the activation of angiotensin and the inactivation of the kinins.

Another important theme is the analogy between the intracellular and extracellular activation of prohormones by proteolytic cleavage. The intracellular mechanism involves the PCs and leads to the secretion of mature hormone; the extracellular mechanism utilizes different proteolytic enzymes, and often involve the cooperation of different organs, such as the kidneys, liver and lungs in the production of angiotensin II.

ing form. ACE is also known as *kininase II* for its essential role in the rapid degradation of *bradykinin* and *kallidin*: 80 to 90% of these kinins are degraded by ACE during a single passage, resulting in a plasma half-life of about 15 seconds. The lungs are also important in the rapid degradation of prostaglandins and other derivatives of arachidonic acid (Box 4-1).

Specialized local circulation is also of importance in endocrine regulation. The general concept is that a cell population produces a hormone, which, because of the direction of blood flow, will reach a target cell population before entering the systemic circulation. In this manner the target cells are exposed to extremely high concentrations of the hormone before the hormone became diluted in the systemic circulation. This arrangement is seen at the following locations:

- Pituitary portal circulation, which connects the median eminence of the hypothalamus (the site of release of hypothalamic releasing and inhibiting hormones) with the adenohypophysis (see Chap. 10)
- Adrenal circulation, in which the medulla receives most of its blood after perfusing the cortex (i.e., the concentrations of cortical hormones are very high in the medulla; see Chap. 12)
- Circulation of the pancreatic islets, where the direction of blood flow is central-to-peripheral in each islet; this assures that the centrally positioned insulin-producers can inhibit the secretory activity of the peripherally located glucagon producers (see Chap. 9).

TRANSPORT THROUGH BARRIERS

The Capillary Endothelium May Limit the Delivery of Hydrophilic Hormones into the Interstitial Fluid Compartment

As mentioned earlier, most endocrine tissues/glands are supplied by fenestrated capillaries, which aids the rapid exchange of hydrophilic signaling molecules between the intravascular and interstitial fluid compartments. In contrast, many target tissues are supplied by capillary beds of continuous, nonfenestrated endothelial lining. The endothelium may either prevent or reduce the penetration of hydrophilic hormones into the interstitial fluid. For example, insulin has a slow transendothelial transport in muscle and adipose tissue, which accounts for the different time-course of insulin action in vitro and in vivo.

Tight Junctions, Low Activity of Transcytosis, and the P-Glycoprotein Contribute to the Protection of Special Transcellular Fluid Compartments

Certain areas of the interstitial and transcellular fluids are separated from the intravascular and general interstitial fluids by barriers typically formed by endothelium *plus* epithelium. These specialized fluid compartments have compositions that are different from the generic interstitial fluid, and these special environments are essential for the normal function of the cells living in these fluid compartments. Note that the barrier for *bone fluid* is provided by bone-lining cells, which are in essence osteocytes and not epithelial cells. From a clinical perspective, three fluid compartments have preeminent importance:

    1. The brain interstitial fluid compartment, which is protected by the *blood-brain barrier* (BBB) and the *blood-cerebrospinal fluid (CSF) barrier*
    2. The luminal compartment of the seminiferous tubules of the testis (the site of sperm development), which is protected by the *blood-testis barrier* (see Chap. 13)
    3. The developing offspring, which is protected by the *placental barrier* in utero, and (in case of breast feeding) by the *mammary epithelium*.

    The BBB is formed by the continuous endothelial lining of brain capillaries. The most important aspect of this barrier is its relative impermeability, which involves:

- highly developed tight junctions, which minimize paracellular transport,
- low endocytotic activity of the brain capillary endothelium, which minimizes transport by transcytosis.

The relative impermeability of the BBB is extremely important in the maintenance of the special composition of brain extracellular fluid (ECF), which is a major determinant of neuronal excitability. It is also important to remember that certain hydrophilic hormones that circulate in plasma are used by the CNS as neurotransmitters: if these (e.g., noradrenaline) had access to the ECF of the brain, they would interfere with the normal signaling processes.

    Note that *the CSF is in an equilibrium with the brain ECF*, mainly because the ependymal lining of the cerebral ventricles, due to the absence of tight junctions, does not represent a significant barrier. Substances penetrating the choroid plexus may therefore reach the neurons in the CNS; however, the kinetics of hormone delivery by this route is different from the direct delivery through the BBB.

    The ability of a substance to cross the BBB is related to several factors. As a first approximation, substances that diffuse through the lipid bilayer of the cell membrane (water, urea, glycerol, lipophilic molecules) will also penetrate the BBB, whereas compounds that cross the cell membrane only with the aid of specific transport proteins (larger polar molecules such as hexoses and charged molecules such as amino acids), will also penetrate the BBB only if these transport proteins are present in the endothelial lining. However, *lipophilic molecules* that have high octanol:water partition coefficients *will not penetrate the BBB if their molecular weight exceeds about 500 Da*. This relative impermeability is due to the presence of the *P-glycoprotein* (Pgp; also known as p170 or MDR1a [*MDR: multidrug resistance protein*]) in the luminal membrane of the brain capillary endothelium. The human genome contains two closely related genes: *MDR-1* and *MDR-3*. The encoded proteins have similar functions but distinct tissue distribution. Pgps are transmembrane proteins, which actively pump out a broad range of large, structurally unrelated compounds from the cell.

Pgp also contributes to the barrier function at sites other than the BBB, including the endothelial cells of the blood-testis barrier, the placental barrier (where Pgp is expressed mainly in the trophoblast cells), and the mammary epithelium. The Pgp protein is highly expressed by certain tumors, such as breast cancer cells, which thus very effectively eliminate anticancer drugs. Pgp in the BBB offers significant protection against the same drugs' neurotoxic side effects. For an effective delivery of anticancer drugs to the CNS (which is often needed for the treatment of brain tumors), the Pgp needs to be bypassed. This can be achieved by an increase in the paracellular transport: tight junctions are transiently disrupted by a sudden increase in plasma osmolality (achieved by mannitol infusion), and the associated shrinkage of the endothelial lining.

Most of the lipophilic hormones are below the 500 Da threshold of Pgp (Table 4-4). Notable exceptions are the thyroid hormones, which nevertheless penetrate the BBB. However, there is evidence that intracellular concentrations of thyroid hormones and cortisol are limited by the function of Pgp in various target cells of these hormones. Thus, Pgp might be involved in the elimination of the hormone signal and/or target cell adaptation.

The Circumventricular Organs of the Brain Are Not Protected by the Blood-Brain Barrier

The CNS is highly dependent on a continuous oxygen supply, and is thus highly vascularized. The capillary bed forms the BBB at most places; however, in the areas of the *circumventricular organs,* the endothelium is fenestrated, thus these areas are *outside of* (meaning not protected by) the BBB

Table 4-4 The Molecular Weights of Selected Lipophilic Hormones

Hormone	MW	Hormone	MW	Hormone	MW
T_4	776.93	1,25(OH)$_2$ VitD3	416.65	Testosterone	288.41
T_3	635.99	Cortisol	362.47	Estradiol	272.37
Retinoic acid	300.42	Aldosterone	060.44	Estrone	270.36
Melatonin	232.27	Corticosterone	346.45	Estriol	288.07
PGF$_{2\alpha}$	354.49	Progesterone	314.45		
PGE$_2$	352.48	Pregnenolone	316.47		

and accessible to hydrophilic signaling molecules. The increased exchange between the vascular fluid and the interstitial fluid of the CNS is also evident by the relative expansion of the interstitial space in these areas of the brain. The following areas of the brain are outside the BBB:

- *Median eminence/neurohypophysis*: the site of release of hypothalamic releasing and inhibiting hormones, and neurohypophyseal hormones into blood; feedback regulation by peptide hormones also targets the axons in this area;
- *Organum vasculosum laminae terminalis (OVLT):* a multifunctional area:
    - It functions as the osmoreceptor, which regulates the secretion of antidiuretic hormone (ADH) from the posterior pituitary;
    - It is the site of action for IL-1-induced febrile response;
    - It is one of the sites of action for angiotensin II-induced drinking.
- *Subfornical organ* (SFO): the main site of action for angiotensin II-induced drinking;
- *Subcomissural organ:* its function is uncertain;
- *Area postrema:* at the floor of the 4th cerebral ventricle; it functions as a chemosensitive trigger zone of vomiting;
- *Pineal gland (epiphysis):* the pineal of most animals has a fenestrated endothelium; however, the human pineal is protected by the BBB.

MECHANISMS OF HORMONE ACTION

OBJECTIVES

1. Define the terms equilibrium dissociation constant (K_d), receptor agonist, antagonist, and partial agonist.
2. Identify the main classes, types, and subtypes of cell surface (membrane) receptors.
3. Define the terms spare receptors and receptor occupancy. Distinguish between decreased sensitivity and decreased responsiveness of target tissues to the action of hormones, and describe the involvement of spare receptors in these phenomena.
4. Discuss the signal transduction pathways utilized by the various types of membrane receptors.
5. Discuss intracellular receptors, with an emphasis on the steroid hormone receptor superfamily. Identify the subfamilies of these receptors, their domains, and mechanisms of action.
6. Discuss the concept and the mechanisms of target cell adaptation.
7. Discuss the integration of multiple hormonal signals.
8. Discuss the potential effect of membrane receptors on gene expression. Discuss cycloheximide-sensitive and -insensitive mechanisms and the kinetics of the response.

HORMONES EXERT THEIR BIOLOGIC ACTION UPON BINDING WITH SPECIFIC RECEPTORS AND ACTIVATING A RECEPTOR-COUPLED EFFECTOR MECHANISM IN THE CELL

Hormone–receptor binding is similar to the binding between the hormone and a carrier protein: it is noncovalent in nature and in principle follows Michaelis–Menten kinetics. The ratio of the rate constants for dissociation and association under equilibrium conditions is called the *equilibrium dissociation constant* (K_d) or *equilibrium association constant* (K_a). We shall discuss the hormone–receptor binding kinetics further as related to hormone measurements (see Chap. 7). At this point it is important to remember that *the lower the value of the K_d, the higher the affinity of the binding.*

Binding affinity does not determine the biologic effect of the ligand. Thus, a ligand that binds to the receptor with high affinity may or may not activate the receptor-coupled effector mechanisms. If a ligand binds to the receptor and activates the effector mechanism, the ligand is called an *agonist.* If the ligand competes for the receptor binding site with an agonist, but does not activate the effector mechanism, it is called a *pure antagonist.* Quite often, however, a ligand may function as an agonist in the absence of a more potent ligand, and as an antagonist in the presence of a more potent ligand: these molecules are termed *partial agonists.*

Mutations of receptors are responsible for several disease states, including endocrine diseases. Two major types of mutations occur.

1. *Gain-of-function (or activating) mutations:* The receptor activates the signaling pathways in the absence of a ligand in a constant fashion. These mutations may imitate the physiologic consequences of hormone overproduction in face of actual normal or subnormal plasma levels of the hormone.

2. *Loss-of-function (or inactivating) mutations:* The receptor is unable to perform its normal function because it is

- absent;
- unable to bind the ligand;
- unable to activate the signal transduction pathway although it binds

the ligand (e.g., a membrane receptor loses its ability to bind with a G-protein or a steroid hormone receptor loses its ability to bind to DNA).

Loss-of-function mutations may imitate the physiologic consequences of the absence of a hormone in face of actual normal or supranormal plasma levels of the hormone.

Both types of mutation may affect molecules of the signal transduction pathway that are downstream of the receptor (e.g., a G-protein). The consequences of these mutations are similar to those of the receptors. However, the clinical picture may be quite varied and often imitates the mutation of multiple receptors because several receptors utilize the same signal transduction machinery.

We will discuss the receptors and the receptor-coupled effector mechanisms as two major groups: plasma membrane receptors, which generally have a preference for hydrophilic hormones, and intracellular receptors, which have a preference for lipophilic hormones. Note that a detailed coverage of signal transduction is beyond the scope of this book. The purpose of this brief discussion is to enable the students to understand interactions between hormones, pathologic processes, and the basis of therapeutic intervention.

CELL SURFACE (PLASMA MEMBRANE) RECEPTORS

In general, hydrophilic hormones and certain lipophilic hormones (melatonin, eicosanoids) exert their action via binding to cell surface receptors. These receptors are proteins having one or several *transmembrane domains,* each of which usually consists of an α-helix of hydrophobic amino acids. The *extracellular domain*(s) of the receptor bind the ligand; upon this binding, the *intracellular domain*(s) transmit the signal to the cytoplasmic compartment thereby activating a *signal-transduction pathway.* The ligand–receptor interaction may alter cellular function by modulating the function of:

- ion-channels (i.e., membrane permeability for an ion), membrane potential and intracellular electrolyte composition, thereby altering protein folding and function in the cell;
- protein kinases (enzymes that transfer a phosphate group from adenosine triphosphatase [ATP] to specific serine, threonine, or tyrosine residues of a protein), which are activated either directly or indirectly. The negatively charged phosphate group alters the charge of proteins, which in turn leads to a conformational change (altered folding) and function.

Thus, protein conformation and function are modulated by altering the composition of the solvent (intracellular fluid [ICF]) and/or altering the structure of the protein. Table 5-1 summarizes the main types of membrane hormone receptors.

The Presence of Spare Receptors Results in a Dissociation Between Receptor Occupancy and the Biologic Response

The concentration of hormones in the extracellular fluid (ECF) is usually lower than the K_d of their receptors. This means that the receptors are not saturated by their ligands; usually the *receptor occupancy* (% of receptors occupied by a ligand) is actually very low. However, this low receptor occupancy may be sufficient to evoke a maximal biologic response. For example, glucose transport into adipocytes is maximally stimulated when insulin occupies as little as 2% of its receptors. This observation would suggest that the rest of the receptors represent a surplus, hence they are called *spare receptors.*

Let us suppose that a cell expresses 10,000 receptor molecules (Fig. 5-1). Under these circumstances, an 18% receptor occupancy evokes a maximal biologic response. It means that the activation of 1800 receptor molecules was necessary to induce the maximal response in this particular cell. In fact, the absolute number of activated receptor molecules determines the response because it determines the activation of second messenger systems. If the cell expresses fewer receptors (e.g., 5000), a higher receptor occupancy (36%) would become necessary to activate 1800 receptors and evoke the same maximal biologic effect. If the total receptor number ex-

Table 5-1   The Main Classes, Types, and Subtypes of Membrane Hormone Receptors

Receptor class	Receptor type	Receptor subtype	Effector	Examples
G-protein linked	Seven transmembrane domain (also known as heptahelical)	$G\alpha_s$, choleratoxin-stimulated mechanism	Stimulation of adenylyl cyclase (increased cyclic AMP), activation of PKA	H_2 histamine receptors, V_2 vasopressin receptors, β-adrenergic receptors, glucagon receptors, hormone receptors potentially involved in the McCune-Albright syndrome: PTH, ACTH, αMSH, FSH, LH, TSH, GHRH
		$G\alpha_i$; pertussis toxin-sensitive mechanism	Inhibition of adenylyl cyclase, and PKA; activation of K^+ channels	Muscarinic cholinergic [(m_2)?] receptors, α_2 adrenergic receptor, D_2 dopaminergic receptor
		$G\alpha_0$; pertussis toxin-sensitive mechanism	Activation of K^+ channels, inactivation of Ca^{2+} channels, activation of PLC-β	
		$G\alpha_q$	PLC-β	H_1 histamine receptors, V_1 vasopressin receptors, α_1 adrenergic receptor, muscarinic cholinergic receptors, Ca^{2+}-sensing receptor
			PLA$_2$	H_1 histamine receptors
Enzyme linked	Single transmembrane domain	Receptor tyrosine kinases (RTKs)	MAPK pathway PI3'K-PKB pathway	Insulin receptor, growth factor receptors: IGFs, EGF, TGF-α, PDGF, neurotrophins
		Serine/threonine kinase receptors		Receptors for the TGF-β superfamily: Müllerian inhibitory hormone, inhibin, activin, BMPs
		Cytokine receptors	Jak—STAT pathway	Receptors for the helix-bundle peptide hormones: most cytokines, erythropoietin, growth hormone/lactogenic hormone family, leptin
		Guanylyl cyclase receptors	Cyclic GMP, PKG	Atrial natriuretic peptide receptors
	Soluble guanylyl cyclase		Cyclic GMP, PKG	Nitric oxide "receptor"
Ion channel linked	Ligand-gated ion channels	Cation channels	Cations (Na^+, K^+, Ca^{2+}): depolarization	Nicotinic cholinergic, serotonin, and glutamate receptors
		Anion channels	Cl^-: hyperpolarization	GABA, glycine receptors
Plasma protein/ transport receptors	Single transmembrane domain		None (?)	LDL receptor, transferrin receptor, mannose-6-phosphate/IGF-2 receptor

ABBREVIATIONS: PTH, parathyroid hormone; ACTH, adrenocorticotropic hormone; αMSH, α melanocyte-stimulating hormone; FSH, follicle-stimulating hormone; LH, luteinizing hormone; TSH, thyroid-stimulating hormone; GHRH, growth hormone-releasing hormone; PLC-β, phospholipase C-β; PLA$_2$, phospholipase A$_2$; IGF, insulin-like growth factor; EGF, epidermal growth factor; TGF-α, transforming growth factor α; PDGF, platelet-derived growth factor; BMP, bone morphogenetic protein; LDL, low density lipoprotein; Jak, Janus kinase; STAT, signal transducer and activator of transcription; MAPK, mitogen-activated protein kinase; PI3'K, phosphotidylinositol 3'-kinase; PKB, protein kinase B; PKG, protein kinase G; PKA, protein kinase A; GABA, gamma aminobutyric acid.

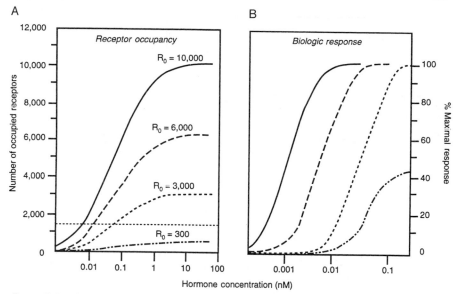

Figure 5-1. The impact of spare receptors on the relationship between receptor occupancy and the biologic response. A. The diagram shows the receptor occupancy as a function of hormone concentration at various total receptor numbers (R_0). The horizontal dotted line indicates the number of occupied receptors minimally required for a maximal biologic response. Note that this threshold is reached at *higher* concentrations of the hormone with decreasing R_0 (decreased *sensitivity*). B. The diagram displays the percent biologic response as a function of hormone concentration at the same set of R_0-s. In B, reaching a 100% biologic response equals with reaching the minimally required number of occupied receptors as symbolized by the horizontal dotted line in A. When the R_0 is lower than this threshold, even a 100% occupancy becomes insufficient to provoke a maximal biologic response (decreased *responsiveness*). (*Source:* Modified from Khan CR, Smith RJ, Chin WW: Mechanism of action of hormones that act at the cell surface. In Wilson JD, Foster DW: Williams Textbook of Endocrinology. Philadelphia, WB Saunders Co., 1992, p. 101.)

pressed by the cell is 1800, the maximal response can be achieved only if saturating concentrations of the hormone are present. This also means that there are no spare receptors expressed by the cell, and that the receptor occupancy and the biologic effect expressed as percentages become numerically identical. Thus, *reductions in the numbers of spare receptors can be compensated for by increasing the hormone concentration*, which also means that *reductions in the numbers of spare receptors equals decreased sensitivity of the cell/tissue to the action of the hormone.*

If, in the above example, the receptor number drops below 1800/cell, the biologic response becomes submaximal, even under maximal receptor occupancy. This means that *reducing the number of receptors when no spare receptors were present equals decreased responsiveness of the cell/tissue to the action of the hormone.* The changes in hormone sensitivity and responsiveness are illustrated in Figs. 5-1 and 5-2.

The concept of spare receptors has major implications in physiologic regulatory mechanisms and in hormone therapy in clinical practice:

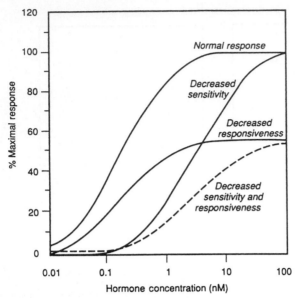

Figure 5-2. Comparison of the types of resistance to hormone action. The biologic response is expressed as a function of hormone concentration. A rightward shift of the dose–response curve indicates decreased sensitivity. A decrease in the maximal response is termed decreased responsiveness. Resistance may be due to the combination of the two mechanisms. (*Source:* Modified from Khan CR, Smith RJ, Chin WW: Mechanism of action of hormones that act at the cell surface. In Wilson JD, Foster DW: Williams Textbook of Endocrinology. Philadelphia, WB Saunders Co., 1992, p. 101.)

- by modulating the receptor numbers expressed by the cells, the biologic response to a given hormone can be influenced even if the concentration of the hormone remained the same (e.g., regulation of β_3 adrenergic receptors in adipose tissue by insulin: insulin decreases the sensitivity of adipocytes to adrenaline/noradrenaline);
- by increasing the dose of a hormone, the therapist may overcome reduced tissue sensitivity (e.g., suppression of prolactin secretion by the dopamine agonist bromocriptine in cases of prolactin-producing pituitary tumors, which do not appropriately respond to the increased endogenous levels of dopamine);
- one may exploit the lack of spare receptors in certain tissues: by exposing these tissues to an appropriate ligand, thereby *downregulating* the receptors (see later), one may achieve decreased tissue responsiveness (e.g., downregulation of gondadotropin-releasing hormone [GnRH] receptors in the pituitary gland by the GnRH agonist leuprolide as a means of inhibiting gonadotropin secretion).

G-Protein-Linked Receptors

All G-Protein-Linked Receptors Are Seven-Pass (Heptahelical) Transmembrane Proteins, Whose Action Is Mediated by G-Proteins to Various Effector Molecules The family of G-protein-linked receptors has the most members of the cell surface receptors. All G-protein-linked receptors are single polypeptide chains and have seven transmembrane α helical domains; the N-terminus is extracellular, the C-terminus is intracellular (Fig. 5-3). The chain forms loops between the transmembrane domains: the intracellular loop closest to the C-terminus is involved in G-protein binding, and the C-terminal portion of the peptide chain is the target of phosphorylation, which in turn results in receptor downregulation (see the subsequent section on "Target Cell Adaptation and Rebound Effect").

The term G-protein refers to the *trimeric guanosine triphosphate (GTP)-binding regulatory proteins*. G-proteins mediate the interaction between the membrane receptor and the effector molecules such as adenylyl cyclase, phospholipase C-β (PLC-β), phospholipase A_2 (PLA$_2$), or an ion channel. The trimeric G-proteins are distinct from the monomeric GTP-binding proteins (GTPases), which are exemplified by the Ras superfamily (see below).

G-proteins under resting conditions are inactive; they do not activate their effector molecules. G-proteins in this inactive state bind guanosine diphosphate (GDP) by their α subunits and their three subunits (α, β and γ designated as G_α, G_β, and G_γ) are assembled into the trimeric protein

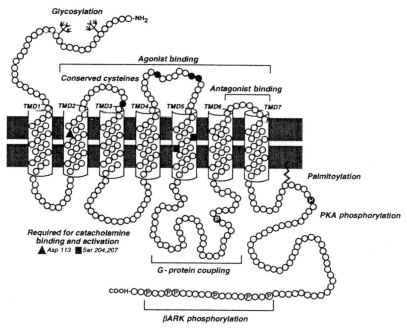

Figure 5-3. Schematic structure of the β-adrenergic receptor as a prototype of the G-protein-coupled heptahelical transmembrane segment receptors. (TMD1-7, transmembrane domains 1 through 7.) After the action of β-adrenergic receptor kinase (βARK), the phosphorylated segment becomes a docking site for arrestin, which results in rapid desensitization of the receptor. The receptors may also become desensitized by a direct action of protein kinase A (PKA). (*Source:* Fig. 9B, p 25, in Chapter 2 of Conn PM, Melmed S: *Endocrinology. Basic and Clinical Principles.* Totowa, New Jersey, Humana Press, 1997.)

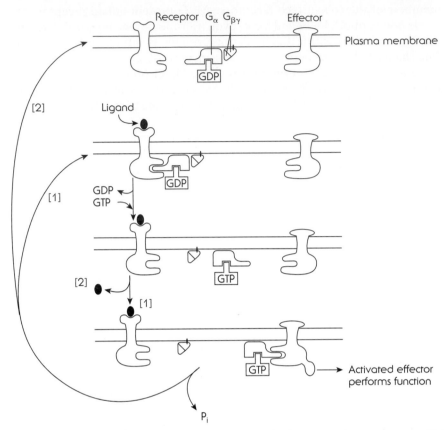

Figure 5-4. The G-protein cycle utilized by heptahelical transmembrane receptors. The cycle either keeps the effector activated in case of continued ligand binding by the receptor (loop 1) or discontinues the activation of the effector upon the dissociation of the ligand from the receptor (loop 2). Note that receptor downregulation mechanisms may interrupt the cycle and deactivate the effector (not shown). The various types of Gα proteins may activate different and often more than one type of effectors such as adenylyl cyclase, phospholipase C-β, phospholipase A$_2$ and ion channels. The effector in certain cases is inhibited rather than stimulated. (*Source:* Modified from Fig. 15-23, p 739 in Alberts B et al: The Molecular Biology of the Cell, 3rd ed. New York, Garland.)

complex. It is this entire complex that binds to the ligand-activated receptor. The *cycle* of signaling cascade includes the following steps (Fig. 5-4):

- the G-protein complex binds with the ligand-activated receptor;
- GDP dissociates from the α subunit and is replaced by GTP. The resulting conformational change leads to dissociation of the α subunit from the other two subunits of the G-protein complex and yields an activated α subunit;
- the activated α subunit binds to the effector molecule and modulates its function;

- the α subunit hydrolyzes its bound GTP into GDP thereby rendering itself unable to maintain binding to the effector molecule (inactivation);
- the GDP-associated α subunit reassembles with the β and γ subunits to form the inactive trimeric G-protein complex.

The activation of the Gα subunit continues in a cyclic fashion as long as the membrane receptor is activated by its ligand *and* the patch of membrane occupied by the receptor remains in the plasma membrane (i.e., not internalized by endocytosis). The latter is required for the association between the activated receptor and the G-protein complex by means of lateral diffusion in the membrane. In the absence of continued activation of the G-protein complex, the signal is short-lived because of the rapid hydrolysis of GTP.

Depending on the nature of the Gα subunit, its activation results in the subsequent activation of different effectors:

- Gα_s, or stimulatory α subunit, activates adenylyl cyclase.
- Gα_i, or inhibitory α subunit, inhibits adenylyl cyclase and/or activates potassium channels resulting in hyperpolarization of the membrane potential.
- Gα_q activates the phospholipase pathways (PLC-β or PLA$_2$). Note that PLC-γ has the same action as PLC-β, but it is activated by different means: by receptor tyrosine kinases. PLA$_2$ is involved in the generation of eicosanoids (see Chap. 12).

These events are confined to the inner surface of the plasma membrane: the tightly associated β and γ subunits are anchored to the membrane by a prenyl-group covalently attached to the γ subunit. The other components of the signaling system are either transmembrane proteins (receptor, adenylyl cyclase, membrane channel) or act on membrane lipids (PLC-β, PLA$_2$).

The Cyclic Adenosine Monophosphatate—Protein Kinase A Pathway Cyclic adenosine monophosphatase (cyclic AMP, or cAMP) is synthesized by adenylyl cyclase from ATP. The activity of adenylyl cyclase can be modulated by two Gα proteins: Gα_s, which stimulates and Gα_i, which inhibits adenylyl cyclase. These Gα protein subunits of the heterotrimeric G-protein complex are associated with different receptors often expressed by the same cell. If the cell is exposed to two hormones activating Gα_s and Gα_i via their respective receptors, the production rate of cyclic AMP will depend on the relative concentrations of the receptors and receptor occupancy.

It is important to remember that both cholera toxin and pertussis toxin increase cyclic AMP production, although their mechanisms of action are different. Cholera toxin permanently activates the Gα_s subunit, while pertussis toxin inhibits the Gα_i subunit. Both toxins achieve their action by inducing adenosine diphosphate (ADP) ribosylation of their targets. The activity of adenylyl cyclase can be experimentally stimulated by the drug *for-skolin*.

Protein kinase A (PKA) is found in the ICF: under resting conditions, its *catalytic subunit* is rendered inactive by the associated *regulatory subunit*. Upon an increased concentration of cyclic AMP, the regulatory subunit binds cyclic AMP, and dissociates from the catalytic subunit thereby activating it. PKA phosphorylates specific serine and threonine residues of target proteins:

- cytoplasmic enzymes involved in metabolism, such as phosphorylase kinase, which ultimately leads to glycogenolysis in the liver (see Chap. 9);
- membrane proteins, such as *cystic fibrosis transmembrane regulator* (CFTR), a chloride channel whose mutation is the cause of cystic fibrosis; and
- transcription factors such as *CREB protein* (see below).

Upon phosphorylation, the CREB protein is transported into the cell nucleus, associates with a coactivator protein termed *CREB-binding protein* (CBP) and binds to the *cyclic AMP response element* (CRE) found in the promoter region of certain genes (hence the name CRE-binding [CREB] protein). This mechanism is utilized for transcriptional regulation by cyclic AMP. There are additional PKA-activated transcription factors, such as CREM and ATF-1.

The $G\alpha_q$ Subunit Activates PLC-β, which in Turn Activates Two Signal Transduction Pathways: The DAG-PKC and the IP$_3$-Calmodulin Second Messenger Systems

The substrates of the enzyme phospholipase C-β (PLC-β) are inositol phospholipids found in the inner leaflet of the cell membrane's lipid bilayer; the most important type contains *phosphatidylinositol 4,5-bisphosphate (PIP$_2$)*. The receptor-activated $G\alpha_q$ subunit activates PLC-β, which in turn cleaves PIP$_2$ from the inositol phospholipid to produce *diacylglycerol (DAG),* which remains anchored in the plasma membrane and inositol 1,4,5-trisphosphate (IP$_3$), which diffuses throughout the cytoplasmic compartment.

DAG is an activator of *protein kinase C* (PKC). The activity of this enzyme is Ca^{2+}-dependent (hence its name). It is distinct from PKA, yet similar to PKA in that it phosphorylates proteins selectively at certain serine and threonine residues. PKC can be experimentally activated by *phorbol esters*. PKC has several major target proteins:

- ion channels in the cell membrane, through which PKC may alter excitability;
- mitogen-activated protein kinase *(MAP-kinase),* which in turn regulates transcription;

• an inhibitory subunit of *nuclear factor-κB* (NF-κB), which upon phosphorylation releases NF-κB from binding; NF-κB enters the nucleus and regulates transcription.

The endoplasmic reticulum (mainly the smooth ER) serves as a calcium storage compartment: although it is inside the cell, its contents are separated from the cytosol (ICF) by a membrane. [One may compare this arrangement with the food that we swallow: it is inside our body, yet it is confined to the lumen of the gut (i.e., the external environment), until being absorbed.] IP_3 binds to the cytoplasmic face of *IP_3-gated Ca^{2+}-channels* of the endoplasmic reticulum and activates these channels. Ca^{2+} enters the ICF driven by its electrochemical gradient (see Table 1-1), and binds to a special calcium-binding protein called *calmodulin*. The *Ca^{2+}-calmodulin complex* serves as an activator of enzymes, most notably *calmodulin-dependent protein kinases* (CaM-kinases), another member of the serine/threonine kinase enzyme family. The increased ICF Ca^{2+} concentration contributes to the activation of PKC as well. Note that CaM-kinases may be activated by signaling cascades not involving PLC-generated IP_3; for example, activation of *voltage-gated Ca^{2+} channels* in the cell membrane during depolarization results in Ca^{2+} influx from the ECF and the rise in ICF Ca^{2+} has the same effect on CaM-kinases. The IP_3 pathway can be simulated experimentally by *Ca^{2+} ionophore drugs*.

Enzyme-Linked Receptors

Enzyme-linked receptors are usually single transmembrane domain proteins which either have intrinsic enzymatic activity in their intracellular domains or are directly associated with an enzyme without an intervening trimeric G-protein. These receptors often form dimers either in the absence of their ligand (insulin receptor) or upon binding their ligand. The latter may include at least three distinct mechanisms:

• Each ligand molecule has a single site for receptor binding, which is exposed even after the ligand forms a dimer with another ligand; the receptors are dimerized by binding with their dimerized ligand. This mechanism is exemplified by *platelet-derived growth factor* (PDGF).
• Each ligand molecule has two binding sites for receptor binding; the receptors are dimerized by binding a single ligand molecule that forms a bridge between the two receptor molecules. This mechanism is exemplified by growth hormone (GH) and the related hormone prolactin (PRL). This binding mechanism explains the bell-shaped (rather than sigmoid) dose-response curve of these hormones: at very high concentrations, receptor-ligand monomers are preferentially formed, which prevents appropriate

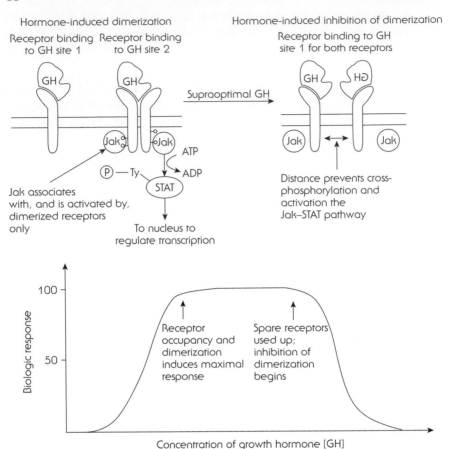

Figure 5-5. Hormone monomer-induced dimerization and signaling. When receptor-ligand complexes have a limited availability of nonliganded receptors for dimerization, signaling becomes inhibited. Abbreviations: GH, growth hormone; Jak, Janus kinase; STAT, signal transducer and activator of transcription. (*Source:* Modified from Fig. 8 A, p 24, in Chapter 2 of Conn PM, Melmed S: *Endocrinology. Basic and Clinical Principles.* Totowa, New Jersey, Humana Press, 1997.)

dimerization of the receptors and activation of the signal-transduction pathway (Fig. 5-5).

• The receptor's extracellular domain changes conformation upon binding its ligand, and the resulting conformation enables the extracellular domains of two separate receptors to bind each other.

Receptor tyrosine kinases (RTKs), which include insulin receptors, are usually growth factor receptors. The closely related receptors of *neurotrophins* (nerve growth factors) are classified as *Trks*. The cytoplasmic domain of RTKs has an intrinsic tyrosine kinase activity. Thus, as opposed to serine/threonine kinases, these enzymes phosphorylate proteins at their tyrosine residues. The first target of these receptors is found within the cytoplasmic domain of the receptor itself. Although this is referred to as *autophosphorylation*, it mainly involves the phosphorylation of each other by the dimerized receptors. The resulting phosphotyrosine residues serve as *docking sites* (binding sites) for proteins containing SH2 domains (Box 5-1). The phosphorylated receptor may bind and activate several of these SH2 domain proteins:

- *PLC-γ* functions similarly to PLC-β (see the section on "G-Protein-Linked Receptors") and activates the PKC and IP$_3$-Ca^{2+} pathways.
- *PI 3'-kinase* (phosphatidylinositol 3'-kinase) and related enzymes such as the normal counterpart of the *ATM (ataxia telangiectasia mutated)* gene.
- *GTPase-activating proteins* (GAPs), which regulate the function of *monomeric GTP-binding proteins* (Ras, Rho, Rac) and in turn the MAP-kinase pathway.

Tyrosine kinase-associated receptors behave similarly to receptor tyrosine kinases, except that they lack the intrinsic tyrosine kinase activity in their intracellular domain. Their associated tyrosine kinases are usually

BOX 5-1   Src Homology (SH) Domains and Adapter Proteins

Retroviruses are enveloped, positive-strand RNA viruses. They contain reverse transcriptase, which generates a DNA copy of the viral genomic RNA; this DNA is inserted into the genomic DNA of the infected cell. During their evolution, some of these viruses have accidentally incorporated permanently active mutants of cell-proliferation-inducing host cell genes (oncogenes), which are not advantageous for the viral replication, but upon infection can cause malignant transformation of the host cell. The first retrovirus that was isolated is the *Rous sarcoma virus* which induces sarcomas in chickens, and malignant transformation of cultured cells. The gene responsible for these effects is an oncogene termed *v-src* (the v-indicates the viral origin); its normal cellular counterpart is the protooncogene *c-src*. The src protein is a tyrosine kinase. Proteins displaying homology with specific regions of src are said to contain src homology (SH) domains. SH2 domains recognize phosphotyrosine residues. Both SH2 and SH3 domains are important in noncovalent protein-protein binding. A number of small *adapter* or *docking proteins* (such as *Grb2* and *Shc*) have been discovered which contain both SH2 and SH3 domains and thus function as bridges between a phosphorylated receptor and other components of the signal transduction pathway. Other adapter and docking proteins may utilize different motifs, such as the *pleckstrin homology (PH) domain* or the *phosphotyrosine-binding (PTB) domain.*

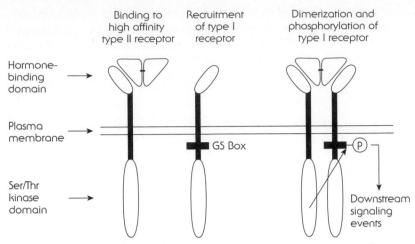

Binding to   Recruitment   Dimerization and
high affinity   of type I   phosphorylation of
type II receptor   receptor   type I receptor

Hormone-
binding
domain

Plasma
membrane
                                              GS Box

Ser/Thr
kinase
domain   Downstream
                                                          signaling
                                                          events

Figure 5-6. Signaling mechanism of the serine/threonine kinase receptors. These receptors are used by members of the transforming growth factor-β (TGF-β) family. TGF-β and the related activins form disulfide-linked dimers, which allow binding two receptors. High affinity binding and specificity are provided by the type II receptor, and the ligand/type II receptor complex recruits the type I receptor. Phosphorylation of the type I receptor by the serine/threonine kinase domain of the type II receptor is a key element in the downstream signaling pathway. (*Source:* Modified from Fig. 7B, p 21, in Chapter 2 of Conn PM, Melmed S: *Endocrinology. Basic and Clinical Principles.* Totowa, New Jersey, Humana Press, 1997.)

members of either the Src family (such as *Fyn*) or the *Janus kinase* (Jak) family (such as Jak1, Jak2, Jak3, or Tyk2). The Jaks often target one or more of the *signal transducer and activator of transcription (STAT)* proteins. This signaling cascade is therefore called the *Jak-STAT pathway.* Most cytokine receptors utilize this mechanism. The ligands of the cytokine receptor superfamily share a similar 3-dimensional structure involving four α-helices *(helix-bundle peptides)*, although their amino acid sequence belongs to diverse subgroups (see Chap. 10).

   Serine/threonine kinase receptors resemble the tyrosine kinase receptors (Fig. 5-6). They have a single transmembrane domain, and are activated upon dimerization. The intracellular domain has an intrinsic serine/threonine kinase enzyme activity. The ligands of these receptors are members of the *transforming growth factor-β* (TGF-β) superfamily. These ligands are either homodimers or heterodimers, and as such have two exposed receptor-binding sites, which promote receptor dimerization. Due to the presence of various receptor subtypes, the dimers may either be homodimers or heterodimers.

   • Receptor types I and II are involved in signaling. Type III receptor *(betaglycan)* may either present the ligand to the type II receptor similar to action of *follistatin* (see Chap. 13) or be involved in its elimination.
   • Type II receptors are responsible for high-affinity and hormone-specific binding of the ligand. Upon binding the ligand, type II receptors may form homodimers.

• Type I receptors are unable to bind the free hormone, but bind to the hormone already associated with the type II receptor, and thus involved in forming heterodimers. They are less specific for the hormone; however, specificity is assured by the prior binding with a type II receptor. The intracellular domain of Type I receptors contains a motif *(GS box)* that is the main target of the serine/threonine kinase activity. The phosphorylated GS box is a presumed target of docking proteins.

The downstream signal-transduction pathway includes the *Smad* family of intracellular proteins. Upon activation of the receptor, Smad2 and/or Smad3 are phosphorylated and complexed with Smad4. The complex is then translocated into the nucleus and regulates gene expression. Disruption of the TGF-β signaling cascade predisposes the individual for the development of colorectal cancer.

Guanylyl cyclase membrane receptors (GCs) and their cytoplasmic counterpart the *soluble guanylyl cyclase* synthesize cyclic GMP from GTP in a manner similar to the biosynthesis of cyclic AMP but without the involvement of G-proteins. The GC membrane receptors which have a single transmembrane domain possess the intrinsic enzyme activity at the C-terminus. The GCs constitute a small family whose members are designated as GCs -A through -F. GCs -D, -E, and -F are orphan receptors expressed in sensory organs. At their extracellular domain, GC-A and GC-B bind *natriuretic peptides* (regulators of ECF volume and blood pressure), whereas GC-C binds heat-stable enterotoxin, which activate the cytoplasmic domain of the receptor. The generated cyclic GMP acts in a fashion similar to cyclic AMP.

The soluble guanylyl cyclase is homologous with the membrane receptor but it is localized mainly in the cytoplasmic compartment, and has a heme group for *nitric oxide* (NO) binding. Although the soluble guanylyl cyclase might be attached to the cytoplasmic face of the membrane (a feature similar to G-protein subunits), it does not have a transmembrane domain. Therefore, due to its location, the soluble guanylyl cyclase cannot be activated by hydrophilic hormones. It is activated by NO, the product of *NO synthase enzymes*. NO is considered to be a second-messenger molecule. However, it is unique in the sense that NO may activate soluble guanylyl cyclase in a cell different from the one that expresses the NO synthase enzyme. NO is a gas that readily penetrates membranes, and thus may reach its target locally by diffusion. A classic example for this signaling pathway is the acetylcholine (ACh)-induced smooth muscle relaxation in the vasculature (Fig. 5-7).

Ligand-Gated Ion Channels (Ion-Channel-Linked Receptors)

The ion channels are multisubunit proteins that form pores in the cell membrane. Upon opening of the pore, flux of specific ions occurs (ions for which the channel is selective). The flux is driven by the electrochemical gradient of each ion involved. Ion channels can be *ligand-gated* or *voltage-*

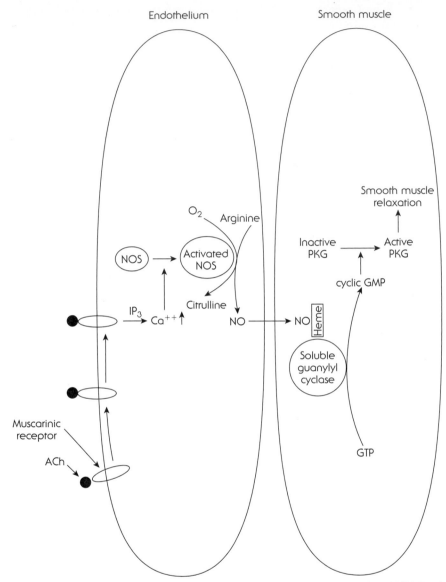

Figure 5-7. The two-cell model of nitric oxide (NO) signaling. Acetylcholine (ACh) binds to its M₃ muscarinic (atropine-sensitive) G-protein coupled receptor in the plasma membrane of the *endothelium*. By activation of the IP₃ pathway and increasing cytosolic concentration of Ca²⁺, ACh activates NO synthase (NOS). The produced NO is a gas that diffuses in every direction, including to the neighboring smooth muscle cells. There it binds to the heme group of the soluble guanylyl cyclase, which in turn generates cyclic GMP. Cyclic GMP activates protein kinase G (PKG) thereby causing smooth muscle relaxation, i.e., vasodilatation.

gated. The ligand-gated ion channels fall into two structural homology groups:

- The first group includes nicotinic cholinergic receptors, serotonin, γ-aminobutyric acid (GABA)- and glycine-gated channels.
- The second group includes the glutamate-gated channels which, based on their ligand selectivity, are further subdivided into
  - *AMPA* (α-amino-3-hydroxy-5methyl-4-isoxazole propionic acid) receptors
  - *NMDA (N methyl-D-aspartate)* receptors
  - *kainate* receptors.

Note that the glutamate-gated ion channels are distinct from the *metabotropic glutamate receptor,* which is a G-protein coupled receptor closely related to the Ca^{2+}-sensing receptor.

Exposure of neurons to high concentrations of glutamate for the duration of a few minutes may result in cell death. This is related to the prolonged influx of Ca^{2+} into the ICF due to stimulation of NMDA receptors. Prolonged stimulation of NMDA receptors in the brain occurs with severe hypoglycemia (drop of plasma glucose concentration) or impaired perfusion of the brain (ischemia). If administered promptly, NMDA receptor antagonist drugs may attenuate the extent of neuronal damage in these pathologic conditions.

Plasma Protein/Transport Receptors

Receptors of this class have a single transmembrane domain. They might not function as signal tranducers; instead they deliver substances from the ECF into the cell by means of *receptor-mediated endocytosis.* Their ligands include low-density lipoprotein (LDL), transferrin, asialoglycoproteins, certain immunoglobulins and other substances. Receptor-mediated endocytosis requires two initial steps:

1. Formation of *clathrin-coated pits* in the cell membrane (the protein clathrin assembles at the cytoplasmic face of the membrane).

2. Association of the receptor-ligand complex with the preformed clathrin-coated pit by lateral diffusion. This involves a binding between the short cytoplasmic domain of the transport receptor and clathrin. Note that ligand binding is not required for the endocytosis of every receptor type. A single clathrin-coated pit may simultaneously associate with several different kinds of receptors.

The clathrin-coated pits are endocytosed as *clathrin-coated vesicles.* Upon losing their clathrin coat, these vesicles join the *early endosomal compartment* of the cell. Due to the ATP-driven proton pump in its membrane, the lumen of this compartment is acidic. The acidic environment induces a conformational change, thereby releasing the ligand from the receptor binding. The contents of these late endosomes merge with *primary lysosomes* to be processed by enzymes. However, the membrane-bound components of the endosomes may have three different fates:

- they may be returned for exocytosis to the membrane surface from which they were derived; this is the mechanism of *receptor recycling;*
- in epithelial cells (such as the vascular endothelium), the endocytosis may occur at the apical membrane, but the exocytosis may occur at the basolateral membrane; this is the mechanism of *transcytosis* (see also Chap. 2);
- some membrane-bound molecules (including the receptors) may merge with lysosomes and thus be broken down. If this pathway is used preferentially by a receptor, the number of receptors at the cell surface decreases. This is one of the mechanisms of *receptor downregulation* (see the section on "Target Cell Adaptation and Rebound Effect").

These cellular mechanisms are utilized by many receptor types, not only by transport receptors. However, quantitative differences exist among the receptor types. For example, the epidermal growth factor (EGF) receptor utilizes the receptor-mediated endocytosis for receptor downregulation (target cell adaptation), whereas transport receptors (such as the *LDL receptor*) uses receptor-mediated endocytosis for delivering cholesterol and fatty acids to the lysosome while the receptor itself is mainly recycled. The lipids liberated from LDL are utilized for membrane synthesis, and in certain cells (such as the trophoblast of the placenta), cholesterol is also used as a precursor of steroid hormones.

One of the transport receptors is referred to as *mannose-6-phosphate/ insulin-like growth factor-2* (M6P/IGF-2) *receptor*. This receptor has multiple ligand binding sites and binds both IGF-2 and several glycoproteins that contain a M6P moiety such as thyroglobulin. This latter feature enables this receptor to bind lysosomal enzymes during vesicular trafficking in the cells. IGF-2 has binding affinity to insulin and IGF-1 receptors, and the latter is the main mediator of its biologic action. The role of binding to the M6P/IGF-2 receptor is the degradation of IGF-2 and protection of the tissues against overexposure to this growth factor (see also in Chaps. 9 and 10).

INTRACELLULAR RECEPTORS

The term intracellular receptor refers to the localization of these proteins: they are not embedded in the plasma membrane to perform binding function at the cell surface, but are found either in the cytoplasm or the cell nucleus and bind ligands that penetrated the cell membrane. The intracellular receptors include three structurally distinct groups of proteins:

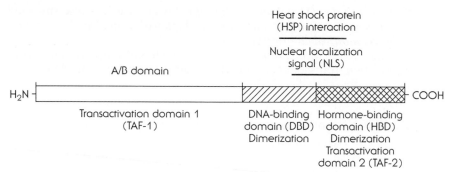

Figure 5-8. Schematic representation of the domain structure of steroid hormone receptors. The size of the DBD and HBD are very similar among the members of the family. Receptors of C21 steroids (progesterone, corticosteroids) have the longest; vitamin D receptors have the shortest A/B domain.

- members of the *steroid hormone receptor superfamily;*
- the *arylhydrocarbon receptor* (AhR);
- *soluble guanylyl cyclase* (see above).

Intracellular receptors were first identified as the receptors of steroid hormones. Several receptors with similar structures and functions were characterized; some of them, however, bound nonsteroidal lipophilic ligands such as thyroid hormones, retinoids, eicosanoids, or long-chain fatty acids. These structurally related receptors are referred to by different names that are interchangeably used in the literature:

- steroid hormone receptor superfamily (although not all ligands are steroids);
- *intracellular receptor superfamily* (meant in a narrow sense, because in a broad sense not all intracellular receptors are structurally related, see above);
- intranuclear or cytoplasmic receptors (a name stemming from initially conflicting observations about the primary localization of these receptors).

In this book, we shall use the term *intracellular receptor superfamily* in its narrow sense, while the AhR and soluble guanylyl cyclase will be referred to by name.

All members of the intracellular receptor superfamily and the AhR bind lipophilic substances and function as *ligand-regulated transcription factors*. The members of the intracellular receptor superfamily are structurally unrelated to the transport proteins of their respective lipophilic hormone ligands. The structure of the intracellular receptors (Fig. 5-8) includes:

- an N-terminal A/B domain of variable size that serves as a *transactivation domain* (TAF-1),

- a *zinc-finger DNA-binding domain* (DBD) which is also involved in receptor dimerization and partially overlaps with a *nuclear localization signal* (NLS) *motif* of the protein, and
- a *hormone-binding domain* (HBD), which is also involved in receptor dimerization, transactivation (TAF-2), and contributes to nuclear localization.

The DBD is both necessary and sufficient to determine target *gene specificity*. The HBD confers the *hormone specificity* to the receptor. Elegant *domain-swap experiments* have demonstrated that the domains function in a modular fashion: hybrid receptors generated by recombinant methods activate genes that contain hormone response elements (HREs) recognized by the DBD module, and the activation requires a hormone which is normally unrelated to the HRE but is specific for the HBD module.

To exert their action, intracellular receptors must be transported into the nucleus through the *nuclear pore complex*. The nuclear pore complex is readily permeable to small molecules, but they perform a gatekeeper function for larger proteins. Thus, only proteins carrying an NLS motif can enter the nucleus. After their synthesis by free cytoplasmic ribosomes, most intracellular receptors are delivered into the nucleus immediately, and their ligand activates them in the nucleus. They are often capable of binding to the DNA in the absence of their ligand, but the ligand is usually required for their full regulatory activity. These receptors are often called *(intra)nuclear hormone receptors*. In certain instances, the expression of these receptors is regulated by their ligands.

Other intracellular receptors reside in the cytoplasm until they bind the specific ligand: these are known as the *cytoplasmic receptors*. While in the cytoplasm, they are associated with a 90-kDa *heat shock protein* (Hsp90) and other proteins such as Hsp70 or immunophilin p59. Zinc is essential for the normal function of these transcription factors. It has been demonstrated that *metallothionein* regulates the availability of zinc, the function of the glucocorticoid receptors, and probably other transcription factors.

The mechanism of action of lipohilic hormones usually involves the following steps (the differences between cytoplasmic and intranuclear receptors are described in parentheses):

- free hormone diffuses through the cell membrane and in most cases (*intranuclear* receptors) through the nuclear membrane;
- the hormone binds with the receptor (the nonactivated *cytoplasmic* receptor molecules exist as hetero-oligomers in association with hsp90);
- the hormone-receptor complex undergoes activation: a conformational change that results in dissociation of the receptor from hsp90 (cytoplasmic receptors);
- translocation of the activated hormone-receptor complex from the cytoplasm into the nucleus (cytoplasmic receptors);

- the activated steroid-receptor complex is either a *homodimer* or a *heterodimer* (involving two different receptors), which binds to specific DNA sequences called *response elements;*
- transcription of specific genes is modified in association with other components of the transcriptional machinery.

The mechanism through which transcription is regulated by these receptors is discussed in Chap. 3.

Some of the intracellular receptors can be activated in a ligand-independent fashion, probably involving receptor phosphorylation. Modulation of PKA activity via cyclic AMP and inhibition of phosphatase activity by okadaic acid have been demonstrated to activate steroid receptors by a ligand-independent mechanism. There are several members of the intracellular receptor superfamily that are orphan receptors, such as *hepatocyte nuclear factor-4α* (HNF-4α) (see Chap. 9). It is quite possible that these are receptor-like transcription factors, which have no physiologic hormone ligands, and are activated by ligand-independent mechanisms similar to those observed in the case of steroid hormone receptors.

Subfamilies of the intracellular receptors have been identified based on the similarities of their DBDs:

- The first four receptors in Table 5-2 (*glucocorticoid receptor* [GR], *mineralocorticoid receptor* [MR], *progesterone receptor* [PR], and *androgen receptor* [AR]) constitute the first subfamily; they are listed in order of decreasing similarity relative to GR. The members of the first subfamily have relatively long A/B domains.
- The second subfamily includes *estrogen receptors* [ERs], *thyroid hormone receptors* [TRs], *retinoid receptors* (*retinoic acid receptor* [RAR] and retinoid X receptor [RXR]), and *vitamin D receptors* [VDRs]. (Some authors designate a separate subfamily for the ERs.) The members of the second subfamily have relatively short A/B domains. Members of this subfamily may bind to the DNA in the absence of their ligand and function as repressors—either binding of the ligand or ligand-independent activation may convert them into activators of transcription.

Note that similar to their affinities for sex hormone binding globulin/testosterone binding globulin (SHBG/TeBG), the potencies of sex steroids on the AR and ERs follow the same order. The DBD of the VDR is most similar to that of TR. The structure of TR is closest to that of RAR. It is important to note that TR and especially RAR are very important in the regulation of embryonic development. This explains the potential teratogenic activity of high doses of vitamin A (a retinoid compound). VDR is not only a regulator of calcium/phosphate homeostasis and bone, but it is also a regulator of cellular differentiation and proliferation. In this capacity, VDR and RAR share similar but distinct functions.

Table 5-2   The Steroid Hormone Receptor Superfamily and
the Arylhydrocarbon Receptor

Receptor	Ligand(s)	Important drugs	Hsp association	Dimer type
1. ("Type II") GR: GR-α: hormone-binding; GR-β: C-terminus-truncated by alternative mRNA splicing, does not bind hormone	Cortisol > corticosterone, aldosterone; partial agonists: progesterone, 11-deoxycortisol, DOC	Agonist: dexamethasone; antagonist: mifepristone (RU486)	Hsp90	Homodimer
2. MR: (also known as type I glucocorticoid receptor)	Aldosterone, DOC, cortisol; antagonist: progesterone	Antagonist: spironolactone	Hsp90	Homodimer
3. PR: A and B isoforms from a single gene	Progesterone	Antagonist/weak agonist: mifepristone	Hsp90	Homodimer
4. AR: gene located on the X chromosome	Dihydrotestosterone > testosterone > androstenedione > DHEA	Antagonist: cyproterone; progesterone (partial agonist?)	Primarily nuclear localization; cytoplasmic too with Hsp	Homodimer
5. ERs: ERα and ERβ	Estradiol > estrone > estriol	Partial agonist, mainly antagonist: tamoxifen	Cytoplasmic receptor associates with Hsps; nuclear localization and DNA binding may occur without ligand	Homodimers and dimers between ERα and ERβ
6. VDR	25(OH)$_2$-Vitamin D$_3$		No association with Hsp90; nuclear localization and DNA binding occurs without ligand	May form heterodimers with RXR
7. TR α and β: separate genes on separate chromosomes; TR-α_2 is a non-hormone-binding inhibitor of T$_3$ action	T$_3$ > T$_4$		"	Homodimer or heterodimer with RXR
8. Retinoid receptors: RAR: RAR α, β and γ; RXR	9-cis retinoic acid	RXR-specific agonists: rexinoids (LGD1069)	"	RAR may form heterodimers with RXR
9. PPAR γ, α, and δ	15Δ-PGJ$_2$, PGI$_2$ (PPAR-γ); DHEAS, long-chain fatty acids (PPARα)	Agonists: troglitazone, rosiglitazone (PPAR γ), gemfibrozil (PPAR α)	—	May form heterodimers with RXR
10. AhR (dioxin receptor): not a member of the steroid hormone receptor superfamily	No known endogenous ligand	Toxic environmental substances such as dioxin-related chemicals	Hsp90	Forms heterodimer with the ARNT protein

ABBREVIATIONS: GR, glucocorticoid receptor; DOC, 11-deoxycorticosterone; MR, mineralocorticoid receptor; Hsp, heat shock protein; PR, progesterone receptor; AR, androgen receptor; ER, estrogen receptor; VDR, vitamin D receptor; RXR, retinoid X receptor; TR, thyroid hormone receptor; T$_3$, triiodothyronine; T$_4$, thyroxine; RAR, retinoic acid receptor; PPAR, peroxisome proliferator-activated receptor; AhR, arylhydrocarbon receptor; ARNT, AhR nuclear translocator.

The members of the first subfamily and ERs tend to form complexes with Hsps and other cytoplasmic proteins, whereas those of the second subfamily (except for ER) are not associated with Hsps. Note that a similar grouping can be observed in the receptors' tendency to form homodimers versus RXR-associated heterodimers (Table 5-2).

Some Intracellular Receptors Share the Same Hormone Response Elements   Because the intracellular receptors bind to the DNA as dimers, the HREs consist of two *half-sites* of six nucleotides, which are separated from each other by a *spacer* of one to five nucleotides. The half-site binds to the *P-box*, a three amino acid segment of the first zinc finger of the DBD: the amino acid sequence of the P-box is specific for the nucleotide sequence of the half-site. The hexameric half-sites maybe either *palindromes* (inverted repeats) or *direct repeats* of DNA (Fig. 5-9).

Among the various intracellular receptors, the following organization can be observed:

- The members of the first subfamily (GR, MR, PR, and AR) of the intracellular receptors share the same palindromic HRE.
- ER recognizes a distinct palindromic HRE.
- The HRE of the second subfamily (TR, retinoid receptors, and VDR, but not ERs) consist of half-sites organized as direct repeats. The nucleotide sequence of the half-site is the same as that of the estrogen-response element (ERE). The binding-specificity of the receptor is determined by the length of the spacer. Note that these are the receptors which act as heterodimers associated with RXR.

These arrangements may explain a number of physiologic observations:

- ERs have weak affinity for thyroid hormone-response elements (TREs) and may act as competitive inhibitors of TR action.
- *Rexinoids* (selective agonist ligands of RXR) are more potent in the prevention and treatment of experimental breast cancer than the ER antagonist tamoxifen, although there is no evidence for RXR:ER heterodimers.
- Progesterone cross-reacts with the HBD of GR and MR. In addition, due to the identical HRE sequences, PR may either mimic or antagonize the action of GR and MR in certain tissues.

Peroxisome Proliferator-Activated Receptors Form Heterodimers with the Retinoid X Receptor (RXR:PPAR Complexes) and Regulate Lipid and Glucose Homeostasis   The *perxosime proliferator-activated receptors* (PPARs) were discovered as orphan receptors. Their name refers to the effect of a number of compounds (such as drugs, industrial chemicals) that induce peroxisome proliferation in the liver of *rodents* involving the activation of PPAR α. Note that activation of PPARs other than PPAR α

A

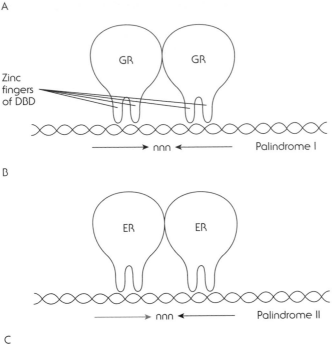

B

C

Figure 5-9. The binding arrangement of steroid hormone receptor dimers to recognition half-sites of hormone response elements (cis acting factors) of the DNA. The binding occurs between DNA and the P-box located on the first zinc finger of each monomeric receptor. Compare with Fig. 3-1. A. The members of the first subfamily of steroid hormone receptors (C21 steroid and androgen receptors) form homodimers that bind to the same palindromic (inverted repeat) half-sites (GR, glucocorticoid receptor). B. Estrogen receptors (ER) bind to a distinct inverted repeat. C. The rest of the second subfamily binds to the same sequence but half-sites are arranged as a direct repeat with variable length of spacer nucleotides (nnn). These receptors (including the thyroid hormone receptor [TR]) often form heterodimers with the rexinoid receptor (RXR), which usually occupies the upstream (5') half-site.

does not cause peroxisome proliferation even in rodents; thus, the term PPAR maybe quite misleading. The peroxisome proliferators (including high doses of DHEAS, a weak androgenic hormone of the adrenal cortex) induce hepatocarcinoma in *rodents*. Humans express significantly lower levels of PPAR α in their liver, and the same compounds do not typically induce peroxisome proliferation or cancer. Yet, activation of PPAR α by certain drugs (the "fibrates," such as *clofibrate* or *gemfibrozil*) can be utilized clinically in the treatment of certain hyperlipidemias. (Note that the fibrates probably do not bind directly to PPAR α but act in an indirect manner.) The terminology of PPARs is somewhat confusing because the ubiquitously expressed PPAR δ is also termed PPAR β and NUC1.

The two isoforms of PPAR γ (PPAR γ_1 and PPAR γ_2) arise from alternative splicing of the same primary transcript and have different expression levels in various tissues. Both isoforms are expressed in adipocytes and skeletal muscle; PPAR γ_2 is also expressed in heart muscle and the liver. Activation of PPAR γ enhances tissue sensitivity and responsiveness to insulin, especially in adipose tissue and in skeletal muscle. PPAR γ agonist drugs (*thiazolidinediones* such as *troglitazone* [Rezulin®] and *rosiglitazone* [Avandia®]) are beneficial in the treatment of type II diabetes mellitus (see Chap. 9).

RXR serves as a partner of several other intracellular receptors in forming heterodimers. RXR:PPAR γ heterodimers are probably the physiologic regulators of insulin sensitivity: synthetic rexinoids in combination with troglitazone are more effective than the drugs are alone, and the combination (but not the stimulation of PPAR γ alone) decreases adiposity. Apparently PPAR α is also active as a RXR:PPAR α heterodimer, because PPAR α requires the presence of RXR and retinoids for mediating the action of peroxisome proliferators. The RXR:PPAR heterodimeric transcription factors usually act together with corepressors and coactivators.

Steroid Hormones May Exert Nongenomic (Nonclassic) Actions   Physiologic concentrations of steroid hormones are sufficient to elicit nongenomic actions. The characteristic features of these nongenomic actions are:

- They are too rapid to allow for transcriptional activation.
- The response is observed in cells, which neither express the appropriate intracellular steroid hormone receptor, nor synthesize RNA and proteins (e.g., spermatozoa).
- Pharmacologic manipulations different from the nuclear receptor-mediated effects interfere with the action.

The best characterized nongenomic actions of steroid hormones have been verified in experiments on spermatozoa, but other sites of action have also been proposed. There is some evidence that androgen-SHBG complexes maybe involved in signaling through cell surface receptors. Metabolites of progesterone and deoxycorticosterone bind to and activate the $GABA_A$ receptor thereby increasing chloride ion flux and resulting in hyperpolarization of the membrane potential. Estradiol, which has been proposed as a protective factor against Alzheimer's disease, acts as agonist on the NMDA receptor in the central nervous system (CNS), including the cortex and the hippocampus. In addition to estradiol, DHEAS and pregenenolone sulfate may also activate NMDA receptors.

The Arylhydrocarbon Receptor:ARNT Protein Heterodimer Regulates the Expression of Enzymes that Metabolize Dioxine-like Environmental Toxins   The AhR has no known endogenous physiologic ligand and is therefore only peripherally related to the endocrine system. Its ligands are environmental substances termed *xenobiotics,* which include toxins, carcinogens, chemicals, and pollutants. The structure of the AhR includes an N-terminal DBD with a helix-loop-helix structure, a ligand-binding domain, and a C-terminal transactivation domain.

The activation of the AhR resembles that of the glucocorticoid receptor. Before it is activated by its ligand, the AhR is complexed with Hsp90 in the cytoplasm. Upon ligand binding, the AhR dissociates from Hsp90, forms a heterodimer with the *AhR nuclear translocator* (ARNT) protein and is translocated to the nucleus. This heterodimer recognizes the *xenobiotic response element* (XRE) of the DNA. Note that ARNT binds with AhR and DNA, but lacks binding affinity for xenobiotics.

The heterodimer induces the transcription of enzymes that metabolize the xenobiotics. Although the mechanism is supposed to protect the organism against toxins, in certain cases the metabolites of xenobiotics may be more dangerous than the original molecule.

ARNT forms heterodimers with other transcription factors, such as the *hypoxia-inducible factor-1α* (HIF-1α, see Chap. 12) and ARNT-related transcription factors are involved in the molecular pacemaker of circadian rhythms (see Chap. 14).

TARGET CELL ADAPTATION AND REBOUND EFFECT

Cellular Signaling Mechanisms Are More Responsive to a Relative Change Rather than the Absolute Composition of the Environment

Obvious everyday examples for this phenomenon are found in the area of special senses. One may smell a gas leak upon entering a building even if the odor is minimal, but within a few minutes of continued exposure, one will not smell the gas any longer, unless its concentration has substantially increased. Switching the lights on at night results in an unpleasant blinding sensation, yet upon continued exposure to the same intensity of light the blinding sensation disappears. Thus, *the change in the environment results in a cellular response, and sustained environmental signal decreases the cellular responsiveness.* This phenomenon is known as *target cell adaptation* or *desensitization.*

Target Cell Adaptation May Involve Relatively Slow Receptor Downregulation and Rapid Modulation of the Receptor's Signal Transducer Function   The endocrine system extensively utilizes various mechanisms for target cell adaptation. The mechanisms can be classified based on their kinetics and the specificity of the desensitizing signal. Based on their kinetic differences, we can distinguish

- *rapid desensitization,* which is effective within seconds to minutes of the exposure; and
- *slow desensitization,* which is effective only after hours of continued exposure.

Based on the specificity of the desensitizing signal, we can distinguish

- *homologous desensitization:* stimulation of the receptor results in desensitization of the same receptor; and
- *heterologous desensitization:* stimulation of the receptor results in desensitization of a different receptor.

The main mechanism of slow desensitization is *receptor downregulation,* which is a decrease in the number of receptors available to the ligand. The foremost mechanism of membrane receptor downregulation is the *internalization* of the receptors by endocytosis (see above). The internalized receptors can be destroyed by lysosomal enzymes. Even if the receptors are recycled to the cell surface, their relative distribution between the cell surface and the endosomal compartment can be shifted to the latter, where they are not exposed to the ECF and cannot sense their hormone ligand. Another important mechanism involves the *inhibition of the synthesis of receptors.* For example, the LDL receptor delivers cholesterol to the cell. If the cellular levels of cholesterol are high, transcription of the LDL receptor decreases. This mechanism protects the cell from cholesterol overload.

A major mechanism of rapid desensitization, at least in case of the heptahelical transmembrane (G-protein linked) receptors, is phosphorylation of the receptor (Fig. 5-3). These receptors have a relatively long C-terminal intracellular domain after their seventh transmembrane helix, which is subject to phosphorylation. In case of the β-adrenergic receptor, there are two phosphorylation sites: one site is targeted by PKA, the other site is targeted by the receptor-specific enzyme *β-adrenergic receptor kinase* (βARK). Both phosphorylations may separately disable the receptor's $G\alpha_s$-activating mechanism. The latter mechanism involves the binding of an inhibitory protein termed *β-arrestin,* which recognizes the βARK-phosphorylated receptor as a docking site. PKA in the cell can be activated by any receptor using the $G\alpha_s$ signaling pathway. As a consequence, phosphorylation of the β-adrenergic receptor by PKA may result from either homologous or heterologous desensitization. In contrast, βARK is activated only by the β-adrenergic receptor upon ligand binding, and therefore the β-arrestin mechanism results only in homologous desensitization.

Cessation of a Prolonged Exposure to Inhibitory Hormones May Result in a Rebound Effect   When the concentration of a hormone suddenly increases in the ECF, the target cell responds to the change, and if the exposure to the hormone is maintained, the target cell adapts by decreasing its responsiveness to the hormone. The same sequence of events can be seen in a reversed fashion when, *after a prolonged exposure to a hormone,* its concentration suddenly decreases in the ECF. The target cell responds to the decrease, and if the reduced hormone exposure is maintained, the target cell adapts by increasing its responsiveness to the hormone. The response to the withdrawal of inhibitory hormones is called the *rebound effect,* which can be demonstrated both in vitro and in vivo.

Examples include the cessation of prolonged exposure of pituitary cells to the growth hormone-inhibiting peptide *somatostatin* (SRIF, or its agonist *octreotide*), the prolactin-inhibiting monoamine *dopamine* (or its agonist *bromocriptine*). When exposure of the pituitary cells is discontinued to SRIF or octreotide, a major surge of growth hormone release is observed even in the absence of the appropriate releasing hormone (GHRH). Similarly, withdrawal of dopamine or bromocriptine leads to an abrupt surge of prolactin release. To avoid the rebound effect in a clinical setting, hormones used as drugs are withdrawn gradually rather than suddenly.

INTEGRATION OF MULTIPLE SIGNALS BY THE CELL

The Main Types of Interaction among Hormones

Hormones Acting on Different Receptors May Be Functional Agonists and Antagonists   All cells are simultaneously exposed to a number of hormones. Although acting on *distinct receptors*, some of the hormones may affect the same cellular function. (It is important to remember that this mechanism is different from the action of receptor agonists and antagonists, which target the *same receptors*.) Hormones may be

- *functional agonists,* if their effects are qualitatively similar (either suppressors or stimulators of the particular function); or
- *functional antagonists,* if their effects are qualitatively opposite of each other (one is a suppressor, the other is a stimulator of the particular function).

For example, in terms of their effects on GH, GH-releasing peptides (*GHRPs;* also known as *GH-secretagogues* [GHS]) are functional agonists of GHRH; *somatostatin* (SRIF) is a functional antagonist of both GHRH and GHRPs. GHRPs, GHRH, and SRIF act on distinct receptors expressed by the GH-secreting pituitary cell (see Chap. 10).

The effect of two functional agonist hormones maybe *additive,* which means that their combined effect equals the sum of their effects achieved separately. The additive effect may have various causes:

- If the two hormones at the concentrations observed (or used experimentally) provoke submaximal biologic effects separately, and the sum of these effects is ≤100% (100% = maximal biologic response), their effects are often additive. However, under these circumstances one cannot draw conclusions about the relationship between the postreceptor mechanisms utilized by the hormones.
- If the two hormones at the concentrations observed (or used experimentally) provoke maximal biologic effects separately, their effects maybe additive if they act via *independent mechanisms*. For example, hormone "A" activates adenylyl cyclase, whereas hormone "B" activates PLC-β. The prerequisites of an additive effect also include that
  - the simultaneous stimulation does not result in a *ceiling effect:* for example, the cellular hormone reserve and the biosynthetic capacity of a GH-producing cell must not be exhausted upon a combined stimulus by GHRH and another stimulus;
  - there is no *cross-talk* between the second messenger systems utilized by the functional agonist hormones.

Because the prerequisites of an additive effect are rarely fulfilled, quantitatively true additive effects are rarely observed. Functional agonists may have combined effects that are different from the additive affect.

- If the combined effect of two functional agonists exceeds the additive effect, it is called *potentiation* or *synergism*. (In a loose sense, the terms synergistic hormones and functional agonist hormones are used interchangeably.)
- The combined effect of the two hormones maybe less than expected from an additive action. This maybe due to a partial overlap of the second messenger systems utilized by the two receptors involved.

If two receptors are coupled with the same second messenger system, which can be maximally stimulated by either of the hormones as ligands, the outcome of combined effect depends on the degree of stimulation as separate effects. For example, hepatic glycogenolysis is stimulated by hormones activating adenylyl cyclase. This mechanism can be activated by several hormones such as adrenaline acting on β-adrenergic receptors and glucagon.

- If these hormones would separately induce submaximal glycogenolysis, their effects maybe additive until the sum of their effects approaches 100%.
- If the sum of their separate effects exceeds 100%, the combined effect will be less than additive.
- If these hormones would separately induce maximal glycogenolysis (100%), their combined effect would be no more than their effects separately.

Permissive Action Is an Important Means of Integrating Multiple Hormonal Signals Permissive action of a hormone means that it has no detect-

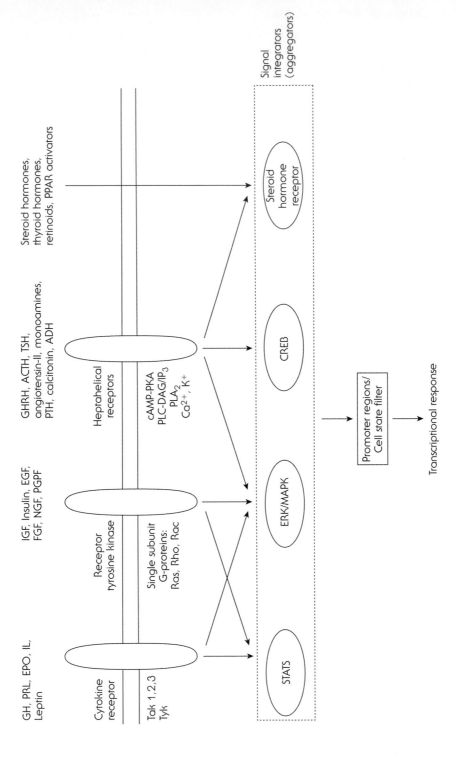

able effect by itself, but permits the action of another. For example, hormone "A" may increase the expression of the receptor for hormone "B" in a particular cell type; however, hormone "A" by itself cannot initiate the postreceptor cascade of hormone "B." In the absence of hormone "B," there is no detectable effect of the increased numbers of hormone "B" receptors. However, upon exposure to hormone "B," the cell may now display an enhanced response, i.e., hormone "A" permitted (enhanced, modulated) the action of hormone B. (See also the concept of modulators in Chap. 2).

This mechanism is utilized extensively in endocrine signaling. Examples include the induction of the β_1 adrenergic receptors of the heart by thyroid hormones (see Chap. 11), or the induction of α_1 adrenergic receptors of vascular smooth muscle cells by glucocorticoids (see Chap. 12). However, the permissive action does not always involve modulation of receptor expression. Induction of an enzyme involved in hormone synthesis may be in effect a permissive action, if the regulation of hormone synthesis and hormone release involves distinct mechanisms (see Chap. 3).

The Signal Transduction Pathways May Produce an Integrated Response to the Multiple Hormonal Input in a Cell-State-Dependent Manner As we have seen, receptors provide cells with the means to respond to hormones with a remarkable ligand specificity. The receptors may either regulate signal transduction pathways or function as transcription factors.

Each cell expresses a number of different receptors, which are simultaneously exposed to various hormones present in the ECF. One could envision that the hormone specificity of the ligand-receptor interaction is matched by the hormone specificity of the postreceptor events. In other words, a given cell responds to hormone "A" via the cyclic AMP-PKA pathway, to hormone "B" via the PKC and calmodulin pathways, and to hormone "C" via the Jak-STAT pathway, and these pathways act in an independent fashion. This would imply that the cellular response would be predictably the same for hormone "A" irrespective of the presence or absence of hormones "B" and "C." This *deterministic model* does not fit well with experimental findings.

The various signal transduction pathways include several shared elements (*convergence points*) resulting in an extensive cross-talk among the second messenger systems (Fig. 5-10). Important examples include the following:

Figure 5-10. Fuzzy logic integration of multiple signals in the regulation of transcription. The parallel processing of multiple inputs leads to convergence points as a part of the cross-talk among second messenger systems. The convergence points function as signal integrators. The signals are "interpreted," meaning that the response will depend on the actual physiologic state of the cell. (*Source:* Modified from Horseman ND et al: The logic of signaling from the cell surface to the nucleus. Trends Endocrinol Metab 8:123–129, 1997.)

- CREB can be activated not only by PKA, but also by CaM-Kinase;
- The MAPK pathway can be activated not only by RTKs, but also by cytokine receptors and by heptahelical receptors via PKC;
- In addition to cytokine receptors, STATs can be activated by RTKs.

The downstream signaling of CREB, MAPK, or STATs will be the same irrespective of the factor that activated them. However, the degree of activation depends on multiple inputs of different intensity. Thus, CREB, MAPK, STATs, and other intracellular signaling molecules act as *signal integrators* (or *aggregators*), which serve as convergence points of various signal transduction pathways.

The effect of any signaling molecule is "interpreted" by the cell, which means that the cellular response to the same signal by a given cell type depends on the current physiologic state of the cell. This also may include the temporal pattern of hormone exposure. For example, prior phosphorylation of a signaling protein at certain sites may prevent phosphorylation of the same protein at other sites (by another kinase), and the activity of the protein is determined by its phosphorylation pattern.

Many signal integrators regulate transcriptional activity and/or cellular growth. As discussed earlier (see Chap. 3), transcription is determined by cellular differentiation: which genes are present in an inducible state as determined by chromatin structure, DNA-methylation, presence of transcription factors, co-activators and co-repressors, etc. Thus, the signal integrators produce a response that depends on the cellular differentiation and the intensity of the integrated signal. A "fuzzy logic" model has been proposed for describing the signaling process from membrane receptors to the cell nucleus.

The signal transduction pathways may also have elements that serve as *divergence (branching) points* of a cascade. For example, PKA not only activates CREB, but also activates several other target proteins unrelated to transcriptional regulation.

The overall cellular response will include some hormone-specific (receptor- or second messenger-specific) elements located upstream of convergence points, and elements that are not specific for hormones but are downstream of convergence points.

Integration of Signaling Pathways in Transcriptional Regulation

Early- and Delayed-Response Genes May Be Induced or Repressed Either Transiently or Stably by the Activation of Cell Surface Receptors

Activation of surface receptors leads to an almost immediate response via the modulation of the function of *preexisting* proteins. A good example for this immediate action is glucagon-induced glycogenolysis in the liver. Such an action involves neither transcription nor translation, and thus it is not inhibited by the protein synthesis inhibitor *cycloheximide.*

However, similar to the typical biologic effects of lipophilic hormones/intracellular receptors, some of the biologic effects of activated cell surface receptors involve transcription (i.e., regulation of gene expression). There are several intracellular cascades that communicate the signal from the membrane to the nuclear DNA. The transcriptional regulation exerted by these cascades has common features:

- the signal may induce *immediate* (or *early response*) *genes,* whose expression is cycloheximide-independent; i.e., the *RNA synthesis* of these genes is performed by preexisting proteins, including trans-acting factors such as STAT proteins, whose activity is usually modulated by phosphorylation;
- the signal may induce *delayed response genes,* whose expression is cycloheximide-sensitive, i.e., requires the *translation* of the mRNA of certain early response genes, which function as trans-acting factors for other genes. Because the synthesis of proteins takes time, the induction of the delayed response genes becomes detectable only at least 30 min after the cell is exposed to the hormone;
- the induction of either the early response or the delayed response genes may follow one of two time-courses: it is either transient or stable. The expression of *transiently induced genes* is usually terminated within 1 to 4 h *in spite of the continued activation of the hormone receptor.* The same transiently induced genes maybe induced by several different hormones (mainly growth factors) and in various cell types. Most transiently induced genes are protooncogenes. In contrast, the expression of *stably induced genes* is *sustained as long as the receptor is stimulated by the hormone;* these genes are usually induced in a more hormone- and cell type-specific manner. The duration and magnitude of gene expression is limited by *counterregulating mechanisms:* e.g., phosphatases, nucleases, and inhibitor proteins located within the cell nucleus. These mechanisms are more effective in terminating the signal of transiently induced genes rather than that of stably induced genes.

Note that although most of the time the regulation refers to induction, in certain cases it involves repression of genes. Table 5-3 provides examples for these types of transcriptional regulation.

Transcriptional Regulation by the MAP-Kinase Pathway Is an Example of Integrated Cellular Response   MAP-kinases (MAPKs; also known as *extracellular-signal-regulated kinases* [ERKs]) are Ser/Thr kinases. To understand their function, we shall discuss two aspects:

- The mechanisms activating MAPKs; and
- The mechanism of transcriptional effects exerted by activated MAPKs.

Table 5-3 Transient and Stable Induction of Early-Response and
Delayed-Response Genes

	Transiently induced genes	Stably induced genes
Early-response genes (cycloheximide-insensitive)	c-fos, c-jun	IGF-1 induced by GH, ca- seins induced by PRL
Delayed-response genes (cycloheximide-sensitive)	c-myc, ODC	Globin (of Hb) induced by EPO

ABBREVIATIONS: IGF-1, insulin-like growth factor 1; GH, growth hormone; PRL, prolactin; ODC, ornithine decarboxylase; EPO, erythropoietin; Hb, hemoglobin.

The activation of MAPKs is achieved by a kinase cascade mechanism,
which is organized in a hierarchy (see Table 5-4 and Fig. 5-11).

For full activity, most MAPKs must be phosphorylated at tyrosine and
threonine residues organized in a *TXY* (Thr-X-Tyr) *motif* (X = any amino
acid). This is accomplished by dual specificity kinases termed *MAP/ERK
kinases* (MEKs). MEKs are specific for their substrates: MEK1 activates
ERK1, MEK2 activates ERK2, etc. MEKs are activated either by MEKK,
Raf, or other members of the MEK kinase family, which are all Ser/Thr

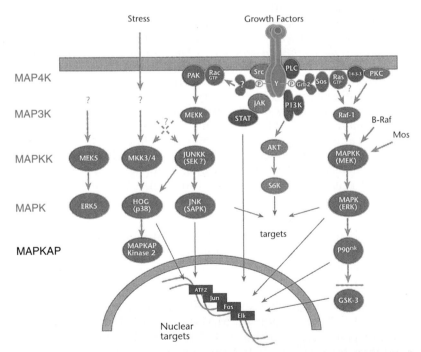

Figure 5-11. The hierarchy of the kinase signaling cascade of the mitogen-activated protein kinase (MAPK) pathway. The steps involved in the hierarchy are highlighted in color.
The position of each step in the hierarchy is shown on the left. (Source: Adapted from Fig.
1 in Seger R: The mitogen-activated protein kinase cascades. Sigma ImmuNotes 14:1–3,
1996.)

Table 5-4 Members of the MAPK Pathway and Their Position in the Hierarchy
of the Kinase Cascade

MAP4K (MAPKKK kinase)	MAP3K (MAPKK kinase)	MAPKK (MAPK kinase)	MAPK (Mitogen-activated protein kinase)
PAK (p21 ras-related protein-activated kinase) PKC	Raf-1	MEKs (MEK1, MEK2, MEK5)	ERKs (ERK1, ERK2, ERK5)
	MEKK (MEK kinase)	MKK3/4 JNKK	HOG JNK (c-Jun amino-terminal kinase) = SAPK (stress-activated protein kinase)
	B-Raf MOS		

kinases. The activated MAPK enters the nucleus and regulates early gene
expression. This involves:

- phosphorylation of the transcription factor *serum response factor*
(SRF)/Elk-1 complex, which in turn induces expression of c-*fos;*
- phosphorylation of the Jun protein (whose expression was induced
by other mechanisms);
- Fos and the phosphorylated Jun form a heterodimer known as
AP–1, which regulates expression of several other genes.

6

ELIMINATION OF THE SIGNAL

OBJECTIVES

1. Discuss the importance and implications of signal elimination.
2. Define the term half-life ($t_{1/2}$). Compare and contrast the definition of the biologic, physical, and effective half-lives of labeled hormones. Be able to perform the essential calculations related to half-life.
3. Discuss the mechanisms of signal elimination at the cellular level.
4. Discuss the mechanisms of signal elimination at the whole-body level.
5. Be able to estimate the molecular weight of polypeptide hormones from the number of their amino acid residues, and to predict their renal clearance.

GENERAL CONCEPTS OF SIGNAL ELIMINATION

Adaptation to Changing Environmental Stimuli Mandate the Signaling Molecules to be Short-Lived

Upon exposure to an adequate stimulus, the cell generates signaling molecules that lead to altered cellular function. The stimulus (i.e., a change in the environment) is typically transient in nature. For example, upon ingestion of a carbohydrate-rich meal, the concentration of plasma glucose increases (hyperglycemia). This leads to changes in cellular signaling in the pancreatic β cells, which in turn release insulin into the circulation. Insulin decreases plasma glucose levels and thereby eliminates the adequate stimulus at the extracellular level (see also under the concept of negative feedback regulation, Chap. 2). However, if the *intracellular* signaling molecules produced within the pancreatic β cell during the transient hyperglycemia were not eliminated, insulin secretion would continue at the enhanced rate, leading to dangerously low levels of glucose (hypoglycemia). The cellular machinery protects against this possibility by the short half-life of most signaling molecules. Another dangerous situation would occur if the insulin secreted in response to the hyperglycemic episode were to remain in the extracellular fluid (ECF) compartment and continue exerting its hypoglycemic effect, even if continued pancreatic insulin release did not occur. Whole-body mechanisms protect against this possibility by the short half-life of insulin in the circulation.

The short-lived nature of the signal is essential for regulation and adaptation to the minute-to-minute needs of the organism. The kinetics of negative feedback regulation are also influenced by the half-lives of the hormones and intracellular signaling molecules involved. In this chapter we shall discuss the main mechanisms responsible for the short-lived nature of the signal. We have already discussed certain mechanisms that are related to signal elimination: target cell adaptation is an attenuation of the signal (see Chap. 5).

The Half-Life of a Molecule Is the Time During which Its Concentration Is Decreased to 50% of the Initial Concentration

The elimination of hormones from the circulation is best described by an exponential function. The half-lives ($t_{1/2}$) of hormones are usually calculated from the *initial* rate of elimination. Quite often, however, the elimination of hormones cannot be accurately described with a single half-life. The second component is typically a longer half-life observed at later stages of hormone elimination, usually at low plasma concentrations of the hormone. This may be due to the presence of a binding protein, which is saturated at low plasma levels of the hormone.

In the absence of binding proteins and secretion of additional quantities of a hormone, its plasma concentration decreases in an exponential manner. The time-course of the elimination can be linearized using a semilogarithmic plot, where the ordinate (y) is the log or ln of the hormone concentration, and the abscissa (x) is the time. The half-life of a hormone in theory can be calculated as:

$$T = \frac{0.693\,t}{\ln x_0 - \ln x_1} \tag{6.1}$$

where T is the half-life of the hormone, t is the time elapsed between the two blood samples that were taken, $\ln x$ is the natural logarithm of the hormone concentration, x_0 is the hormone concentration at time point zero, x_1 is the hormone concentration at the time point corresponding with t, and 0.693 is a constant (ln 2).

Occasionally, concentrations of endogenous hormones decline according to this *biologic half-life*. Certain hormones, such as luteinizing hormone (LH), are secreted in a pulsatile manner. The mechanism involves synchronized exocytosis of LH from the pituitary gonadotroph cells resulting in a surge of plasma hormone levels. The sudden and coordinated exocytosis is followed by an abrupt cessation of hormone release, and LH is not secreted for several minutes. During this period, LH declines in plasma according to its biologic half-life.

The biologic half-life of a hormone can be experimentally determined from the rate of elimination of exogenously administered radioactive hormone. The labeled hormone is infused at a constant rate and its plasma concentration reaches an equilibrium determined by the elimination of the hormone and the rate of infusion. The equilibrium is verified by multiple blood samples. At this point the infusion is stopped, and several blood samples are drawn. From the time-dependent decrease of the labeled hormone, its *effective half-life* can be calculated. The effective half-life is determined by two components: the biologic half-life and the physical half-life. The *physical half-life* is the half-life of the radioactive isotope used for labeling the hormone: the decrease of radioactive signal within the labeled hormone does not indicate elimination of the hormone. The relationship between the effective, biologic, and physical half-lives can be calculated as

$$\frac{1}{T_{biol}} = \frac{1}{T_{eff}} - \frac{1}{T_{phys}} \tag{6.2}$$

The elimination/termination of the intracellular signal is typically an active process regulated by enzyme reactions.

The elimination of the extracellular signal (the hormone per se) may involve:

- cellular internalization and degradation of the hormone by the target cell;
- degradation of hormones by specific organs such as the liver, kidney, or lung (intracellular and ectoenzymes);
- excretion of chemically modified (inactivated) and/or native hormone by the kidneys (and other organs such as the liver, sweat glands, salivary glands, etc.); and
- degradation of the hormone within the circulation by plasma enzymes.

ELIMINATION OF THE SIGNAL AT THE CELLULAR LEVEL

Membrane Receptors

The Cytoplasmic Concentration of a Signaling Molecule Is Determined by Its Production as well as Its Elimination One of the best characterized second messengers is cyclic adenosine monophosphate (cyclic AMP). Its cytoplasmic concentration is determined mainly by the activity of adenylyl cyclase and its degradation by *cyclic phosphodiesterases* (cyclic PDEs), which hydrolyze cAMP into 5'-AMP. The cyclic PDEs can be inhibited by *methylxanthine drugs,* such as *caffeine, theophylline,* and *theobromine.* Thus, cyclic AMP concentration in the intracellular fluid (ICF) can be increased either by inducing the adenylyl cyclase and/or by inhibiting the degradation of cAMP by methylxanthines. The methylxanthines in a clinical setting exert most of their effects by acting as antagonists on *adenosine receptors;* concentrations sufficient to inhibit cyclic PDE are near-toxic, mainly because of their effects on the central nervous system (CNS).

Another cyclic nucleotide second messenger is *cyclic guanosine monophosphatase* (cyclic GMP), which is produced either by guanylyl cyclase membrane receptors or the nitric oxide- (NO)-stimulated soluble guanylyl cyclase. The cyclic GMP is also hydrolyzed by cyclic PDE enzymes. There are at least seven types of cyclic PDEs, which show varying degrees of substrate specificity for cyclic AMP and/or cyclic GMP, different regulatory characteristics, and tissue distribution. Selective inhibition of the cyclic GMP-specific *type 5 cyclic PDE* with the drug *sildenafil citrate* (Viagra®) is used for the treatment of erectile dysfunction: the increased concentration of cyclic GMP in penile vascular smooth muscle cells causes relaxation and thus vasodilation and erection. It is easily understandable that sildenafil is contraindicated in patients taking *NO-donor drugs* (organic nitrates such as *nitroglycerine* or *nitroprusside*) for certain heart conditions; this drug combination may cause life-threatening generalized vasodilation (and drop of blood pressure). NO, which is a second messenger itself, is very labile; it *is mainly eliminated by its binding to hemoglobin.*

Several signal transduction pathways include activation of ion channels either directly (ligand-gated ion channels) or indirectly (IP$_3$-activated Ca^{2+}-channels, phosphorylation of ion channels by protein kinase A [PKA], protein kinase C [PKC], etc.), thereby altering membrane potential and/or activating calcium-dependent mechanisms. Opening of the channels enables ion flux according to the electrochemical gradient. The elimination of this signal means restoration of the ion distribution normally found under resting conditions—this process involves adenosine triphosphate- (ATP)-driven ion pumps.

Phospholipase C (PLC) liberates two second messengers: inositol 1,4,5-triphosphate (IP$_3$) and diacylglycerol (DAG). IP$_3$ is mainly inactivated by *phosphatase* enzymes. DAG is also rapidly inactivated by further cleavage eventually yielding fatty acids and glycerol.

The most widely utilized second messenger mechanism is phosphorylation of various target proteins. Although degradation of cyclic AMP prevents further PKA function, and degradation of DAG prevents further PKC function, the targets of these kinases could continue functioning according to their phosphorylated state. However, the effects of these and other protein kinases are normally short-lived because the phosphate groups are continuously eliminated by specific *protein phosphatase* enzymes. These enzymes have different

- specificities for Ser/Thr-phosphate and/or Tyr-phosphate residues;
- types of regulatory subunits;
- cellular localizations (cytoplasmic, nuclear; there are also membrane receptors that have a phosphatase activity in their cytoplasmic domain); and
- sensitivities for phosphatase inhibitor drugs (such as *okadaic acid*, *cyclosporin A*, *FK506*, *tautomycin*, *vanadate*, and others).

A well-known example is *protein phosphatase 2B*. This enzyme, which is present in the CNS in high concentrations, is regulated by calmodulin (hence its other name: *calcineurin*). It is localized both in the cytoplasm and in the nucleus. It is inhibited by FK506 and cyclosporin A; these drugs are best known for their immunosuppressive effects. Although phosphatases show a significant basal activity, their activity is a regulated (and not a constitutive) function.

Intracellular Receptors

Although it is obvious that the signals of intracellular (steroid) receptors need to be eliminated, relatively little is known about the process. These ligand-regulated transcription factors are phosphoproteins. Certain members of this superfamily can be activated by phosphorylation in a ligand-independent fashion (see Chaps. 5 and 12). Thus, it is plausible that their inactivation could involve phosphatases.

Another consideration is related to the dynamic changes in the concentration of the ligand. When the plasma level of the free hormone decreases below its concentration in the cell, diffusion may occur in the reverse orientation. The hormone dissociates from its receptor, and is carried away from the tissue by its binding protein in plasma. This diffusion-based mechanism of intracellular signal elimination is tied to the elimination of the hormone from the circulation, and thus correlates with the half-life of the hormone. Thus, this mechanism is considerably slower than the signal elimination by cPDE, protein phosphatases or ion pumps. The P-glycoprotein (see blood-brain barrier, Chap. 4) may also limit the intracellular concentration of lipophilic hormones by an active pumping mechanism.

DEGRADATION AND EXCRETION OF HORMONES

The elimination of hormones from the circulation may involve various mechanisms. Hormone degradation may involve multiple steps; in most cases the first step eliminates the biologic activity of the hormone. Certain degradation products of the hormones (such as the amino acids of polypeptide hormones) are partially recycled. However, most hormones are ultimately excreted from the body mainly in the urine by the kidneys and in the bile by the liver. Hormones are also excreted in milk by the lactating mammary gland, in sweat by the eccrine and apocrine sweat glands, and in saliva.

Hormones maybe excreted either as intact molecules or after chemical modification (usually enzyme-dependent inactivation). Hormones and their metabolites in urine are routinely measured in clinical practice (see Chap. 7).

The Estimated Molecular Weight of a Hormone often Provides Insight about Its Half-Life in the Circulation

As a rule of thumb, the approximate molecular weight of a (nonglycosylated) polypeptide can be estimated by multiplying the number of its amino acid residues by 100. This helps in finding out whether the hormone can be filtered by the renal glomerulus, which may be a determining factor in the clearance of the hormone. Although the lipophilic hormones are small molecules, most of them are bound to carrier proteins (see Chap. 4) increasing their effective size above the cutoff limit of the glomerular filter. However, the free hormone is readily filtered by the glomerulus.

The *effective pore size* of the glomerular filter (a basement membrane) is such that it normally retains proteins of about 70 kDa or larger. Albumin, which is the most important plasma protein in the maintenance of oncotic pressure has a molecular weight of 66 kDa, yet it is retained because its negative charge is repelled by the negatively charged basement membrane proteins that form the filter. Understanding of this pore size is important for several reasons:

- Knowing the size of the hormone and the characteristics of the glomerular filter will allow us to predict the renal clearance and the half-life of the hormone.
- We can use the same conceptual framework for understanding penetration of the hormones through the basement membranes of exchange vessels in tissues.
- It helps us understanding some of the pathophysiologic consequences of increased effective pore size of the basement membranes under conditions such as diabetes mellitus.

Polypeptide Hormones Are Degraded by Circulating Enzymes and Membrane-Anchored Ectoenzymes within the Circulation, and by Lysosomal Enzymes upon Receptor-Mediated Internalization

As discussed earlier (Box 4-1), the autacoids bradykinin and kallidin are degraded by the same enzyme which activates angiotensin I (angiotensin converting enzyme [ACE]). Most of the ACE activity is membrane anchored in the pulmonary endothelium, but some is cleaved and circulates in an active form in plasma. Similar to this example, most polypeptide hormones are rapidly degraded by various peptidase/protease enzymes. Polypeptide hormones bound to carrier proteins (growth hormone, insulin-like growth factor-1 [IGF-1], etc.) are typically protected against proteolytic cleavage. Glycosylation may confer partial protection against cleavage; thus, glycoprotein hormones usually have longer half-lives than simple peptides. Much of the degradation of polypeptide hormones occurs in lysosomes after receptor-mediated internalization.

The degradation of other hormones (e.g., steroids, thyroid hormones and monoamines) includes well-characterized and often substrate-specific enzymes. Thus, similar to their synthesis, their degradation will be discussed elsewhere in this book.

7

LABORATORY EVALUATION OF THE ENDOCRINE SYSTEM

OBJECTIVES

1. Compare and contrast the characteristics of binding between a hormone and its binding protein, receptor, or antibody. Discuss the principles of competitive and noncompetitive binding assays. Be able to draw conclusions from Scatchard plots.
2. Compare and contrast the terms immunoreactive and bioactive hormone.
3. Discuss the meaning of the "normal range" of laboratory values.
4. Discuss the importance of association between laboratory values, especially as the association relates to negative feedback regulation. Define "primary," "secondary," and "tertiary" dysfunctions of a hormone system.
5. Identify the types of secretory patterns of hormones, and the impact of these patterns on the clinical interpretation of hormone levels in plasma samples.
6. Discuss the benefits and drawbacks of urine samples versus plasma samples in the evaluation of the endocrine system. Be familiar with the impact of renal function on urinary hormone and metabolite *concentrations* and *amounts*. Discuss creatinine clearance and its importance in the interpretation of urinary hormone excretion.
7. Discuss endogenous and exogenous factors that may affect hormone levels and interfere with the interpretation of laboratory results.
8. Discuss the physiologic background of stimulation (provocation) and suppression tests, and the rationale for using them in clinical practice.
9. Discuss false laboratory results.

MEASUREMENT OF HORMONES

Immunologic Methods Meet Most Requirements for Measuring Hormones with High Specificity and at Low Concentrations Found in Bodily Fluids

Any laboratory measurement must have

- high accuracy (which indicates how well the calculated values fit the nominal concentrations of the hormone);

• high precision (which indicates the reproducibility of individual measurement points; high precision means low variability);
• low intraassay and interassay variation coefficients (reproducible assay characteristics).

Under physiologic conditions, signaling molecules are present in very low (usually around nanomolar) concentrations in bodily fluids, and many hormone molecules have closely related structures. Therefore, measurement of hormones requires very high sensitivity (the detection limit must be low) and high specificity.

The high affinity and specificity of the hormone-receptor interaction is closely paralleled by those of the antigen-antibody interaction. Both types of interaction rely on high-affinity noncovalent binding. Thus, immunologic methods are potentially suitable for hormone measurements. (Note that antibodies may bind the hormone at sites different from the one involved in receptor binding.)

Highly specific *antibodies* (*immunoglobulins*) can be developed against most if not all hormones. Polypeptide hormones usually display species-specific differences in their amino acid sequences in spite of the conserved overall structure of homologous hormones. To be recognized as foreign, a peptide also needs to have a large enough size: about 5 kDa or above. Thus, polypeptides containing about 50 or more amino acids are potentially immunogenic, as long as they display foreign *epitopes* (*antigen determinant groups* that direct the immune reaction and bind the antibodies) that are different from the epitopes of the host's own hormone. Antibody production in animals against human hormones (e.g., growth hormone [GH], β-hCG, etc.) is widely used in the development of clinical laboratory assays for the hormones. The flip side of the coin is that treatment of patients with hormones purified from animal sources can provoke antibody production. For example, type I diabetic patients will develop specific antibodies if treated with *bovine* insulin. These antibodies in turn will prevent the biologic action of the injected bovine insulin.

Molecules smaller than 5 kDa are not immunogenic. In addition, many small hormone molecules (thyroid hormones, monoamines, steroids, melatonin, cyclic adenosine monophosphate [cyclic AMP] and even peptides like thyrotropin-releasing hormone [TRH], etc.) display no species specificity. However, these small molecules may function as *haptens:* they can serve as epitopes if they are conjugated with a large carrier protein. The carrier protein provides the size necessary for provoking the immune reaction; the hapten directs the specificity of the reaction. Once the antibody is developed, it may bind with both the conjugated and the unconjugated hapten.

Mainly *immunoglobulin G (IgG)* antibodies are utilized in immunoassay procedures (Fig. 7-1). During immunization, several different clones of IgG-producing B lymphocytes develop, which all contribute to the pool of different antibodies in the *antiserum* (the serum of immunized animals).

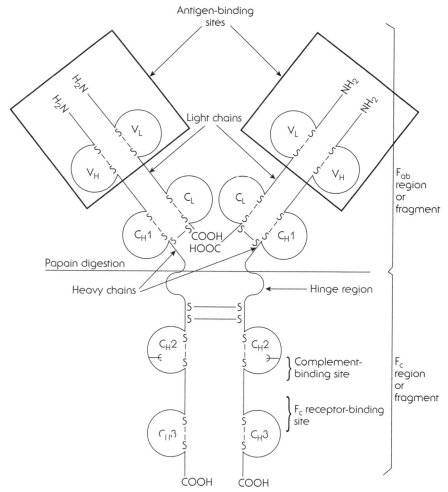

Figure 7-1. Schematic structure of immunoglobulins (Igs). The molecule consists of two *light chains* and two *heavy chains*, which are held together by interchain disulfide bonds (S-S). Intrachain disulfide bonds (S--S) form loops with variable (V) or constant (C) amino acid sequences. Based on the C-terminal *constant region* (C) of the light chain, κ and λ chains are distinguished. Based on the constant region of the heavy chain five main types of heavy chain are identified (α, δ, ε, γ, and μ), which correspond with IgA, IgD, IgE, IgG, and IgM, respectively. The constant region of the heavy chain determines the *isotype* of the antibody. Papain digestion cleaves the antibody in the *hinge region*, yielding a *crystallizable fragment* (F_c) and two *antigen-binding fragments* (F_{ab}). Different portions of the heavy chain constant region are responsible for complement fixation and binding to the F_c receptors of macrophages. The epitope specificity is determined by the antigen-binding sites found within each F_{ab} fragment, which consist of the variable regions (V) of both heavy and light chains. The variable regions shared by antibodies belonging to various isotypes are termed *idiotypes*. These may serve as antigen determinant groups directing antibody production in the same individual. The resulting immunoglobulins are known as *antiidiotype antibodies*, which modulate the immune response.

Thus, the antiserum contains *polyclonal antibodies*. These antibodies are heterogenous in terms of their types (their light chains may either be κ or λ, their γ heavy chain may be of several subtypes), their epitope recognition, and their affinities, even if they recognize the same epitope.

As seen earlier, carrier proteins and receptors are not absolutely specific for a single ligand, and may bind related hormones, usually with lower affinity. Antibodies often exceed the specificity of hormone receptors and carrier proteins. The receptors and carrier proteins were used in radioligand assays (protein or receptor binding assays) similar to *radioimmunoassays* (RIA), but they have been replaced by the more specific immunoglobulins. Nevertheless immunoglobulins may sometimes bind antigens different from their specific ligand: this phenomenon is termed *cross-reactivity*. Characterization of an antiserum or immunoglobulin includes tests of cross-reactivity with compounds that are structurally related to the antigen. Another important aspect of characterization is the *avidity* of the antibody. The terms *affinity* and avidity are sometimes used interchangeably. They both refer to the strength of binding between the ligand and its binder (receptor, immunoglobulin, etc.); however, affinity is a property of the ligand as it binds to a receptor or antibody, whereas avidity is a property of the binder as it binds a ligand.

Today many immunoassays rely on the use of *monoclonal antibodies*. These antibodies represent a homogenous population, and are synthesized by the descendents of a single B lymphocyte (hence their name). B lymphocyte clones can be isolated from the spleen of immunized mice and fused with B-lymphoma cells, which by themselves are unable to produce antibodies. The population of fused cells is called a *hybridoma*. Hybridoma cells obtain their ability to produce a specific antibody from the B lymphocyte of the immunized mouse, and their immortality from the lymphoma cell. Colonies are then derived from single hybridoma cells, and their (obviously) monoclonal antibodies are characterized. Appropriate clones are selected, and propagated either in culture and/or as *ascites*-producing tumors injected into the peritoneal sac of mice. *The monoclonal method is suitable for generating antibodies specific for selected epitopes of a polypeptide hormone.*

To measure antibody-antigen binding at very low concentrations, one must

- introduce a highly detectable tag (label) either into the antigen or the antibody; this is achieved by radioactive isotopes, chemiluminescent compounds, enzymes, etc.; and
- be able to separate the labeled material which is in a bound form from that in the free (unbound) form.

Several similar assays have been developed and are being utilized that rely on these principles. We shall discuss two prototypes: the RIA and the *immunoradiometric assay* (IRMA).

Most Hormones Are Measured by Radioimmunoassay

The principle of RIA is the competition between a nonlabeled ("cold") and a radiolabeled ("hot") antigen for the antigen-binding sites of immunoglobulins. Competition is assured if the antibodies' binding sites are already saturated by the hot antigen. The hot antigen can be displaced from binding by increasing concentrations of cold antigen.

In practice, each assay tube in a RIA has the same standardized amount of immunoglobulin and hot antigen. The *calibration tubes* of the assay also contain known amounts of cold antigen (standardized hormone preparation). According to the laws of mass effect, *the binding sites of antibodies will be occupied by cold and hot antigens in proportion with the ratio of their molar concentrations in solution.* The calibration includes extremes of the possible ratios:

- B_0 (B zero) or *total bound* (TB) is the binding of hot antigen at zero concentration of cold antigen;
- *Nonspecific binding* (NSB) is the binding of hot antigen in the absence of the antibody, which theoretically approximates the binding of hot antigen in the presence of overwhelming concentrations of cold antigen.

Total count (TC) is determined with tubes that only contain the hot antigen. Antibody concentrations are usually adjusted to yield a 30 to 50% specific binding of TC in the B_0 tubes:

$$\frac{B_0 - \text{NSB}}{\text{TC}} \approx 0.5, \tag{7.1}$$

which means that 50% of the hot antigen is sufficient to saturate the binding sites of the antigen. The rest of the RIA tubes contains the samples ("unknown") instead of the standard ("known") hormone preparation.

Once an equilibrium of binding is achieved, the *bound hormone* (immune complexes) are separated from the *free* (unbound) *hormone fraction.* Several methods are being used for this separation. In certain methods, the antibody is chemically bound to a particle by its Fc portion; the particle can be pelleted by centrifugation or a magnetic field. Alternatively, antibodies in solution can be precipitated. This may be done by various means such as *Staphylococcal protein A* or a second antibody. In the double antibody method, for example, if the *primary antibody* (targeting the hormone) was raised in mice, the *secondary antibody* raised in sheep targets the F_c region of murine IgG. The precipitated immunocomplexes are pelleted by centrifugation, and the radioactivity in the precipitate is measured.

The calculated response parameter is the relative specific binding of the hot antigen at each concentration of cold antigen:

$$\frac{B - \text{NSB}}{B_0 - \text{NSB}} \tag{7.2}$$

the value of which may range between 0% (if B = NSB) and 100% (if B = B_0).

The relationship between the concentration of cold hormone (abscissa) and the relative specific binding (ordinate) is typically a negative sigmoid curve (Fig. 7-2). Various mathematical methods are used for linearization of this curve. Using the equation and the measured/calculated value of $(B - \text{NSB})/(B_0 - \text{NSB})$ for each sample, the cold hormone concentrations can be calculated.

A typical RIA is most reliable near the inflection point of the sigmoid curve, and its precision decreases toward the upper and lower plateaus. This may influence the interpretation of laboratory data.

Scatchard Plot Calculated from Equilibrium Binding Assays Is Used for Determining the Affinity and the Ligand-Binding Capacity of Antisera and Receptors As shown, the appropriate dilution of the antiserum (i.e., concentration of the antibody) yields about a 50% specific binding as "total bound." The concentration of the labeled ligand should be near the average concentration of the cold hormone in the samples; this will assure that competition can be demonstrated between the varying concentrations of

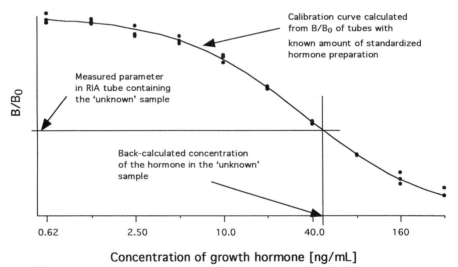

Concentration of growth hormone [ng/mL]

Figure 7-2. The principle of radioimmunoassay (RIA) calculations. A calibration curve is obtained with tubes containing a dilution series of a known amount of standardized hormone preparation. This is used for calculating an equation (calibration curve) that describes the relationship between the hormone concentration in the tube and the response parameter (B/B_0). In the same RIA, tubes are included with unknown concentrations of the hormone. The response parameter is measured directly, and the concentration can be back calculated from the equation. In this example, the 50 μL of serum included in the sample RIA tube resulted in a displacement that fell within the useful range of the calibration curve. The back calculated concentration was 43 ng/mL. The black dots around the calibration curve are replicate measures obtained with the same concentration of standard hormone. The replicates of the 'unknown' sample are not shown.

cold hormone and the constant concentration of hot hormone. Using the standard hormone preparation, one can find (or calculate) the concentration that results in a 50% *displacement* of the labeled hormone:

$$\frac{B - NSB}{B_0 - NSB} = 0.5 \tag{7.3}$$

which means that 50% of the antibodies were occupied by labeled hormone, while the other 50% were occupied by the cold hormone. This also means that the concentrations of the hot and cold hormones were equal. The concentration of the cold hormone was known (it was the standard), the radioactivity of the hot ligand was directly measured. Thus, the *specific activity* of the radiolabeled hormone can be calculated. The value may be expressed, for example, as Ci/mmol.

Once we know the total (labeled + cold) hormone concentrations in each RIA tube, we can calculate the impact of increasing ligand concentration on the binding characteristics. This can be used for the determination of the binding avidity (affinity) and the binding capacity of the antiserum. The same calculations apply to other competitive binding assays as well, and can be used for the characterization of plasma binding proteins and hormone receptors. This has practical consequences: the higher the affinity of the antibody-ligand interaction, the lower the detection limit (i.e., the higher the sensitivity) of the assay.

The details of the reasoning that leads to the Scatchard plot are beyond the scope of this text; however, the Scatchard plot itself is relevant:

$$\frac{[L]_b}{[L]_f} = -\frac{1}{K_a}[L]_b + \frac{n[B]_t}{K_a} \tag{7.4}$$

where $[L]_b$ is the concentration of the bound ligand, $[L]_f$ is the concentration of the free ligand, K_a is the association constant, $[B]_t$ is the total concentration of the binder (antibody, receptor, carrier protein), and n is the *valence* of the binder (number of identical independent binding sites of each binder molecule).

One may easily recognize that the above equation is describing a straight line:

$$y = ax + b \tag{7.5}$$

where y is the ratio of the bound and free concentrations of the ligand, a (the slope of the line) is $-1/K_a$, and b (a constant) is $n[B]_t/K_a$. Indeed, in any given assay, this latter component is a constant because all tubes contain the binder at the same concentration, and the valence and K_a are attributes of the binder. The *slope* of the Scatchard plot *is the affinity* (avidity) of the antibody-hormone interaction; the unit of the affinity is usually expressed as L/mol. High affinity yields a steep slope; low affinity yields a shallow slope in Scatchard plot. Because the value of a is negative, the equation becomes:

$$y = b - ax \hspace{4cm} (7.6)$$

which means that the ratio of the bound and free concentrations of the ligand equals zero when $b = ax$ or $[L]_b$ equals $n[B]_t$. The *intercept* of the Scatchard plot *with the abscissa is the binding capacity* of the antiserum; its unit is usually expressed as mol. Figure 7-3 shows a standard curve and its linearized Scatchard plot. It must be emphasized that these calculations are valid only under equilibrium conditions.

For most RIAs the Scatchard plot does not yield a perfectly straight linear but a curvilinear relationship. This is due in part to the heterogeneity of antibodies in polyclonal antisera. Under these conditions, two equations are calculated at low and high concentrations of the bound ligand, respectively.

The Noncompetitive Immunoradiometric Assay Exceeds the Sensitivity of RIA and May Differentiate between Intact and Cleaved Hormones The principle of IRMA is the binding between a nonlabeled ("cold") antigen and two antibodies that recognize two different epitopes. Both antibodies are used in molar concentrations exceeding that of the

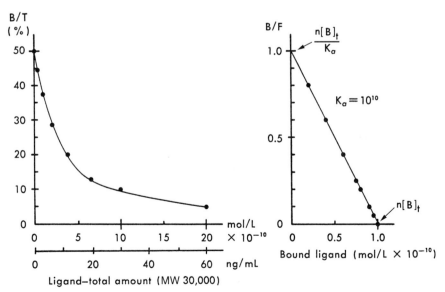

Figure 7-3. Standard curve and its corresponding Scatchard plot. The intercept with the abscissa is the binding capacity of the antiserum; the slope of the line describes the affinity of the hormone-antibody interaction ($1/K_a$). (*Source:* Modified from Fig. 2-4 in Thorell JI, Larson SM: *Radioimmunoassay and Related Techniques. Methodology and Clinical Application.* St. Louis, Mosby, 1978.)

antigen; thus, the assay is noncompetitive. One of the antibodies is conjugated through its Fc region with a particle that can be sedimented by centrifugation or magnetic field. The other antibody carries a radioactive label. The radiolabeled antibody can be sedimented only if it is bound to the particle via the bridge formed by the antigen. This system is often compared to a sandwich: the two slices of bread are the two antibodies, the meat in the sandwich is the antigen (Fig. 7-4).

The sensitivity of IRMA typically exceeds that of the RIA. However, the assay requires that the antigen have two epitopes that are both accessible for simultaneous binding of antibodies. Thus, small antigens (such as steroid hormones) are not suitable for detection by IRMA.

On the other hand, IRMA is the choice of assay for certain polypeptide hormones, which are

- near the detection limit of a RIA;
- found in the circulation both as an intact, biologically active form and as a partially cleaved, biologically inactive form, and the two forms need to be distinguished;
- difficult to label.

A good example is the rationale of measuring *parathyroid hormone* (PTH) by IRMA in clinical practice. The N-terminal epitope of PTH is needed for receptor binding and biologic activity. In plasma, PTH is cleaved very rapidly at its N-terminal, rendering the hormone biologically inactive. As a consequence, the normal concentration of intact PTH is extremely low, near the detection limit of the RIAs utilizing N-terminal epitope-specific antibodies. In addition, this region of PTH is identical with that of *PTH-related protein* (PTHrP), a hormone often elevated in patients suffering from certain types of cancers *(humoral hypercalcemia of malignancy* [HHM]). Thus, N-terminal epitope-specific RIAs are neither sensitive nor specific enough. RIAs utilizing C-terminal specific antibodies do not recognize PTHrP, and reveal higher values because the cleaved PTH has a longer half-life than the intact hormone. Although the cleaved PTH is more readily detectable than intact PTH, this value does not necessarily reflect biologic activity. IRMA targets both the N-terminal and the C-terminal epitopes. The bridge is formed by PTH between the two antibodies only if both epitopes are present. The C-terminal epitope-specific antibody assures that PTHrP is not recognized by the assay. The N-terminal epitope-specific antibody assures that only biologically active PTH is measured. The inherently superior sensitivity of IRMA over RIA assures that either normal, or subnormal concentrations of intact PTH are well above the detection limit of the assay.

The Immunoreactivity of a Hormone May Be Different from Its Biologic Activity   When the concentration of a hormone is measured by an immunoassay, it is often assumed that the values obtained reflect biologically active

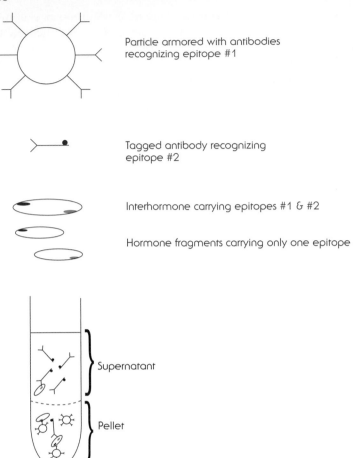

Particle armored with antibodies recognizing epitope #1

Tagged antibody recognizing epitope #2

Interhormone carrying epitopes #1 & #2

Hormone fragments carrying only one epitope

Supernatant

Pellet

Figure 7-4. The principle of the immunoradiometric (IRMA)-type assay. A monoclonal antibody recognizing a selected (such as an N-terminal) epitope of the hormone is covalently bound through its Fc region to a particle that can be sedimented by centrifugation. A second monoclonal antibody recognizing a different (for example C-terminal) epitope is labeled with radioiodine. The radiolabeled antibody cannot be pelletted under the conditions used for the centrifugation step, and it has no binding affinity for the particle or the particle-bound antibody. Standard hormone preparation (for calibration curve) and patient plasma ('unknown') are incubated in separate tubes together with both types of antibodies. The incubation is followed by centrifugation, after which the supernatant is decanted. Radioactivity is measured in the pellet. Only the intact hormone will form such a sandwich (or bridge) that results in sedimentation of the radiolabeled antibody. The pellet also contains particles armored with antibodies binding hormone fragments and free epitope #1-specific binding sites; however, these do not contribute to the sedimented radioactivity, because they are nonlabeled. The supernatant contains some labeled antibodies with free binding sites and some binding with hormone fragments carrying epitope #2. However, these do not contribute to the sedimented radioactivity because they are decanted. Thus, the radioactivity in the pellet is positively related to the concentration of intact hormone carrying both epitopes.

levels of the hormone. However, as also seen in the above example, this assumption may be incorrect. The discrepancy between immunoreactivity and bioactivity may stem from several factors:

- The presence of *binding proteins* in plasma limits the availability of the free hormone to the tissues. Most of the time, the free hormone carries the biologic activity, yet the *RIA usually measures both free and bound hormones together*, which is referred to as the *total hormone* concentration. Various methods have been developed for either the direct measurement or the estimation of free hormone levels for better assessment of biologically relevant concentrations. A good example for this is the measurement of thyroid hormones (see Chap. 11).
- Protein hormones often have more than one epitope. *During the degradation of a polypeptide hormone, the receptor binding activity may be lost (i.e., the hormone is rendered biologically inactive), but the epitope recognized by the antibody of the RIA is still retained.* This problem may be circumvented either by the use of epitope-specific antibodies (see above) or by bioassay of the hormone in the sample.
- Certain hormones display molecular *microheterogeneity* due to posttranslational modifications. This *may differentially affect the immunoreactivity and biologic activity of the hormone.* For example, a portion of the lactogenic hormone prolactin (PRL) may become glycosylated. Glycosylation will reduce both the immunoreactivity and the receptor-binding activity of PRL, and may influence its half-life. Because the reduction of immunoreactivity and biologic activity are disproportional, the bioactivity to immunoreactivity (B/I) ratio of the hormone is affected by glycosylation. Different sources of PRL produce different proportions of nonglycosylated and glycosylated PRL; pituitary PRL is mainly nonglycosylated, while decidual PRL is to a great extent glycosylated. Both sources of PRL contribute to plasma PRL during pregnancy, and differentially influence the assay results.

INTERPRETATION OF LABORATORY RESULTS

Comparison of the Patient's Values to the "Normal Range" and Association of Laboratory Findings

Laboratory reports display a reference range of values, which is typically seen in healthy individuals using a particular method for measurement. The variability stems from individual biologic differences and the less than perfect reproducibility of the assay. The normal values of hormones reported by various clinical laboratories may be quite different because of the use of different assay methods and/or standard (reference) hormone preparations. *The patient's laboratory results must be interpreted using the normal range reported by the same laboratory that performed the assay for the patient.*

The normal value of certain laboratory tests displays a broad range. In this case, *attention must be paid to low-normal and high-normal values.* For example, the normal range of alkaline phosphatase in serum of 1- to 12-year-old boys is normally <350 U/L by the Bowers–McComb method. A 4-year-old boy having GH deficiency may present at the time of diagnosis with 150 U/L alkaline phosphatase; after 1 year of therapy with human recombinant GH, the serum levels increase to 320 U/L. Both values are normal, but the more than twofold increase is a good indication of increased bone growth because most of serum alkaline phosphatase activity in children (unlike in adults) is derived from bone (see Chap. 10).

There are laboratory values that are tied to each other by regulatory processes, and their interpretation requires association. For example, a patient's urine sample has a specific gravity of 1.003 (very dilute urine, which is normal after excessive consumption of water), and a simultaneously collected serum sample has a sodium concentration of 145 mmol/L (high end of normal spectrum). Although both values are within their respective normal ranges, their association raises the possibility of *diabetes insipidus* (usually due to antidiuretic hormone [ADH] deficiency; see Chap. 10) because high normal sodium means relatively high plasma osmolality, which should activate ADH; therefore, the patient should be producing a highly concentrated urine.

The Concept of Negative Feedback Can Be Utilized in the Laboratory Differential Diagnosis of Endocrine Diseases   Feedback mechanisms imply that the concentrations of a regulator (hormone) and its regulated substance (either a hormone or another parameter) do not change independently, but their values are interrelated. These laboratory values should be monitored and interpreted together. This approach enables the clinician to deduce the nature of the endocrine disease. Two generic examples will be used here to introduce the concept: regulation of plasma Ca^{2+} by PTH and regulation of thyroxine by thyroid stimulating hormone (TSH). Although the basic concept in the two examples is the same, the conventional nomenclature describing the functional disturbances is different because the target of the regulator in case of TSH is an endocrine gland.

The PTH-Ca^{2+} Feedback Loop: An Example of Nonendocrine Target of the Regulator Hormone   Under normal conditions, PTH increases plasma Ca^{2+} by several mechanisms (see Chap. 8). The stimulus for increased PTH secretion is subnormal concentration of plasma Ca^{2+}. Supranormal levels of plasma Ca^{2+} suppress PTH secretion to yield plasma PTH concentration below the normal range. This constitutes a negative feedback loop (see Fig. 2-4A). If a patient presents with *hypercalcemia* (supranormal concentration of Ca^{2+}), its cause must be identified. One possibility is that PTH is overproduced, which also implies that the elevated Ca^{2+} is unable to suppress PTH secretion. This condition is known as *primary hyperparathy-*

roidism, which can be caused by a hyperplasia or a tumor of the parathyroids. The laboratory values show an association of elevated PTH with elevated Ca^{2+} (Table 7-1A). However, if the hypercalcemia is associated with subnormal levels of PTH, the conclusion is *secondary hypoparathyroidism,* which can be caused by excessive ingestion of calcium *(milk alkali syndrome)* or vitamin D *(hypervitaminosis D).* (Note that demonstrating suppression of PTH would be practically impossible with RIA because the detection limit of the assay is near the normal value.) In this case, the feedback mechanism is operational and suppresses PTH.

If the plasma Ca^{2+} is normal (or subnormal) and PTH is elevated, then the plasma Ca^{2+} is maintained by an increased PTH output. This condition is known as *secondary hyperparathyroidism,* which maybe caused, for example, by increased urinary Ca^{2+} losses. Finally, if both PTH and Ca^{2+} are subnormal, then one must conclude that the hypocalcemia is unable to induce increased PTH secretion, and actually the hypocalcemia is caused by inadequate PTH production. This is known as *primary hypoparathyroidism,* which may be due to inadvertent surgical removal of the parathyroid glands during thyroidectomy, an autoimmune disease that gradually destroys the parathyroid glands or congenital absence of the parathyroid glands.

Table 7-1   Association of Laboratory Values in the Diagnosis of Endocrine Disorders

A: The Target of Hormonal Regulation Is Not a Hormone

| | | Target (Ca^{2+}) | |
		Low	High
Regulator (PTH)	High	Secondary hyperparathyroidism	Primary hyperparathyroidism
	Low	Primary hypoparathyroidism	Secondary hypoparathyroidism

B: The Target of Hormonal Regulation Is a Hormone

| | | Target (T_4) | |
		Low	High
Regulator (TSH)	High	Primary failure of the target gland (primary hypothyroidism)	Autonomous secretion of the tropic hormone or resistance to the action of the target gland's hormone (secondary hyperthyroidism)
	Low	Deficiency of the tropic hormone (secondary hypothyroidism)	Autonomous secretion of the target gland's hormone or its secretion is maintained by factors other than the tropic hormone (primary hyperthyroidism)

Compare Table 7-1B with Table 11-6.

Note that the term *primary* refers to dysfunction of the regulator gland and/or its hormone. This terminology is used for those hormones whose target (which provides the feedback) is not a hormone. In contrast, in case of hormones whose target (which provides the feedback) is a hormone, the term *primary* refers to the dysfunction of the regulated endocrine gland. We shall use the regulation of the thyroid gland to illustrate this point.

The TSH-T$_4$ Feedback Loop: An Example of Endocrine Target of the Regulator Hormone

The hormones of the thyroid gland (thyroxine [T$_4$] and triiodothyronine [T$_3$]) are important regulators of other hormones (such as GH, ADH), the Na$^+$/K$^+$-ATPase, basal metabolic rate, growth, cardiovascular function, gastrointestinal motility, and myelinization and function of the CNS. A complex regulatory circuitry is involved in the maintenance of the *euthyroid state*, which means normal levels of *free* thyroid hormones (discussed in detail in Chap. 11). Here only a simplified mechanism is presented for illustrating the feedback mechanisms and their laboratory interpretation.

The immediate regulator of thyroid hormone secretion is TSH *(thyrotrop(h)in)*, a glycoprotein dimer produced by the anterior pituitary gland. In turn, secretion of TSH is stimulated by *thyrotropin releasing hormone* (TRH, *thyroliberin*), a tripeptide produced by the hypothalamus and released into the pituitary portal circulation.

The TRH-TSH-T$_4$ axis is a good example of the *hypothalamus-pituitary-target gland* arrangement. The feedback mechanisms regulating the secretion of anterior pituitary hormones include long-loop, short-loop, and ultra-short-loop feedbacks (Fig. 7-5). The discussion of the thyroid hormones is simplified by the fact that only the long-loop feedback plays a clinically significant role in their regulation. The *long-loop feedback* means that the hormone of the target endocrine gland (in this case the thyroid gland) provides negative feedback at the level of the hypothalamus and/or the pituitary gland.

Deranged hormone levels due to a dysfunction of the target endocrine gland per se are referred to as *primary,* those due to the dysfunction of the pituitary gland are referred to as *secondary* (Table 7-1B), and those due to hypothalamic dysfunction are referred to as *tertiary.*

TSH levels are normally low, and close to the detection limit of RIAs. Thus, suppression of TSH can be verified only by IRMA-type assays. Note that both the biologic activity and the feedback action are the properties of *free* thyroid hormones, which constitute only a small proportion of the *total* plasma thyroid hormone levels (see Chap. 11). We also must differentiate between clinical and laboratory euthyrodism. For simplicity, we shall assume that the laboratory and clinical findings are in harmony.

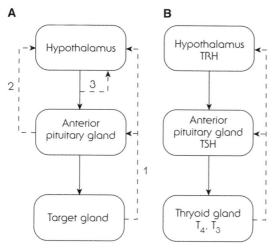

Figure 7-5. Basic negative feedback mechanisms of endocrine regulation by the hypotha-lamo–hypophyseal system. Solid lines and dashed lines indicate stimulation and inhibition, respectively. A. General scheme. The feedback provided by target gland to the pituitary gland and the hypothalamus is *long-loop feedback* (1). The arrows involved in this feedback in effect indicate the systemic circulation. The pituitary may feedback to the hypothalamus usually at the median eminence; this is known as *short-loop feedback* (2), which involves either systemic or retrograde flow in the pituitary portal circulation. The hypothalamic releas-ing and inhibiting hormones may regulate their own secretion by *ultrashort-loop feedback* (3) that is comparable to autocrine and paracrine mechanisms. B. Simplified diagram showing the regulation of thyroid hormone secretion. Note that of the three types of feed-back, only long-loop feedback is significant in the regulation of thyroid hormones. Thyroid hormones directly suppress both TRH and TSH secretion.

Primary hypothyroidism can be recognized by low levels of thyroid hormones associated with high levels of TSH. It is caused by the dysfunction of the thyroid gland per se: agenesis of the thyroid gland during embryonic life, destruction of the thyroid tissue by an autoimmune disease, lack of iodine (an essential component of thyroid hormones) in the diet, or ablation of the thyroid gland by surgery or treatment with radioactive iodine.

Secondary or tertiary hypothyroidism is suspected if low levels of thy-roid hormones are associated with low levels of TSH. Low levels of thyroid hormones are expected to raise TRH and TSH secretion. In case of second-ary hypothyroidism, TSH remains low in spite of an increased hypothalamic TRH output. In case of tertiary hypothyroidism, hypothalamic TRH secre-tion is abnormally low. It would be difficult to measure TRH in the portal circulation; instead, TRH is injected intravenously as a bolus, and its effect on plasma TSH is evaluated. If exogenous TRH stimulates TSH, the low TSH is due to the lack of endogenous TRH, and tertiary hypothyroidism can be diagnosed. If exogenous TRH is not (or subnormally) effective, the damage is suspected in the pituitary gland. This means that the association of spontaneous laboratory values (T_4, TSH) is insufficient to distinguish between secondary and tertiary types of hypothyroidism, and the diagnosis necessitates a *provocation test*: an intravenous bolus injection of TRH (see the section on Provocation Tests). Secondary hypothyroidism may be a part of congenital panhypopituitarism (subnormal production of most pituitary hormones), destruction of normal pituitary architecture by a pituitary tumor, or other causes. Tertiary hypothyroidism "normally" occurs in prematurely born infants, and under certain pathologic conditions such as hypothalamic tumors.

The hallmark of *primary hyperthyroidism* is the association of elevated thyroid hormone and suppressed TSH levels. In addition, the TRH provocation test would yield a subnormal TSH response, indicating that pituitary responsiveness to TRH is reduced by the hyperthyroid state. This maybe due to a hormone-secreting tumor of the thyroid gland, an activating mutation of the TSH receptor's signaling system, or an overdose of thyroid hormone medication, but most often it is the result of an autoimmune disease known as *Graves'* (also known as *Basedow's*) *disease*. In Graves' disease, the autoantibodies bind to a specific epitope of the TSH receptor and imitate the biologic action of TSH. Although the underlying pathology is immunologic in nature, the rest of the regulatory system acts as if the pathological change was in the thyroid gland per se.

Secondary hyperthyroidism is deduced from the association of elevated thyroid hormone and elevated TSH levels, which can be caused by a TSH-secreting pituitary adenoma (an *adenoma* is a glandular tumor). In rare cases, the elevated TSH may arise from an ectopic (extrapituitary) source. Among the anterior pituitary hormones, ectopic production is most often encountered with ACTH, which can be produced by small-cell bronchial cancers.

The differential diagnosis of the hormonal dysfunction as outlined above has a profound consequence on the treatment and the prognosis of the patient.

Secretory Profiles of Hormones

Hormones are usually secreted both by means of constitutive and regulated secretion. Certain hormones are often secreted as episodic bursts or as pulses at regular intervals *(pulsatile secretion)*. A randomly taken plasma sample may have either trough or peak levels of the hormone (or anything in between), that can make the laboratory value difficult to interpret. This problem is usually encountered with hormones that have very short half-lives. There are several approaches to evaluate the levels of these hormones:

• repeated collection of samples suitable to ascertain the endogenous secretory profile; e.g., luteinizing hormone (LH) (see Chap. 13);

• stimulation and inhibition tests during which the plasma hormone levels follow a predictable timecourse (see the section on Stimulation and Suppression Tests);

• measurement of a more stable laboratory parameter that is influenced (almost) exclusively by the hormone in question. For example, while GH secretion shows large fluctuations, plasma concentration of insulin-like growth factor-1 (IGF-1), whose secretion is regulated by GH, is relatively stable;

• measurement of the hormone and/or its metabolites in urine (see the section on Urine Samples and Evaluation of Renal Function).

Another important secretory profile is related to the time of day when the blood sample is collected. The secretion of many hormones follows a *circadian rhythm*. A well-known example for a circadian rhythm is the ACTH-adrenal cortex axis. ACTH and cortisol levels peak early morning. Thus, *the time of day is crucial for collecting the blood samples*. An early symptom of Cushing's disease (ACTH overproduction by a pituitary adenoma) is the loss of the circadian rhythm: the morning values of ACTH and cortisol maybe within the normal range, but unlike in healthy individuals they fail to decrease by the afternoon.

The word circadian refers to the Latin *circa diem* ("approximately a day"). In the absence of photic cues (sunrise, sunset), *the population average* of the endogenous daily rhythm is approximately 24 h, but each individual displays a very reproducible daily rhythm that is slightly different from 24 h. Photic cues reset the biologic clock on a daily basis and synchronize the individual endogenous rhythms (see Chap. 14). The *entrainment of the circadian rhythm* of the ACTH-cortisol axis also involves the timing of meals. Thus, these *environmental factors must be controlled* for a proper interpretation of the data that display a circadian pattern.

Urine Samples and Evaluation of Renal Function

The kidney plays a major role in the maintenance of homeostasis. Renal function usually influences plasma and urine levels of hormones, metabolic products, and electrolytes. As will be discussed later, renal function has an especially important role in calcium homeostasis, osmotic regulation, and acid-base balance. Therefore, interpretation of the laboratory values requires an assessment of renal function. In addition, urinary excretion of hormones is more comparable to normal values, if the values are standardized by parameters of renal function: usually urinary values of hormone metabolites and other solutes are compared to urinary creatinine. Urine production involves the function of *renal corpuscles* and *renal tubules* (Fig. 7-6).

• *Ultrafiltration* is the function of renal corpuscles. The entire glomerular capillary functions as the arterial end of a systemic capillary (see Chap.

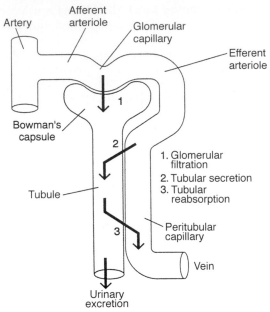

Figure 7-6. The fundamental renal processes. The figure illustrates only the directions of fluid and solute movements, not the specific sites, order of occurrence or anatomical arrangements. (*Source:* Fig. 1-8, p. 17, in Vander AJ: *Renal Physiology,* 5th ed. New York: McGraw-Hill, 1995.)

2, Fig. 2-3). Indeed, the efferent vessel of the glomerulus is not a vein but an arteriole. The hydrostatic pressure in the glomerular capillaries exceeds the colloid osmotic pressure of plasma, which forces low molecular weight plasma constituents through the glomerular membrane (a specialized basal lamina) into the lumen of *Bowman's capsule.* The glomerular filtrate is drained from the Bowman's capsule by the renal tubules.

   • The *renal tubules* modify the composition of the ultrafiltrate by two mechanisms:

   1. *Transporting solutes,* which (depending on the direction of transport) is referred to as *reabsorption* or *secretion.* Most of the reabsorption and secretion is performed by specific transporter and ion-channel membrane proteins. Filtered proteins are reabsorbed by endocytosis. These mechanisms favor reabsorption of "useful" compounds (such as glucose, amino acids, or electrolytes), while "useless" and/or toxic byproducts of metabolism (such as urea, creatinine, or degradation products of hormones) are destined for excretion due to not being reabsorbed and/or being actively secreted. In connection with renal function, the term *excretion* refers to the appearance of solutes in the final urine, irrespective of the mechanisms involved (filtration and/or secretion).

   2. *Transporting water,* by regulated changes in the water permeability of the collecting ducts that allows (or denies) water to follow the movement of solutes.

In clinical practice, urine samples may offer certain advantages over plasma samples. Excretion of a hormone and/or its metabolites in urine over a 24-hour period *(24-hour urine samples)* gives a more stable estimate of hormone production than a plasma value. The wide fluctuations of plasma values are translated into an "area under the curve" by urine; this is known as the (mathematical) "integrator" function of the kidney. For example, adrenaline and noradrenaline (mediators of stress responses secreted by the sympathoadrenal system) display wide fluctuations throughout the day under normal circumstances. In the diagnosis of *pheochromocytoma* (a tumor of the adrenal medulla), plasma levels are not informative enough because levels may also fluctuate in pheochromocytoma patients, and one may obtain a "normal" value. However, the amount of catecholamines and their metabolites (metanephrines and vanillylmandelic acid [VMA]) in 24-hour urine samples is a sensitive measure and useful in establishing the diagnosis.

In other cases, plasma values remain unaltered in the patient, yet urinary excretion may be markedly altered. For example, excessive glucocorticoid production (e.g., Cushing's disease) does not elevate serum concentrations of calcium, but results in serious hypercalciuria. Obviously, in this condition the serum calcium determination *in itself* is not informative.

Creatine phosphate is used as a rapidly mobilizable, high-energy phosphate store in muscle tissue. *Creatinine* is derived from creatine phosphate by nonenzymatic cyclization. The production of creatinine is proportionate to muscle mass, and is a relatively stable parameter for each adult individual; its normal plasma value in adults is 0.6 to 1.3 mg/dL, its 24-hour urinary excretion is approximately 0.6 to 2.0 g/d. Meat is an important dietary source of plasma creatinine; however, diet has less influence on creatinine than on *blood urea nitrogen* (BUN, see below). Plasma levels of creatinine are mainly determined by its elimination by the kidney. For each 50% reduction in *glomerular filtration rate* (GFR), serum creatinine doubles. Because of its steady production, urinary creatinine is used for assuring the accuracy of 24-hour urine sample collection.

Urea is primarily derived from protein catabolism, and is generated in the liver by the *urea cycle (ornithine cycle)*. About 80% of nitrogen is excreted as urea; 24-hour urinary excretion of urea is approximately 12 to 20 g/d in an adult, who is in the state of nitrogen balance. *BUN* is a function of both the amount of urea produced in the liver and the amount excreted by the kidney. BUN increases with age and is sensitive to dietary protein content. Its normal range in adults is about 6 to 20 mg/dL serum. Similar to creatinine, it is increased in renal failure. However, unlike creatinine, it is increased upon dehydration or any other cause of reduced renal perfusion. It is useful to calculate the *BUN:creatinine ratio*. In *prerenal azotemia* (accumulation of nitrogenous waste products under conditions not related to kidney damage, but to the reduced perfusion of an otherwise normal kidney) this ratio is increased, usually above 10:1 or 12:1 (mass ratio; the molar ratio is about fourfold higher than the mass ratio).

In clinical practice, the *endogenous creatinine clearance* (C_{Cr}) is used as a routine estimate of GFR. Although creatinine is mainly filtered by the glomerulus, secretion by renal tubules contributes to its excretion. Thus, C_{Cr} is an overestimate of GFR. The tubular secretion of creatinine is inhibited by certain drugs, which may result in falsely low estimates of GFR. Creatinine clearance is calculated as

$$C_{Cr} = (U_{Cr} \cdot V)/(P_{Cr} \cdot 1440) \qquad (7.7)$$

where U_{Cr} and V are the concentration of creatinine in and the volume of the 24-hour urine sample, and P_{Cr} is the plasma concentration of creatinine. The plasma sample is collected at midpoint of the 24-hour urine collection period. In other words, the amount of creatinine excreted in urine over 24 hours is divided by its concentration in plasma and 1440 (to convert the GFR/24h to GFR/min). This gives the virtual plasma volume cleared of creatinine, or the GFR. GFR is proportionate with body surface area. If the patient is an adult (i.e., has a body surface area close to the average 1.73 m²), correction of the C_{Cr} for body surface is not routinely done. However, correction is needed for children. The normal value of endogenous creatinine clearance in adults is approximately 60 to 140 mL/min/ 1.73 m².

Factors Affecting Hormone Levels

Hormones in the course of their normal function react to environmental and intrinsic factors, which can influence laboratory values and interfere with their interpretation. Some of the major factors include

- meals; for example, *postprandial* (after meal) collection of samples will influence plasma glucose, lipids, insulin, glucagon, GH, cortisol, and other laboratory parameters;
- stress of any kind (such as related to hospital environment, blood sampling, or traffic in case of ambulatory patients); there are a number of stress-responsive hormones, for example, cortisol, adrenaline/noradrenaline, GH, PRL, etc;
- circadian rhythms (see above);
- reproductive stage (prepubertal, pubertal, stage of menstrual cycle, pregnancy, lactation, or menopause); and
- renal function (see above).

Stimulation (Provocation) and Suppression Tests

As mentioned, interpretation of spontaneous hormone levels may be difficult. Difficulties may arise from factors and differential diagnostic problems in addition to those already discussed.

Normal hormone levels may be close to the detection limit of the assay. This makes detection of a decreased hormone level extremely difficult. Under these circumstances, stimulation tests can be performed, which may determine the *reserve capacity* of an endocrine gland. For example, in a suspected case of GH deficiency, one may estimate pituitary GH reserves by stimulating GH secretion with insulin-induced hypoglycemia, arginine infusion, or a bolus injection of GH-releasing hormone (GHRH).

Conversely, in suspected cases of GH overproduction, the presence of normal regulation of GH secretion can be verified by oral administration of glucose: the resulting hyperglycemia suppresses plasma GH levels. Pituitary tumors escape the normal regulatory processes, and their GH production will not be suppressed.

These tests evaluate the pathophysiologic behavior of the endocrine dysfunction, which often has implications in the treatment of the disorder.

False Laboratory Results

False laboratory results may stem from endogenously produced or exogenous compounds (such as certain meals and drugs), which may interfere with the laboratory tests. For example, *ketone bodies,* which are dramatically increased in blood during diabetic ketoacidosis may result in falsely elevated serum creatinine levels. This may be of importance especially because diabetes mellitus may cause impairment of renal function. Another example is the determination of urinary *5-hydroxy-indoleacetic acid* (5-HIAA), which is used in the diagnosis of carcinoid tumors: several foods have high hydroxyindole content that will result in falsely elevated 5-HIAA values (e.g., avocado, banana, pineapple, plum, tomato, and walnut). Steroids found in contraceptives or the potassium-sparing diuretic spironolactone may interfere with cortisol RIA and lead to a false diagnosis of Cushing's syndrome. Reference manuals on clinical laboratory tests need to be consulted for the potential chemical interferences.

Part 2
System-Based
Endocrinology

8

THE PHYSIOLOGY OF BONE AND THE HOMEOSTASIS OF CALCIUM AND PHOSPHATE

OBJECTIVES

1. Describe bone tissue. Identify the proportion of cellular components and the extracellular matrix. Discuss the cell types of bone, their origins and main functions. Define *basic multicellular units*. Discuss bone as an organ. Compare and contrast the features of *compact* versus *cancellous* bones. Discuss the relationship between bone tissue and bone marrow. Describe the innervation, blood supply, and the concept of centrifugal perfusion of bones.

2. Compare and contrast *endochondral* and *intramembranous* mechanisms of ossification. Identify *periosteal* ossification as a subtype of intramembranous ossification. Discuss the nature and functions of *bone morphogenetic proteins* (BMPs). Define the terms *epiphyseal growth plate, epiphyseal closure*, and *dysplasia segments*. Discuss the main factors regulating growth and closure of the epiphyseal plates. Discuss assessment of skeletal development and its endocrine regulation: *bone age, upper-to-lower body segment ratio*, fontanels, and tooth development. Compare and contrast the features of *woven* versus *lamellar* bones. Describe the synthesis, the nature and degradation of bone proteins.

3. Discuss the main biologic functions of calcium and phosphate. Identify their chemical and physical forms. Compare and contrast their distribution among the fluid compartments of the body. Discuss the effect of plasma protein concentration and pH on plasma levels of ionized calcium. Discuss the concept of *solubility product*. Discuss *matrix vesicles* and the mechanism and phases of mineralization. Describe the symptoms of hypocalcemia and hypercalcemia, and the relationship between calcium in plasma and in cerebrospinal fluid (CSF). Be aware of the *recommended dietary allowance* (RDA) for calcium. Discuss the quantitative aspects of calcium and phosphate fluxes between fluid compartments, and identify the main regulators of these fluxes.

4. Discuss the *calcium-sensing receptor* (CaR): its tissue distribution, physiologic functions, ligand-binding properties, and possible second messengers. Discuss the consequences of receptor dysfunction in *benign familial hypocalciuric hypercalcemia, neonatal severe hyperparathyroidism*, and *autosomal dominant hypocalcemia*.

5. Discuss the histogenesis of the parathyroid glands and the regulation of their tissue mass. Describe the biosynthesis, regulation of secretion, and degradation of *parathyroid hormone* (PTH). Discuss the role of magnesium in the regulation of PTH secretion. Discuss the effects of PTH. Distinguish PTH-dependent and PTH-independent reabsorption of calcium. Discuss hyperparathyroidism, its types, and the potential association of primary hyperparathyroidism with *multiple endocrine neoplasia* (MEN) syndromes. Compare and contrast PTH and *PTH-related protein* (PTHrP): the structure of the hormones, their tissue distribution/source(s), physiologic targets, receptors, actions, and regulators. Discuss the second messengers of their receptors and receptor-related disease states, such as *McCune–Albright syndrome* and the various types of *pseudohypoparathyroidism*.

6. Discuss the relationship between dietary and endogenously synthesized vitamin D. Be aware of the RDA of vitamin D. Discuss the biosynthesis of vitamin D, the regulation of its activation, plasma transport and degradation. Compare the biologic activity of various vitamin D derivatives. Identify the targets of vitamin D derivatives: organs, cells types, and receptors. Discuss the physiologic actions of vitamin D derivatives; compare and contrast direct and indirect effects on bone/bone minerals. Distinguish vitamin D-dependent and -independent absorption of dietary calcium. Discuss *vitamin D-resistant (type II) rickets* and *hypervitaminosis D*.

7. Discuss the source, biosynthesis, regulation of secretion, and degradation of *calcitonin* (CT). Discuss the embryologic origin of the C-cells, *medullary thyroid cancer*, its diagnosis by provocative tests, and the peptides measured. Compare the receptor of CT with that of PTH/PTHrP. Identify the potential targets of CT, and the difference in the effects of endogenous versus exogenous CT in states of health and disease.

8. Describe the involvement of other hormones in the regulation calcium and phosphate: estrogens, prolactin (PRL), growth hormone (GH)/insulin-like growth factor-1 (IGF-1), thyroid hormones, and glucocorticoids. Identify the mechanisms that support skeletal development of the fetus or neonate, and protect against maternal bone and mineral losses.

9. Discuss the local factors in the regulation of bone remodeling. Discuss the coupling of mechanical stress with the activity of basic multicellular units. Identify the relationship between mechanical load and bone structure. Discuss the local circuitry of cytokines in the balanced function of *osteoblasts* and *osteoclasts*, and the systemic hormones as modulators of the local circuitry. Discuss the basis of the requirement for cell-to-cell contact in the recruitment, maturation, and activation of osteoclasts, and the concept of *decoy receptors*.

10. Discuss the integrated endocrine regulation of plasma ionized calcium, bone structure, and bone minerals. In this context, discuss hypercalcemic and hypocalcemic conditions, *renal osteodystrophy* (as a hyperphosphatemic condition), and *hypophosphatemic rickets*.

11. In addition to those listed above, be familiar with salient aspects of selected disease states: *osteoporosis, osteomalacia/rickets, milk-alkali syndrome, Paget's disease, osteopetrosis, osteogenesis imperfecta, achondroplasia, Jansen's* and *Blomstrand chondrodysplasias,* and *DiGeorge's syndrome*.

12. Identify clinical laboratory parameters useful in the assessment of osteoclastic activity, osteoblastic activity, and degradation of bone matrix. Define the laboratory criteria for hypercalcemia, hypocalcemia, and hypercalciuria.

THE STRUCTURE OF BONE

Most of the calcium and phosphate content of the body is found in bones. Accordingly, bone is a major determinant of calcium and phosphate homeostasis. The compartmentalization of calcium in bone is an important component of physiologic regulation. Thus, before we discuss these homeostatic mechanisms, we need to understand the structure of bone.

Anatomically, each bone is composed of a blend of tissues, and thus constitutes an *organ.* The bulk of bone consists of a mineralized and highly vascular *bone tissue,* which is surrounded by a connective tissue sheath known as the *periosteum.* The periosteal sheath is missing at the joints, where bones are usually covered by cartilage.

Bones are heterogenous in their structural features and histogenesis (Table 8-1). Macroscopically, bones are classified based on their shapes and dimensions. *Long bones* are divided into three portions (see also Fig. 8-1):

- *diaphysis* (shaft), a cylinder-shaped structure that mainly consists of thick *compact bone* surrounding a medullary cavity;
- proximal and distal *epiphyses,* which are typically covered by *articular cartilage* (a specialized *hyalin cartilage* lacking a perichondrium) and primarily consist of *spongy bone* with a thin shell of compact cortex;
- *metaphyses,* which are found between the diaphysis and the epiphyses; they have a structure similar to the epiphysis, but (in a growing individual) are separated from the adjacent epiphysis by the cartilagineous *epiphyseal growth plate.*

Table 8-1   Classification of Bones

The basis of classification	Types of bone
Gross anatomic appearance/relative dimensions	Long, flat, cuboidal
Relative contribution of bone tissue and vasculature/marrow *by volume*	*Compact (cortical) bone:* <10% soft tissue *Trabecular (cancellous, spongy) bone:* approximately 75% soft tissue
Histogenesis of bone	*Endochondral ossification* *Intramembranous ossification* (including *periosteal ossification*)
Organization of the collagen fibers	*Woven bone* (primary, immature): haphazard orientation of collagen fibers *Lamellar bone* (secondary, mature): parallel bundles of collagen oriented according to mechanical stress

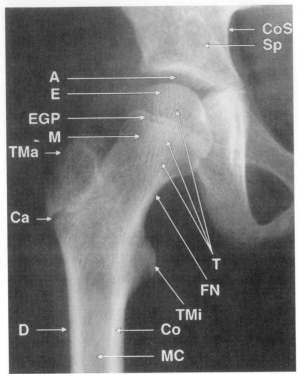

Figure 8-1. Anteroposterior x-ray image of the hip region of an 11-year-old boy. Because x-ray photographs are negative images, the white areas are the dense radiation-absorbing tissues, i.e., calcified material. The femur seen in this image is an example of long bones: the diaphysis (D) is characterized by a thick cortical bone (Co) surrounding the medullary cavity (MC). At the metaphysis (M), the cortical bone is thinner, and the trabeculae (T) of cancellous bone structure are apparent. Note that the pelvis is also formed by cancellous (spongy) bone (Sp), which is surrounded by a thin cortical shell (CoS) typical of cuboidal and flat bones. Several empty-looking areas are filled with noncalcified cartilage. These include the articular cartilage (A), the epiphyseal growth plate (EGP) separating the metaphysis from the epiphysis (E), and a similar cartilage (Ca) connecting the trochanter major (TMa) to the metaphysis. Note that the metaphyseal trabeculae seem to transverse the EGP and continue into the epiphysis. Although the trabeculae are interrupted, they follow the trajectories of mechanical stress forces. Additional anatomic landmarks are the trochanter minor (TMi) and the femoral neck (FN).

The Calcified Extracellular Matrix of Bone Is Maintained by the Balanced Function of Bone-Depositing Osteoblastic and Bone-Resorbing Osteoclastic Cells

Bone tissue is a specialized supporting/connective tissue. As is the case with any connective tissue, the mechanical function of bone is fulfilled by its extracellular matrix, which is quantitatively dominant over its cellular components. The unique and common feature of all bone tissues is that their extracellular matrix is highly mineralized. Due to their mineralization, bones absorb x-rays more than soft tissues; the difference in the x-ray absorbance of tissues is the basis of clinical radiologic imaging.

The extracellular matrix of bone is de novo deposited, remodeled, and constantly adapted to the needs of the body by various types of *bone cells* that belong either to the *osteoblastic* (bone-depositing) or the *osteoclastic* (bone-resorbing) *lineage*. Table 8-2 describes the main types of bone cells. In a healthy adult individual who is on an appropriate diet, active bone deposition and resorption occur even though these actions are not accompanied by a net change in bone mass or composition. The turnover, which is much needed for adaptive bone remodeling, prevention of *osteopetrosis* (see Box 8-1), and the minute-to-minute maintenance of Ca^{2+} in the extracellular fluid (ECF), is due to the balanced function of the bone cells. The osteoblastic and osteoclastic cells, which constitute a local functional unit are referred to as a *bone remodeling unit* or *basic multicellular unit* (BMU). The bone cells are subject to humoral regulation by systemic hormones as well as local factors (see details in the sections on the endocrine regulation of calcium and phosphate and the integrated regulation of calcium and phosphate).

The Two Main Types of Mature Bone Tissue Are the Compact and the Cancellous (Trabecular or Spongy) Bone

Compact bone tissue constitutes about 80% of bone mass. It is best exemplified by the diaphysis of long bones such as the femur, but it actually *forms the outer shell of all bones*. An important example of the compact bone shell is the *lamina dura* of teeth, which is often utilized in the radiologic diagnosis of endocrine disorders that impact bones.

Mature compact bone is organized as *lamellae*. The innermost layers of periosteum contain *osteoprogenitor cells* that differentiate into osteoblasts and are responsible for the *appositional growth* of bone by means of *periosteal ossification*. These periosteal cells deposit the *circumferential lamellae* that encircle the entire perimeter of the diaphysis. The medullary cavity of the diaphysis is lined by *endosteum,* which is in essence a layer of bone-lining cells. The endosteal cells may be displaced by *osteoclasts* that resorb bone. Bone resorption at the endosteal surface and bone deposition at the periosteal surface are coordinated components of bone growth. This explains how the medullary cavity as well as the thickness of cortical bone increase in diameter during growth. The process can be visualized by understanding that the outer diameter of the thin-walled neonatal femur is smaller than the diameter of the medullary cavity of the thick-walled adult femur. This indicates that the entire thickness of the compact bone is achieved by appositional growth, which would imply that the entire thickness should be occupied by circumferential lamellae.

Table 8-2 The Origins, Types, Main Functions, and Regulators of Bone Cells

Cellular origin	Cell type and location	Main functions	Regulators of function
Osteoprogenitor cells (committed mesenchymal stem cells): all derivatives are mononuclear cells	Osteoblasts (found on bone surfaces)	Depositing new bone: secretion of type I collagen and other bone proteins, mineralization of the deposited osteoid seams	Stimulation of growth: GH, IGF-1, FGFs Inhibition of growth: glucocorticoids Stimulation of differentiation: BMPs
	Bone-lining cells (synonyms: resting [non-protein-secreting] osteoblasts, surface osteocytes): found on bone surfaces including the endosteum; form the interface between bone fluid and general ECF	Regulation of recruitment, differentiation and stimulation of osteoclasts by surface expression and secretion of cytokines (ODF, OPG, M-CSF, IL-11, IL-6)	Stimulation of cytokine production: PTH, calcitriol, IL-1 and TNF-α Inhibition of cytokine production: estrogens
	Osteocytes: resting osteoblasts entrapped within the bone matrix; connected to each other and bone lining cells via processes and gap junctions	Regulate the flux of minerals between bone fluid and general ECF	Stimulation of mineral resorption: PTH
			Stimulation of mineral resorption: PTH
Osteoclast precursors: CFU-GM and probably PBM; while the precursors are mononuclear, their mature osteoclastic derivatives are always multinuclear	Osteoclasts: multinuclear (i.e., "giant") cells: replace bone-lining cells and excavate bone in areas termed Howship's lacunae	Bone resorption: liberation of soluble minerals from hydroxyapatite crystals by acidification and hydrolysis of the organic matrix	Simulation: cytokines (ODF, OPG, M-CSF, IL-11, IL-6); PTH acts only indirectly via mobilization of cytokines from osteoblasts Inhibition: CT, estrogens, IFN-γ, IL-18

ABBREVIATIONS: GH, growth hormone; IGF, insulin-like growth factor; FGF, fibroblast growth factor; BMP, bone morphogenetic proteins; PTH, parathyroid hormone; TNF-α, tumor necrosis factor α; ODF, osteoclast differentiation factor; OPG, osteoprotegerin; M-CSF, macrophage colony-stimulating factor; ECF, extracellular fluid; CFU-GM, granulocyte, macrophage colony forming units; PBM, peripheral blood monocytes; CT, calcitonin; IFN, interferon; IL, interleukin.

BOX 8-1   Osteopetrosis (Albers–Schönberg disease)

Osteopetrosis (also known as *marble bone disease*) is the consequence of dramatically reduced or absent osteoclastic activity, which results in diffuse symmetric skeletal sclerosis. The reduced bone turnover causes the increased formation of pyridinium crosslinks in the bone, increased bone mass and increased bone density. The bones assume a stone-like quality, yet they are abnormally brittle. Osteopetrosis has at least four subtypes, and different etiologies.

Most of the thickness of compact bone, however, is occupied by the *Haversian systems* also known as *osteons:* lamellae concentrically arranged around a central *Haversian canal* (Fig. 8-2). The osteons are the products of *bone remodeling.* The circumferential lamellae and the lamellae of older osteons are destroyed by osteoclasts. The surface of the resulting *resorption cavity* is invaded by osteoprogenitor cells that deposit the lamellae of a new osteon. The remnants of the prior circumferential and Haversian lamellae are called *intercalated lamellae,* which fill the space between the new osteons.

The Haversian canal is lined by bone-lining cells, and not by the capillary endothelial cells, which are more centrally located in the canal. The osteocytes are found in the *lacunae*, which are concentrically arranged around the central canal. The lacunae are connected by tiny tunnels called *canaliculi*. The processes of osteocytes occupy the canaliculi. This extensive network of cells is in contact with *bone fluid*, which is a specialized ECF separated from the general ECF compartment by the bone-lining cells.

The Haversian canal contains blood vessels and nerves. These communicate among the adjacent Haversian canals and with the bone surface through the *Volkmann's canals* that are approximately perpendicular to the Haversian canals. Some of the nerves are sympathetic and regulate blood flow. Others stain positive for *substance P* or *calcitonin gene-related peptide* (CGRP) and constitute the pain sensors of bone. Except for the dense connective tissue of the periosteum, *there are no lymphatic vessels within bone*. This explains why *primary bone tumors such as osteosarcoma spread by a hematogenous and not by a lymphatic route.*

Cancellous bone constitutes about 20% of the total bone mass. It is found in several locations, such as the epiphyses and metaphyses of long bones, in flat bones (such as the bones of the *skull vault,* the *sternum,* the *iliac bone*), and in cuboidal bones (such as the *vertebral bodies* and carpal and tarsal bones). The lamellae of cancellous bone are organized as *trabeculae* (beams, spicules) that typically have a diameter too small to house a Haversian system. The trabeculae contain entrapped osteocytes, and their surface is covered by bone-lining cells. The *intertrabecular space* is occupied by bone marrow, quite often by the hematopoietically active *red bone marrow.* In the case of long bones, the intertrabecular space of the epiphyses

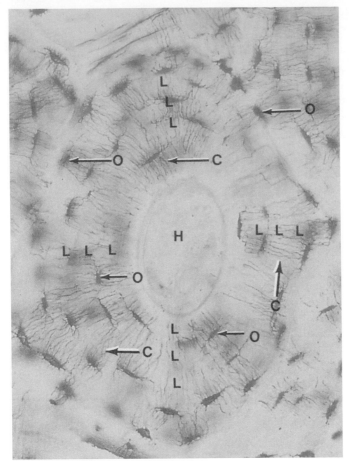

Figure 8-2. Histologic section of bone depicting an osteon (Haversian system) in compact bone. The lamellae (L) are arranged concentrically around the Haversian canal (H). The osteocytes (O) occupy the lacunae; the osteocyte processes communicate with each other via the canaliculi (C). (*Source:* Fig. 4-4, p. 41, in Berman I: *Color Atlas of Histology,* Stamford, CT. Appleton & Lange 1993.)

is continuous with the marrow cavity of the diaphysis, which in adults is occupied by the fatty *yellow bone marrow.*

Bone marrow consists of two compartments:

- The *vascular compartment* contains blood, and is bordered by a vascular wall that consists of an endothelial lining, a basal lamina, and a layer of adventitial cells. The circulation of the marrow is "closed," meaning that the arteries are connected to the veins directly via the sinusoids. The *sinusoids* are the sites where newly formed blood cells may enter the vascular compartment via apertures through (and *not* between) endothelial cells.
- The *hematopoietic compartment* is extravascular. It is found between the vascular wall and the bone-lining cells covering the trabeculae.

The hematopoietic tissue found in this compartment contains the precursor cells of both the osteoblastic and osteoclastic lineages. The fatty connective tissue (which is more characteristic of yellow marrow) is also found within this compartment.

Cancellous bone has a larger *surface-to-mass ratio* than compact bone. Thus, *cancellous bone is more actively involved in the exchange of minerals between bone and the ECF* than compact bone is. In adults, the renewal rate of cancellous bone by remodeling is about 20% per year, as opposed to compact bone which is renewed at a rate of only about 4% per year. As a consequence, cancellous bone is generally more sensitive to an imbalance in the endocrine regulation of calcium homeostasis and bone remodeling. The consequence of this is often seen in clinical practice: compression fractures of vertebral bodies are often the first signs of *osteoporosis* (reduced bone mass; Fig. 8-3).

The Extracellular Space of Bone Tissue Is Occupied by Bone Fluid and an Organic Matrix that Is Impregnated with Precipitated Bone Minerals

The nonmineralized organic matrix called *osteoid* and minerals account for about 35% and 65% of bone tissue mass, respectively. The mineralization of the osteoid usually occurs 12 to 15 days after its deposition. Hence, the newly deposited unmineralized matrix found as a layer between mineralized bone and the osteoblasts is referred to as the *osteoid seam*. Most of the calcium and phosphate content of the body is found in bone minerals mainly in the form of poorly crystallized *hydroxyapatite* $[Ca^{2+}_6(H_3O^+)_2 \cdot (PO_4^{3-})_{10}(OH^-)_2]$. *Bone hydroxyapatite is relatively calcium deficient and may contain other constit-*

A   **B**

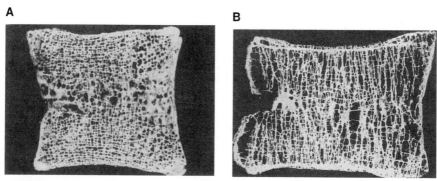

Figure 8-3. Osteoporosis in cancellous bone. Two to three mm thick sagittal sections of lumbar vertebral bodies. (a) The cancellous bone of an 18-year-old male shows no sign of osteoporosis. (b) The vertebral body of an 80-year-old female shows postmenopausal osteoporosis. The spacing between the trabeculae is enlarged, the horizontal elements are greatly reduced in numbers. (Courtesy of J.S. Arnold.) (*Source:* Fig. 7-44, p 245, in Webster SSJ, Chapter 7 in Weiss L: *Cell and Tissue Biology*, 6th ed. Urban & Schwarzenberg, 1988.)

uents such as carbonate (which makes the crystals smaller) *and fluoride* (which may promote formation of larger and more stable crystals). It must be emphasized that the hydroxyapatite crystals are found in the ECF compartment, but not in the fluid per se. Unlike calcium and phosphate ions present in solution, their *crystals are osmotically inactive.*

The mineral content is important for the mechanical function of bone. Moreover, this bone mineral is utilized as a calcium store that is mobilized to maintain Ca^{2+} concentration in the ECF. Because *hypocalcemia* (the subnormal concentration of Ca^{2+} in blood plasma) is a potentially life-threatening condition, normocalcemia is maintained even at the expense of losing bone *mineral content* (as seen in *osteomalacia* and *rickets*) or losing bone mass (losing *organic matrix plus minerals* as seen in *osteoporosis*).

Bone fluid occupies the space

- between the mineralized bone and the bone lining cells;
- between the osteoid seam and the osteoblasts;
- in the lacunae and the canaliculi surrounding the osteocytes and their processes.

Bone fluid has several physiologic functions:

- It contains a *rapidly accessible pool* of calcium utilized in the maintenance of normocalcemia (most of the crystalline calcium is only slowly accessible).
- It provides the crucial microenvironment for the process of the mineralization of the osteoid.
- Its flow is a physiologic signal in the process of adaptive bone remodeling.

Blood Perfuses Bones from the Endosteal Toward the Periosteal Surface

The hemodynamics of bone determines both intravascular and interstitial fluid movements through bone tissue. Under resting conditions, bones are perfused by about 200 to 400 mL/min of blood, which is about 4 to 8% of the cardiac output. The blood supply of long bones is provided by three types of arteries:

- *nutrient arteries*
- *metaphyseal-epiphyseal arteries*
- *periosteal arteries.*

The diaphysis and metaphysis receive the bulk of their arterial supply from the nutrient arteries, which penetrate the cortical bone and branch only in the medullary cavity. The branching provides a *parallel* (as opposed to a serial) *supply* of bone marrow and cortical bone tissue. The perfusion rate of the marrow is about 10 to 20% higher than that of cortical bone.

The *nutrient veins* (which run antiparallel with the nutrient arteries) drain the sinusoids of the marrow. In contrast, *the blood supply of cortical bone is drained by periosteal vessels*. The intravascular hydrostatic pressure in endosteal vessels is about 60 mmHg, whereas that in the periosteal vessels is about 15 mmHg. The pressure gradient maintains the *centrifugal perfusion* of bone, i.e, from the endosteal toward the periosteal surface.

Macromolecules (such as albumin) may leave the intravascular compartment and enter the interstitial ECF compartment of bone. The interstitial ECF of bone is compartmentalized by the bone-lining cells, which form a barrier between the general ECF and bone fluid. Even though bone-lining cells are asymmetrical ("polarized"), they are not epithelial in nature and thus not joined by tight junctions that could significantly limit the paracellular route of transport. This leads to albumin and other plasma proteins reaching the bone fluid. The arrangement has major consequences:

- Some of the albumin entering bone fluid binds to the mineralized bone surface, thereby altering the solubility and surface charge of bone minerals.
- Extravasation of albumin in every tissue necessitates a lymphatic drainage, which allows albumin to reenter blood plasma. Bone, however, lacks lymphatic vessels; lymphatic drainage starts at the blind endings of lymphatic capillaries in the periosteum. Therefore, similar to the direction of blood flow, the extravascular ECF of bone displays an *overall* centrifugal orientation of flow. The flow of bone fluid occurs via the lacunae and canaliculi of lamellar bone.
- The shear stress generated by the flow of bone fluid is a signal to osteocyte function that is essential for the maintenance of bone mass (see the section discussing The Local Factors in the Regulation of Bone Remodeling).

Due to the particularly rich capillarization of the vessels, blood flow slows down in the metaphyseal region, which predisposes it to inoculation by hematogenously spreading bacteria and tumors. The metaphysis is therefore often involved in *osteomyelitis*, abscess development, and tumor metastases. In adults, due to the lack of an epiphyseal growth plate, the infection or tumor spreads into the adjacent epiphysis.

THE DEVELOPMENT OF BONE

Bone Tissue Is Formed by Two Major Mechanisms: Intramembranous Ossification and Endochondral Ossification

Intramembranous ossification utilizes direct bone deposition by osteoblastic cells derived from the mesenchymal stem cells *(osteoprogenitors)*. *Periosteal ossification* (see above) is a type of intramembranous bone formation. In contrast, during *endochondral ossification* (Fig. 8-4) the mesenchyme first develops a *cartilaginous anlage*, which is subsequently transformed into bone tissue.

Most bones develop and grow by utilizing both mechanisms. For example, long bones such as the femur initially form, and grow longitudinally, by endochondral ossification, but grow in diameter by periosteal ossification. Although most of the cartilagineous anlage of the long bone is transformed into bone early in life, a special cartilage is retained near the epiphyses. These are known as the *epiphyseal growth plates*. Epiphyseal plates are also found in other types of bones, such as the upper and lower laminae of the vertebral bodies.

In long bones, the proximal and distal epiphyseal growth plates grow at different rates. In the lower limb, the epiphyseal plates close to the knee grow faster. In contrast, in the upper limb, the epiphyseal plates farther from the elbow grow faster. The regions of fast growing epiphyseal plates are the predilecting sites of certain primary bone tumors, such as *osteosarcoma,* that develop from transformed stem cells.

The growth plates are responsible for continued longitudinal growth mainly under the influence of local factors, systemic humoral regulators such as the GH/IGF–1 axis, thyroid hormones and, during puberty, sex steroids mainly acting via stimulating the GH/IGF–1 axis. Stimulation of estrogen receptors in the epiphyseal growth plate ultimately results in the conversion of the cartilage into bone. This event, known as the *epiphyseal closure,* terminates further *longitudinal* growth. The normal time of epiphy-

A

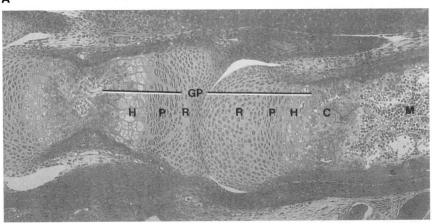

Figure 8-4. Endochondral ossification of long bones. A. The epiphyseal growth plates of two adjacent long bones are shown by the horizontal bars. The zone of resting (R), proliferating (P), hypertrophied (H), and calcified (C) cartilage are labeled. The space between the calcified cartilage spicules formerly occupied by hypertrophied cartilage is connected to the medullary (marrow) cavity (M).

B

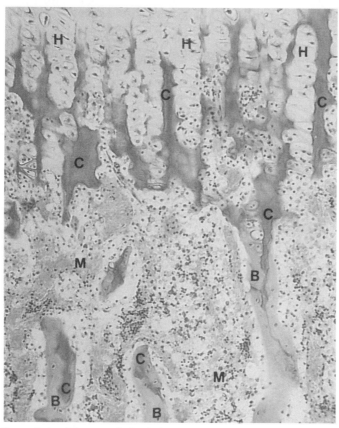

Figure 8-4. (*Continued*) B. At higher magnification, it is clear that the hypertrophied chondrocytes (H) form rows like corn on the cob. The dark stained areas between them are spicules of the calcified cartilage matrix (C). In the medullary cavity (M), bone tissue (B) is deposited onto the surface of the spicules, which shows as lighter stained (eosinophilic) material surrounding a dark (basophilic) core. (*Source:* Figs. 5-2 and 5-4, pp 47, 49, in Berman I: *Color Atlas of Histology*, Stamford, CT: Appleton & Lange 1993.)

seal closure varies with the bone, the location of the growth plate within the bone, and is influenced by the gender and pubertal developmental stage of the individual. In general, pubertal growth and epiphyseal closure occur earlier in females than in males. The slow-growing cartilagenous growth plates of the vertebral bodies are among the last to fuse at about the age of 25 years.

The vertebral column and the bones of the limbs develop and grow longitudinally by an endochondral mechanism. These structures are the main determinants of statural growth and final height. Therefore, *statural growth and height are mainly determined by the growth of cartilage.*

Body Proportions Are Mainly Determined by the Relative Growth of the Trunk and the Limbs

The *upper to lower (U/L) body segment ratio* is a useful clinical measure for the evaluation of skeletal development, and the endocrine function regulating it.

- The *lower body segment* is defined as the distance between the sole of the foot and the symphysis pubis.
- The *upper body segment* is defined as the height (or length) of the individual minus the lower body segment. In pediatric practice it is often directly measured in infants as *head to rump length*.

Infants are born with a relatively large head and a long trunk. In contrast, their limbs (especially the lower limbs) are relatively short. As a consequence, their U/L body segment ratio is relatively high, about 1.7. During normal development, the limbs (especially the lower limbs) grow faster than the trunk. Thus, the U/L body segment ratio decreases, and reaches approximately 0.97 in adults. This pattern implies that under normal endocrine influences, relatively more growth occurs in the limbs than in the vertebral column. Because both the limbs and the vertebral column develop and grow in length by endochondral ossification, their different rates of growth reflects the impact of local factors (such as BMPs; Box 8-2) and different sensitivities to the regulating mechanisms. *Any dysfunction leading to altered rate of growth in the epiphyseal cartilages impacts both the height and the body segment proportions of the individual.* This is well exemplified by the effect of sex steroids on body proportions.

As mentioned earlier, stimulation of estrogen receptors is mainly indirectly responsible for the pubertal growth spurt and directly responsible for the fusion of epiphyseal growth plates (termination of statural growth).

- Individuals suffering from *hypogonadism* (production of subnormal levels of male or female sex steroids) present with a delayed epiphyseal closure. As a consequence, these individuals are tall as adults. Because their U/L body segment ratio continues the normal decreasing trend for a prolonged time, they have disproportionately long limbs and a low U/L body segment ratio (usually below 0.9).
- In contrast, *precocious puberty* leads to a premature pubertal growth spurt and a premature epiphyseal closure. As a consequence, these individuals are tall for their age as children, but short as adults. Because their U/L body segment ratio proceeds with the normal decreasing trend for a shortened time, they have disproportionately short limbs and a high U/L body segment ratio.

Cartilage Is Used Both as an Anlage and as a Template

Achondroplasia is a genetic disease that causes hypoplasia of cartilage. This is due to the gain of function mutation of *fibroblast growth factor* (FGF)

BOX 8-2   Bone Morphogenetic Proteins and Growth and Differentiation Factors

Bone morphogenetic proteins (BMPs) and *growth and differentiation factors* (GDFs) are members of the transforming growth factor β (TGF-β) family of proteins. BMPs were discovered by their ability to induce ectopic de novo bone formation, when implanted in extraosseal connective tissue. This action, a combination of *osteoinduction* and *osteogenesis,* results in the development of mesenchymal stem cells into all cellular components of bone, including bone marrow. BMPs are locally acting substances, which is indicated by the close spatial distribution of BMPs and their receptors in tissues. For example, *ALK–6,* a type I TGF-β receptor mediating the actions of BMP2 and BMP4, displays a tissue distribution that matches that of BMP2 and BMP4.

The physiological actions of BMPs are varied and occur at three distinct periods of life:

• *Early stages of embryogenesis:* BMPs are generally involved in the formation of body plan, the specification of axes and tissue types.
• *Organogenesis during embryonic development:* Specific BMPs and GDFs selectively induce formation of skeletal stuctures.
• *In adults:* BMPs are involved in bone repair after fractures.

The functions of BMPs indicate their intimate relationship with homeobox genes. In general, BMPs induce bone and its precursor cartilage, whereas GDFs (mainly GDFs 5, 6, and 7) induce joint-related tissues (including cartilage and ligaments) and tendons. Experiments with mutant, transgenic, and knockout mice indicate specific functions performed by specific BMPs. For example, absence of BMPs 2 and 4 (which are key elements for bone fracture repair in adults) is lethal during early embryonic life due to mesoderm, heart, or amnionic developmental defects. In contrast, BMP7 knockout mice are born live but with kidney and eye defects, and die shortly after birth. The mutant *short-eared mouse* is a proof that BMP5 is not essential for life, but is required for the proper development of the ribs, sternum, and ears. The GDF5-deficient *brachyospodism mouse* displays dysmorphogenesis of joints primarily in the elbows and knees.

3 receptors *(FGFR3).* FGFs acting on the normal counterpart of these receptors would cause *inhibition of chondroblast proliferation.* Thus, the mutation does not affect intramembranous ossification. The growth of the vertebral column and, even more severely, that of the long bones is impaired in achondroplastic patients. The consequence is a disproportionate dwarfism that includes short stature and a high U/L body segment ratio.

The growth retardation mainly involves the proximal limbs *(rhizomelic shortening;* Box 8-3).

Achondroplastic patients present with a large forehead *("frontal bossing")* because the bones of the calvaria develop by intramembranous ossification. In contrast, these patients have a *hypoplastic mandible,* although except for its condylar process, the mandible also develops by an intramembranous mechanism. However, the developing mandible uses the cartilage of the first branchial arch *(Meckel's cartilage)* as a template: the bone is deposited *onto the surface* of the cartilage by intramembranous ossification. The hypoplastic Meckel's cartilage therefore leads to a reduced mandibular size.

Bone Age, Closure of Fontanels, and Tooth Development Are Used to Assess Maturation of Bones and to Evaluate the Impact of Certain Endocrine Disorders on the Skeletal System

Maturation of bones (bone growth and ossification of the cartilagineous anlage) is influenced by several hormones:

- stimulatory hormones include GH/IGF-1, thyroid hormones, PTH (by indirect action), vitamin D, and sex steroids (mainly estrogens);
- inhibitory hormones include PTHrP that retards cartilage maturation but not cartilage growth, and excessive concentrations of glucocorticoids that retard both maturation and growth of cartilage.

Clinically, the maturation of bones is assessed as the *bone age.* The left wrist is x-rayed, and the pattern of ossification centers of bones of the hand and the epiphyseal plates of the forearm bones are compared to the gender-specific normal developmental pattern. In a healthy individual, the age estimated from the bone structure (bone age) generally agrees with his or her chronological age. However, in certain disease states the bone age and the chronological age may be quite different. For example, children with glucocorticoid excess (such as Cushing's disease, or glucocorticoid therapy for asthma), GH deficiency, or hypothyroidism have a bone age younger than their chronological age. In contrast, precocious puberty results

BOX 8-3 Dysplasia Segments

A differential involvement of the proximal (femur, humerus), middle (tibia/fibula, radius/ulna), and distal (feet, hands) portion of the limbs are referred to as *rhizomelic, mesomelic,* and *acromelic* shortening, respectively. The differential involvement of these *dysplasia segments* is typical for the dysfunction of locally acting factors such as BMPs, growth factors, and/or their receptors.

in an advanced bone age. Bone age is also important for the prognosis of GH therapy: it predicts the timing of epiphyseal closure, after which GH therapy is unable to increase the height of the patient.

Hormones also affect the maturation of bones that develop by intramembranous ossification, including those of the calvaria. Palpation of the fontanels may provide insight about the skeletal development of an infant. *The timely closure of the fontanels requires normal intracranial pressure and normal skeletal maturation.* Term infants are born with two fontanels.

- The *posterior fontanel* (found at the junction between the occipital and parietal bones) is very small (barely allows the insertion of a fingertip), and becomes closed (nonpalpable) by the 6th to 8th week postpartum.
- The *anterior fontanel* (found at the junction between coronal and sagittal sutures) is about 2×2 cm in size at birth, and its closure occurs at about 18 months of age.

Persisting fontanels may indicate increased intracranial pressure (such as in *hydrocephalus*) or slow bone growth and skeletal maturation such as seen in *congenital hypothyroidism* or in *rickets* (e.g., vitamin D deficiency).

Teeth have a structure similar to bone, and their development requires almost the same set of systemic hormones: GH, thyroid hormones, PTH, and vitamin D. Teeth develop in two waves: *primary (decidual) teeth* and *secondary (permanent) teeth*. The development of teeth can be monitored by timing of:

- the beginning and completion of their calcification as seen on x-rays;
- their eruption; and
- the shedding of the decidual teeth.

The timing of tooth eruption is the most often utilized parameter. *Delayed tooth eruption* may indicate hypothyroidism, dysfunction of the GH/IGF-1 axis, and/or that of calcium homeostasis (PTH/vitamin D regulatory system). Dysfunction of calcium homeostasis may also lead to mineralization defects of the enamel, which may result in extensive *caries*.

The Initially Deposited Woven Bone Is Replaced by the More Organized and Resilient Lamellar Bone

Thus far we have discussed the structure of mature bone and the means of the ossification process. However, it must be emphasized that during embryonic development, bone is first deposited in a less organized manner *(immature* or *woven bone),* and this bone is replaced by mature bone in the process of remodeling.

Woven and lamellar bones differ mainly in the organization of their collagen fibers. *Woven bone* is deposited rapidly due to the involvement of abundant osteoblasts. As a consequence, relative to the amount of bone matrix, many entrapped osteocytes are found in woven bone. Because its collagen fibers are deposited in a haphazard orientation, woven bone is a weak structure that can resist moderate forces equally in any direction. *Lamellar bone can resist strong mechanical forces in preferential directions because its collagen fibers are organized as parallel bundles that follow the trajectories of stress lines.* The deposition of lamellar bone is performed by fewer osteoblasts. Therefore, lamellar bone is deposited more slowly, and its bone matrix contains fewer entrapped osteocytes.

Woven bone is found in the fetus and in broken bones of adults during the early stages of repair *(early bony callus).* Lamellar bone is the characteristic type in adults both in compact and in cancellous bones.

While the Synthesis of the Main Bone Protein, Type I Collagen, Is Vitamin C-Dependent, Some of the Noncollagenous Matrix Proteins Are Vitamin K-dependent

Type I collagen, a major determinant of the mechanical properties of bone, accounts for about 90% of the protein mass in the extracellular organic matrix of bone. Various mutations affecting type I collagen lead to four different major types and clinical manifestations of *osteogenesis imperfecta,* which are characterized by reduced mechanical resistance ("brittle bone disease") and reduced bone mass. Thus, osteogenesis imperfecta constitutes a subtype of osteoporosis.

Collagen contains a large number of proline and lysine residues that are posttranslationally hydroxylated in a *Vitamin C*-dependent manner. During the degradation of collagen, *hydroxyproline* is liberated and excreted in the urine. More than 90% of the hydroxyproline in urine is excreted in the form of small peptides. Urinary hydroxyproline is in part derived from extraosseal connective tissues, mainly the skin. *Pyridinoline* and *deoxypyridinoline* are referred to as *pyridinium crosslinks.* They are derived from lysine and hydroxylisine residues that crosslink adjacent collagen fibrils into *mature* fibers. *Urinary excretion of pyridinium crosslinks is a sensitive and specific marker of bone resorption.* Pyridinium crosslinks are absent from skin; in addition to bone, they are derived from cartilage and dentin.

Most noncollagenous matrix proteins are the products of osteoblasts. The noncollagenous matrix proteins include

- cell adhesion molecules (such as *osteopontin*);
- calcium binding-proteins (such as *osteonectin*);
- regulators of mineralization *(osteocalcin);*
- growth factors (including cytokines);

• enzymes liberated from osteoblasts *(alkaline phosphatase)* and osteoclasts *(proteases, tartrate-resistant acid phosphatase* [TRAP]); and
• proteins incorporated from blood plasma (mainly albumin).

About 30% of the noncollagenous matrix proteins is *osteocalcin* (also known as *bone Gla protein* [BGP]), which is the only protein unique to bone tissue. *Gla* refers to *γ-carboxylated glutamic acid residues* found in certain proteins, including BGP, matrix Gla protein (MGP, whose function is unknown), and clotting factors II, VII, IX, and X. The posttranslational modification process involving the γ-carboxylation of glutamic acid residues requires *vitamin K,* a lipid-soluble vitamin.

We shall discuss the calcification of the osteoid matrix in the context of the homeostasis of calcium and phosphate.

COMPARTMENTALIZATION OF CALCIUM AND PHOSPHATE, AND FLUXES OF CALCIUM AND PHOSPHATE BETWEEN COMPARTMENTS

Calcium and phosphate play important roles in various physiologic and biochemical processes (Table 8-3). Before discussing the endocrine regulation of calcium and phosphate homeostasis, we need to be aware of the following core information:

• The distribution of calcium between its various *chemical forms* (ionized, protein bound, or complex);

Table 8-3   Functions of Calcium and Phosphate

Calcium	Phosphate
A major component of bone mineral content	A major component of bone mineral content
Second messenger (intracellular signal)	Second messenger (intracellular signal)
• Influx through Ca^{2+} channels:	• Regulation of protein function by kinases and phosphatases
• IP_3-gated	• Component of second messengers such as cyclic AMP, cyclic GMP, or IP_3
• voltage-gated	
• stretch-activated	
• Calmodulin pathway	
• Activation of muscle contraction	
• Release of neurotransmitters	
• Involvement in exocytosis	
Regulation of membrane excitability as an extracellular signal	A component of membrane phospholipids
Clotting factor (factor IV)	Energy storage and utilization (high-energy phosphate compounds such as ATP, creatine phosphate; phosphorylation of glucose for metabolism)

ABBREVIATIONS: AMP, adenosine monophosphate; GMP, guanosine monophosphate; ATP, adenosine triphosphate.

• The distribution of calcium and phosphate among the various *fluid compartments* of the body;
• The fluxes of calcium and phosphate.

While Most of the Extraosseal Calcium Is Extracellular, Most of the Extraosseal Phosphate Is Intracellular

About 1.6% of the body weight of adult humans is calcium (1.1 kg in a 70-kg adult). Less than 0.1% (900 mg) of the total bodily calcium is found in the general ECF, 0.1 to 0.2% is found in the intracellular fluid (ICF), and the rest of the calcium is sequestered in bone as crystals. Calcium is found in various forms in biologic fluids (Table 8-4). The concentration of *ionized calcium*, the form that is responsible for most biologic actions, is tightly regulated in both the ECF and the ICF. This means that the concentration of ionized calcium normally ranges about ±6.5% around the average concentration (average concentration being considered as 100%). Note that most of the intracellular calcium is not in an ionized form (see Table 1-1).

Total calcium levels are significantly influenced by changes in plasma protein concentration. *A change of 1 g/dL of albumin concentration corresponds with a change of about 0.8 mg/dL (0.2 mM) total calcium concentration.* For example, in a *nephrotic syndrome,* which is characterized by urinary loss of albumin and consequent hypoalbuminemia, total calcium is subnormal; however, ionized calcium may remain normal. Conversely, *multiple myeloma* (a B-cell lymphoma overproducing a light chain of immunoglobulins), which causes hyperproteinemia, results in elevated *total* calcium levels. Thus, in the clinical laboratory evaluation of calcium homeostasis it is important to measure plasma proteins simultaneously with calcium and phosphate concentrations.

Complexed calcium includes calcium complexed mainly with phosphate, lactate, or citrate. Unlike protein-bound calcium, ionized and complexed calcium readily penetrate capillary walls and the glomerular filter.

Table 8-4   Calcium Pools in Adult Human Serum (between the ages of 18 and 60 years)

Calcium pool in serum	Concentration (mg/dL)	Concentration (mM)
Total serum calcium	8.6–10.0	2.15–2.50
Ionized calcium	4.64–5.28	1.16–1.32
Protein-bound calcium		
• Total protein (6.4–8.3 g/dL)[a]	~4.64	~1.16
• Albumin (3.4–4.8 g/dL)[a]	~3.68	~0.92
Complexed calcium	~0.64	~0.16
(phosphate, lactate, citrate)		

Conversion of units: Divide concentration in mg/dL by 4 to obtain mM.
[a] The concentrations in parentheses are the normal ranges of protein concentrations; the corresponding normal protein-bound calcium concentrations apply only if serum protein concentrations are normal.

Hypocalcemia (subnormal levels of *ionized* calcium in plasma) can be a life-threatening situation *due to the increased membrane excitability* (Box 8-4). It is important to remember that hypocalcemia in vivo never results in clotting problems: plasma levels of ionized calcium during a fatal hypocalcemic crisis are still sufficient to support appropriate clotting. The manifestations of *hypercalcemia* are discussed in Box 8-4. Further details of hypercalcemia are discussed under primary hyperparathyroidism (Box 8-5).

The total phosphorus content of the adult human body is about 0.5 to 0.8 kg. About 85 to 90% of the phosphorus is found in bones. Most of the extraosseal phosphorus is in the form of *inorganic phosphates* (P_i: PO_4^{3-}, HPO_4^{2-}, $H_2PO_4^-$), and is confined to the ICF. Under pathologic conditions such as crush injuries of muscles *(rhabdomyolysis)*, the intracellular phosphate pool can be suddenly dumped into the ECF. This may result in a sudden decrease in plasma levels of ionized calcium (see *solubility product*) and a life-threatening hypocalcemic tetany.

The concentration of P_i in adults normally ranges between 2.7 and 4.5 mg/dL (0.87 to 1.45 mM), most of which is in a free form (Table 8-5). Thus, the concentration of P_i normally ranges $\pm 25\%$ around the average concentration, which means that the plasma levels of P_i are not as tightly regulated as those of ionized calcium. Plasma phosphate concentration displays a *circadian rhythm:* peak levels are observed during late morning hours, lowest levels in the evening. The circadian rhythm of plasma calcium is approximately the opposite: peak levels occur in the evening, trough levels occur early in the morning. Plasma phosphate concentrations show a *circannual rhythm* (in the USA and Europe, peak levels occur in May and June, trough levels in the winter).

The plasma concentrations of both calcium and phosphate vary with age. They are highest during the neonatal period, when intensive bone growth and mineral deposition occur.

The Concentration of Ionized Calcium in the ECF Is Influenced by Acute Changes of pH

The charge of proteins is pH dependent. Due to their dicarboxylic amino acid content, most proteins are negatively charged at physiologic pH. With

Table 8-5   Phosphate Pools in Adult Human Serum

Phosphate pool in serum	Relative contribution (%)	
Free phosphate	82	
• HPO_4^{2-}		• 44
• $H_2PO_4^-$		• 10
• $NaHPO_4^-$		• 28
Protein-bound phosphate	12	
Complexed phosphate (with calcium, magnesium)	6	

BOX 8-4 Clinical Manifestations of Abnormal Ionized Plasma Calcium Levels

The increased membrane excitability due to *hypocalcemia* manifests as *paresthesia* (tingling sensation usually felt in the fingers) and as *hypocalcemic tetany,* which is a tendency for developing involuntary muscle contractions and spasms. Note that muscle contraction requires an increase in cytoplasmic Ca^{2+} as a signal; however, this is derived from the endoplasmic (sarcoplasmic) reticulum, and not directly from the ECF. The signs of tetany include

- *Chvostek's sign:* tapping on the facial nerve (as it emerges from the parotid gland) causes twitching or spasm of the ipsilateral facial muscles;
- *Trousseau's sign:* latent tetany can be demonstrated by inflating a blood pressure cuff on the arm, which results in carpal spasm or on the thigh, which causes pedal spasm;
- *laryngospasm,* which can be fatal.

The main manifestations of *hypercalcemia* may include:

- *nephrogenic diabetes insipidus:* hypercalcemia, due to its direct renal action, causes polyuria and secondary polydypsia;
- *urolithiasis:* calcium stones in the urinary tract;
- *peptic ulcer disease:* direct stimulation of gastric parietal cells to secrete hydrochloric acid;
- *neurologic disturbances:* weakness, hyporeflexia, muscle twitching due to an increased calcium influx in motor nerve terminals leading to the release of larger *quanta* of acetylcholine;
- *psychiatric disturbances:* difficulty in concentration, confusion, lethargy, psychosis, coma and death.

About 90% of CSF calcium is ionized, mainly because of the low protein concentration of CSF. The concentration total and ionized calcium in the CSF is approximately 47% and 85% that of plasma, respectively. *During hypercalcemia, the gap widens between plasma and CSF calcium concentrations* as an indication of blood brain barrier (BBB) function. The psychiatric manifestations imply that the increased concentrations of ionized calcium in plasma lead to increased concentrations of ionized calcium in the CSF. Such a positive correlation has been demonstrated in patients suffering from primary hyperparathyroidism. The increased concentration of ionized calcium in the ECF of brain alters membrane excitability, the synthesis and release of neurotransmitters.

Disturbances of plasma calcium also manifest in cardiac function and *electrocardiograms (EKG).* Hypocalcemia causes a prolonged Q–T interval, may result in bradycardia or even in a first-degree heart block. In contrast, hypercalcemia shortens the Q–T interval because it enhances the process of ventricular repolarization.

BOX 8-5   Primary Hyperparathyroidism

Primary hyperparathyroidism is a consequence of parathyroid gland hyperplasia, adenoma, or carcinoma. The manifestations of the disease are due to the unregulated hypersecretion of PTH. Some of the symptoms are related to the direct actions of PTH, while others are directly related to hypercalcemia (see Box 8-3). The effect of PTH on bone is hyperstimulated osteoclastic activity that may result in the development of cystic lesions. Due to today's early diagnosis, the classic presentation of *osteitis fibrosa cystica generalisata of von Recklinghausen* and *brown tumors* (hemorrhagic lesions infiltrated by reactive fibrotic tissue and macrophages) are rarely encountered. The osteoclastic activity is a major contributor of hypercalcemia. The renal effects of PTH result in increased urinary cyclic adenosine monophosphate (cyclic AMP) excretion and increased *fractional* reabsorption of calcium by the distal renal tubule. Although this contributes to hypercalcemia, it is insufficient to prevent hypercalciuria, which is due to increased glomerular filtration of calcium. (The increased filtration is secondary to the increased ionized plasma calcium concentration.) The hypercalciuria often leads to the development of *urolithiasis*, usually in the form of calcium oxalate stones. The effect of PTH on the proximal tubules is to increase 1α-OHase activity and to inhibit phosphate reabsorption. The former effect is responsible for the increased efficiency of intestinal calcium (and phosphate) absorption, and the activation of osteoclasts synergistic with PTH. The clinical manifestations of primary hyperparathyroidism are often recalled as "*stones, bones, abdominal groans, and psychic moans.*"

increasing pH *(alkalosis)*, the negative charge of plasma proteins increases. In contrast, a decrease in pH *(acidosis)* suppresses the dissociation of H^+ ions of dicarboxylic amino acids, and the negative charge of plasma proteins decreases.

Ca^{2+} ions are bound to plasma proteins by ionic interaction. Thus, acidosis impairs the ability of Ca^{2+} to bind with the proteins, and Ca^{2+} is liberated from the protein-bound pool as ionized Ca^{2+}. In contrast, alkalosis results in an increased Ca^{2+} binding capacity of plasma proteins, and Ca^{2+} shifts from the ionized pool to the protein-bound form. *If plasma protein levels are normal, a shift of 0.1 pH results in a change of about 0.16 mg/dL (0.04 mM) of ionized calcium concentration.*

Because the excitability of membranes is regulated by the concentration of *ionized* calcium in the ECF, *acute alkalosis* (such as hyperventilation-induced alkalosis during a hysteric attack) *may provoke hypocalcemic tetany.* The acute nature of the shift in pH is important: although Ca^{2+} is tightly regulated, the endocrine regulation is too slow to counteract the sudden shift of calcium between its various plasma pools.

At Physiologic Concentrations, Plasma Is a Saturated Solution of Calcium and Phosphate Ions

Calcium phosphate is poorly soluble in water and precipitates at relatively low concentrations. Calcium phosphate is ideal for mineralization because it becomes insoluble at low osmolality, and does not expose the tissues to severe osmotic challenges.

In general, crystallization is promoted if a solution is not stirred. In addition, the presence of crystals and certain charged surfaces being in contact with the solution enhance the crystallization process because they serve as nuclei for *crystal proliferation (mineral propagation)*. Calcium and phosphate (PO_4^{3-}) ions in plasma are present at saturation concentrations: a significant portion of complexed calcium is in the form of phosphate, and close to 6% of P_i is complexed with calcium. However, a generalized precipitation of calcium phosphate is prevented by several factors:

- *pyrophosphate* ions in ECF;
- absence of crystallization nuclei; and
- movement of plasma/ECF.

In other words, the saturation conditions in the ECF are sufficient to *maintain* the structure and proliferation of preformed hydroxyapatite crystals, but insufficient to *initiate* crystallization.

If a saturated solution of calcium phosphate is in contact with the precipitated form of the same compound, the concentrations of Ca^{2+} and PO_4^{3-} multiplied by each other ($[Ca^{2+}] \cdot [PO_4^{3-}]$) yield a constant, known as the *solubility product*. The concept of solubility product implies that whenever the concentration of Ca^{2+} increases (e.g., by adding $CaCl_2$ to the solution), the concentration of PO_4^{3-} must decrease, and *vice versa*. As stated above, plasma (and thus ECF in general) contains calcium phosphate at saturating concentrations. The ECF is in contact with the precipitated form of calcium phosphate: hydroxyapatite in bone. Therefore, the concentrations of calcium and phosphate ions in the ECF are interdependent.

Note that PTH, the primary regulator of ionized calcium concentrations in plasma, increases plasma calcium and decreases plasma phosphate levels. Because PTH influences the concentrations of these ions in an opposite direction, $[Ca^{2+}] \cdot [PO_4^{3-}]$ does not increase. Thus, PTH *in itself* does not promote bone mineralization. In contrast, *calcitriol* (active vitamin D) promotes mineralization because it enhances the intestinal absorption of both calcium and phosphate, thereby increasing $[Ca^{2+}] \cdot [PO_4^{3-}]$ in the ECF.

The solubility product and therefore the precipitation of calcium phosphate and the solubility of hydroxyapatite are pH dependent: *alkaline pH promotes precipitation, while acidic pH increases solubility. Nucleation* is important in the physiologic mineralization of bone matrix. Most nucleation occurs in *matrix vesicles* (see below). However, under certain circumstances proteins may serve as nuclei for calcification because of the pattern of their surface charge. Therefore, local changes of pH influence the nucleation process.

Matrix Vesicles Serve as the Initial Sites of Calcification in All Skeletal Tissues

Matrix vesicles are membrane-invested structures and as such are similar to secretory vesicles. They are located extracellularly, indicating that they cannot be released by exocytosis, which would result in fusion of the vesicle membrane with the cell membrane. Instead, *matrix vesicles are released by budding* from the surfaces of chondrocytes, osteoblasts, and odontoblasts. These cells are asymmetrical ("polarized") and deposit the vesicles in an oriented manner.

• The biogenesis of matrix vesicles in the epiphyseal growth plates is linked to the stage of maturation and apoptosis of chondrocytes, and the vesicles are localized in the longitudinally oriented "septal" extracellular matrix.
• In newly deposited bone and dentin, the vesicles are localized within the osteoid seams.

Mineralization has two discernible phases:

• *Phase 1* of mineralization *(crystal initiation, nucleation)* occurs within the sap of matrix vesicles *only after* their release from their parent cells. This process is controlled by
    • *phosphatases* (including *alkaline phosphatase, pyrophosphatase,* and *adenosine triphosphatase),* which are mainly membrane associated and increase the concentration of PO_4^{3-} in the sap;
    • calcium binding molecules (such as *calbindin, annexins II and V*) and calcium ion channels, which promote calcium uptake and increase the concentration of Ca^{2+} within the sap. *Type X collagen,* which is found exclusively in the growth plates in the mineralizing matrix of hypertrophic cartilage, and *type II collagen* appear to regulate the function of matrix vesicles, probably by stimulating calcium uptake.
The increased $[Ca^{2+}] \cdot [PO_4^{3-}]$ in the sap first leads to precipitation of *octacalcium phosphate* $(Ca_8H_2(PO_4)_6 \cdot 5H_2O)$, a metastable crystal that transforms into hydroxyapatite. During hydroxyapatite formation protons accumulate in the vesicle. Their elimination is a crucial step in the crystallization process, which is made possible by *carbonic anhydrase II,* an enzyme also important in osteoclast function. Thus, the high $[Ca^{2+}] \cdot [PO_4^{3-}]$ and the appropriate pH required for the initiation of crystallization are achieved extracellularly, yet within an environment separated from the ECF by a lipid bilayer.

BOX 8-6   Pathologic Calcification

Pathologic calcification is usually classified as

- *metastatic calcification*, which occurs in a previously uninjured tissue due to an increase of $[Ca^{2+}] \cdot [PO_4^{3-}]$;
- *dystrophic calcification*, which occurs in an injured tissue when $[Ca^{2+}] \cdot [PO_4^{3-}]$ is normal.

The mechanism of both types of pathologic calcification is similar to that of physiologic calcification of skeletal tissues. Fragmentation of necrotic cells may yield *matrix vesicle-like structures*. Such a mechanism is important in the development of calcified atherosclerotic plaques, where alkaline phosphatase-rich vesicles are generated during the demise of smooth muscle cells.

Crystal formation may also occur intracellularly upon accumulation of calcium and phosphate by cell organelles, mainly by mitochondria. Mitochondria actively accumulate calcium and phosphate, and events leading to an overload of the cytoplasmic concentration of these ions (such as their increased concentrations in the ECF, plasma membrane injuries due to ischemia or toxic substances) may result in crystallization of calcium phosphate in the mitochondrial matrix. Once the crystal perforates the mitochondrial membranes, the cell breaks up, and the mineral propagation may proceed by the phase 2 mechanism.

- *Phase 2* of mineralization *(mineral propagation)* begins when the growing crystal perforates the membrane of the matrix vesicle. The crystal exposed to bone fluid serves as a nucleus, or a template for *epitaxial* (appositional) *crystal proliferation*. Epitaxial crystal proliferation is regulated directly by the composition of bone fluid, including $[Ca^{2+}] \cdot [PO_4^{3-}]$, pH, the concentrations of anionic proteoglycans, and other matrix proteins. Although collagens (type I in bone, types II and X in the growth plates) are not the sites of crystal nucleation, they regulate the rate of mineral propagation into the osteoid matrix. *Osteocalcin* is nonessential in this process. Its function appears to be the development of larger sized and more stabile (mature) crystals in *cortical* bone.

Pathologic calcification of tissues relies on a similar two-phase process (see Box 8-6).

Plasma Calcium Concentration Is Influenced by Absorption in the Gut, Reabsorption in the Kidneys, and Resorption of Bone

The terms *absorption, reabsorption,* and *resorption* have similar meanings but they refer to different sites:

- *absorption* refers to the uptake of dietary calcium and phosphate from the gut;
- *reabsorption* refers to the renal tubular uptake of calcium and phosphate filtered by the glomeruli;
- *resorption* refers to mobilization of calcium and phosphate from bone either by osteocytic or by osteoclastic osteolysis.

These three processes determine the fluxes of calcium and phosphate among the various fluid compartments (Figs. 8-5 and 8-6).

The RDA of calcium in adults is 1 g/d. For lactating and pregnant women, the RDA is 1.2 g/d. In the average adult, who is in the state of calcium and phosphate balance, a *net* 200 mg of the 1000 mg/d dietary calcium, and a *net* 900 mg of the 1500 mg/d dietary phosphate are *absorbed;* the rest is excreted in the feces.

The calcium and phosphate balance implies that the quantities of these compounds leaving the body equal their total dietary intake. Thus, the total quantities of *absorbed* calcium and phosphate must leave the body (mostly) in the urine. The urinary losses of calcium and phosphate appear to be similar to their fecal losses. However, this is due to the extensive reabsorption of both calcium and phosphate. In fact, if it were not for the reabsorption, urinary loss of calcium would be about 10 g/d, which is more than 11 times more calcium than the total calcium pool of the ECF and about 50 times more the actual normal urinary loss.

Calcium and phosphate balance also implies that neither net bone resorption nor net bone deposition occurs. However, the lack of net change is the result of an equilibrium between the opposite fluxes of calcium phosphate between bone and the ECF. Note that the 500 mg/d flux of calcium between these compartments is quantitatively significant compared to the 900 mg total calcium content in the ECF.

It is important to understand that the hydroxyapatite crystals are in the extracellular space *within* the bone fluid compartment. As noted above, the *bone fluid* compartment is separated from the general ECF by the bone-lining cells.

Calcium in bone exists as two pools:

- *readily exchangeable pool* (approximately 4 g calcium; 0.4% of total bone calcium);
- *stable pool* (approximately 1 kg; 99.6% of total bone calcium).

The readily exchangeable pool of calcium is mainly found in bone fluid and the hydroxyapatite crystals that are directly exposed to bone fluid. Since the exchange occurs between bone fluid and the general ECF, this process is regulated by the bone-lining cells. Mobilization of calcium from the readily exchangeable pool is termed *osteocytic osteolysis.*

The stable pool is exchanged very slowly in the process of *bone remodeling.* This process involves the function of phagocytic osteoclast cells.

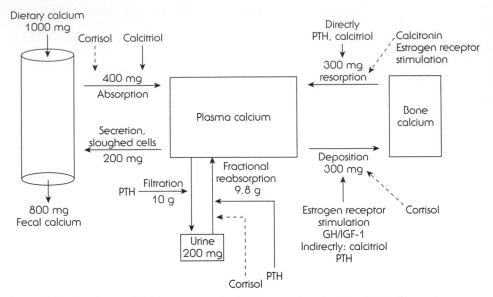

Figure 8-5. The fluxes of calcium among the fluid compartments of the body. The main regulators of calcium fluxes are also shown. Solid lines: stimulation/increase of flux; dashed lines; inhibition/decrease of flux; PTH, parathyroid hormone; GH, growth hormone; IGF-1, insulin-like growth factor-1.

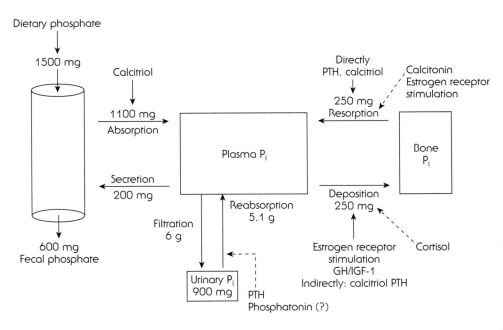

Figure 8-6. The fluxes of inorganic phosphate (P$_i$) among the fluid compartments of the body. The main regulators of phosphate fluxes are also shown. Solid lines, stimulation/increase of flux; dashed lines, inhibition/decrease of flux; PTH, parathyroid hormone; GH, growth hormone; IGF-1, insulin-like growth factor-1.

Osteoclasts not only liberate bone minerals but also *break down the organic matrix*. This mechanism, termed *osteoclastic osteolysis,* is also an important component of calcium mobilization. PTH and calcitriol (active vitamin D) are among the main *systemic* stimulators of both osteocytic and, through indirect mechanisms, osteoclastic osteolysis.

THE ENDOCRINE REGULATION OF CALCIUM AND PHOSPHATE

The Main Physiologic Regulators of Calcium *Fluxes* Are Parathyroid Hormone (PTH) and Calcitriol (Active Vitamin D), Whose Productions Are Regulated by the *Concentration* of Ionized Calcium in the ECF

Plasma levels of calcium and phosphate ions are interdependent, and the regulation of ionized calcium is far more tightly controlled than that of P_i. This is due to the fact that the hormones which regulate plasma P_i primarily regulate ionized calcium, and receive feedback *mostly* from ionized calcium. A notable exception is the role of P_i as a suppressor of active vitamin D synthesis in the kidney (see below).

The tight feedback control of plasma-ionized calcium concentration implies that it is monitored by cellular mechanisms. This is accomplished by the CaR, a member of the G-protein coupled heptahelical receptor family, which binds $[Ca^{2+}]_{ECF}$ as a ligand in a concentration-dependent fashion. The CaR intervenes at multiple sites of the normal regulatory process. PTH and vitamin D are the main regulators of calcium fluxes. Because the CaR regulates production of PTH and active vitamin D, and also regulates PTH-induced reabsorption of calcium, *the fluxes of calcium are regulated by the concentration of ionized calcium in the ECF*, and the calcium fluxes attempt to normalize the concentration of ionized calcium. *The fluxes of P_i mainly depend on the relative activities of PTH and active vitamin D*. Although both of these hormones are hypercalcemic, their actions on plasma P_i is opposite: PTH decreases and active vitamin D increases plasma P_i levels. The relative activities of PTH and *active* vitamin D mainly depend on the dietary availability of calcium and the *vitamin D status* of the individual (dietary and endogenously produced vitamin D and its 25-hydroxylated form).

The main hormones involved in the feedback-based regulation of plasma ionized calcium are listed in Table 8-6. It must be noted, however, that several other hormones have significant impact on calcium/phosphate homeostasis without receiving a significant direct feedback from plasma levels of ionized calcium (see the section on Other Hormones Involved in the Regulation Calcium and Phosphate). These hormones are listed in Table 8-7.

Table 8-6 Hormones Involved in the Feedback-Based Regulation of Plasma Concentrations of Ionized Calcium

Hormone	Source	Target(s)	Action
Ca^{2+} in ECF (not a true hormone but has a similar receptor-mediated action)	Absorption from diet; resorption from bone; reabsorption from glomerular filtrate	Chief cells of the parathyroid glands	Inhibits every step of PTH production and the proliferation of the chief cells
		C-cells of the thyroid gland	Stimulates calcitonin secretion
		Proximal renal tubules	Inhibits 1-hydroxylation of 25(OH) vitamin D$_3$
		Thick ascending limb of the loop of Henle	Inhibits NaCl, Ca^{2+}, and Mg^{2+} reabsorption, decreases cyclic AMP, and reduces the action of ADH
PTH	Parathyroid glands: chief cells	Osteoblastic lineage	Acute: Increased osteocytic osteolysis
			Chronic: recruitment and stimulation of osteoclasts via increased production of cytokines (ODF, M-CSF, IL-11, IL-6)
		Proximal renal tubules	Stimulates 1α-hydroxylation of 25(OH) vitamin D$_3$; inhibits phosphate reabsorption; increases cyclic AMP in tubular fluid and urine
		Distal renal tubules	Stimulates Ca^{2+} reabsorption

Hormone	Site of production	Target tissue	Action
$1,25(OH)_2$ vitamin D_3 (active vitamin D_3)	Proximal tubule of the kidney (the prior 25-hydroxylation of dietary or endogenous vitamin D by the liver is required)	Intestinal epithelium	Stimulates Ca^{2+}, Mg^{2+}, and phosphate absorption by inducing *calbindins* and by other mechanisms
		Osteoblasts	Activation similar to that by PTH; increased synthesis of osteocalcin and other proteins
		Osteoclast precursors (but not mature osteoclasts)	Stimulates recruitment and maturation of osteoclast precursors
		Chief cells of the parathyroid gland	Inhibition of PTH gene expression, synthesis, and secretion, inhibition of cell proliferation
		Kidney (minor action)	Increased Ca^{2+} reabsorption by inducing calbindin
		Many tissues	Induction of differentiation, inhibition of cell proliferation (e.g., antipsoriatic action in skin)
$24,25(OH)_2$ vitamin D_3 (another vitamin D_3 derivative active on an unidentified receptor)	Mainly in the proximal tubule of the kidney using $25OHD_3$ as c substrate	Osteoblasts (?)	Stimulates intramembranous (including periosteal) ossification, promotes maturation of chondrocytes, stimulates mineralization of osteoid, promotes fracture repair
CT (has only vestigial physiologic functions in humans)	C-cells of the thyroid gland	Osteoclasts	Direct inhibition
		Kidney	Transient increase of calcium and phosphate clearance

ABBREVIATIONS: ECF, extracellular fluid; PTH, parathyroid hormone; AMP, adenosine monophosphate; ADH, antidiuretic hormone; ODF, osteoclast differentiation factor; M-CSF, macrophage colony-stimulating factor; CT, calcitonin; IL, interleukin.

Table 8-7 Hormones Involved in the Regulation of Calcium/Phosphate Homeostasis without Receiving a Direct Feedback from Plasma Concentrations of Ionized Calcium

Hormone	Source	Target(s)	Action
PTHrP	Most tissues, especially epithelia	Mesenchyme adjacent to developing epithelial organs	Regulation of mesenchyme-epithelium interaction in development, growth and/or branching of epithelial organs (e.g., hair, mammary, and other glands)
	Pancreatic islets (most cell types)	Pancreatic β cells	Increase of pancreatic β cell mass
	Perichondrium	Chondrocytes in growth plates	Retards chondrocyte maturation during endochondral ossification
	Fetal parathyroid gland, placenta, mammary epithelium	Epithelia (trophoblast, mammary, renal tubules)	Drives the placental Ca^{2+} pump, stimulates transepithelial Ca^{2+} transport
		Smooth muscle	Causes vascular and visceral smooth muscle relaxation
Estrogens (and androgens mainly after local aromatization into estrogens)	Ovary (preovulatory and luteinized granulosa and theca interna cells), testis (Leydig cells), adrenal cortex (mainly zona reticularis)	Osteoblasts	Inhibition of TNF-α- and IL-1-induced production of IL-6 and other cytokines (M-CSF, GM-CSF)
		Peripheral blood monocytes, (bone tissue) macrophages	Inhibition of TNF-α- and IL-1 production; overall bone effect—inhibition of bone resorption
		Proximal renal tubules	Increase of vitamin D 1α-OHase expression, increased production of calcitriol
		C-cells of the thyroid gland	Increased production of calcitonin

GH/IGF-1	GH: somatotroph acidophils of the pituitary gland; IGF-1: hepatocytes, fibroblasts	Chondroblasts and chondrocytes in endochondral bone formation, periosteal osteoblasts	Increased proliferation and synthesis of extracellular matrix
		Proximal renal tubules	Increase of vitamin D 1α-OHase expression, increased production of calcitriol
PRL	Mammotrope acidophils of the anterior pituitary	Mammary gland	Increased calcium loss via milk (joint action with PTHrP to support neonatal bone growth)
		Proximal renal tubules	Increase of vitamin D 1α-OHase expression, increased production of calcitriol (weak action)
Excessive cortisol (glucocorticoids)	Adrenal cortex (mainly zona fasciculata); exogenously administered steroids	Intestine	Inhibition of Ca^{2+}, Mg^{2+}, and phosphate absorption by antagonizing calcitriol
		Kidney	Inhibition of Ca^{2+} reabsorption
		Osteoblasts	Inhibition of collagen and OPG synthesis
Thyroid hormones (T_4, T_3)	Thyroid gland	Bone remodeling units (osteoblasts and osteoclasts)	Increased bone turnover with a shift toward bone resorption

ABBREVIATIONS: PTH, parathyroid hormone; PTHrP, PTH-related protein; TNF, tumor necrosis factor; IL, interleukin; M-CSF, macrophage colony-stimulating factor; GM-CSF, granulocyte-macrophage only-stimulating factor; GH, growth hormone; IGF, insulin-like growth factor; PRL, prolactin; OPG, osteoprotegerin; OHase, hydroxylase.

Calcium-Sensing Receptor, Parathyroid Hormone, and PTH-Related Protein

The Chief Cells of the Parathyroid Glands Are the Sources of Parathyroid Hormone The thymus, thyroid, and parathyroid glands develop mainly from the pharyngeal endoderm, with contributions from neural crest cells in the pharyngeal arches and (mainly placodial) ectoderm. As a consequence, both type 1 and type 2 *MEN syndromes* may include parathyroid tumors (see Chaps. 10 and 12). Homozygous mutations of the *Hoxa3* homeobox gene result in developmental defects in all three organs.

There are two pairs of parathyroid glands: superior and inferior. The superior parathyroids develop from the fourth pharyngeal pouch, and the inferior parathyroids and the thymus develop from the third pharyngeal pouch. A protrusion of the fourth pharyngeal pouch (sometimes called the fifth pharyngeal pouch) housing neural crest-derived cells gives rise to the C-cells of the thyroid gland (see Fig. 11-2). The developmental aberration of the third and fourth pharyngeal pouches around the 8th gestational week results in *DiGeorge's syndrome,* which involves a combined agenesis or hypoplasia of the thymus (leading to impaired T-cell mediated immunity), the parathyroid glands (leading to tetany), and the calcitonin-producing C-cells of the thyroid.

Each normal parathyroid gland is a lentiform, pea-sized, compact epithelial structure weighing about 3 to 50 mg. The total parathyroid tissue mass is an important determinant of plasma PTH concentration. The pathohistologic differentiation of parathyroid hyperplasia from adenoma is difficult. As their name indicates, the parathyroid glands are anatomically closely associated with the thyroid gland (see Fig. 11-1). A clinically important consequence of this anatomic relationship is the inadvertant removal of the parathyroid glands during surgical thyroidectomy. The location of the inferior parathyroids is especially variable; it is not uncommon to find them in the anterior mediastinum, to where they migrate with the thymus. Localization of adenomatous *ectopic parathyroid glands* may require radiological imaging such as *technetium (Tc 99m) sestamibi scintigraphy.*

Microscopically, the parathyroid glands consist of highly vascularized cords of epithelial cells. The fenestrated endothelium aids the diffusion of PTH from the interstitial fluid into plasma. Most epithelial cells are *chief cells,* which actively secrete PTH. During fetal life, the chief cells secrete PTHrP, which drives the placental calcium pump. The active calcium transport is essential for the maintenance of the physiologic hypercalcemia of the fetus, which is required for appropriate bone development. *Oxyphil cells* appear in the parathyroid gland around puberty and increase in numbers with age. The cytoplasm of oxyphil cells is packed with mitochondria but the PTH-containing secretory granules are usually scanty or absent. The specific function of oxyphil cells (if any) is unknown. Although the overall weight of the parathyroid glands normally remains constant during adult life, the relative contribution of stromal adipocytes increases with age. Thus, there is an age-related decrease in the mass of chief cells.

Mature PTH consists of a single polypeptide chain of 84 amino acids. PreproPTH contains a 23-amino acid signal peptide and a 6-amino acid N-terminal extension. This latter is completely cleaved by *furin* (see Chap. 3) in the Golgi complex. Thus, secretory vesicles contain only the mature peptide.

Concentration of Ionized Calcium in the ECF Regulates the Function of Chief Cells via Calcium-Sensing Receptors The CaR is a member of the G-protein coupled heptahelical receptor family. The inverse relationship between the concentration of ionized calcium in the ECF and PTH secretion by the chief cells is *steeply* sigmoidal. This means that a minor decrease in $[Ca^{2+}]_{ECF}$ leads to a marked increase in PTH secretion. The inflection point of this negative sigmoid curve (i.e., where PTH secretion is half-maximal) is found at a $[Ca^{2+}]_{ECF}$ slightly lower than the normal plasma value of $[Ca^{2+}]_{ECF}$. Thus, under resting conditions, PTH is secreted at rates of only 2 to 25% of the maximal output. This observation implies that PTH secretion is under a tonic inhibitory control by $[Ca^{2+}]_{ECF}$, which indicates that CaRs are not downregulated by the chronic exposure to their ligand.

The CaR may be coupled to effectors by various G-proteins. In some cell types, it is mainly coupled by $G\alpha_i$ and inhibits adenylyl cyclase. In the chief cell, increased $[Ca^{2+}]_{ECF}$ induces phospholipase C (PLC) activity via a coupling mechanism that involves a member of the $G\alpha_q$ family. PLC in turn activates protein kinase (PKC) and IP_3, and increases intracellular Ca^{2+} both by releasing Ca^{2+} from the endoplasmic reticulum, and by increasing influx of Ca^{2+} from the ECF. As shown, *exocytosis of secretory vesicles is typically induced by an increase of intracellular Ca^{2+}. The chief cell is unusual in this regard because the increased intracellular Ca^{2+} results in an inhibition of PTH release.* In the chief cell, stimulus–secretion coupling is performed by intracellular Mg^{2+} rather than by Ca^{2+}. Thus, *depletion of magnesium stores can lead to hypoparathyroidism.* Note that hypermagnesemia (increased concentration of ionized magnesium in the ECF) also inhibits PTH secretion due to its binding to the CaR. When exocytosis is inhibited, secretory vesicles are fusing with lysosomes, and their stored PTH degrades intracellularly.

In addition to the secretion of PTH, CaR also regulates the transcription and biosynthesis of PTH. Hypocalcemia may therefore lead to *secondary hyperparathyroidism,* which is characterized by an attempt to normalize plasma ionized calcium at the expense of supranormal PTH secretion (see also Chap. 7).

CaR also signals to the nucleus as an inhibitor of cell proliferation. Chronic hypocalcemia reduces the inhibitory signal and results in parathyroid hyperplasia. Chronic hypocalcemia may eventually cause the development of autonomous inappropriate hypersecretion of PTH. This condition is known as *tertiary hyperparathyroidism*. Although the pathogensis is different, this condition is similar to *primary hyperparathyroidism* in that the hypercalcemia is associated with hypersecretion of PTH (see Box 8-5).

Calcimimetic drugs act by activating the CaR. NPSR-568, a small organic molecule, suppresses PTH secretion and decreases plasma calcium levels. Calcimimetic drugs are promising for the palliative treatment of metastatic parathyroid cancer.

The Main Targets of Circulating PTH Are the Cells of the Osteoblastic Lineage and the Renal Tubules   The secreted PTH circulates in plasma as a free hormone with a *half-life of up to about 4 minutes,* which is comparable with that of insulin. PTH is cleaved mainly by the liver and the kidney. The resulting C-terminal fragment has a longer half-life than intact PTH, accumulates in plasma, and is eventually filtered by the kidney. The N-terminal fragment cannot be detected in blood. The difference in the half-lives between intact PTH and its C-terminal fragment accounts for the higher plasma concentrations of immunoreactive PTH obtained with C-terminal specific than with N-terminal specific antibodies (see also Chap. 7). The initial cleavage inactivates PTH: its N-terminal portion is essential for receptor binding.

PTH has two important physiologic actions (see also Table 8-6):

- *increases plasma calcium* by
    - immediate mobilization of calcium from bone via stimulating osteocytic osteolysis;
    - mobilization of calcium from bone by recruiting osteoclast precursors and by activating mature osteoclast, thereby stimulating osteoclastic osteolysis via indirect mechanisms involving osteoblasts;
    - immediately increasing the reabsorption of calcium from the distal renal tubules;
    - activating vitamin D by inducing 25(OH)D-1α-hydroxylase; the activated vitamin D in turn increases absorption of calcium and synergizes with PTH in bone (see below);
- immediately *decreases plasma phosphate* by inhibiting phosphate reabsorption from the proximal renal tubules *(phosphaturic action).*

The two functions tend to leave plasma $[Ca^{2+}] \cdot [P_i]$ unaltered.

About 90% of the calcium filtered by the glomeruli is reabsorbed in a PTH-independent manner. This reabsorption is coupled with sodium reabsorption and occurs mainly in the proximal tubules. Under physiologic conditions, about 10% of the filtered calcium reaches the distal nephron. This calcium is reabsorbed in the distal tubules by a PTH-regulated, low-capacity, saturable active transport mechanism. Normally this is responsible for the reabsorption of up to 8% of the filtered calcium.

It is important to note that PTH increases the *fractional reabsorption* of calcium, which also means that PTH decreases the *fractional excretion* of calcium. Thus, by definition, the *percentage* of the excretion of the filtered calcium, and not necessarily its absolute quantity, is decreased by PTH. There are important implications of this effect:

• Only the non-protein bound fraction of plasma calcium is filtered. If the concentration of ionized and/or complexed calcium is elevated, the filtration rate of calcium is increased.
• Due to the low capacity of the PTH-stimulated calcium transport mechanism, the increase in the amount of calcium filtered may not be compensated for by the increase in its fractional reabsorption. Therefore, although the fractional reabsorption is increased, *hypercalciuria* occurs. This is the case in, for example, primary hyperparathyroidism.

Hypercalciuria is diagnosed either as a supranormal amount of calcium in a 24-h urine specimen (>0.3 g/d) or as a supranormal *calcium/creatinine ratio*. This ratio is normally <0.14 (w/w) or <0.40 (mol/mol). Values above 0.20 (or 0.57) suggest hypercalciuria.

The effect of PTH on bone depends on its concentration and duration of exposure. Prolonged hypersecretion of PTH results in bone resorption mainly in compact bones by osteoclastic activation. However, small doses of exogenously administered PTH may increase bone deposition and has potential in the treatment of osteoporosis.

The Calcium-Sensing Receptor Is a Direct Regulator of the Renal Handling of Divalent Cations   Elevated peritubular, but not luminal, concentrations of Ca^{2+} directly inhibit accumulation of cyclic AMP in the *thick ascending limb* of the loop of Henle. This results in an inhibition of several transport functions, such as reabsorption of Ca^{2+}, Mg^{2+}, and NaCl, and reducing the action of vasopressin (antidiuretic hormone). This latter effect of hypercalcemia is a subtype of *nephrogenic diabetes insipidus* (see Chap. 10).

In the case of primary hyperparathyroidism, the fractional reabsorption of Ca^{2+} is increased by PTH. The calcium retention is attenuated by the increased concentration of plasma Ca^{2+} by its direct action on the thick ascending limb. In addition, stimulation of CaR in the proximal tubules antagonizes the action of PTH in inducing 25(OH)D-1α-hydroxylase. Through this action, plasma Ca^{2+} attenuates the production of active vitamin D and intestinal absorption of calcium/phosphate. Thus, *the renal action of Ca^{2+} can be viewed as an emergency break of calcium homeostasis protecting against hypercalcemia.*

Not only elevated, but also physiologic, concentrations of plasma Ca^{2+} are involved in the regulation of Ca^{2+} and Mg^{2+} reabsorption. *Familial hypocalciuric hypercalcemia (FHH, formerly referred to as familial benign hypercalcemia*) is due to a loss of function mutation of the CaR in *heterozy-gous* patients. The reduced CaR function in the parathyroid gland causes mild hypersecretion of PTH that is partially responsible for the moderate (usually <12 mg/dL) asymptomatic hypercalcemia. Another cause of hyper-calcemia is the reduced inhibitory effect of plasma Ca^{2+} on calcium reabsorp-tion. The reduced renal action is important in the differential diagnosis of FHH from primary hyperparathyroidism. Whereas FHH is characterized by hypocalciuria, primary hyperparathyroidism presents with hypercalciuria.

The *fractional excretion* of calcium (FE_{Ca}) is calculated as

$$FE_{Ca}(\%) = \frac{U_{Ca}/P_{Ca}}{U_{Cr}/P_{Cr}} * 100 = \frac{U_{Ca}}{P_{Ca}} * \frac{P_{Cr}}{U_{Cr}} * 100 \qquad (8.1)$$

where U refers to urinary and P refers to plasma concentrations of creatinine (Cr) and (filterable) calcium (Ca). Its normal value is approximately 2 to 4%. A value <1% supports the diagnosis of FHH.

The homozygous form of the loss-of-function mutation of CaR results in *neonatal severe hyperparathyroidism,* a life-threatening condition that usually presents at birth or the first postpartum week with extremely high (usually 14 to 20 mg/dL) plasma calcium. Activating mutations of CaR cause *autosomal dominant hypocalcemia.*

PTH and PTH-Related Protein Share Structural Similarities and a Receptor which Is Coupled to Adenylyl Cyclase by a $G\alpha_s$ Protein   The N-terminal 13 amino acids of PTH and PTHrP are highly homologous. This explains why both peptides are physiologic ligands of a PTH receptor, which is also known as the *PTH/PTHrP receptor* (or *PTH1 receptor*).

The activated PTH/PTHrP receptor is coupled with effectors through two G-proteins: $G\alpha_s$ (cyclic AMP–PKA pathway) and $G\alpha_q$ (PLC pathway). In clinical practice, the measurement of urinary cyclic AMP can be used for the diagnosis of hyperparathyroidism and *humoral hypercalcemia of malignancy* (HHM): the only significant determinant of urinary cyclic AMP is the stimulation of the PTH/PTHrP receptors in the proximal renal tubules either by PTH and/or by PTHrP. Cyclic AMP is transported from the cytoplasm of proximal renal tubular cells into the lumen by the *probenecid-sensitive organic anion transporter.* The normal urinary cyclic AMP output ranges between 100 to 723 μmol/mol creatinine (0.29 to 2.10 mg/g creat-inine).

Another clinically important consequence of the second messenger coupling is related to *mutations of the gene encoding the $G\alpha_s$ subunit*:

• Gain-of-function mutation during the early stages of embryonic development results in a ligand-independent activation of adenylyl cyclase. The affected individual is a genetic mosaic for the mutation. This is known as *McCune–Albright syndrome* (see Fig. 13-51). Because the $G\alpha_s$ subunit is shared by several receptors, the syndrome has a pleiomorphic presentation that, depending on the tissue distribution of the mutation, may include:

- osteolytic bone lesions and hypercalcemia imitating hyperparathyroidism;
- *café au lait* spots due to mimicking the activation of α-melanocyte stimulating hormone (α-MSH) receptors in epidermal melanocyte clusters;
- precocious puberty in either sex due to mimicking the activation of follicle stimulating hormone (FSH) and luteinizing hormone (LH) receptors;
- thyroxine-secreting adenomas of the thyroid gland due to mimicking the activation of the TSH receptor;
- acromegaly due to mimicking the activation of growth hormone-releasing hormone (GHRH) receptors in the pituitary gland and consequent overproduction of GH;
- adrenocortical hyperplasia due to mimicking the activation of the adrenocorticotroph hormone (ACTH) receptor.

- The usually inherited loss-of-function mutation of the Gα$_s$ subunit yields a clinical picture that typically mirrors that of the McCune–Albright syndrome, and results in an attenuated tissue response to the normal hormone ligand. This condition may present as *pseudohypoparathyroidism* (Box 8-7).
- A unique temperature-sensitive mutation of the Gα$_s$ subunit acts as a loss-of-function mutation at the core body temperature (37°C) but as a gain-of-function mutation in the testis, which is at a cooler scrotal temperature (30 to 33°C). The mutation results in a combination of pseudohypoparathyroidism and LH-independent testosterone overproduction by the Leydig cells (see Chap. 13).

Unlike the PTH1 receptor, the *PTH2 receptor* does not bind PTHrP, and has a more restricted tissue distribution than the PTH/PTHrP receptor. PTH2 receptor is abundant in the brain and the pancreas, but it is absent in the conventional target tissues of PTH, such as bone and the kidney. The physiologic function of the PTH2 receptor is currently unknown.

PTHrP, the Agent Responsible for Humoral Hypercalcemia of Malignancy, Mainly Functions as a Physiologic Growth Factor   PTHrP is a product of a single multiexonic gene, which is organized similar to that of PTH. Due to alternative splicing, three initial translation products are synthesized. The shortest of these, PTHrP(1-139) is present in all three products, whereas their C-terminal extensions are different. The functional domains of PTHrP are depicted in Fig. 8-7. The initially synthesized peptides undergo post-translational processing that can yield various secretory forms:

- PTHrP(1-36) is homologous with PTH and acts on
  - the PTH/PTHrP receptor and

BOX 8-7   Pseudohypoparathyroidism

Pseudohypoparathyroidism (PHP) mimics PTH deficiency and results in hypocalcemia and hyperphosphatemia. However, circulating PTH levels are high. The usually maternally inherited loss of function mutant $G\alpha_s$ subunit (encoded by the *GNAS1* gene) is the cause of PHP type 1A, which presents in clinical symptoms in a heterozygous individual. The symptoms also include *Albright's hereditary osteodystrophy* (AHO–short stature, short digits and fourth metacarpal bones, short neck, round face, and subcutaneous ossifications). The causes of this inheritance pattern are genomic imprinting (which preferentially silences the paternal allele in certain tissues, such as the kidney and endocrine glands; see Chap. 3), and that the affected males are infertile, which precludes their passing on the mutated gene. Because the affected $G\alpha_s$ subunit is shared by several receptors, PHP type 1A is often associated with resistance to TSH, LH, and FSH. The condition known as *pseudo-pseudohypoparathyroidism (PPHP)* presents with AHO, but normal calcium homeostasis and normal endocrine and reproductive function. PPHP also involves the *GNAS1* gene. Note that *GNAS1* expression is not paternally imprinted in bones and PPHP can be transmitted from either parent.

 PHP type 1B is the other end of the spectrum presenting with an isolated renal PTH resistance, without other endocrine abnormalities or AHO. The inheritance shows paternal imprinting similar to that of PHP type 1A, and maps to a small telomeric region of chromosome 20q, which includes *GNAS1*. The identity of the affected gene, however, is uncertain at this time.

- an as yet undefined, N-terminal PTHrP-specific receptor;
- *Midregion PTHrP* [PTHrP(38-94), (38-95) and (38-101)] apparently acts on its own (as yet undefined) cognate receptor;
- C-terminal PTHrP(107-139) is termed *osteostatin* for its direct osteoclast-inhibiting action, which again involves a distinct receptor.

PTHrP is expressed by several tissues and mainly acts in a paracrine fashion. The actions of PTHrP fall into three broad categories (see also Table 8-7):

- *Growth factor functions:* regulation of cell proliferation, differentiation and apoptosis;
- *Stimulation of calcium transport* through epithelial barriers (renal tubules, placental trophoblasts, and mammary epithelium);
- *Smooth muscle relaxation* in both visceral (uterus, urinary bladder, gastrointestinal tract) and vascular smooth muscles via increasing cyclic AMP and endothelium-independent production of nitric oxide (NO). Note that the gene of a functional antagonist of PTH, calcitonin, also encodes for CGRP, and CGRP is a potent smooth muscle relaxant.

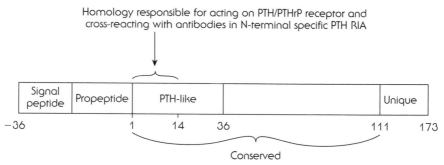

Figure 8-7. The functional domains of parathyroid hormone-related protein (PTHrP). Three initial translational products are generated due to alternative RNA processing. The longest of the three products is depicted; all products are identical in the region of PTHrP(1-139). Note that the numbering starts after the removal of the signal peptide and the prohormone peptide (propeptide). The conserved domain [PTHrP(1-111)] differs only in 3 amino acids between humans and rodents. PTHrP, the agent responsible for humoral hypercalcemia of malignancy, is derived from the N-terminal portion of the conserved domain. The midregion peptides arise from the C-terminal part of the conserved domain [PTHrP(38-101)]. The amino acid sequence of the unique domain is not as conserved among various species as that of PTHrP(1-111). The unique domain contains most of the osteostatin sequence, and sequences unique to primates (hence the name). (*Source:* Adapted from Fig. 1 in Wysolmerski JJ, Stewart AF: The physiology of parathyroid hormone-related protein: An emerging role as a developmental factor. Annu Rev Physiol 60:431–460, 1998.)

The PTH/PTHrP receptor and PTHrP ligand is among the first hormone systems during ontogeny: they are expressed as early as the morula stage of development. Loss-of-function mutations of the PTH/PTHrP receptors in homozygous forms are lethal: these infants either die shortly after birth or are stillborn. The condition is know as *Blomstrand chondrodysplasia,* which involves premature differentiation of chondrocytes and premature calcification of the cartilage leading to short bones with a high mineral density. The condition is due to the lack of PTHrP action and not that of PTH.

Gain-of-function mutations of the PTH/PTHrP receptor lead to *Jansen's metaphyseal chondrodysplasia,* a condition that is the mirror image of Blomstrand chondrodysplasia. Jansen's metaphyseal chondrodysplasia mimicks the effects of PTHrP overproduction. PTHrP normally retards chondrocyte differentiation and prevents chondrocyte apoptosis before appropriate calcification of the extracellular matrix is achieved. Thus, the condition results in a prolonged retention of cartilage, and consequential deformities of skeletal development. Maturation of cartilage is ultimately achieved during the second decade by sex steroids acting on estrogen receptors. The biochemical abnormalities are comparable with those of HHM: hypercalcemia, hypophosphatemia, and hypercalciuria, but without an increased concentration of plasma PTHrP or PTH.

The PTHrP pool that is responsible for affecting the chondrocytes is synthesized by the perichondrium. Perichondrial PTHrP secretion is stimulated by *Indian hedgehog,* a protein secreted by the prehypertrophic chondrocytes of the growth plate. PTHrP targets the prehypertrophic and hypertrophic chondrocytes. This arrangement is a paracrine *positive* feedback loop, whose function is to maintain the chondrocyte population as a target of GH/IGF-1 and other regulators of skeletal growth. Note that Indian hedgehog is stimulated by other factors, most notably BMPs.

For normal skeletal development, PTHrP is essential not only because of its action on cartilage but also because of its *hypercalcemic effect*. PTHrP (derived in part from the fetal parathyroid gland and in part from the placenta) acts upon the *midregion-specific* PTHrP-receptors of *placental trophoblast* cells to promote active calcium transport from the maternal into the fetal ECF. After birth, the appropriate dietary calcium supply to the neonate is assured by the PTHrP-stimulated active calcium transport from the maternal ECF into milk by the lactating *mammary epithelium*.

The intimate relationship between PTHrP and the mammary gland is reflected by the need of a paracrine PTHrP action for *the branching morphogenesis during normal mammary gland development*. The mechanism of the branching morphogenesis also includes *relaxin* (see Chap. 13). Another skin appendage, the *hair follicle,* utilizes PTHrP as a regulator of its development and life cycle.

PTHrP is produced by all endocrine cells of the pancreatic islets, and targets the insulin-producing β-cells. The N-terminal segment of PTHrP is responsible for the effect; however, the effect is not mediated by cyclic AMP. PTHrP does not interfere with the set point of the glucose sensor in the pancreatic β-cells, but increases the number of β-cells, which leads to hyperinsulinemia and hypoglycemia (see Chap. 9).

Vitamin D Derivatives

Vitamin D Is Obtained from the Diet and from Endogenous Synthesis in the Epidermis upon Its Exposure to Ultraviolet Light   Vitamin D was originally discovered as the substance, whose absence was responsible for *rickets (rachitis,* Box 8-8). Although it was originally termed as a vitamin, vitamin D is in effect a steroid hormone. The vitamin D added to dairy products, *ergocalciferol (vitamin D_2),* is produced by the ultraviolet (UV) irradiation of plant-derived ergosterol. Similarly, the endogenously produced vitamin D, *cholecalciferol (vitamin D_3),* is synthesized from *7-dehydrocholesterol* by the keratinocytes of the *stratum spinosum* and *stratum basale* of the epidermis in a photochemical reaction upon exposure to suberythemal doses of UVB light. The reaction yields a 9-10 secosterol *(previtamin D_3)* by opening the B ring of the steroid precursor, which is followed by a thermally induced isomerization (Fig. 8-8). Note that there is no vitamin D_1; the biologic activity originally described as vitamin D_1 was due to a mixture of antirachitic substances.

BOX 8-8   Osteomalacia and Rickets

Defective mineralization of the osteoid matrix is the cardinal feature of both osteomalacia and rickets. The cause of the disease is varied, but usually involves a deficiency of vitamin D availability, biosynthesis, metabolism, or action. *The difference between osteomalacia and rickets is the timing of the mineralization defect relative to epiphyseal closure*: osteomalacia develops if the defect occurs after bone development is complete, whereas rickets develops if the defect occurs before epiphyseal closure. The defective mineralization impairs the mechanical resistance of bones and leads to bone deformities such as

- *craniotabes* (softening of the skull and consequent deformities),
- chest deformities including *rachitic rosary* (tissue overgrowth at the junction of cartilaginous and bony parts of ribs) and *pigeon-breast,* and
- *bowing* of the legs.

The predilecting sites of the deformities depend on mechanical forces and thus are influenced by the onset of walking during infancy.

The UV spectrum of solar light affecting the skin includes the long-wave UVA (λ = 320 to 400 nm) and the short-wave UVB (λ = 290 to 320 nm). Both UVA and UVB are melanogenic, but 1000-fold more UVA than UVB energy is required to produce the same effects (see also Chap. 12). *Melanin,* which is produced by melanocytes mainly in response to UVB exposure is transferred to the keratinocytes and shields the cells of the stratum basale (the site of stem cells and melanocyte cell bodies) from UVB. This mechanism is needed for the prevention of various types of skin cancers, such as carcinomas, basalioma, and melanoma. However, the increased pigment shield reduces the production of cholecalciferol. Thus, dark-skinned populations, such as African Americans, enjoy protection from UV-induced skin malignancies, but need either longer exposure to sun or more dietary intake to meet vitamin D requirements.

The RDA of dietary vitamin D in the USA is 200 IU. The RDA for infants, children, and pregnant and lactating women is 400 IU. One IU equals 40 μg vitamin D. It is important to realize that the vitamin D requirements are typically met from both dietary sources and endogenous synthesis. Because exposure to sunlight is needed for the synthesis, production of cholecalciferol varies with the season, latitude, altitude, and pigmentation of the skin. Oversupply of vitamin D (*hypervitaminosis D*) may lead to severe consequences, such as pathologic calcification of soft tissues. To avoid hypervitaminosis, the daily dietary intake of vitamin D must match the demand defined as the difference between the total need for vitamin D minus the actual endogenous synthesis. Vitamin D is a prohormone,

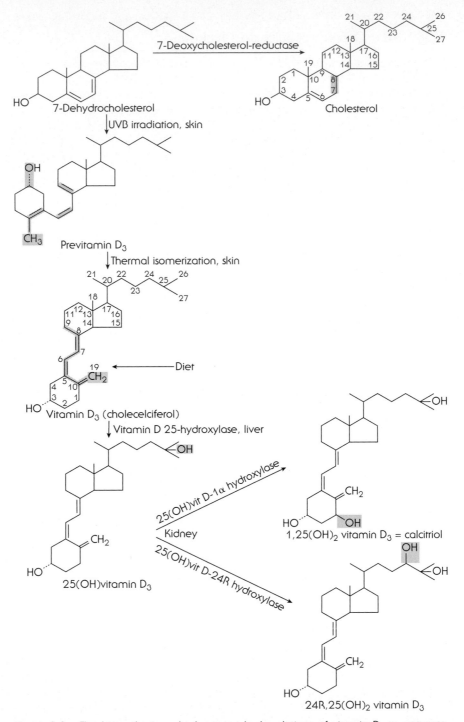

Figure 8-8. The biosynthesis and subsequent hydroxylations of vitamin D₃ to generate active forms of vitamin D₃. The numbers in the structures refer to the conventional numbering of carbonic atoms in cholesterol and cholecalciferol. The highlighted areas display the change in molecular structure in a given step.

and its activation is a regulated process. Mildly insufficient intake or mild oversupply of vitamin D can be compensated for by increased or decreased activation of the prohormone, respectively.

Calcitriol (1,25(OH)$_2$D) and 24R,25(OH)$_2$D Are Steroid Hormones Involved in the Regulation of Calcium and Phosphate Homeostasis, Bone Mineralization, Intramembranous Ossification and Fracture Repair   Cholecalciferol and ergocalciferol are equipotent, activated and metabolized in an identical fashion (Fig. 8-9). Thus, although cholecalciferol is used as an example, the following discussion applies to both compounds. Cholecalciferol is transported in blood to the liver, where it is hydroxylated at the C$_{25}$ position (*calcifediol* or 25(OH)D$_3$). This reaction is not tightly controlled. The resulting 25(OH)D$_3$ is the best clinical indicator of the overall vitamin D status. A significant proportion of 25(OH)D$_3$ is excreted in the bile and recycled by the *enterohepatic circulation*. Mainly via enterohepatic recycling, 25(OH)D$_3$ reenters the circulation and is transported mainly bound to *vitamin D-binding protein* (DBP, see Chap. 4) to the kidney. In the proximal tubules of the kidney, 25(OH)D$_3$ becomes 1α-hydroxylated in a regulated fashion, yielding *calcitriol* (1,25(OH)$_2$D$_3$). The regulators of the renal *1α-hydroxylase* (1α-OHase) enzyme are shown in Table 8-8. Calcitriol is the main biologically active derivative of vitamin D.

The liver and the kidney are not the only organs that metabolize cholecalciferol. Although most of the cholecalciferol leaves the epidermis as such, some is locally converted to calcitriol by hydroxylase enzymes of the epidermal cells. Calcitriol has a well-documented *antipsoriatic action*. The epidermal synthesis of cholecalciferol and its metabolization into calcitriol may be responsible for the antipsoriatic action of suntanning.

Several organs have limited 1α-OHase activity. However, other than the kidney the placenta is the only organ that significantly contributes to the circulating pool of calcitriol. The physiologically increased levels of calcitriol during pregnancy target both the mother to increase calcium absorption and the fetus to promote bone development. Under pathologic conditions, such as *granulomatous diseases* (sarcoidosis, tuberculosis, etc.)

Table 8-8   The Main Regulators of 25-Hydroxyvitamin D-1α-Hydroxylase

Stimulators	Inhibitors
PTH/PTHrP receptor activation	Activation of the CaR (increased Ca^{2+} in the ECF)
Decrease of P$_i$ in the ECF	Increase of P$_i$ in the ECF
Dietary deficiency of vitamin D	1,25(OH)$_2$ vitamin D$_3$ and dietary oversupply of vitamin D
Growth hormone	Cortisol(?)
Prolactin (weak action)	
Estrogens	

ABBREVIATIONS: PTH: parathyroid hormone; PTHrP, PTH-related protein; CaR, calcium-sensing receptor; ECF, extracellular fluid; P$_i$, inorganic phosphate.

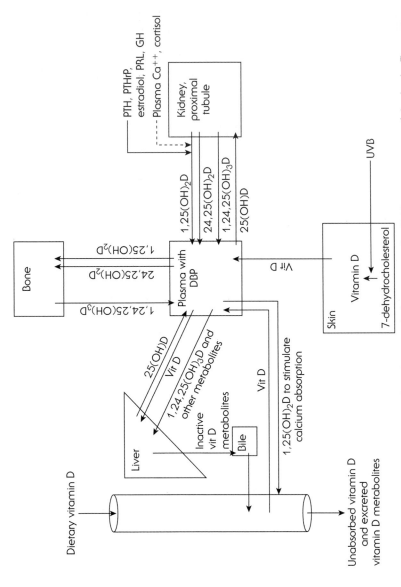

Figure 8-9. The fluxes of vitamin D and its metabolites among the fluid compartments of the body. The main regulators of the conversions are also shown. Solid lines, stimulation/increase of flux; dashed lines, inhibition/decrease of flux; DBP, vitamin D-binding protein; PTH, parathyroid hormone; PTHrP, PTH-related protein; GH, growth hormone; PRL, prolactin; UVB, ultraviolet B radiation.

high levels of 1α-OHase in the granuloma tissue may result in an increase of circulating calcitriol and cause hypercalcemia.

Both $25(OH)D_3$ and $1,25(OH)_2D_3$ may be hydroxylated at the 24th position. The reaction, which is not specific for the kidney but performed by several target tissues of vitamin D (intestine, bone, macrophages, skin, placenta), reduces the biologic activity of $1,25(OH)_2D_3$ by converting it into $1,24,25(OH)_3D_3$. The action of 24-hydroxylase (24-OHase) on $25(OH)D_3$ is not necessarily inactivation. The resulting $24R,25(OH)_2D_3$ displays unique biologic actions distinct from those of $1,25(OH)_2D_3$, although its specific (probably membrane-bound) receptor has not yet been identified. It is hotly debated whether $24R,25(OH)_2D_3$ has a physiologic function. Recent experiments with 24-OHase knockout mice support such a physiologic function of $24R,25(OH)_2D_3$. At sites of *intramembranous (including periosteal) bone formation,* the osteoid matrix of 24-OHase knockout mice displays a severe defect of mineralization. In addition, $1,25(OH)_2D_3$ by itself is insufficient for proper healing of fractured bones. Physiologic concentrations of $24R,25(OH)_2D_3$ are needed for appropriate *fracture repair.* This activity of $24R,25(OH)_2D_3$ might be related to its action on chondrocytes. The pharmacologic activity of $24R,25(OH)_2D_3$ is clearly established; in hypophosphatemic mice (a model for human *familial X-linked hypophosphatemic rickets*) $24R,25(OH)_2D_3$ increases bone formation in a dose-dependent manner without inducing excessive bone resorption.

The plasma concentration of $24R,25(OH)_2D_3$ (5 to 10 nM) is usually 10 times lower than that of $25(OH)D_3$ but exceeds that of $1,25(OH)_2D_3$ by about one hundredfold. Under normal circumstances, the biosynthesis of $1,25(OH)_2D_3$ and $24R,25(OH)_2D_3$ *in the renal tubules* is regulated reciprocally because PTH inhibits the transcription of 24-OHase and stimulates expression of 1α-OHase. Thus, in the renal tubules PTH allows the biosynthesis of $1,25(OH)_2D_3$ and minimizes its degradation into $1,24,25(OH)_3D_3$. In addition, $1,25(OH)_2D_3$ induces the expression of 24-OHase. This mechanism prevents overt production of $1,25(OH)_2D_3$.

The effect of PTH on the catabolism of $1,25(OH)_2D_3$ varies with the target cell. In contrast with the renal action, PTH synergizes with $1,25(OH)_2D_3$ to induce 24-OHase in osteoblasts. PTH does not modulate 24-OHase activity in the intestinal epithelium because these cells do not have PTH/PTHrP receptors. This also indicates that PTH has only indirect action on the intestinal absorption of calcium.

Vitamin D-Binding Protein Is a High-Capacity Carrier System, which Also Functions as an Actin-Scavanger and as a Co-chemotaxin   As discussed in Chap. 4, DBP is an albuminoid carrier protein produced by the liver. Each DBP protein has a single binding site for vitamin D derivatives. Plasma DBP has a high binding capacity: approximately 5% of the vitamin D binding sites are occupied by a ligand. The binding preference of DBP for its ligands is best described as $25OHD_3 = 24,25(OH)_2D_3 =$

$25,26(OH)_2D_3 > 1,25(OH)_2D_3 \gg$ vitamin $D_3 >$ vitamin D_2. Due to the differences in binding affinity, relatively more $1,25(OH)_2D_3$ than $25OHD_3$ or $24,25(OH)_2D_3$ circulates in a free form, which effectively decreases the half-life from 12 days ($25OHD_3$, $24,25(OH)_2D_3$) to a mere 6 h ($1,25(OH)_2D_3$). DBP plays the major role in the egress of endogenously synthesized vitamin D from skin, and appears to restrain D-sterols from too rapid/excessive cell entry. Most of dietary vitamin D is transported by chylomicrons to the liver, where it is efficiently taken up and hydroxylated at its 25th carbon. However, about half of the dietary vitamin D may be stored in the lipid droplets of adipocytes.

Although estrogens increase plasma concentrations of DBP, DBP is not influenced by disorders of mineral homeostasis.

Along with plasma *gelsolin,* DBP comprises the plasma *actin-scavenger* system that facilitates removal of G-actin (which is liberated from lysed cells) by prevention of its polymerization into F-actin. Recently, the DBP has been shown to behave as a co-chemotaxin of the complement peptide C5a. A unifying hypothesis suggests that *DBP might provide vitamin D delivery to cells to aid the resolution of tissue injuries during inflammation.*

Active Vitamin D Increases Plasma Concentrations of Both Calcium and Phosphate, and Thus Promotes Mineralization   The target cells and actions of $1,25(OH)_2D_3$ are listed in Table 8-6. A major determinant of mineral homeostasis is the intestinal action of $1,25(OH)_2D_3$. In spite of the identification of *calbindins* (calcium binding proteins), which are induced by $1,25(OH)_2D_3$ in the small intestine, the molecular mechanism of enhanced calcium absorption is poorly understood. It has been suggested that $1,25(OH)_2D_3$-induced changes in *plasma membrane phospholipase activity* are necessary for initiating the calcium transport.

The *absorption of phosphate* involves two mechanisms:

• a passive movement of phosphate following calcium, and
• a $1,25(OH)_2D_3$-stimulated active phosphate transport mechanism.

If dietary calcium load is low, the initial hypocalcemia results in increased PTH secretion, which increases the production of $1,25(OH)_2D_3$. In contrast, increased dietary calcium load results in a decrease of PTH secretion and, as a cosequence, a decrease of $1,25(OH)_2D_3$. This mechanism is a negative feedback loop, which regulates the efficiency of calcium absorption and keeps it within a narrow range in spite of significant changes in the dietary availability of calcium. Note that this mechanism is efficient only in the range between 500 and 1100 mg/d dietary calcium intake.

• In case of a daily intake below 500 mg, the increased efficiency of calcium absorption will be unable to compensate, and the patient shifts into a negative calcium balance.

• In case of a daily intake over 1100 mg, a positive calcium balance (calcium retention) occurs. It is important to recognize that if the dietary calcium load is sufficiently high, the absorption of calcium proceeds in a *vitamin D-independent* manner. This may result in hypercalcemia, such as seen in *milk-alkali syndrome*, a condition usually caused by excessive intake of milk and/or antacids that contain absorbable calcium.

The direct action of $1,25(OH)_2D_3$ on bone is counterintuitive for understanding its antirachitic action: it synergizes with PTH to induce *bone resorption*. This action involves activation of osteoblasts, which in turn recruit and activate osteoclasts. In addition, osteoclast *precursors* require $1,25(OH)_2D_3$ for their maturation process. The overall direct action on bone is an increased bone remodeling activity. The *antirachitic activity* of $1,25(OH)_2D_3$ can mainly be attributed to an indirect mechanism: the increased intestinal absorption of calcium and phosphate raises $[Ca^{2+}] \cdot [P_i]$, thereby promoting precipitation of calcium phosphate. The direct bone effect of calcitriol appears to be nonessential for proper mineralization. In fact, the mineralization defect of children suffering from *vitamin D–resistant rickets* (see below) can be corrected by calcium infusion.

The *renal actions* of $1,25(OH)_2D_3$ include inducing the transcription of 24-OHase, and increasing *proximal* tubular reabsorption of calcium and phosphate. The increased reabsorption of phosphate is partly due to an indirect mechanism: $1,25(OH)_2D_3$ suppresses production of PTH, a phosphaturic hormone, in the *parathyroid glands*.

Calcitriol is a potent inhibitor of PTH production in the chief cells of the parathyroid glands. In addition, calcitriol exerts an antiproliferative action on chief cells that may prevent parathyroid hyperplasia. The antiproliferative and differentiation-inducing activities of $1,25(OH)_2D_3$ are utilized in the treatment of psoriasis. However, an analog of $1,25(OH)_2D_3$, *calcipo triol*, is used because it is less prone to induce hypercalcemia.

Most Actions of Vitamin D Are Due to Calcitriol's Action on the Vitamin D Receptor   Vitamin D receptor (VDR) is a member of the streroid hormone receptor superfamily (see also in Chap. 5). VDR forms a heterodimer with retinoid X receptor (RXR), and binds to the *vitamin D response element* (VDRE). RXR and VDR bind the 5'- and 3'-VDRE repeat, respectively. VDRE acts as an enhancer of certain genes, such as osteocalcin or 24-OHase, and as a suppressor for others, such as PTH. VDR displays allelic heterogeneity. Up to 75% of the genetic determination of *peak bone mass* (see Box 8-9) is related to allelic variants of VDR. Note that the consequences of hypervitaminosis A include hypercalcemia (an effect similar to hypervitaminosis D) and midshaft hyperostosis of the long bones.

The notion that calcitriol's main action is mediated by the intracellular VDR is supported by the clinical picture associated with loss-of-function mutations of VDR. These mutations result in *hereditary vitamin D–resistant*

BOX 8-9 Peak Bone Mass

During the normal life-span, three phases of changes in bone mass can be identified:

- *Attainment* of peak bone mass: until about epiphyseal closure;
- *Consolidation and maintenance* of peak bone mass;
- Slow, age-dependent bone *loss,* which starts between the ages of 30 to 40 years.

Bone mass peaks in the third decade of life, and is determined by genetic and environmental factors. These include:

- *Gender:* males have a higher peak bone mass than females.
- *Race:* African Americans have a higher peak bone mass than Caucasians or Asians.
- *Inheritance:* allelic variants of VDR and estrogen receptors.
- *Physical activity:* the mechanical stress related to exercise directly stimulates bone deposition and helps to attain and retain peak bone mass.
- *Nutrition:* calcium supplementation, especially during adolescence, helps to attain peak bone mass. Increased dietary calcium helps to reduce the rate of bone loss during the third phase.

As discussed earlier, osteoporosis is a significant loss of bone mass. The rate of bone loss during the third phase appears to be steady. Therefore, *the higher the peak bone mass, the later in life will bone loss reach the degree of osteoporosis.* Stimulation of estrogen receptors is protective against age-dependent bone loss.

(often, but misleadingly, termed vitamin D-*dependent*) *rickets type II.* (The hereditary vitamin D-dependent rickets type I is due to renal 1α-OHase deficiency.) The consequences of vitamin D resistance are practically the same as those of vitamin D deficiency, i.e., severe defect of bone mineralization, although laboratory measurements of $25(OH)D_3$ and $1,25(OH)_2D_3$ clearly distinguish these two causes of rickets.

VDR may be stimulated by supranormal concentrations of $25(OH)D_3$ thereby causing hypercalcemia, hyperphosphatemia, and pathologic calcification. This mechanism is important in vitamin D intoxication. Because 25-hydroxylation of vitamin D is not tightly regulated, oversupply of dietary vitamin D yields supranormal plasma levels of $25(OH)D_3$.

Some actions of vitamin D, however, may include mechanisms too rapid for a transcriptional regulation. For example, $1,25(OH)_2D_3$ has been shown to exert an immediate type of action on calcium absorption by intestinal epithelial cells. This mechanism maybe operational only if the intracellular VDR is intact because its mutation impairs regulated calcium absorption in spite of supranormal plasma levels of $1,25(OH)_2D_3$. The biologic action of $24,25(OH)_2D_3$ is apparently mediated by a receptor distinct from VDR (see above).

Vitamin D Metabolites Are Primarily Eliminated in the Bile   The degradation of vitamin D may include multiple hydroxylation and oxidation steps. Although renal 24-OHase is a major determinant of vitamin D degradation, the urinary excretion of vitamin D and its metabolites are minimal. The liver is involved in several important steps of vitamin D metabolism:

- It converts D_3 into $25(OH)D_3$, which is the main circulating form of vitamin D. The concentration of this metabolite is the best indicator of vitamin D supply.
- It excretes biologically active vitamin D metabolites (including $25(OH)D_3$) with bile in the process of enterohepatic circulation.
- It excretes degradation products of vitamin D (such as *calcitroic acid*) into bile.
- It conjugates some of the metabolites with glucuronide or sulfate. This minor pathway yields more water-soluble products that are excreted in the urine.

Calcitonin

Calcitonin Has Minimal Physiologic Role in the Regulation of Plasma Calcium, but Acts as a Powerful Protector of Bone Mass   Calcitonin (CT) has been discovered as a hormone that reduces plasma concentrations of ionized calcium. This 32-amino-acid-long peptide hormone is secreted by the *parafollicular cells* (also known as the *C cells*) of the thyroid gland. However, either surgical or raidothyroidectomy, which eliminates CT from the circulation, does not result in a hypercalcemic state. This indicates that CT is not a major factor in the physiologic regulation of *plasma* calcium in humans. CT is utterly important for maintaining normal plasma calcium in saltwater fish, which are exposed to the high ambient concentration of calcium in sea. Humans normally face the opposite challenge of maintaining their plasma (and bone) calcium in face of a limited availability of dietary calcium.

The physiologic function of CT is most likely limited to its osteoclast-inhibiting action that protects against excessive bone resorption. While the importance of this action as a physiologic regulator of bone mass is an unsettled issue, it is clear that exogenously administered CT (either as nasal spray or as injection) is an effective treatment of osteoporosis and Paget's disease (see later).

Calcitonin Secretion Is Stimulated by Hypercalcemia, Incretins, and Estrogens   As shown, the C-cells of the thyroid gland are derived from the neural crest and develop in the last pharyngeal pouch. In several sub-mammalian vertebrates, such as salmonids, the C-cells are not dispersed among the thyroid follicles but form a distinct *ultimobranchial organ*. The embryonic origin of the C-cells explains why their tumors (*medullary thyroid cancer* [MTC]) are often associated with *pheochromocytoma* (tumors of the adrenal medulla, another neural crest-derived endocrine tissue), in the MEN type 2a syndrome. The cells of MTC secrete CT and katacalcin in an unregulated fashion. *Katacalcin* is a polypeptide flanking CT at its C-terminal within their common precursor (see Fig. 3-2). The physiologic significance of katacalcin (if any) is unknown. However, measurements of katacalcin may corroborate the diagnosis of MTC.

Normal C-cells secrete CT, equimolar quantities of katacalcin, and trace quantities of CGRP. Secretion of CT is stimulated by

- hypercalcemia;
- incretins: *gastrin* (a hormone produced by gastric mucosal cells) and related hormones that share the same 4-amino-acid N-terminal sequence, such as *cholecystokinin* or *glucagon;*
- estrogens and lactation.

The C-cells express calcium-sensing receptors. However, the coupling of the $[Ca^{2+}]_{ECF}$ with the secretory process in the C-cell is fundamentally different from that observed in the parathyroid chief cells. CT is stored in secretory granules, which are exocytosed upon the increase of cytosolic concentration of Ca^{2+}. The increase in cytoplasmic Ca^{2+} is attained by the activation of voltage-gated Ca^{2+} channels, which means that the Ca^{2+} is derived from extracellular, rather than intracellular (endoplasmic reticulum) sources.

It has been proposed that certain gastrointestinal hormones referred to as *"incretins"* induce CT secretion in a manner similar to their effect on insulin secretion (see Chap. 9). This is an anticipatory mechanism: the increased CT inhibits osteoclastic activity, and thus *attenuates postprandial hypercalcemia* even before the influx of dietary calcium into the circulation. The physiologic relevance of this mechanism is uncertain. However, it is important to remember that gastrin-induced CT secretion is a provocative test used in the diagnosis of MTC.

Estrogens and lactation increase plasma CT. This mechanism appears to be important as a protection of bone mass

- in pregnancy and postpartum, when the calcium demand of the fetus or the infant must be met without losing maternal skeletal minerals. Note that estrogens also protect bone mass by other mechanisms (see Table 8-7).
- in premenopausal women in general. After menopause plasma CT decreases, which may contribute to postmenopausal osteoporosis.

Both basal and stimulated levels of plasma CT are higher in men than in women. The basal levels in heparinized plasma are ≤ 19 and ≤ 14 pg/mL, respectively; these values, however, are influenced by the specificity of the antibody. CT circulates in plasma as a free hormone with a half-life of about to 10 min. It is primarily degraded and eliminated by the kidney. Some degradation products of CT are recognized by various antibodies used in clinical laboratories.

Calcitonin Inhibits Osteoclasts via a G-Protein-Coupled Receptor   The main effect of CT is the direct inhibition of osteoclasts. Exogenously administered CT results in a rapid inhibition of osteoclastic activity. In patients who are in the osteolytic stage of Paget's disease (see below), but not in healthy adults, the acute inhibition of octeoclastic activity by parenteral administration of CT is accompanied by a decline in plasma concentration of calcium. Long-term administration of CT decreases the number of osteoclast cells. However, exogenous CT may lose its effectiveness due to receptor downregulation.

CT slightly decreases calcium and phosphate reabsorption, probably by acting on the proximal tubules of the kidney. In MTC, when hypersecretion of CT occurs, renal CT receptors are apparently downregulated and the calciuric effect of CT cannot become prominent.

The CT receptor is closely related to the PTH receptor and apparently utilizes the same second messenger systems, i.e., mainly $G\alpha_s$-coupled stimulation of adenylyl cyclase and $G\alpha_q$-coupled stimulation of PLC. The primarily opposing effects of PTH and CT are achieved by the differential receptor expression of their target cells.

Other Hormones Involved in the Regulation Calcium and Phosphate

As mentioned, several hormones have significant impact on calcium homeostasis without receiving a direct feedback signal. Most of these hormones make calcium available for essential physiologic processes, such as bone growth, pregnancy, and lactation. In the latter two cases the hormones must support the mineralization of growing fetal and infant bones, and also protect maternal bone mass.

The main regulators of bone growth are the GH/IGF-1 axis and, during the pubertal growth spurt, sex steroids (androgens and estrogens). Androgens are locally converted into estrogens by *aromatase*, and the sex steroid-induced bone maturation is mainly mediated by estrogen receptors. The increased demand for calcium and phosphate for mineralizing the newly deposited osteoid is supported by GH- and estrogen-induced renal 1α-OHase activity, and the increased plasma level of calcitriol.

PRL, the main regulator of lactation, is a hormone structurally related to GH. PRL increases intestinal absorption of calcium and phosphate mainly by inducing renal 1α-OHase activity. The absorbed minerals, how-ever, are destined to leave the body with milk. From the mother's perspec-tive, milk secretion is mainly a PRL-regulated loss of fluids. Calcium is transported into milk due to the action of PTHrP on the mammary epithe-lium. Casein, a major protein in milk synthesized under the influence of PRL, is highly phosphorylated and thus binds much of the transported calcium. Phosphate and the bound calcium are liberated from casein during digestion and absorbed from the infant's GI tract. Thus, milk provides sufficient quantities of both minerals for skeletal tissues in the breast-fed infant. Because PRL is a weak inducer of 1α-OHase, lactating women are almost invariably in the state of secondary hyperparathyroidism. This condition can be attenuated by increased dietary calcium intake.

Estrogens protect bone mass involving several sites of action (see Table 8-7). The loss of this protection results in an accelerated development of bone loss known as *postmenopausal osteoporosis*. Postmenopausal osteopo-rosis is not associated with detectable changes in plasma calcium, PTH, or hypercalciuria. It develops very slowly, but once developed, it appears to be irreversible; even exogenously administered estrogens are unable to restore bone mass. Estrogens also play a role in providing minerals for the developing bones of the fetus by inducing renal 1α-OHase activity. Remember, however, that the placenta is a major site of extrarenal 1α-OHase activity, and thus is a significant contributor to circulating calcitriol. Similar to its role in the mammary epithelium, PTHrP (of fetal and placental origin) is driving the calcium pump in the placenta.

Thyroid hormones regulate the metabolic rate. The increased meta-bolic rate seen in *hyperthyroidism* favors catabolic over anabolic processes. In line with this general theme, patients with hyperthyroidism have in-creased bone turnover and a concomitant loss of bone mass caused by thyroxine-stimulated osteoclastic activity. The loss of bone mass may amount to *osteoporosis*. The *negative calcium balance* during hyperthyroid-ism is due to a mild initial hypercalcemia, which suppresses PTH secretion. The resulting secondary hypoparathyroidism results in reduced fractional reabsorption of calcium, reduced production of calcitriol, and reduced intes-tinal absorption of calcium and phosphate.

Excessive levels of *glucocorticoids* also result in negative calcium bal-ance by multiple sites of action. Glucocorticoids antagonize the intestinal action of calcitriol and may inhibit renal 1α-OHase expression. Due to the *direct inhibitory action of cortisol on renal reabsorption of calcium*, the urinary loss of calcium is increased *(hypercalciuria)*. Thus, glucocorticoids inhibit both absorption and reabsorption of calcium. The resultant initial hypocalcemia is corrected by elevated PTH via increased osteoclastic activ-ity. Glucocorticoids inhibit collagen synthesis, and therefore osteoid pro-duction by osteoblasts. Thus, the balance between osteoblasts and osteo-clasts is shifted toward bone resorption. The combined action of supranormal levels of glucocorticoids (such as seen in Cushing's disease) may result in rapidly developing osteoporosis. In adrenal insufficiency, hypercalcemia may occur, suggesting that physiologic levels of glucocorticoids contribute to the maintenance of normocalcemia.

Local Factors in the Regulation of Bone Remodeling

Bone turnover is achieved in the process of bone remodeling by BMUs. The coupling of osteoblastic and osteoclastic function is crucial in the maintenance of bone mass. The *basis of this coupling is the cell-to-cell interaction between osteoblasts and osteoclast progenitors*. The coordinated function of BMUs is under the control of

- the direct shear stress exerted by the movement of bone fluid;
- systemic hormones; and
- locally acting humoral factors such as cytokines, prostaglandins, and NO.

Osteoclastic Bone Resorption Is a Two-Step Process Involving Demineralization of the Matrix and Subsequent Degradation of the Osteoid

The prerequisite of bone deposition during bone remodeling is the resorption of preexsisting bone by osteoclasts. Mature osteoclasts attach to the bone surface with an *adhesion ring*. At the adhesion ring, the cytoplasm of the osteoclast is devoid of organelles, and contains numerous actin filaments. For this reason, the cytoplasmic side of the adhesion ring is called the *clear zone*. The actin filaments bind to transmembrane proteins called *integrins*. The extracellular domains of the integrins bind to bone matrix proteins. The integrins include *integrin αVβ3*, which regulates adhesion of osteoclasts to bone extracellular matrix proteins, such us osteopontin. The *vitronectin receptor,* an integrin expressed by phagocytic cells, is highly expressed by osteoclast and is used as a diagnostic marker protein.

The adhesion ring thus becomes the lateral barrier of a fluid compartment between the plasma membrane of the osteoclasts and the surface of bone matrix. *This sealed fluid compartment* (the *resorptive compartment*) *is functionally analogous to a secondary lysosome.* The large patch of osteoclast membrane that is encircled by the adhesion ring and forms the dome of the resorptive compartment becomes highly folded. This is known as the *ruffled border*.

The ruffled border provides an increased membrane surface. The membrane incorporates *proton pumps,* mainly H^+-*ATPase*. The proton pumps acidify the fluid in the resorptive compartment. The low pH (pH 3 to 4) greatly increases the solubility of calcium phosphate, the hydroxyapatite crystals are dissolved, and the osteoid becomes demineralized.

The protons are generated by the zinc metalloenzyme *carbonic anhydrase II,* which is also found in the renal tubules (see Chap. 12) and in osteoblasts. *Acetazolamide,* a diuretic drug that inhibits carbonic anhydrase,

inhibits osteoclastic bone resorption. Congenital absence of carbonic anhydrase II results in osteopetrosis (see Box 8-1).

The digestion of the osteoid matrix involves the release of lysosomal
hydrolases into the resorptive compartment. Several proteases break down
the organic matrix: *matrix metalloproteinase 9* (MMP-9), *cathepsin O* (also
known as *cathepsin K*), and *cathepsins B* and *L*.

TRAP is a tyrosine phosphatase present in the lysosomes of osteoclasts
at high levels. Plasma concentration of TRAP is a useful marker enzyme
in clinical laboratory assessment of osteoclastic activity. TRAP is needed
for the normal process of endochondral bone formation, but does not
appear to play a significant role in bone resorption during remodeling.

Osteoclasts have a limited life span and are eliminated by apoptosis.
The disintegration of osteoclasts liberates the contents of the resorptive
compartment, which joins the general ECF via the movement of bone fluid.

**An Important Local Signal for Adaptive Bone Deposition Is the Direct
Shear Stress Exerted by the Movement of Bone Fluid**   Bone tissue responds
to mechanical stress with adaptive changes in mass and structure. Mechanical force applied to bone produces two localized mechanical signals on the
cell: deformation of the extracellular matrix *(substrate strain)* and ECF flow
(movement of bone fluid). The movement of bone fluid occurs in the lacunar-
canalicular pore space. Bone fluid is propelled by two main forces: the
centrifugal perfusion of bone and by mechanical stress *(squeeze flow)*. If
the canaliculi have diameters of about 0.2 μm, squeeze flow can nourish
four to five concentric layers of osteocytes in an osteon. The movement of
bone fluid has two effects:

• It generates an electrokinetic force (known as *stress-generated potentials* [SGP]) by the flow of mobile ions in bone fluid over the charged surfaces.
• The movement of fluid exerts a *direct shear stress* force on the cells.
The magnitude of the fluid-induced shear stresses is in the range of 8 to
30 dyn/cm^2.

Although bone cells are sensitive to electric fields and may respond
directly to SGP, *the physiologically important signal is the shear stress of
fluid flow*. When bone is subjected to bending loads, interstitial fluid in
the bone matrix flows away from regions of high compressive stress. The
interstitial fluid flow, the shear stress and the SGPs in the lacunar-canalicular
network are strongly influenced by the load. The fluid flow induces the
following cellular responses in the cells of the osteoblastic lineage:

• specific activation of *gadolinium-sensitive stretch-activated Ca^{2+}-
channels* (but not of the voltage-gated Ca^{2+}-channels), which increases influx
of Ca^{2+} from the ECF.
• the expression of *cyclooxygenase-2* (*COX-2*, also known as "inducible COX" or *prostaglandin H synthase-2* [PGHS-2]), but not that of COX-1

(PGHS-1). The production of prostaglandins (mainly PGE_2 and $PGF_{2\alpha}$) remains enhanced for at least 1 h after the cessation of stimulation. The role of prostaglandins is to amplify the cellular response to mechanical stress by

- stimulation of cyclic AMP production.
- activation of the inositol trisphosphate (IP_3) pathway, which leads to release of Ca^{2+} from the endoplasmic reticulum.

The signaling results in increased protein synthesis and secretion by the cells of the osteoblastic lineage (deposition of osteoid). The accumulation of calcium in the cytosol also heralds the production of membrane-bounded *matrix vesicles,* which are deposited by budding and pinching off either into the lacunar-canalicular space and/or into the space between bone and the bone-lining cells. The deposition of matrix vesicles is phase 1 of the calcification process of the newly deposited osteoid.

Stress-induced flow is important in bone remodeling, and lack of such flow may be one cause for producing *osteoporosis* and *hypercalcemia during prolonged immobilization.* As pointed out, interstitial fluid flow is strongly influenced by load. This explains the well-established observation that regular weight-lifting exercise improves bone mass development and retention if the weight (load) is increased, and not if the same small weight is lifted repeatedly. Local pressure exerted by tumors (such as those of the pituitary gland) may impair the flow of bone fluid and result in bone resorption, thereby providing space for further growth of the tumor.

Systemic Hormones and Locally Produced Cytokines Regulate Osteoclast Function Mainly by Modulating the Osteoblastic Production of Osteoclast Differentiation Factor and Its Decoy Receptor, Osteoprotegerin

Osteoclasts are derived from granulocyte-macrophage colony forming units (CFU–GM) and possibly also from peripheral blood monocytes (PBM). The still mononuclear *committed osteoclast precursors* are the first to express calcitonin receptor and are already postmitotic. The committed osteoclast precursors fuse to form the multinucleated *immature osteoclasts.* The *mature osteoclasts* are terminally differentiated, activated cells.

Osteoclast differentiation *and activity* depends on a membrane-anchored cytokine expressed by bone marrow stromal cells and osteoblasts. This cytokine is the *osteoclast differentiation factor* (ODF), a member of the membrane-associated tumor necrosis factor *ligand* family. ODF is identical with SOFA *(stromal osteoclast-forming activity),* and *tumor necrosis factor-related activation-induced cytokine* (TRANCE), also known as *RANK-ligand* (RANKL), which enhances T-cell growth and dendritic cell function in the immune system. The ODF receptor (ODF-R, also known as TRANCE-R or *receptor activator of NF-κB* [RANK]) is expressed by osteoclast precursors, peripheral blood monocytes and also by mature osteoclasts. Stimulation of ODF-R is essential for the *recruitment, differentiation, survival, and activation* of osteoclasts. ODF-R activates NF-κB (a transcription factor) by mechanisms involving members of the *TNF receptor-associated factor* (TRAF) family of signal transducers.

Osteoblasts not only express ODF on their plasma membranes, but also secrete a protein termed *osteoprotegerin* (OPG). OPG is a non-membrane-anchored member of the TNF *receptor* superfamily. OPG functions as a *decoy receptor* of ODF (see Box 8-10), and inhibits osteoclastogenesis by interrupting the cell-to-cell interaction between osteoblasts and osteoclast precursors. Hence OPG is also known as *osteoclastogenesis-inhibitory factor* (OCIF). The unusual feature in this system is that a hormone-like ligand (ODF) is membrane-anchored, and a receptor (OPG) is the secreted soluble protein.

When injected, OPG has an acute hypocalcemic effect without increasing urinary calcium excretion. OPG blocks ovariectomy-associated bone loss in rats. Either administration of recombinant OPG into normal mice or hepatic expression of OPG in transgenic mice results in a profound yet nonlethal *osteopetrosis,* coincident with a decrease of osteoclast differentiation. Ablation of OPG in knock-out mice leads to severe *osteoporosis* due to enhanced osteoclastogenesis. The marked bone loss is accompanied by destruction of the growth plate and the lack of trabecular bone in the femur. OPG-deficient mice also exhibit calcification in the *tunica media* of the aorta and renal arteries, suggesting that regulation of OPG, or its ligand(s) may play a role in the clinically observed association between osteoporosis and vascular calcification.

The final common pathway in the regulation of bone remodeling is the modulation of the interaction between ODF and its receptor. The main target of both *local and systemic factors* involved in this modulation is the osteoblast. These factors may *alter the expression of ODF, OPG, and/or alter the ODF:OPG ratio,* thereby modulating osteoclastogenesis and osteoclast function.

The cells of both osteoblastic and osteoclastic lineages produce cytokines, which serve as important local paracrine/autocrine regulators of the basic multicellular units. In addition, mobile transient cell populations of bones such as PBMs and lymphocytes may contribute to the local cytokine environment both under physiologic and pathologic conditions (Table 8-9).

BOX 8-10   Decoy Receptors

Soluble decoy receptors are used by the immune system to prevent binding of ligands to their functional membrane-anchored receptors. Decoy receptors inhibit the activation of the functional receptors by competing for the ligand. *TRAIL* is a tumor necrosis factor-related ligand that induces apoptosis upon binding to its *death domain-containing* (apoptosis-inducing) *receptors, DR4* and *DR5.* Two additional TRAIL receptors, TRID/DcR1 and DcR2, lack functional death domains and function as decoy receptors for TRAIL. Osteoprotegerin (OPG) also functions as a receptor for the cytotoxic ligand TRAIL.

Table 8-9 Cytokines Involved in the Regulation of the Basic Multicellular Units

Source	Cytokine	Target	Function
Local stimulators of bone resorption			
Marrow stromal cell, osteoblast	**ODF** (synonyms TRANCE, RANKL SOFA)	CFU-GM, peripheral blood monocyte (?) osteoclast precursor, osteoclast	Performs obligatory cell-to-cell interaction to recruit osteoclast precursors, induce their differentiation, and activation; binds to ODF-R (synonyms: TRANCE-R, RANK)
Marrow stromal cell, osteoblast, endothelium	M-CSF, osteoblast	CFU-GM, osteoblast	Recruits osteoclast precursor cells and induces their differentiation
Marrow stromal cell and osteoblast	IL-11, osteoblast	CFU-GM, osteoblast	Recruits osteoclast precursor cells and induces their differentiation via prostaglandins
Tissue macrophage, peripheral blood monocyte	IL-1, TNF-α	Bone marrow stromal cell, osteoprogenitor, osteoblast, osteoclast	Potent inducers of bone resorption via activation of osteoblasts and by direct action on osteoclasts
Tissue macrophage, peripheral blood monocyte, marrow stromal cell, osteoblast, and osteoclast	IL-6	Bone marrow stromal cell, osteoprogenitor, osteoblast, osteoclast	Recruits osteoclast precursor cells, induces their differentiation and activation; involved in the pathomechanism of Paget's disease
Local inhibitors of bone resorption			
Marrow stromal cell, osteoblast	OPG (synonym: OCIF)	Autocrine: marrow stromal cell, osteoblast	Antagonizes obligatory cell-to-cell interaction between osteoblasts and osteoclast precursors serving as a decoy receptor
Marrow stromal cell, osteoblast	TGF-β and TGF-β precursor	Osteoclast precursor, osteoclast	Inhibits proliferation and fusion of osteoclast precursors, inhibits osteoclast activity; osteoclasts may activate secreted TGF-β precursor
Marrow stromal cell, osteoblast	IL-18	Osteoclast precursor	Inhibits proliferation and fusion of osteoclast precursors
NK cells, T lymphocytes	IFN-γ	Osteoclast precursor	Inhibits IL-1 and TNF-α induced proliferation and fusion of osteoclast precursors by overt stimulation of NO production

ABBREVIATIONS: ODF, osteoclast differentiation factor; TRANCE, tumor necrosis factor-related activation-induced cytokine; RANKL, receptor activator of NF-κB ligand; SOFA, stromal osteoclast-forming activity; ODF-R, ODF receptor; TRANCE-R, TRANCE receptor; M-CSF, macrophage colony-stimulating factor; CFU-GM, granulocyte, macrophage colony forming unit; TNF, tumor necrosis factor; IL, interleukin; OPG, osteoprotegerin; OCIF, osteoclastogenesis-inhibitory factor; TGF, transforming growth factor; NK, natural killer; IFN, interferon; NO, nitric oxide.

The main systemic factors influencing this local circuitry are depicted in Fig. 8-10.

PTH, 1,25-$(OH)_2D_3$ and IL-11 increase the ODF:OPG ratio. Anti-ODF polyclonal antibody, which neutralizes ODF activity (i.e., acts similar to OPG), prevents bone resorption induced by PTH, 1,25-$(OH)_2D_3$, or prostaglandin E_2 (PGE_2). PGE_2 downregulates the expression of OPG mRNA in bone marrow stromal cells, probably via an increase in cyclic AMP. This mechanism might also be involved in PGE_2-induced bone resorption. OPG mRNA levels are decreased by glucocorticoids. The reduced production of OPG from osteoblasts and/or marrow stromal cells is in part responsible for glucocorticoid-induced bone resorption.

Paget's disease of bone *(osteitis deformans)* is the result of the dysregulation of bone remodeling units either in several bones *(polyostotic form)*, or more rarely in a single bone *(monostotic form)*. Mounting evidence supports that Paget's disease is caused by *canine distemper* viral infection of osteoclasts. Pagetic osteoclasts secrete supranormal amounts of IL-6, which appears to activate the bone remodeling units partly via an autocrine

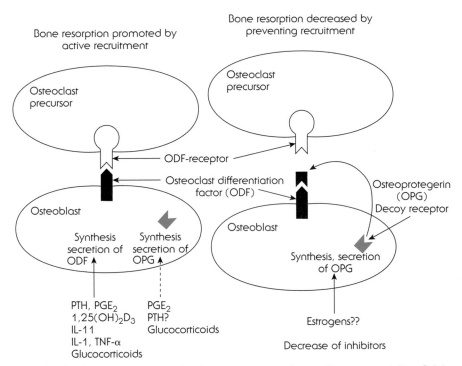

Figure 8-10. Interaction between local and systemic regulators of bone remodeling. Solid lines indicate stimulation/increase; dashed lines indicate inhibition/decrease. A. Direct cellular contact via osteoclast differentiation factor (ODF) and ODF-receptor, and its inhibition by the decoy receptor osteoprotegerin (OPG). Systemic hormones and local factors may alter the ODF:OPG ratio and modulate recruitment of osteoclast precursors.

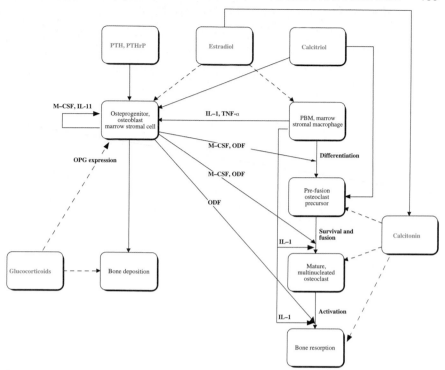

Figure 8-10. (*Continued*) B. The systemic hormones (highlighted in color) modulate bone remodeling mainly acting via the osteoblasts. Calcitonin, however, acts via osteoclast precursors and their descendents. Locally acting mediators (secreted and membrane-anchored cytokines) are produced by osteoprogenitors, osteoblasts and peripheral blood monocytes (PBM)/tissue macrophages. Osteoclasts, especially in Pagetic bone produce IL-6 (not shown). PTH, parathyroid hormone; IL, interleukin; TNF, tumor necrosis factor; PGE$_2$, prostaglandin E$_2$; M-CSF, macrophage colony-stimulating factor; PBM, peripheral blood monocytes.

mechanism, partly via acting on osteoblasts. The disease presents in three stages:

- *Osteolytic stage,* which is characterized by agressive osteoclastic bone resorption;
- *Mixed osteoclastic-osteoblastic stage,* during which thick but structurally unsound bone is deposited by osteoblasts.
- *Burned out stage:* the osteoclastic hyperactivity and eventually the overtaking osteoblastic activity subside.

Depending on the stage of the disease, marker enzymes in serum (osteoblast-derived alkaline phosphatase and osteoclast-derived tartrate-resistant acid phosphatase) are preferentially elevated. After osteoporosis, Paget's disease is the second most common geriatric bone disease. The most serious but rare complication of Paget's disease is osteosarcoma.

INTEGRATED REGULATION OF CALCIUM AND PHOSPHATE

Regulation of Plasma Calcium

The most important components of the complex regulatory circuitry that regulates plasma concentrations of ionized calcium are shown in Fig. 8-11. We have already discussed all elements displayed, and the following discussion is intended to give examples for using this flowchart. Here we shall discuss the possible causes of, and responses to, three conditions that are frequently encountered in clinical practice: hypercalcemia, hypocalcemia, and renal osteodystrophy. Selected causes of hypercalcemia and hypocalcemia are given in Table 8-10. The causes determine how the entire regulatory circuitry responds. This differential response is utilized in the differential diagnosis of the conditions.

Note that *secondary hyperparathyroidism* is not shown in Table 8-10 because in this case plasma calcium levels are within the normal range. The normal plasma calcium, however, is achieved at the expense of excessive production of PTH, a consequent mobilization of calcium from bones and a negative calcium balance. As discussed earlier, this situation occurs in cases of excess glucocorticoids. In adults, insufficient dietary intake or absorption of vitamin D may yield in osteomalacia that is associated with similar laboratory findings.

Hypercalcemic Conditions   As discussed, *primary hyperparathyroidism* is an unregulated hypersecretion of PTH. The consequences and laboratory profile that were discussed earlier (see Boxes 8-4 and 8-5) can be deduced from Fig. 8-11.

In HHM, hypersecretion of PTHrP results in overstimulation of the PTH/PTHrP receptors. Therefore, other than immunoreactive PTH, the laboratory findings are qualitatively the same as in primary hyperparathyroidism. Immunoreactive PTH is suppressed because of the elevated plasma levels of both ionized calcium and $1,25(OH)_2D$.

In case of *vitamin D intoxication,* due to the unregulated nature of hepatic 25-OHase activity, plasma 25(OH)D increases. Although this compound is less active than $1,25(OH)_2D$, when it is present in high concentrations, it may activate VDR. This results in a direct inhibition of PTH secretion and a direct stimulation of intestinal calcium (and phosphate) absorption. The increased intestinal calcium absorption is the main cause of hypercalcemia, which occurs in spite of low levels of PTH and a decreased fractional reabsorption of calcium. In addition, both the low levels of PTH and hypercalcemia directly decrease 1α-OHase activity in the proximal tubules.

In *milk-alkali syndrome,* the dietary calcium overload results in vitamin D-independent absorption and hypercalcemia. The plasma 25(OH)D is

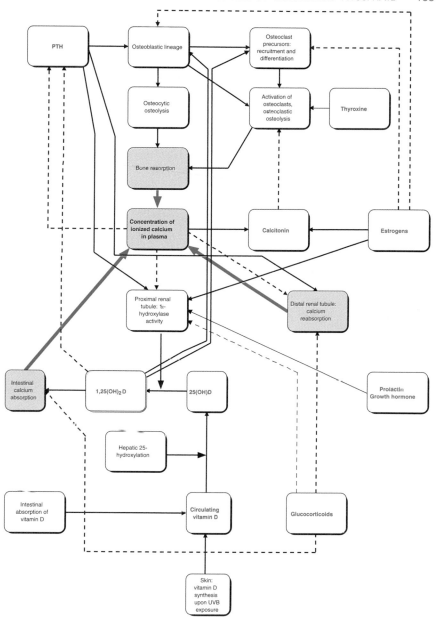

Figure 8-11. Hormonal regulation of plasma concentrations of ionized calcium. Solid lines indicate stimulation/increase; dashed lines indicate inhibition/decrease. The three thick lines indicate the three main sources of plasma calcium (i.e., absorption, resorption and reabsorption). The main active hormones are highlighted in color. Note that ionized calcium functions as a hormone-like signal on calcium-sensing receptors. The regulation of bone deposition is not included in the figure.

Table 8-10   Selected Causes of Hypercalcemia and Hypocalcemia

Hypercalcemia	Hypocalcemia
Immobilization	Hypoparathyroidism (congenital, surgical, autoimmune, hypomagnesemic)
Primary hyperparathyroidism (adenoma, carcinoma, possible association with MEN1 or MEN2a)	Pseudohypoparathyroidism types 1A and 1B
Tertiary hyperparathyroidism	1α-OHase deficiency (vitamin D-dependent rickets type 1)
Humoral hypercalcemia of malignancy (overproduction of PTHrP)	VDR mutations (vitamin D-dependent rickets type 2 = vitamin D resistance)
Osteolytic malignancies: breast cancer lymphomas, including metastatic multiple myeloma and leukemia	Advanced stages of malabsorption of lipids (steatorrhea)
Loss of function mutations of the CaR: familial hypocalciuric hypercalcemia and neonatal severe hyperparathyroidism	Rhabdomyolysis and other causes of rapid phosphate influx into plasma
Vitamin intoxication (vitamin D and/or vitamin A)	
Granulomatous diseases (1α-OHase activity)	
Dietary oversupply of calcium (milk-alkali syndrome)	
Endocrine diseases: thyrotoxicosis, adrenal insufficiency, acromegaly (overproduction of growth hormone)	

ABBREVIATIONS: MEN, multiple endocrine neoplasia; VDR, vitamin D receptor; PTHrP, parathyroid hormone related protein; CaR, calcium-sensing receptor; OHase, hydroxylase.

normal. The other features are similar to vitamin D intoxication (PTH, 1α-OHase activity are suppressed).

Hypocalcemic Conditions   In *pseudohypoparathyroidism* (types 1A and 1B), the renal actions of PTH are blunted. This results in lower reabsorption of calcium, increased reabsorption of phosphate, and decreased 1α-OHase activity. A general feature of hormone resistance syndromes is that, due to the loss of negative feedback, the secretion of the hormone per se is increased. Both the hypocalcemia and the decreased levels of $1,25(OH)_2D$ mean lack of negative feedback to PTH secretion. Thus, immunoreactive PTH is high, yet urinary cyclic AMP is low. The decreased levels of $1,25(OH)_2D$ result in decreased calcium and phosphate absorption. Plasma levels of phosphate are high because of the lost phosphaturic action of PTH. The high concentration of phosphate may keep the $[Ca^{2+}] \cdot [PO_4^{3-}]$ high enough to prevent demineralization of bone (osteomalacia/rickets).

   Vitamin D–resistant rickets (type II) is a hormone resistance syndrome. Accordingly, plasma levels of $1,25(OH)_2D$ are high. Plasma levels of $25(OH)D$ are normal because this is determined only by dietary intake and UVB-dependent endogenous production of vitamin D. The lack of

1,25(OH)$_2$D's action and hypocalcemia result in secondary hyperparathyroidism, which causes excessive bone resorption. This is unable to increase plasma levels of calcium, but very effectively induces phosphaturia thereby decreasing plasma levels of phosphate. There is a severe decrease in [Ca^{2+}]·[PO$_4^{3-}$] that results in demineralization of bone. The *1α-OHase deficiency* (vitamin D-dependent rickets type I) is similar to vitamin D-resistant rickets, except that plasma levels of 1,25(OH)$_2$D are extremely low.

Malabsorption of lipids (such as in *celiac disease*) results in osteomalacia by two mechanisms:

- Fatty acids liberated from lipids by lipase form nonabsorbable salts with calcium ("soap scum"), which contributes to the characteristically pale color of stool.
- Absorption of all lipid-soluble vitamins (D, E, K, and A) is impaired. Thus, absorption of dietary vitamin D, and the enterohepatic recycling of 25(OH)D are impaired. The decrease in circulating 25(OH)D is dramatic, and in spite of the increased renal expression of 1α-OHase, plasma levels of 1,25(OH)$_2$D are low. A minor confounding factor is that osteocalcin production may become impaired due to the associated vitamin K deficiency.

The reduced absorption of calcium is initially compensated by PTH-induced bone resorption. However, the hypersecretion of PTH exaggerates the hypophosphatemia, thereby yielding osteomalacia. During advanced stages of the disease, the compensatory mechanisms become insufficient and hypocalcemia develops.

Regulation of Plasma Phosphate

Hyperphosphatemia and Renal Osteodystrophy   Renal osteodystrophy refers to skeletal disorders of patients with *chronic renal failure:* osteitis fibrosa, osteomalacia, osteosclerosis, osteoporosis, and extraskeletal calcifications. The two main factors responsible for the presentation are:

- phosphate retention due to reduced filtration;
- reduced production of 1,25(OH)$_2$D$_3$.

At least initially, the reduced production of 1,25(OH)$_2$D$_3$ is caused by phosphate retention, and hyperphosphatemia acting upon the proximal tubules of functioning nephrons. Phosphate retention becomes significant when the creatinine clearance (a measure of *glomerular filtration rate* [GFR]) drops below 40 mL/min.

The decreased plasma 1,25(OH)$_2$D$_3$ results in decreased absorption of calcium and decreased negative feedback to PTH either by Ca^{2+} or by 1,25(OH)$_2$D$_3$ itself. The resultant secondary hyperparathyroidism corrects plasma levels of Ca^{2+} by inducing bone resorption. However, the normalized calcium concentration is associated with hyperphosphatemia, and the increased $[Ca^{2+}] \cdot [PO_4^{3-}]$ results in *metastatic extraosseal calcifications*. The extraosseal calcifications occur at the expense of bone mineral losses. Depending on the stage of the disease, the osteitis fibrosa cystica (which is due to PTH-induced osteoclastic activity) may be associated with osteomalacia. Therapy for the condition includes administration of $1,25(OH)_2D_3$, limiting dietary phosphate and its absorption, and dialysis of plasma.

Hypophosphatemic Rickets

A Putative Phosphate-Regulating Hormone Might Be Responsible for X-Linked Hypophosphatemic Rickets and Oncogenic Osteomalacia *X-linked hypophosphatemic rickets* (XLH) and *oncogenic osteomalacia* share several common features such as that the normal concentrations of plasma PTH and Ca^{2+} are associated with severe hypophosphatemia which is due to reduced reabsorption of phosphate from the proximal tubules. The decreased $[Ca^{2+}] \cdot [PO_4^{3-}]$ is the immediate cause of osteomalacia. Plasma levels of $1,25(OH)_2D_3$ are usually in the low-normal range in XLH, which is inappropriately low for the plasma phospate levels. Plasma levels of $1,25(OH)_2D_3$ are usually suppressed in oncogenic osteomalacia.

It has been proposed that the altered function of a hormone regulating renal phosphate handling and 1α-OHase activity is responsible for both pathologic conditions. XLH is caused by a loss of function mutation of the *PEX* gene (*p*hosphate-regulating gene with homologies to *e*ndopeptidases found at the HYP locus on the *X* chromosome). *PEX* is normally expressed in several extrarenal tissues, especially in osteoblasts, but not in the kidney. The gene product PEX is a membrane-anchored endopeptidase, which normally *inactivates* the putative hormone *phosphatonin*. Phosphatonin inhibits sodium-dependent phosphate transport and 1α-OHase in the proximal tubule.

Phosphatonin-like bioactivity is produced by osteoblasts, hepatocytes and tumors that cause oncogenic osteomalacia. These tumors have been described as "strange tumors in strange places." Most of these are obscure, slow-growing benign tumors of mesenchymal origin. The suggested mechanism of oncogenic osteomalacia is such an oversupply of phosphatonin that exceeds the degrading-capacity of PEX.

9

THE ENDOCRINE PANCREAS

OBJECTIVES

1. Discuss the cell types of the pancreas, their arrangement in the gland and within the *islets of Langerhans*. Identify the hormones produced by these cells. Be familiar with the blood supply (especially the venous drainage) of the pancreas and the perfusion of the pancreatic islets. Discuss the involvement of IDX-1/IPF-1 in the embryonic development of the pancreas, in the neogenesis of islet cells, and in the regulation of hormone production.

2. Discuss the definition of *diabetes mellitus* and the etiologic background of its various types. Define the terms *euglycemia, hypoglycemia, hyperglycemia, impaired glucose tolerance, insulin sensitivity,* and *insulin resistance.* Identify hypoglycemic and hyperglycemic hormones, and discuss in which ways these hormones function as functional antagonists or agonists.

3. Discuss the main determinants of plasma glucose concentration and glucose fluxes. Define the terms *glucose disposal* and *hepatic glucose output* (HGO), and discuss their constituents. Discuss the various types of *glucose transporters,* their physiologic roles and regulation.

4. Discuss *glucagon* and the *glucagon-related peptides.* Identify the sources of these hormones, their receptors, physiologic function and circulating half-life. Discuss the molecular and biochemical mechanisms involved in the actions of glucagon. Identify steps antagonized by insulin. Discuss the regulation of glucagon secretion and the concept of *insulin:glucagon ratio.*

5. Discuss the biosynthesis, molecular structure and secretion of *insulin, proinsulin,* and the *C-peptide.* Discuss insulin in the circulation: sites of degradation, half-life, and penetration of endothelial barriers in target tissues. Identify the main biologic actions of insulin. Discuss the insulin receptor, the postreceptor mechanisms of insulin signaling, and the molecular mechanisms of insulin action.

6. Discuss the molecular mechanism of glucose-induced insulin secretion. Identify stimulators, amplifiers, and inhibitors of insulin secretion. Describe the involvement of *glucose transporter 2* (GLUT2), *glucokinase,* mitochondrial function, the *sulfonylurea receptor,* and the *adenosine triphosphate (ATP)-sensitive potassium channel.* Identify mutations causing various dysfunctions of the pathway, including the types of *maturity-onset diabetes of the young* (MODY).

7. Discuss the regulation of insulin secretion at the whole-body level. Describe the two phases of insulin response to a sustained glucose stimulus, the *ultradian rhythm* of insulin secretion, and the concept of *entrainment*. Discuss the *single gateway hypothesis*. Describe the relationship between insulin secretion and insulin sensitivity in health and disease. Identify determinants of glucose sensitivity/resistance. Discuss *leptin*, the *peroxisome proliferator activated receptors*, *syndrome X, fatty acyl translocase*, tumor necrosis factor α (TNFα), and the central role of free fatty acids in the development of type II diabetes.

8. Identify the complications of diabetes and discuss their pathogenesis. Discuss the development of *diabetic ketoacidotic coma* and the derangements of electrolyte homeostasis. Explain the *honeymoon period* of insulin-dependent diabetes mellitus. Explain the *Somogyi effect*, and contrast its mechanism with those of the *dawn phenomenon* and *waning of circulating insulin levels*. Discuss *nonenzymatic glycosylation* of proteins, its deleterious consequences and its laboratory evaluation as a measure of glycemic control. Describe the *polyol pathway*, its activation in hyperglycemia, and identify the resulting pathologies. Describe the basic features of lipoprotein metabolism, its derangement in diabetes, and the development of *macroangiopathy*.

9. Describe the other normal and abnormal (tumor-derived) hormones of the pancreas, their physiologic roles, and the manifestations of their endocrine tumors.

THE STRUCTURE AND DEVELOPMENT OF THE ENDOCRINE PANCREAS

The pancreas functions both as an exocrine and an endocrine gland. The *exocrine pancreas* is a compound tubuloalveolar salivary gland, which is histologically similar to the parotid gland and consists of serous secretory acini and a duct system. It produces digestive enzymes (mainly amylase, trypsin, and lipase) and a bicarbonate-rich fluid, which are delivered into the lumen of the duodenum. The *endocrine pancreas* consists of the *pancreatic islets (islets of Langerhans)* and serves as a major regulator of glucose, lipid, and protein homeostasis. All major pancreatic hormones are polypeptides. The pancreatic islets contain a heterogenous population of cells, which are unevenly distributed in the pancreas (Table 9-1).

The various cell types are not randomly located within the islets: typically the *β cells* occupy the central portion of the islet, whereas *α- and δ cells* are mainly found at the periphery of the islets and form a mantle (Fig. 9-1). The islets are richly vascularized by fenestrated capillaries, and their perfusion rate is severalfold higher than that of the surrounding exocrine pancreas. The direction of perfusion within the islets is preferentially *central to peripheral.* This aids inhibition of *glucagon* secretion by locally high concentrations of *insulin* and *gamma aminobutyric acid* (GABA) acting in part by a paracrine mechanism before they would enter (and become diluted in) the systemic circulation. The lack of this β cell-mediated inhibition explains the high circulating levels of glucagon in type I diabetes. GABA

Table 9-1   Cell Types of the Human Pancreas

| Cell type | Relative contribution to islet cell volume (%) | | Secretory products |
	Anterior head, body, tail (derivatives of the dorsal bud)	Posterior head (derivative of the ventral bud)	
α (A) cell	10	<0.5	Glucagon, proglucagon, GLP-1 and GLP-2
β (B) cell	70–80	15–20	Insulin, proinsulin, C-peptide, amylin, GABA, PTHrP
δ (D) cell	3–5	<1	Somatostatin (SRIF, mainly SRIF-14)
F (PP) cell	<2	80–85	Pancreatic polypeptide

ABBREVIATIONS: GLP, glucagon-like peptide; GABA, gamma aminobutyric acid; PTHrP, parathyroid hormone related protein; SRIF, somatostatin.

is synthesized by two isoforms of *glutamic acid decarboxylase* (GAD), which are designated by the molecular weight of the isoenzymes in kilodaltons as GAD65 and GAD67. It appears that GAD65 is a main target of the autoimmune reaction that destroys pancreatic β cells in type I diabetes (see Box 9-1).

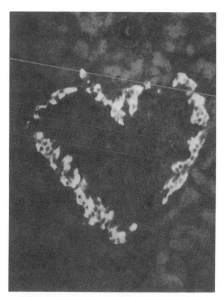

Figure 9-1. Immunofluorescent staining for glucagon in the pancreatic islet. The glucagon-producing α cells are located at the peripheral rim of the islet. The islet is surrounded by nonstaining cells of the exocrine pancreas. The central nonstaining area mainly consists of insulin-producing β cells. Due to the preferentially central to peripheral perfusion of the islet, the glucose-induced secretory products of β cells effectively inhibit glucagon secretion. This accidentally heart-shaped islet appeared in a St. Valentine's day issue of the New England Journal of Medicine. (Source: Bosco D, Meda P: Cellular aggregation in the pancreas. Images in Clinical Medicine, NEJM 138:435, 1998.)

BOX 9-1   Diabetes Mellitus

Type I (insulin-dependent) diabetes mellitus (IDDM) is due to the T-cell mediated progressive autoimmune destruction of the pancreatic β cell population. Most of the α, δ, and F cells are spared. IDDM becomes symptomatic when over 70% of the β cells are destroyed. The disease usually presents at a young age. IDDM is a consequence of absolute insulin deficiency. Untreated patients typically have little body fat (Fig. 9-2). IDDM is associated with certain *histocompatibility locus* or *human leukocyte antigen* (HLA) *haplotypes,* mainly DR3 and DR4; its development requires environmental factors. It might be triggered by an infection with the common Coxsackie B enteroviruses (especially B4), which have a protein motif displaying homology with GAD65. Although the autoimmune reaction targeting GAD65 is mainly a T lymphocyte-mediated response, B lymphocytes may produce GAD65-specific antibodies, which are detectable in more than 95% of IDDM patients. Other early antigens targeted in IDDM are *insulin* and islet cell antigen 512 (ICA512, a tyrosine phosphatase-like protein). The autoimmune reaction against these antigens develops sequentially, with GAD65 being most often the first target. Although the antibodies are not causative agents, their demonstration in plasma is useful in the diagnosis of the disease process even before the development of extensive β cell destruction. IDDM can be transferred by bone marrow transplantation from IDDM donors into previously non-diabetic recipients, indicating that the primary derangement is in the immune system. IDDM is associated with celiac and Addsion's disease in 5 and 0.5% of IDDM patients, respectively. IDDM may be the manifestation of type II multiple endocrine glandular failure (Schmidt's syndrome), which may also involve Addison's disease, hypothyroidism, pernicious anemia, and vitiligo.

   Most diabetics (80 to 90%) have *Type II (non insulin-dependent) diabetes mellitus* (NIDDM). It is a heterogenous group of diseases. NIDDM usually presents first in middle-aged individuals; it is a relative (rather than absolute) deficiency of insulin, which involves both β cell dysfunction and *insulin resistance.* Eighty-five percent of NIDDM patients are obese; obesity plays a significant role in the decompensation of metabolic regulation. Most patients are hyperinsulinemic; their hyperinsulinemia does not meet their tissue demand for insulin-dependent glucose uptake because of insulin resistance. Insulin resistance is primarily due to an impaired postreceptor signaling mechanism of the insulin receptor. NIDDM has strong but, except for MODY (see the section on the regulation of insulin secretion), unidentified multigenic cause. NIDDM is not associated with HLA haplotype and noxious environmental factors. According to the *thrifty genotype hypothesis,* the insulin resistance genes have protected individuals during long periods of starvation by an enhanced ability of storing energy as fat. Western diet (processed

BOX 9-1 (*Continued*)

food, high caloric intake that includes a simultaneous consumption of carbohydrates and disproportionately large amounts of fat) has made these ancestral protective genes deleterious, suggesting that these individuals are not equipped with the metabolic machinery to handle overeating.

Secondary diabetes is caused by various factors, including overproduction of insulin-antagonist hormones (such as growth hormone, cortisol, adrenaline, thyroxine, or glucagon) and mutations of the insulin receptor.

Gestational diabetes mellitus (GDM; see details in Chap. 13) is in part due to overproduction of certain insulin-antagonist hormones and thus similar to secondary diabetes. However, 98% of pregnant women remain euglycemic in spite of the same increase in their insulin-antagonist hormones. GDM indicates that the patient is unable to maintain glucose homeostasis under these conditions; thus, a possible underlying defect is brought to the surface by pregnancy. Indeed, approximately 60% of patients diagnosed with GDM will develop type II diabetes within 15 years.

Anatomically the pancreas is a large retroperitoneal gland, which consists of a head, a body, and a tail. The pancreatic head fits into the horseshoe formed by the duodenum; the tail is found at the hilus of the spleen. The arterial blood supply of the pancreas is provided mainly by branches of the *splenic artery* (a direct branch of the *celiac trunk,* running along the length of the pancreas to the splenic hilus), and of the *superior and inferior pancreaticoduodenal arteries* (branches of the *gastroduodenal* and *superior mesenteric arteries,* respectively). *The venous blood of the pancreas carrying all pancreatic hormones is drained into the hepatic portal vein.* This arrangement is important because the liver is a target of pancreatic hormones (in case of glucagon it is the main target), and the liver is exposed to the high hormone concentrations of portal blood before the hormones can be diluted by joining the systemic circulation. It is also important that a first passage through the liver eliminates a significant portion of these hormones from blood. The pancreas is innervated by sympathetic (from the *celiac ganglion*) and parasympathetic *(vagal)* nerve fibers, which contribute to the regulation of islet cell function (see Chap. 12 and The Regulation of Insulin Secretion in this chapter).

The parenchyma of the pancreas develops from the *dorsal and ventral buds* of the foregut endoderm. *The ventral bud* (which develops next to the *hepatobiliary bud*), due to the rotation of the duodenum to the right, becomes posteriorly positioned and *develops as the posterior portion of the pancreatic head*. Most islet cells in this portion of the pancreas are *F cells,* producing *pancreatic polypeptide*. All the rest of the pancreatic parenchyma develops from the *dorsal bud*; insulin-producing β cells predominate in

BOX 9-2   The APUD Concept

Several hormone-producing cells scattered throughout the body (especially the visceral canals) belong to the *diffuse endocrine system* and display similar ultrastructural and biochemical properties. They contain round secretory granules with an inner core of variable electron density, active in uptaking biogenic amine precursors, such as dihydroxyphenylalanine (DOPA) and 5-hydroxytryptophan (5-HTP), and synthesize peptide hormones. In 1966, Pearse coined the term *APUD cells* referring to the cells' ability of *amine precursor uptake and decarboxylation.* The APUD cells include all peptide hormone-producing cells of the gastrointestinal tract and the pancreatic islets, the adrenal medulla and the paraganglia, the adenohypophysis, the parafollicular cells of the thyroid gland, the Kulchitsky's cells of the bronchial tree, endocrine cells in the urogenital system, the dark cells in eccrine sweat glands, and the melanocytes. Although their biochemical character is different, the parathyroid chief cells are often classified as APUD cells in part because they may be involved in multiple endocrine neoplasia (MEN) syndromes (see Boxes 10-3 and 12-2). None of the steroid hormone-producing cells belong to the APUD system. Although the APUD concept originally postulated that all of its constituent cells are derived from the neural crest or the neuroectoderm, overwhelming evidence indicates that the APUD cells of the gastrointestional tract and the pancreatic islets originate from the endoderm. Thus, the acquisition of the biochemical features of APUD cells (referred to as *neuroendocrine programming*) occurs during differentiation of endodermal as well as neural crest-derived cells.

Tumors of APUD cells are often called *APUDomas.* APUDomas may be benign, such as most *carcinoid tumors* of the gut and the lung, pituitary, pancreatic islet, and parathyroid adenomas (MEN type I) and most *pheochromocytomas* of the adrenal medulla and paraganglia. Certain types of *thymomas* (tumors of the epithelial cells of the thymus) are also classified as APUDomas. APUDomas may be malignant, such as *medullary thyroid carcinoma* (MTC), *neuroblastoma, oat cell (small cell) bronchial cancer,* and the less frequently encountered malignant forms of carcinoid, pituitary, parathyroid, and other APUD cell tumors. These hormone-secreting APUDomas may produce more than one hormone and manifest as a *paraneoplastic syndrome.* APUDomas may appear as "ectopic" sources of hormones; although the normal APUD cells might secrete minute quantities of the hormone responsible for the paraneoplastic syndrome, the normal APUD cells (unlike the cell of the APUDoma) are not the determinant sources of the hormone in the circulation. Unlike the eutopic sources of hormones, APUDomas are usually not subject to negative feedback regulation. Most APUDomas express high levels of *somatostatin receptors* that can be exploited for diagnostic and often for therapeutic purposes.

these islets. The development of the pancreas and the hormone production of islet cells are under the influence of IDX-1 (also known as *insulin promoter factor-1* [IPF-1]), a master regulator homeodomain protein of about 280 amino acids encoded by chromosome 13q12.1. The absence of IDX-1 results in *pancreatic agenesis*. IDX-1 is expressed in the developing pancreatic ductal epithelium, which serves as a precursor for the endocrine stem cells of the islets. The pancreatic islet cells belong to the *amine precursor uptake and decarboxylation (APUD) system* (see Box 9-2). Unlike most APUD cells, which are derived from the neural crest, islet cells are of endodermal origin. Nevertheless, pancreatic islet cells display neuron-like characteristics (e.g., they are electrically excitable, may develop neurite-like processes in vitro, and express several antigens normally found in neurons).

The expression of IDX-1 is stimulated by glucose (moderate, *acute* hyperglycemia), transforming growth factor β (TGFβ) and activin, and inhibited by glucose (extreme, *sustained* hyperglycemia) and basic fibroblast growth factor (bFGF). Pancreatic islet development is promoted by parathyroid hormone-related protein (PTHrP) and, via inducing the expression of preadipocyte factor-1 (Pref-1, see Chap. 15), by the hormones of the lactogenic family, mainly placental lactogen, however, their relationship with IDX-1 is currently unknown. In adults, IDX-1 is mainly expressed in pancreatic β cells (the source of insulin), and to a lesser extent in subpopulations of ductal epithelium and α- and δ-islet cells. IDX-1 regulates the expression of insulin, glucokinase, and GLUT2, all of which are essential in the maintenance of euglycemia (normal levels of blood glucose, see below).

The cells of the pancreatic islet have a limited lifespan (about 30 days in rats); thus, in adults the islet cells are continuously replenished in part by a limited proliferative capacity of islets cells and in part from precursor cells located in the ductal epithelium. This *islet cell neogenesis* is mediated by IDX-1. Sustained hyperglycemia downregulates IDX-1 leading to a reduced neogenesis, accelerated apoptosis of β cells, and a reduced β cell mass. In addition, insulin expression in existing β cells becomes suppressed. The dysregulation of β cell function in response to sustained hyperglycemia is known as *glucose toxicity*.

INTRODUCTION TO THE REGULATION OF CARBOHYDRATE METABOLISM

The endocrine regulation of glucose, lipid, and protein homeostasis is extremely complex. Although insulin plays a pivotal role in all of them, several other pancreatic and non-pancreatic hormones such as glucagon, glucocorticoids, adrenaline, noradrenaline, growth hormone, insulin-like growth factors (IGFs), and TNF-α are involved in the process. Moreover, the metabolites regulated by these hormones (especially glucose and free fatty acids [FFA]) also serve as important signals in the regulation of metabolism. We shall first introduce the basic metabolic parameters and pathways regulated by insulin and its functional antagonists.

Fasting Glucose Levels and Oral Glucose Tolerance Tests Are Routine Tools in the Assessment of Glucose Homeostasis

For an initial evaluation of a patient's metabolic profile, venous blood sample is taken *after an overnight fast*. Under these conditions, the serum levels of glucose in an adult individual normally range between 74 and 106 mg/dL (4.1–5.9 mM), which is referred to as *euglycemia*. Glucose levels above and below this range are called *hyperglycemia* and *hypoglycemia*, respectively. Note that these values are given for venous blood; because tissues take up glucose from arterial blood, venous blood plasma glucose levels are about 20 mg/dL lower than the levels in arterial blood plasma.

A *fasting serum glucose* level of 126 mg/dL (7.0 mM) or above is diagnostic for *diabetes mellitus* (see Box 9-1), a disease affecting up to 3 to 5% of the population in developed countries. The term refers to sweet [-tasting] "passing through" (i.e., urine) as opposed to *diabetes insipidus* (diuresis without a taste; see Chap. 10); these terms are reminders of the ancient "laboratory test": physicians used to taste their patients' urine. Diabetes mellitus is a prevalent metabolic disorder, which is due to either absolute or relative insulin deficiency and/or insulin resistance. Although its cardinal symptom is hyperglycemia, it affects not only carbohydrate but also lipid and protein homeostasis. The fasting serum glucose of 126 mg/dL is an arbitrary cutoff limit, which is based on epidemiologic studies: fasting serum glucose levels reaching this limit in the long run are associated with diabetic complications, such as coronary heart disease, diabetic nephropathy, angiopathy, and neuropathy (see Diabetic Complications in this chapter).

Hyperglycemia in itself does not necessarily indicate abnormal glucose homeostasis: upon ingestion of a meal or during stress the patient may normally display transient hyperglycemia. The quantitative analysis of the plasma glucose profile upon a glucose load is utilized in clinical medicine as the *oral glucose tolerance test* (OGTT) and the less often used intravenous glucose tolerance test (IVGTT).

OGTT imitates *postprandial* (after meal) *hyperglycemia* under standardized conditions. OGTT is a routine procedure used for the early diagnosis of diabetes mellitus and especially *gestational diabetes mellitus* (see Chap. 13). After an overnight fast, the patient consumes glucose orally (75 g for nonpregnant adults; 50 or 100 g for pregnant women). Blood samples are withdrawn at specific timepoints before and after the oral glucose load (Fig. 9-3). If the hyperglycemia exceeds the normal range *and* the defined

A   **B**

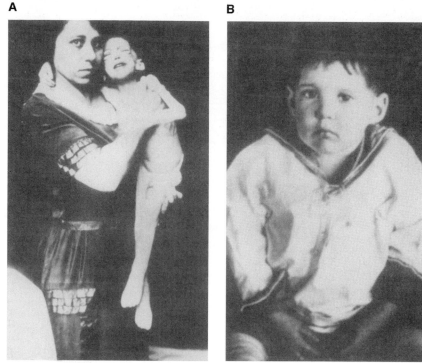

Figure 9-2. A piece of medical history. A. On the brink of death: type I diabetes results in muscle wasting and severe depletion of fat stores. B. The child seen in Fig. 9-2A was among the first patients saved by insulin therapy shortly after its discovery in the 1920s. (Source: Eli Lilly and Co.)

diagnostic thresholds, either *impaired glucose tolerance* (IGT) or diabetes mellitus can be diagnosed. IGT is diagnosed if the fasting plasma glucose is <126 mg/dL, and 2 h after the oral load plasma glucose is ≥140 mg/dL (7.8 mM) but <200 mg/dL (11.1 mM). A 2-h postload plasma glucose of ≥200 mg/dL may indicate diabetes mellitus. The diagnosis requires confirmation on a subsequent day. The OGTT is a more accurate assessment of glucose homeostasis than the measurement of fasting glucose because it provokes an adaptational response, which reflects both *insulin secretion* and *insulin sensitivity*. By the same token, OGTT is more liable to yield a false positive diagnosis of diabetes mellitus than fasting glucose alone.

Consumption of refined sugar yields higher postprandial glucose levels than the consumption of the same amount of complex carbohydrates. The difference stems from the gradual release of glucose from the complex carbohydrate during intestinal digestion. In the treatment of non-insulin-dependent diabetes mellitus (NIDDM), this gives the rationale for the use of the intestinal striated border *alpha-glucosidase inhibitors* such as *acarbose*. The attenuated postprandial hyperglycemia decreases the demand for insulin.

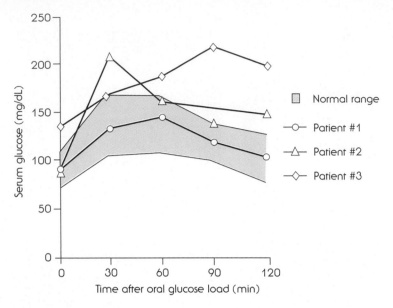

Figure 9-3. Oral glucose tolerance test (OGTT). After consuming 75 g of glucose, plasma glucose should remain within the range shown as a shaded area. Plasma glucose in patient #1 follows the predicted normal course. Plasma glucose of patient #2 was within the normal range before the oral glucose load. Upon glucose ingestion his plasma levels exceeded the normal range; nevertheless an antihyperglycemic response was evident (impaired glucose tolerance). Patient #3 had frank diabetes mellitus: his fasting plasma glucose was above 126 mg/dL, and his antihyperglycemic response was practically ineffective.

Insulin, the Only Important Hypoglycemic Hormone, Antagonizes Several Hyperglycemic Hormones

The hormones involved in the regulation of plasma glucose can be grouped as *hyperglycemic* (the ones increasing plasma glucose) and *hypoglycemic* (the ones lowering plasma glucose) agents. From a physiologic standpoint, insulin is the only important hypoglycemic agent (see Box 9-3), and practically all other hormones affecting plasma glucose are hyperglycemic; therefore *in that regard* they are antagonists of insulin. Because of the redundancy of hyperglycemic agents, their deficiencies may sometimes be masked by compensatory increases in the production of (or responsiveness to) others. For example, glucagon deficiency rarely manifests as a disease. In contrast, lack of insulin will manifest as diabetes mellitus.

To understand the metabolic regulation by insulin, the three main target organs of insulin must be taken into consideration. *The main target organs of insulin are the liver, adipose tissue, and muscle tissue.* Because the liver plays a central role in glucose homeostasis, muscle and adipose tissues are often referred to as peripheral sites of action for insulin as well as the hyperglycemic hormones.

BOX 9-3 Hypoglycemic Hormones

Serum contains insulin-like activity that can be detected by bioassay but not by radioimmunoassay (RIA). Immunoneutralization of insulin by adding excess antibodies to serum revealed that part of the insulin-like bioactivity remained unaffected. This bioactivity is termed *nonsuppressible insulin-like activity* (NSILA). NSILA was later chemically identified as *insulin-like growth factors* (IGFs): *IGF-1* (also known as *somatomedin C*) and *IGF-2 (somatomedin A)*. The IGFs are important regulators of growth and protein metabolism (see Chap. 10), but their insulin-like hypoglycemic action is insufficient to compensate for insulin-deficiency. Overproduction of IGF-2 by certain tumors, however, may result in *non-islet-cell tumor-induced hypoglycemia* (NICTH).

Growth hormone (GH) is mainly an insulin antagonist in terms of its effects on glucose and lipid homeostasis. However, when a GH-deficient patient is started on GH substitution therapy, GH has a transient hypoglycemic effect known as the *early insulin-like action of GH*.

The relationship between insulin and the hyperglycemic hormones is complex:

- the antagonism in terms of carbohydrate metabolism involves all three main target tissues;
- the antagonism is also observed in terms of lipid metabolism;
- in terms of protein/amino acid metabolism, insulin antagonizes the action of most hyperglycemic hormones, but synergizes with growth hormone.

Euglycemia Is a Result of the Balance between Glucose Disposal (Uptake and Utilization by Tissues) and Glucose Input [to Plasma]

Before we discuss insulin and its actions in detail, we need to understand the various mechanisms of glucose disposal (from blood) and how insulin fits into an overall scheme of glucose homeostasis. Figure 9-4 provides a purposefully simplified diagram of the regulation of plasma glucose. The diagram neglects tissue sensitivity to insulin and the precise mechanisms of action of hyperglycemic hormones and insulin. The maintenance of euglycemia can be compared to a bathtub in which the level of water is determined by the influx of water from two taps and the efflux of water via two sinks and an overflow safety valve. The efflux through one of the sinks can be regulated with a tap, whereas the other sink is always open and the efflux through it is relatively stable. Obviously, water levels can increase by two main mechanisms or their combination:

A

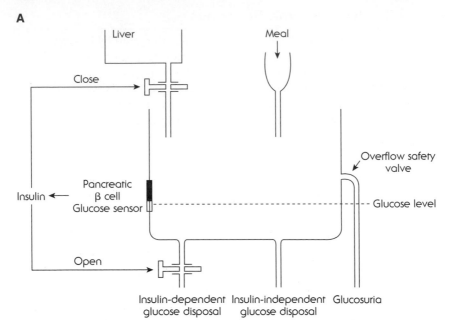

Figure 9-4. The overall scheme of glucose homeostasis. A. Mechanistic model of glucose homeostasis. The fluid level in the tank represents plasma glucose concentration. The insulin secretion of β cells is activated when the fluid level stimulates the glucose sensor (glucoki-nase). Insulin closes the "liver tap" and opens a "glucose-disposal sink." These mechanisms normalize the fluid level in the tank. When the fluid levels reach very high (i.e., insufficient insulin), the overflow safety valve attempts to ameliorate further increase (glucosuria). B. The same regulation shown as a flowchart of the process makes it clear that the arrangement is built on negative feedback. This diagram of plasma glucose regulation is an expanded version of Fig. 2-4B. The solid arrows indicate stimulation/increase, the dashed arrows indicate inhibition/decrease. GLUT, glucose transporter.

- the influx of water is increased, and the efflux is unaltered;
- the influx of water is unaltered, and the efflux is reduced.

Similarly, hyperglycemia may result from increased glucose input to blood and/or from reduced glucose disposal.

There are two major sources of *glucose input:*

- *dietary carbohydrates,* which serve as the postprandial glucose source for about 2 h after a meal, and
- *hepatic glucose output* (HGO), which serves as the glucose source during fasting *(postabsorptive state).* Hepatic glucose output initially relies on *glycogenolysis* (the breakdown of glycogen), but prolonged hepatic glucose output requires *gluconeogenesis* (usually from glucogenic amino acids, such as alanine).

A major purpose of the *postprandial* regulatory processes is *to replenish* the carbohydrate resources of the liver and muscle. The regulatory processes

B

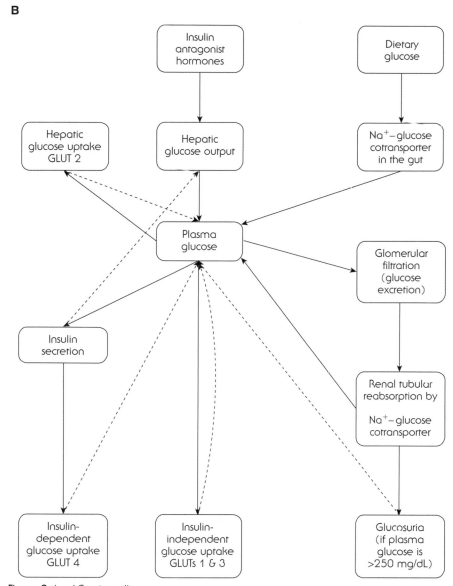

Figure 9-4. (*Continued*)

during *fasting mobilize* these resources; however, only the liver and to a minimal degree the kidney are involved in maintaining euglycemia. Thus, the regulatory processes of the *well-fed* and the *fasting state* are different. Diabetes mellitus may be viewed as a fasting state in face of hyperglycemia ("starvation amidst of plenty").

Glucose disposal is achieved by the following mechanisms:

• *insulin-dependent glucose disposal* involving GLUT4-mediated cellular uptake of glucose and its utilization (see the section on GLUTs), which serves as the regulated sink in the analogy;
• *insulin-independent glucose disposal* involving mainly GLUT1- and GLUT3-mediated cellular uptake of glucose and its utilization, and also GLUT2-mediated uptake mainly by the liver during postprandial hyperglycemia;
• *glucosuria* (urinary loss of glucose) if the renal threshold of glucose reabsorption is exceeded by the glucose filtered through the renal glomeruli. Glucosuria is not a physiologic regulator of plasma glucose, but becomes important in diabetic patients (overflow safety valve function). Glucosuria causes osmotic diuresis (*polyuria*) and *secondary polydipsia* (see also Chap. 10).

It is important to note up front that the hypoglycemic effect of insulin involves two major mechanisms:

• Insulin inhibits hepatic glucose output during postprandial hyperglycemia. This is in part a direct hepatic action of insulin. However, an indirect mechanism predominates: insulin inhibits lipolysis in adipose tissue, and the decrease in circulating FFAs inhibits hepatic glucose output (see at the single gateway hypothesis, later in this chapter).
• Insulin increases glucose uptake mainly in muscle and adipose tissue. The mobilization of GLUT4 in muscle tissue becomes more responsive to insulin when plasma FFA is decreased via the antilipolytic action of insulin on adipose tissue.

The Mechanisms of Cellular Glucose Uptake Include Facilitated Diffusion by GLUTs and Secondary Active Transport by the Sodium-Glucose Cotransporters

Glucose is a hydrophilic (relatively large, uncharged polar) molecule, and as such cannot penetrate the cell membrane. Cellular uptake of glucose is achieved either by *secondary active transport* (Na^+-glucose cotransporters) or by *facilitated diffusion* utilizing different glucose transporter proteins (GLUTs; see Table 9-2). All GLUTs belong to the 12-transmembrane segment transporter superfamily.

For the purpose of delivering glucose to the intracellular compartment, the facilitated diffusion carried out by any GLUT is sufficient because upon entering the cell, glucose is phosphorylated either by high-affinity *hexokinase* (in most tissues) or by low-affinity *glucokinase* (in the liver, kidney and pancreatic β cell). The conversion of glucose into glucose-6-phosphate (glucose-6-P) lowers intracellular glucose levels, which maintains the concentration gradient between extracellular (plasma, interstitial fluid) and intracellular glucose. In addition, glucose-6-P is unable to leave the cell because it cannot bind to GLUTs and is even less able to penetrate the lipid bilayer of the membrane than glucose.

Table 9-2 Transport Proteins Involved in Cellular Glucose Uptake

Transporter	Major sites of expression	Affinity for glucose (or fructose)	Regulation
GLUT4	Muscle adipocytes	Medium (K_m = 2.5–5 mmol/L)	Mobilized by insulin and in muscle also by exercise (contraction pathway)
GLUT1	Endothelium in general, including brain capillaries, red blood cells, placenta, all tissues	High (K_m = 1 mmol/L)	Increased by growth factors and hypoglycemia; decreased by hyperglycemia
GLUT3	Brain neurons, all tissues	High (K_m < 1 mmol/L)	?
GLUT2; bidirectional transporter	Pancreatic β cell, liver, basolateral surface of the intestinal epithelium and proximal tubules of the kidney	Low (K_m = 15–20 mmol/L)	?
GLUT7; confined to endoplasmic reticulum	Liver, other gluconeogenic tissues (?)	Similar to GLUT2 (?)	None
GLUT5; mainly a fructose transporter	Spermatozoa, jejunum, liver	Medium (K_m = 6 mmol/L)	?
Na$^+$-glucose (2:1) cotransporter (SGLT1)	Apical surface of the intestinal epithelium and proximal tubules of the kidney	High	Thyroid hormone (T_3) stimulates; CCK-8 inhibits
Na$^+$-glucose (1:1) cotransporter (SGLT2)	Proximal tubules of the kidney	Low	?

ABBREVIATIONS: GLUT, glucose transporter; SGLT, sodium-glucose cotransporter; CCK, cholecystokinin.

Glucose Disposal Is in Part Insulin-Dependent and in Part Insulin-Independent

Insulin-dependent glucose uptake involves the mobilization of GLUT4. GLUT4 in the absence of insulin is located in intracellular vesicular membranes, and thus is inaccessible for glucose in the extracellular fluid (ECF). Insulin activates second messengers that result in translocation of GLUT4 to the surface of the cell (see the section on insulin action). Impaired mobilization of GLUT4 results in cellular starvation in adipose tissue and mainly in muscle, and is sufficient to cause hyperglycemia even under resting conditions. *Insulin-dependent glucose uptake accounts for approxi-*

mately 40% of the total glucose disposal; about 80% of this is performed by muscle tissue. Either upon postprandial hyperglycemia or stress-induced mobilization of hepatic carbohydrates, the relative importance of GLUT4 in glucose disposal becomes exaggerated.

Exercise aids the mobilization of GLUT4 directly acting on muscle by a mechanism distinct from the insulin signaling pathway. Hypoxia and N-(6-aminohexyl)-5-chloro-1-naphthalenesulfonamide (W-7) are stimulators of the *contraction pathway* of GLUT4 mobilization. Exercise also improves the efficacy of insulin-dependent GLUT4 mobilization. As a consequence, exercise improves the control of plasma glucose in diabetic patients, while a sedentary lifestyle worsens the control. A 30-min exercise improves GLUT4-mediated glucose-disposal as well as insulin-sensitivity for approximately 48 h.

Under resting (euglycemic, fasting) conditions, when insulin secretion proceeds at a basal rate, about 60% of the tissue glucose uptake is performed by the ubiquitous GLUT1 and GLUT3. It is important to remember that GLUT1 is expressed in muscle and adipose tissue, and it contributes to the low basal levels of glucose uptake (insulin-independent glucose disposal) by these tissues. GLUT1 mediates glucose transport through the placenta into the fetus. GLUT1 is present in red blood cells (RBCs), and in vivo the glucose concentrations in plasma and in the cytoplasm of RBCs are equal. RBCs lack mitochondria and thus rely on anaerobic glycolysis for ATP production. RBCs also require glucose for their active hexose monophosphate shunt. Their glucose uptake and utilization continues after a blood sample is taken; therefore, delayed separation of serum from RBCs may yield artifactually low levels of serum glucose.

GLUT1 and GLUT3 are crucial for glucose to permeate the blood-brain barrier (BBB) and for neuronal glucose uptake, respectively. The brain (except for certain cells in the ventral hypothalamus) does not require insulin for glucose uptake. The brain cannot utilize fatty acids as a fuel. Although after several days of fasting the brain will start utilizing *ketone bodies* (see Glucagon), it always utilizes glucose. Because the brain does not store glucose, it requires a continuous supply from plasma. Although the K_m values of GLUT1 and GLUT3 are low (i.e., their affinities are high), due to the structure of the blood-brain barrier, the apparent K_m of glucose transport is about 7 to 11 mmol/L. Compared to this, even the normal level of plasma glucose (4.1 to 5.9 mmol/L) is low. Hence, brain function is sensitive to hypoglycemia, and severe *acute* hypoglycemia may result in a life-threatening coma, such as during an overdose of insulin in a diabetic patient.

GLUT1 expression is highly regulated. In general, *GLUT1 is increased by most stimuli that induce cell proliferation (mainly growth factors),* which may reflect the energy requirement of the growth process. GLUT1 expression is decreased in skeletal muscle of NIDDM patients and is stimulated by activators of PPAR γ such as troglitazone and rosiglitazone. GLUT1 expression of the brain capillary endothelium is inversely related to the chronic glycemic state:

- GLUT1 is upregulated in chronic hypoglycemia, thereby decreasing the apparent K_m of glucose transport into the brain. This condition may lead to *hypoglycemia unawareness.*
- In contrast, chronic hyperglycemia downregulates GLUT1, thereby increasing the apparent K_m of glucose transport into the brain. In this condition, a decrease of plasma glucose to the euglycemic range may provoke hypoglycemic symptoms and activation of the sympathoadrenal adrenergic response.

The ventral hypothalamus is important in the regulation of appetite (see Chap. 15). In this region of the brain, insulin-dependent glucose uptake functions as a signal of glycemic status. In the absence of GLUT4 mobilization, these neurons "starve," which contributes to the sensation of hunger.

GLUT2 Is a Low-Affinity Bidirectional Glucose Transporter, which Is Crucial in Normal Glucose Homeostasis

The low affinity of GLUT2 ensures that glucose uptake by the pancreatic β cells is increased only during hyperglycemia; the increased uptake of glucose in the β cells is crucial in the signaling process that results in the release of insulin (see the Regulation of Insulin Secretion). Thus, the low affinity of GLUT2 prevents *inappropriate* insulin release.

The liver is an "altruistic" organ: it takes up glucose only during postprandial hyperglycemia and provides glucose to other tissues under fasting conditions. GLUT2 is essential for these functions of the liver. The low affinity of GLUT2 prevents hepatic uptake of glucose under fasting conditions, thereby sparing glucose for glucose-dependent tissues such as the brain.

During fasting, euglycemia is maintained by hepatic glucose output. For the intracellular glucose (i.e., glucose-6-P) to become able leaving the cell, it must be dephosphorylated by the enzyme *glucose-6-phosphatase.* This enzyme is present only in a few cell types (liver, kidney, intestinal epithelium); however, the liver is the only significant glucose donor for the circulation during fasting. During fasting, intracellular concentration of glucose generated by glucose-6-phospatase exceeds plasma levels, which provides the gradient necessary for transport. Thus, the transport facilitated by GLUT2 is bidirectional.

GLUT7 is a recently discovered and poorly characterized member of the GLUTs. It shows the highest homology with GLUT2. It was originally cloned from hepatocytes, but it is probably expressed in other gluconeogenic tissues as well. Its C-terminus contains a 6-amino-acid extension corresponding with the consensus motif for retention of membrane proteins in the endoplasmic reticulum. Its proposed function is transporting free glucose out of the endoplasmic reticulum after glucose was liberated from glucose-6-P by microsomal glucose-6-phosphatase.

GLUT5 Is Mainly a Fructose Transporter

Fructose is produced by the seminal vesicles and is the main fuel for spermatozoa, which take it up via GLUT5. The presence of GLUT5 in the jejunum explains why absorption of oral fructose (as opposed to glucose) does not require energy. A significant portion of dietary fructose is obtained from the intestinal digestion of sucrose.

There is no GLUT6 protein, but there is a *GLUT6* pseudogene. *Pseudogenes* are unexpressed portions of the genomic DNA that typically arise during evolution by the duplication of a functional gene followed by mutations. The mutations disable the expression of the gene. The surplus nonfunctional DNA is not necessarily eliminated from the genome.

The Transepithelial Transport of Glucose Involves the Sodium-Glucose Cotransporter (SGLT1) and GLUT2 in the Intestine, and SGLT1, SGLT2 and GLUT2 in the Kidney

The intestinal absorption of glucose is performed by the Na^+-glucose cotransporter (SGLT1) in concert with GLUT2 (Fig. 9-5). The renal reabsorption of glucose involves SGLT1, the high-capacity/low-affinity cotransporter SGLT2 and GLUT2.

Glucose transport across these epithelia occurs against a concentration gradient, and thus requires energy. The SGLT1 mechanism is a secondary active transport. Na^+ and glucose bind to the same carrier protein at a molar ratio of 2:1 and enter the cell together. The electrochemical gradient of Na^+ provides the driving force for glucose to enter the cell against a higher *cytoplasmic* glucose concentration. The energy is directly utilized for maintaining the electrochemical gradient of sodium: the Na^+ entering the cell by means of the cotransporter is pumped out by the Na^+/K^+-ATPase.

This mechanism delivers large quantities of glucose into the cytoplasmic compartment of the intestinal epithelium or the epithelium of the proximal renal tubules. Delivery of glucose from the epithelial cytoplasm into the interstitial fluid is achieved by facilitated diffusion mediated by GLUT2. Glucose follows the concentration gradient generated by the Na^+-glucose cotransporter: the cytoplasmic concentration of glucose exceeds its extracellular (plasma) concentration. Because GLUT2 is a low-affinity bidirectional transporter, it prevents uptake of glucose by these cells from the interstitial fluid under euglycemic and hypoglycemic conditions.

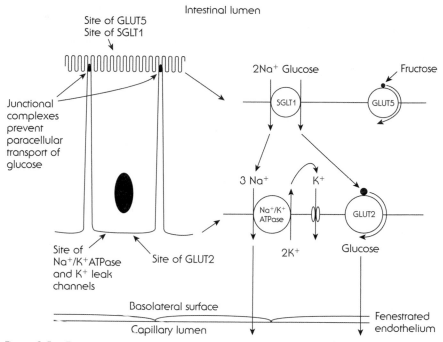

Figure 9-5. Transepithelial transport of glucose in the small intestine. The intestines are lined by a simple columnar epithelium. The epithelial cells are connected by junctional complexes, which include tight junctions that prevent paracellular transport of solutes. The absorptive enterocytes have apical microvilli (striated border) for increasing their surface. The proteins performing the transport are embedded in the apical and basolateral membranes. Glucose uptake via SGLT1 is driven by the electrochemical gradient of sodium. The sodium entering the cell is removed from the ICF by the 3Na⁺/2K⁺-ATPase. Thus, glucose absorption is a secondary active transport. The excess potassium entering the cell may leave via potassium leak channels. Glucose crosses the basolateral membrane by facilitated diffusion via GLUT2, and enters the circulation. Fructose absorption is a passive transport aided by GLUT5. Similar mechanisms function in the kidney to effect the reabsorption of filtered glucose.

The major reabsorptive mechanism for glucose in the kidney is *SGLT2*, which is located in the early proximal convoluted tubule (segment S1). In contrast to SGLT1, SGLT2 has a Na^+ to glucose coupling ratio of $1:1$ and does not transport D-galactose. The plant glucoside *phlorhizin* inhibits both intestinal absorption and renal reabsorption of glucose by competing for the glucose-binding site of SGLT1 and SGLT2.

Glucosuria Is a Type of Glucose Disposal by the Kidney

Glucose freely penetrates the renal glomerular filter. Under normal circumstances, the *glomerular filtration rate* (GFR) is approximately 125 mL/min (180 L/d). Calculating with a plasma glucose concentration of 80 mg/dL, the kidneys filter approximately 144 g glucose per day. Nearly all of this glucose is reabsorbed by the proximal tubules; the amount of glucose in urine collected over a 24-h period is normally less than 0.5 g (i.e., less than 0.35% of the filtered amount).

The renal tubular reabsorption mechanism becomes saturated if the glucose load exceeds the capacity of the Na^+-glucose cotransporters (*tubular transport maximum, T_m*). The T_m for glucose is approximately 375 mg/min in men and 300 mg/min in women. The *renal threshold* for glucose is different from the T_m, and it is defined as the plasma concentration above which urinary glucose increases. The renal threshold is lower than calculated from T_m and GFR; its normal range is between 160 and 240 mg/dL.

THE HORMONES OF THE ENDOCRINE PANCREAS

The two main pancreatic hormones acting via the systemic circulation are glucagon and insulin. First we shall discuss glucagon, which has a relatively simple mechanism of action and limited target tissues.

Glucagon

Proglucagon Is a Polyprotein that Gives Rise to the Insulin-Antagonist Glucagon, the Insulinotropic/Appetite Suppressant Glucagon-Like Peptide-1 (GLP-1), and the Intestinal Growth Factor GLP-2

The gene encoding *proglucagon* found on chromosome 2q36 is expressed in the pancreatic α cells, the intestinal *L cells* (an enteroendocrine/APUD cell), and in the brain. The cell type-specific posttranslational processing of proglucagon by proprotein convertases yields several biologically active peptides (Fig. 9-6).

Glucagon, the main product of the pancreatic α cells, is a member of the *secretin family* of polypeptide hormones, which also includes glucagon-like peptides (GLPs) -1 and -2, vasoactive intestinal polypeptide (VIP), peptide hystidyl-methionine-27 (PHM-27), pituitary adenylyl cyclase activating peptide (PACAP), gastric inhibitory peptide (GIP), and growth hormone-releasing hormone (GHRH). The receptors of these peptides all belong to the G-protein-linked heptahelical transmembrane receptor family. The *glucagon receptor* (encoded by chromosome 17q25) is coupled by $G\alpha_s$ and stimulates adenylyl cyclase. Glucagon circulates in plasma as a free hormone with a half-life of about 6 minutes. About 80% of glucagon is broken down by the liver during the first passage. Depending on the specificity of the antiserum, varying proportions of plasma glucagon-like immunoreactivity belong to *glicentin* and other intestinally produced peptides derived from proglucagon. The average fasting plasma level of glucagon is 75 pg/mL (normal range: 20 to 100 pg/mL). Glucagon is a major functional antagonist of insulin.

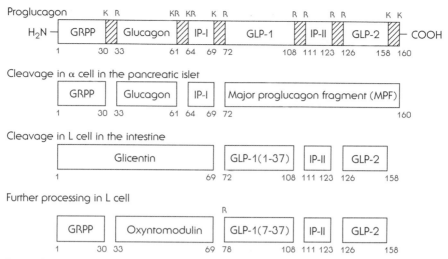

Figure 9-6. Tissue-specific posttranslational processing of proglucagon. The numerals of amino acid residues in the proglucagon sequence and the basic amino acids at the cleavage sites (lysine [K], arginine [R]) are displayed. In the pancreatic α cell, proglucagon is cleaved into glicentin-related pancreatic polypeptide (GRPP), glucagon, intervening peptide-I (IP-I), and major proglucagon fragment (MPF). In the intestinal L-cell, proglucagon is cleaved into glicentin, GLP-1(1-37), IP-II and GLP-2. Glicentin is further processed into GRPP and oxyntomodulin, but IP-I is not liberated. GLP-1(1-37) is truncated to yield GLP-1(7-37), the most important incretin.

Glucagon-like peptide-1[7-37] (GLP-1[7-37]) is the most potent insulinotropic hormone known and functions as the main *incretin* hormone. It is produced by the intestinal L cells in response to increased *luminal* glucose concentration. The incretin mechanism is the enhancement of the insulin response to glucose by intestinal hormones (mainly GLP-1[7-37] and GIP), and explains why the insulin response is higher to oral than to intravenous glucose. GLP-1[7-37] acts on its cognate receptor (encoded by chromosome 6p21.1). The physiologic involvement of GLP-1[7-37] in the attenuation of postprandial hyperglycemia has been verified with the GLP-1 receptor antagonist *exendin(9-39)*, a peptide fragment of *exendin-4* found in the venom of the lizard *Gila monster*. In addition to enhancing insulin secretion, GLP-1[7-37] stimulates proinsulin synthesis and is trophic for pancreatic β cells. The L cell-derived GLP-1[7-37] is a potent inhibitor of glucagon secretion from pancreatic α cells. GLP-1[7-37] slows gastric emptying, thereby decreasing the rate of glucose absorption after carbohydrate-rich meals. Its physiologic functions include mediation of the *ileal-brake effect*, the inhibition of upper gastrointestinal functions elicited by the presence of unabsorbed nutrients in the ileum. GLP-1[7-37] may completely normalize blood glucose levels in type II diabetic patients. In the brain, GLP-1 decreases food and fluid intake. Leptin-induced appetite suppression is in part mediated by GLP-1. GLP-1[7-37] is rapidly eliminated from the circulation by the ubiquitous *dipeptidyl peptidase IV*. Inhibitors of dipeptidyl peptidase IV alone and in conjunction with GLP-1[7-37] are being tested as a potential treatment of type II diabetes.

GLP-2 appears to promote proliferation of the intestinal epithelial lining as a locally acting hormone of the gut.

Glucagon Is a Catabolic Hormone, which Stimulates Lipolysis in Adipose Tissue, Glycogenolysis, Gluconeogenesis, VLDL, and Ketone Body Production in the Liver Glucagon has two direct target tissues: the liver and the adipocytes. Glucagon has no direct action on muscle. The actions of glucagon are listed in Table 9-3. In both target tissues its action is mediated by increased intracellular levels of cyclic adenosine monophosphate (cyclic AMP) and activation of protein kinase A (PKA). Glucagon secretion is high during fasting, starvation, and in (especially type I) diabetes mellitus. Its function is to mobilize energy. Thus, *glucagon-dependent phosphorylation activates catabolic and inhibits anabolic enzymes*. In addition, the gene expression of certain enzymes is regulated by glucagon via the PKA–CREB pathway. Again, the expression of catabolic enzymes is induced, while the expression of anabolic enzymes is suppressed.

Glucagon stimulates lipolysis in adipose tissue by PKA-mediated activation of *hormone-sensitive lipase* (Fig. 9-7). Note, however, that other hormones (such as noradrenaline, adrenaline, and GH aided by the permissive action of cortisol) are quantitatively more important regulators of lipolysis. The term "sensitive" usually refers to inhibition; the hormone-sensitive lipase was named as such because it is inhibited by the action of insulin. Hormone-sensitive lipase converts triglycerides (i.e., triacyl glycerols) into FFAs and diacyl glycerol. Diacyl glycerol is further processed by other lipases into FFA and glycerol.

- Glycerol cannot be utilized by the *adipose tissue* because it *lacks glycerol kinase*. Glycerol is delivered by the circulation to the liver, where (after being phosphorylated by hepatic glycerol kinase) it can be used either for gluconeogenesis, glycolysis, or re-esterification (triglyceride synthesis). Note that the glycerol phosphate for triglyceride synthesis in adipocytes is

Table 9-3   The Biologic Actions of Glucagon

Target	Action
Liver	Stimulates glycogenolysis and inhibits glycogen synthesis
	Stimulates gluconeogenesis and inhibits glycolysis
	Stimulates β oxidation of fatty acids, increases ketone body production
	Stimulates production of VLDL mainly indirectly by mobilizing free fatty acids from adipose tissue
	Inhibits cholesterol synthesis
Adipose tissue	Stimulates lipolysis by activating hormone sensitive lipase

ABBREVIATION: VLDL, very low density lipoprotein.

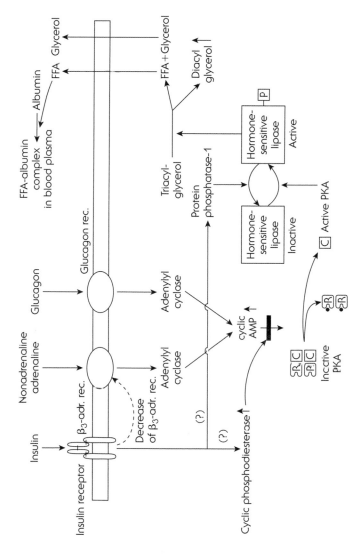

Figure 9-7. Activation of hormone-sensitive lipase in adipose tissue by glucagon and β_3-adrenergic receptor stimulation. When the cytosolic cyclic AMP concentration is low, protein kinase A activity is inhibited by regulatory subunits (R). Upon cyclic AMP-binding, the regulatory subunit detaches from the catalytic subunit (C), which becomes active. PKA activates hormone-sensitive lipase by phosphorylation of serine/threonine residues. Triacylglycerol (neutral lipid) molecules are cleaved into free fatty acid (FFA) and diacylglycerol. Diacylglycerol is further cleaved by other lipases present in the adipocyte. The FFA released from the cell is transported in plasma by albumin. Glycerol is transported in the aqueous phase of plasma. Insulin inhibits the lipolytic activity. Its mechanism may involve elimination of cyclic AMP by activating cyclic phosphodiesterases.

derived from glycolysis. Thus, storage of lipids depends on glucose uptake by the adipocytes.

  • FFAs move through the cell membrane and the capillary wall, and bind to albumin. Except for nervous tissues, the adrenal medulla (a modified nervous tissue) and RBCs, all tissues take up and use FFAs as a major energy source. The quantitatively most important targets of FFAs are skeletal muscle and the liver. In the liver, FFA not only serves as a fuel (which supports gluconeogenesis), but may become re-esterified with glycerol. The supply of FFA is the main determinant of the production rate of very low density lipoprotein (VLDL).

The liver is the quantitatively most important target of glucagon, where it regulates amino acid, carbohydrate, and lipid metabolism. Glucagon stimulates hepatic glucose output (Figs 9-8 and 9-9). This action involves the following targets:

  • Glucagon via the PKA–CREB pathway and cortisol via the glucocorticoid receptor increase gene expression of *glucose-6-phosphatase,* thereby converting glucose-6-phosphate into glucose, which can leave the hepatocyte by GLUT2. At the same time, glucagon suppresses the expression of glucokinase, thereby inhibiting the reverse pathway.
  • Glucagon stimulates *glycogenolysis* by PKA-mediated phosphorylation, which ultimately activates *glycogen phosphorylase.* PKA directly inactivates *glycogen synthase.*
  • Glucagon inhibits *glycolysis* and stimulates *gluconeogenesis.* Gluconeogenesis utilizes glycerol, lactate *(Cori cycle),* glucogenic amino acids (such as alanine; see Box 9-4) and pyruvate for ATP-dependent glucose synthesis. When amino acids are the main substrates of gluconeogensis, their processing usually starts with deamination; the amino group is processed in the hepatic *urea cycle,* and excreted in the urine. Gluconeogenesis cannot use acetyl-CoA as a substrate because *the action of the mitochondrial pyruvate dehydrogenase (PDH) complex,* which catalyzes the conversion of pyruvate into acetyl-CoA, *is irreversible.* However, acetyl-CoA derived from β-oxidation of FFA is an important fuel of gluconeogenesis. The main targets of glucagon in the gluconeogenic pathway include:
      • Glucagon and cortisol stimulate the expression of *cytoplasmic phosphoenolpyruvate carboxykinase* (PEPCK), the rate-limiting enzyme of gluconeogenesis. Glucagon also suppresses the expression as well as the activity of *pyruvate kinase,* a glycolytic enzyme that converts phosphenolpyruvate into pyruvate.
      • Glucagon regulates the activity of the *PFK-2/FBP-2 enzyme.* This enzyme has two catalytic centers: its *phosphofructokinase-2 (PFK-2) activity* generates fructose-2,6-bisphosphate (F-2,6-bisP) from fructose-6-phosphate. F-2,6-bisP is a strong activator of PFK-1, thereby enhancing glycolysis. The *fructose-bisphosphatase-2 (FBP-2) activity* of the enzyme catalyzes the opposite reaction, and enhances gluconeogenesis. By phosphorylating PFK-2/FBF-2, glucagon inactivates the PFK-2 and activates the FBP-2

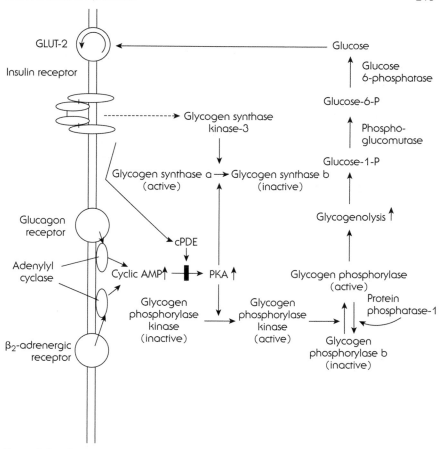

Figure 9-8. The regulation of glycogen metabolism by glucagon and adrenaline in the liver. By activating PKA, these hormones inhibit glycogen synthesis and stimulate glycogenolysis. The mobilized glucose-phosphate is ultimately dephosphorylated and delivered to the ECF by facilitated diffusion via GLUT2. Stimulation of the insulin receptor antagonizes these actions. In the human liver, insulin does not inhibit glycogen phosphorylase. The dashed arrow indicates inhibition.

activity, thereby inhibiting glycolysis and stimulating gluconeo-genesis.

Glucagon regulates the fate of fatty acids in the liver. As mentioned above, the increased supply of FFA from adipose tissue is a direct determinant of VLDL production. In addition, glucagon promotes *keto-genesis* (synthesis and secretion of *ketone bodies*) and inhibits the biosynthesis of cholesterol (Fig. 9-10). In these actions, *3-hydroxy-3-methyglu-taryl-CoA* (HMG-CoA) plays a central role. This metabolite is either converted into acteoacetate by *HMG-CoA lyase* (ketogenesis in mitochondria), or into mevalonate by *HMG-CoA reductase* (cholesterol synthesis in the cytosol).

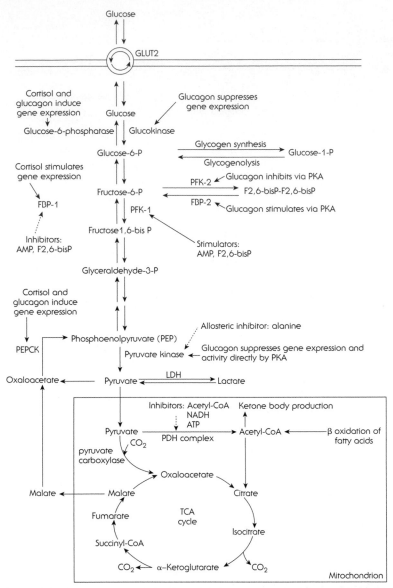

Figure 9-9. The regulation of glycolysis and gluconeogenesis in the liver. Cortisol (a glucocorticoid) by increasing enzyme mRNA levels, and glucagon also by inducing enzyme activity via PKA-mediated phosphorylation stimulate gluconeogenesis. Glucagon inhibits glycolysis both by decreasing enzyme mRNAs and enzyme activities. Adrenaline, by activating the same signal transduction pathways, shares the activities of glucagon (not shown). PFK, phosphofructokinase; FBP, fructose bisphosphatase; PEPCK, phosphoenolpyruvate carboxykinase; LDH, lactate dehydrogenase; PDH, pyruvate dehydrogenase; TCA, tricarboxylic acid.

BOX 9-4 The Cori Cycle and the Alanine Cycle

Both cycles involve the muscle as a source of substrate and the liver as the site of gluconeogenesis. In the *alanine cycle,* alanine is either derived from the glycolysis or mobilized by the degradation of muscle proteins mainly by the *ubiquitine-proteasome pathway* (see Chap. 12). The glycolytic pathway may produce alanine by the *transamination* of pyruvate. Alanine, the main glucogenic amino acid, is delivered for gluconeogenesis to the liver. The liver supplies the muscle with glucose via the circulation. In addition to being converted by a transaminase into alanine, pyruvate may have a different fate in muscle: it may be reduced to lactate by *lactate dehydrogenase.*

In the *Cori cycle,* mainly *type II skeletal muscle fibers* (see Chap. 11) degrade glucose by anaerobic glycolysis and generate lactate. Lactate is delivered to the liver, which converts it into glucose by gluconeogenesis. The liver then supplies the muscle with glucose.

- Due to the absence of *thiophorase* (succinyl-CoA:acetoacetate-CoA transferase), acetoacetate cannot be coupled with CoA in the liver. Therefore, unlike muscle and (after at least 2 days of fasting) the brain, the liver itself cannot use ketone bodies as fuel. Ketone bodies (*acetoacetate* and its reduced derivative, *3-hydroxybutyrate*) are delivered by the hepatocytes into the ECF, taken up and utilized by most cells *except RBCs, which do not have mitochondria.* Acetoacetate is also converted into *acetone* by nonenzymatic decarboxylation. Acetoacetate and 6-hydroxybutyrate may accumulate in blood during starvation and in (mainly) type I diabetic patients, and are responsible for *anion gap acidosis* (see Box 1-2). All ketone bodies appear in urine. Acetone is volatile; thus it is also exhaled. Acetony (also called fruity) breath is a typical symptom of starving and diabetic ketotic conditions.
- Glucagon causes PKA-mediated phosphorylation and inactivation of HMG-CoA reductase, the rate-limiting step of cholesterol biosynthesis. Insulin prevents the inactivation of HMG-CoA reductase probably by promoting the breakdown of cyclic AMP. In addition, insulin as well as thyroid hormones stimulate the gene expression of HMG-CoA reductase. Thus, in type I diabetes (absolute insulin deficiency and elevated levels of glucagon), one would expect decreased plasma levels of cholesterol. In actuality, plasma cholesterol is increased in type I diabetes mainly for two reasons:
  - Plasma clearance of VLDL is decreased. This is in part explained by a decreased lipoprotein lipase activity in the absence of insulin. Low density lipoprotein (LDL) clearance is also decreased due to the downregulation of LDL receptors. Thus, in spite of decreased HMG-CoA reductase activity, cholesterol accumulates in plasma.
  - In the absence of insulin, adipose tissue lipolysis (by hormone-sensitive lipase) is overtly active, and FFA stimulates VLDL production.

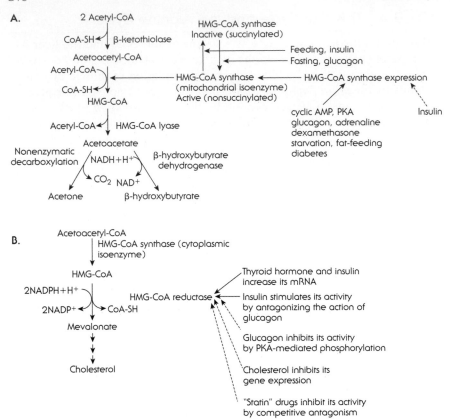

Figure 9-10. The regulation of ketone body production and cholesterol biosynthesis in the liver. A key metabolite in both pathways is HMG-CoA (3-hydroxy-3-methyglutaryl-CoA). Note that the HMG-CoA synthase involved in ketone body production is a mitochondrial enzyme, whereas the HMG-CoA synthase involved in cholesterol synthesis is cytoplasmic. The two enzymes are encoded by two separate genes. A. Mitochondrial HMG-CoA synthase is the main regulated step in ketone body production. Both its gene expression and its activity are stimulated by glucagon and fasting. B. The rate-limiting step of cholesterol synthesis is HMG-CoA reductase. Its expression and activity are regulated by multiple factors. Whereas insulin stimulates, glucagon inhibits cholesterol synthesis. "Statin" drugs include simvastetin, tovastatin, and related compounds.

Type II diabetes (NIDDM) is associated with even higher plasma cholesterol because the *relative* insulin-deficient state continues to stimulate
HMG-CoA reductase activity.

Glucagon Secretion Is Stimulated by Fasting, Stress, and Protein-Rich Meals, and Inhibited by Carbohydrate-Rich Meals and Free Fatty Acids

The main regulators of glucagon secretion are shown in Table 9-4. Most
regulators of glucagon secretion also regulate insulin secretion (see Table
9-7 for comparison) but in an opposite manner. This results in the modulation of the insulin:glucagon ratio. Because insulin and glucagon oppose
each other's actions, the insulin:glucagon ratio is an important determinant
of the net metabolic response.

A carbohydrate-rich meal suppresses glucagon secretion, mainly via indirect mechanisms: mobilization of GLP-1[7-37] from the intestinal L cells,
and insulin and GABA from the pancreatic β cells. The postprandial decrease
of glucagon decreases hepatic glucose output, and allows insulin-supported
storage of fuel in the liver (glycogen synthesis) and in adipose tissue (lipogenesis). Lipogenesis also occurs in the liver: meals rich in simple carbohydrates
promote hepatic triglyceride synthesis and the production of triglyceride-
rich VLDL. Triglycerides are mobilized from VLDL by lipoprotein lipase in
adipose (and muscle) tissue and delivered to the intracellular compartment.
Thus, *a high insulin:glucagon ratio results in an anabolic state.*

Although stimulation of β_2-adrenergic receptors increases the secretion
of both glucagon and insulin, sympathoadrenal activation increases only
glucagon secretion because in the β cells the inhibitory α_2-adrenergic receptors predominate. Thus, stress results in a low insulin:glucagon ratio, which
is responsible for hyperglycemia, ketogenesis, and increased plasma VLDL.

Glucagon as well as insulin secretion is stimulated by certain amino
acids, and the hyperaminoacidemia following protein-rich meals. If only
insulin were released upon a protein-rich meal, hypoglycemia would ensue;
the concomitant release of glucagon prevents hypoglycemia by increasing
hepatic glucose output.

Table 9-4   Regulators of Glucagon Secretion

Stimulators	Inhibitors
Decrease in plasma glucose (e.g., fasting, starvation)	Hyperglycemia mainly via β cell products: insulin, GABA
Increase in plasma amino acids (arginine, alanine but not leucine)	GLP-1[7-37]
Sympathoadrenal activation, increased sympathetic outflow via β_2-adrenergic re- ceptors	High levels of free fatty acids
Parasympathetic (vagal) activation (mus- carinic cholinergic)	

ABBREVIATION: GLP, glucagon-like peptide.

Insulin

The Synthesis and Degradation of Insulin

After Cleavage of Proinsulin by Proprotein Convertases and Carboxypeptidase H, Mature Insulin Is Stored in Secretory Granules as Osmotically Inactive Zinc-Insulin Crystals   The gene encoding insulin is located on chromosome 11p15. The signal peptide of *pre-proinsulin* is cleaved in the lumen of the endoplasmic reticulum and yields proinsulin. *Proinsulin* is homologous with IGFs 1 and 2 (Fig. 9-11). Proinsulin folds up and its N-terminus (which becomes the *B-chain* of 30 amino acids) lines up parallel with the C-terminus (the *A-chain,* 21 amino acids). This arrangement is stabilized by two disulfide bonds that become interchain bridges upon proteolytic cleavage of the middle piece known as the *connecting peptide* (C-peptide). The cleavage, which yields *insulin,* is performed at adjacent positively charged amino acids by three enzymes: *proprotein convertases* PC3/PC1 and PC2, which cut at the B/C and C/A chain junctions respectively, and *carboxypeptidase H,* which removes the two adjacent positively charged amino acids from the C termini of the B- and C-chains. This proteolytic process occurs mainly in the cisternae of the rough endoplasmic reticulum (ER) and in the Golgi apparatus. Thus, secretory granules contain insulin and small quantities of proinsulin. Insulin in the secretory granules is tightly associated with zinc, and forms crystals that are identical with those of commercially available crystalline zinc insulin. This renders insulin osmotically inactive and chemically stable in the granule. Upon stimulation of the β cell, insulin, equimolar quantities of the C-peptide, and up to 15% proinsulin are released into the interstitial fluid compartment by means of exocytosis.

In insulin-dependent diabetes mellitus (IDDM), the epitope specificity of about 93% of the insulin-specific T-cell clones is directed against amino acid residues 9-23 of the B-chain and the remainder against residues 7-21 of the A-chain. Low-dose insulin treatment, which serves as an antigen exposure, alters the course of the autoimmune reaction by decreasing the T-cell-mediated reaction and may prevent the development of IDDM. The same effect may be achieved either by subcutaneous or by intranasal administration of the B:9-23 peptide.

Insulin Is Rapidly Cleared from the Circulation Mainly by the Liver, Kidney, and Placenta   Insulin circulates in plasma unbound and has a half-life of about 3 to 5 min. The short half-life of insulin is related to cellular uptake by endocytosis and destruction by *insulin protease (insulinase).* The degradation of insulin takes place in all insulin-sensitive tissues; however, most of the insulin degradation is performed by the liver (60%, mainly as first passage) and the kidneys (30%). The renal handling of insulin involves filtration, reabsorption in the proximal tubules, followed by degradation.

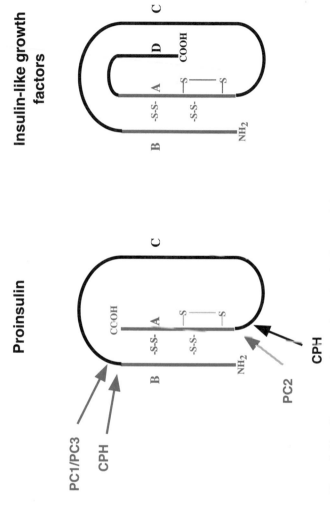

Proinsulin

Insulin-like growth factors

Figure 9-11. The structure of proinsulin and insulin-like growth factors (IGFs, also known as somatomedins). *Left:* Schematic presentation of the folding of the proinsulin polypeptide chain. The domains contributing to mature insulin are shown in color; chains A and B remain tied together by disulfide bridges. The connecting peptide (C) is removed by the sequential action of proprotein convertases (PCs) and carboxypeptidase H (CPH). *Right:* The folding of mature IGFs displayed to emphasize the similarity between insulin and IGFs. The insulin-like regions are highlighted in color. The C-domain of IGFs corresponds with the C peptide of proinsulin. Note the D domain, which is unique for IGFs. The C and D domains of IGFs are not cleaved.

219

Only minute quantities of intact insulin appear in the urine. The rest of insulin degradation mainly occurs in muscle. Interestingly, adipose tissue is less capable of internalizing and degrading insulin. The placenta is very active in insulin degradation. This may contribute to the enhanced insulin requirement during pregnancy.

The C-peptide Is a Reliable Measure of Endogenous Insulin Secretion   Insulin and C-peptide are released by the pancreatic β cells in equimolar quantities. Due to negligible hepatic extraction, the C-peptide has a longer half-life than insulin, which results in a plasma C-peptide:insulin molar ratio of >5. Although C-peptide is probably biologically inactive, its measurement is a useful tool in the assessment of β cell function of diabetic patients even in the presence of exogenous insulin or anti-insulin antibodies. The measurement of C-peptide is useful in the differential diagnosis of the various types of diabetes mellitus (see below), and in the diagnosis of insulin overdose because commercial preparations do not contain the C-peptide.

The Molecular Mechanisms of Insulin Action

The Insulin Receptor Is a Heterotetrameric Receptor Tyrosine Kinase   The insulin receptor gene on chromosome 19p consists of 22 exons and spans a region of greater than 120,000 base pairs. The insulin receptor is structurally related to receptor tyrosine kinases (such as the epidermal growth factor receptor) and the cytokine receptor superfamily (tyrosine kinase-associated receptors). As such, one would expect that the receptor consists of a single polypeptide chain with a single transmembrane domain and that ligand-induced dimerization and subsequent autophosphorylation of the receptor on tyrosine residues activate the intracellular signaling cascade. This generic mechanism, however, is somewhat modified in the case of the insulin receptor and its closest relative, the type 1 insulin-like growth factor receptor (IGF-1R):

• The single polypeptide chain of the receptor is posttranslationally cleaved to yield an α and a β *subunit,* which remain bound to each other by a disulfide bond. The α subunit binds the ligand. The β subunit contains the transmembrane domain and the tyrosine kinase catalytic activity.
• The insulin receptor is dimerized by a disulfide bond formed between two α subunits in the absence of the ligand. The dimer of two α and two β subunits is referred to as a *heterotetramer.* In certain cases, the insulin hemireceptor (i.e., a single α/β subunit) may form a *hybrid heterotetramer* with an IGF-1 hemireceptor (see also Chap. 10).
• The two α subunits bind a single ligand, which alters the conformation of the entire receptor leading to autophosphorylation of the β subunit. In effect, the autophosphorylation means that the two β subunits phosphorylate each other.

Table 9-5   Tissue-Specific Actions of Insulin

Effect	Target tissue
Stimulation of glucose uptake	Muscle, adipocyte
Stimulation of the Na$^+$/K$^+$-pump	Muscle, adipocyte
Inhibition of glycogenolysis[o]	Liver, muscle
Stimulation of glycogen synthesis	Liver, muscle
Inhibition of gluconeogenesis	Liver
Stimulation of cholesterol synthesis	Liver, adrenal cortex, gonad
Inhibition of lipolysis	Adipocyte, liver
Stimulation of fatty acid synthesis and ester-ification	Adipocyte, liver
Enhancement of glucose-induced insulin secretion	Pancreatic β cell
Stimulation of lipoprotein lipase	Mainly in the capillary beds of adipose tissue and skeletal muscle
Stimulation of milk production	Mammary gland
Suppression of appetite	Insulin-mediated glucose uptake in the ventral hypothalamus
Regulation of the expression of over 100 genes	Cell type-specific variations
Stimulation of amino acid uptake	All cells
Stimulation of protein synthesis	All cells
Inhibition of protein degradation	All cells
Stimulation of DNA synthesis and cell-cycle progression	All cells
Inhibition of apoptosis	All cells

[o]Recent evidence suggests that insulin does not inhibit glycogen phosphorylase in human liver.

These initial events of receptor activation exert a pleiotropic effect on cellular function (Table 9-5) mediated by a complex second messenger system that displays some variations depending on the cell type.

Mutations of the insulin receptor are rare. The mutation of the α subunit of the insulin receptor results in *Mendenhall syndrome*, which includes severe insulin resistance with diabetes mellitus and multiple somatic abnormalities such as *acanthosis nigricans* (a typical cutaneous manifestation of insulin resistant states, Fig. 9-12), hyperandrogenic state, pineal hyperplasia and dental dysplasia.

The Insulin Receptor Expressed in Muscle, Adipose Tissue, Liver, and Pancreatic β Cells Has Tissue-Dependent Impact on Glucose Homeostasis   Insulin receptor knockout (IRKO) mice have been generated, in which the insulin receptor is ablated in a cell-type specific manner. Depending on the targeted tissue, these animals are referred to as MIRKO (muscle), FIRKO (fat), LIRKO (liver), and BIRKO (beta cell) mice. These knockout mice have been instrumental for the characterization of tissue involvement in the pathogenesis of NIDDM (type II diabetes). The key findings with these mice include:

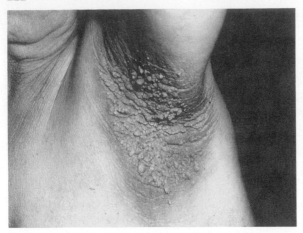

Figure 9-12. Acanthosis nigricans. The thickened, warty appearance is due to hyperkeratosis (resulting in a dirty brown to black color) and epidermal folding. This is a typically smooth/velvety cutaneous manifestation that is often observed in insulin-resistant states. It has been treated by dermatologists with retinoid ointments well before the discovery of the RXR : PPAR heterodimer intracellular receptor and its role in mediating rexinoid- and troglitazone-induced improvement of tissue insulin sensitivity. Note that severe forms of acanthosis nigricans may accompany various malignant tumors. (Source: Ackerman AB, Niven J, Grant-Kels JM: *Differential Diagnosis in Dermatopathology*. Volume I, p 95. Lea & Febiger, 1982.)

- MIRKO mice have normal glucose tolerance because glucose shifts to adipose tissue, where the action of insulin is normal, including the anti-lipolytic action. These animals develop "central obesity," have an about 80% increase in plasma triglycerides, but only a 20% increase in FFAs.
- FIRKO mice have supranormal glucose tolerance because of the normal insulin action on muscle. These mice are very lean and protected against the development of obesity.
- LIRKO mice display hyperinsulinemia because the receptor-mediated insulin uptake is important in the hepatic clearance and first passage phenomenon of insulin. These animals are mildly hyperglycemic and mildly glucose intolerant because of sustained gluconeogenesis. The mild hyperglycemia results in islet cell hyperplasia that contributes to hyper-insulinemia.
- BIRKO mice lack the first phase insulin response to an acute glucose challenge, yet respond with normal insulin release to arginine (see regulation of insulin secretion below). The loss of glucose-induced release of insulin results in a significant impairment of glucose tolerance that progressively worsens with age.

These findings suggest that NIDDM involves a more severe insulin resistance in muscle than in adipose tissue. Insulin resistance in adipose tissue manifests primarily as unsuppressed lipolysis, whereas glucose uptake and incorporation into triglycerides are retained. The mechanism of NIDDM appears to include impaired insulin receptor signaling in the pancreatic β cell, even though these cells do not require insulin for glucose uptake.

The Second Messengers of the Activated Insulin-Receptor Are Mainly Recruited by a Class of Docking Proteins Known as Insulin Receptor Substrates The postreceptor signaling cascade of insulin is only partially understood. However, this area is extremely important because the etiology of type II diabetes includes decreased tissue responsiveness to insulin due to impaired postreceptor mechanisms. Figure 9-13 provides a model of insulin signaling.

By autophosphorylation, receptor tyrosine kinases typically generate docking sites for second messenger proteins containing Src homology 2 (SH2) domain (see also Chap. 5). Although the insulin and IGF-1 receptors undergo autophosphorylation, their phosphotyrosine residues do not comprise docking sites for SH2 domains. Instead, they phosphorylate NPXY (Asn-Pro-X-Tyr) motifs, which bind proteins containing *pleckstrin homology* (PH) or the closely related *phosphotyrosine binding* (PTB) domains. The *insulin receptor substrate* (IRS) proteins (IRS-1 through IRS-4) contain a PH and a PTB domain in tandem near their N-terminus. During a *transient* binding via the PH and PTB domains, the activated insulin receptor phosphorylates the IRS proteins at multiple tyrosine residues, thereby generating docking sites for proteins with SH2 domains. This arrangement has certain characteristics:

• Because the tyrosine-phosphorylated IRS dissociates from the insulin receptor, a single activated insulin (or IGF-1) receptor may activate multiple copies and multiple forms of IRS molecules, and/or the distantly related insulin receptor substrates *Gab-1* and *p62^dok*. This eliminates the stoichiometric constraints of direct SH2 domain-mediated activation seen in the case of receptor tyrosine kinases, and leads to an enhanced signal amplification. The activity of the different IRSs varies with the cell type. For example, IRS-3, a strong activator of the PI3-K pathway, appears to be limited to adipocytes. The differential usage of docking proteins explains in part the pleiotropic effects of insulin in various tissues.

• The IRS molecules can be activated by receptors other than the insulin or IGF-1 receptors. In fact, IRS-2 was originally discovered as a second messenger of interleukin-4 (IL-4) receptors. IRS can be activated by receptor tyrosine kinases (such as EGF or the vascular endothelial growth factor [VEGF] receptor) and tyrosine-kinase associated receptors such as the members of the cytokine receptor family, including GH and prolactin (PRL) receptors. This explains the early insulin-like effect of GH.

• A single activated IRS docking protein may bind multiple second messengers via SH2 domains, such as the SH2/SH3 adapter proteins *Grb-2, nck, crk,* the tyrosine kinase *fyn,* the serine/threonine kinase protein kinase C zeta *(PKCζ)* and, most importantly, *phosphatidylinositol 3-kinase* (PI3-K).

• Upon ligand-binding, receptors typically undergo internalization and join the endosomal compartment of the cell. The receptor tyrosine kinases recruit SH2 domain proteins directly, and thus these second messengers follow the intracellular trafficking of the receptor. In contrast, IRSs

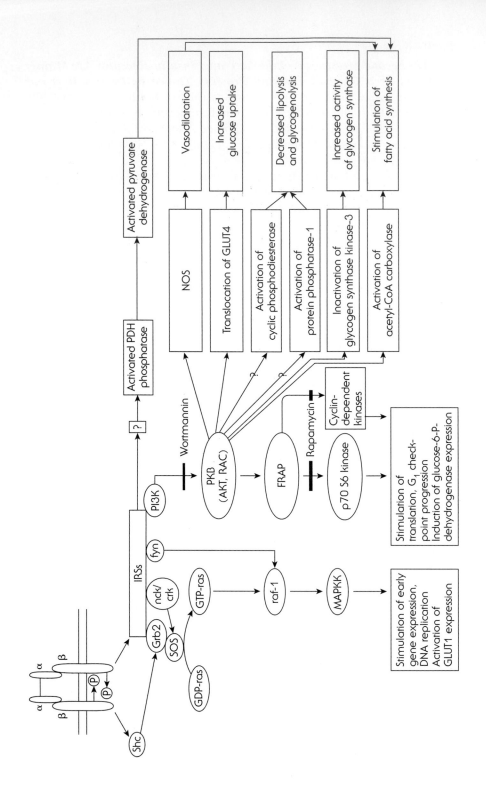

dissociate from the activated insulin receptor and may join other cellular compartments. This appears to be essential in the mobilization of GLUT4; the insulin receptor per se, unlike IRS-1, never colocalizes with GLUT4.

• IRS molecules are subject to serine/threonine phosphorylation at multiple sites, which decreases their insulin signal-transducing function in a quantitative manner in part by inhibiting subsequent tyrosine phosphorylation. This mechanism is used as a cross-talk between signaling systems (such as the PKC or TNF-α pathways), and also as a feedback by serine/threonine kinases located downstream of the IRS in the insulin signal cascade, such as PI3-K or MAPK (see below).

IRS-1 and IRS-2 are encoded by chromosomes 2 and 13q, respectively. Experiments with knockout mice indicate a more significant role of IRS-1 in mediating the growth factor functions of insulin, whereas IRS-2 appears to be more significant in whole-body glucose control. Nevertheless, IRS-1 is the main mediator of insulin action in skeletal muscle. Skeletal muscle of IRS-1 knockout mice retains only about 20% insulin response in terms of glucose uptake, glycogen, and protein synthesis. IRS-1 knockout mice display severe growth retardation. In spite of their relative insulin resistance, they do not develop NIDDM, probably because of appropriate compensation by IRS-2 that leads to normal insulin-induced suppression of hepatic gluconeogenesis. In contrast, IRS-2 knockout mice proceed to develop NIDDM in an age-dependent manner, yet their growth defects are minimal.

Mutations of IRS-1 in humans are rare, and are definitely not among the leading causes of NIDDM. As we shall see, the main causes of NIDDM include a multitude of conditions resulting in high circulating levels of FFA, such as undefined postreceptor defects of insulin signaling mainly affecting *adipocyte* function. This is consistent with an indirect (FFA-mediated), rather than direct (e.g., IRS-1 mutation-related), insulin resistance of skeletal muscle in NIDDM.

The IRS–PI3-K–Protein Kinase B Pathway Is a Major Mechanism of Insulin Receptor Signal Transduction A major pathway activated by IRS molecules involves *PI3-K,* a dimer composed of a 110-kDa catalytic subunit, which is associated with one of five different SH2 domain protein regulatory subunits (p555^{PIK}, p55$^\alpha$, p50$^\alpha$, p85$^\alpha$, p85$^\beta$). The regulatory subunits

Figure 9-13. A model for the signaling cascade of insulin. Insulin receptor substrates (IRSs) are docking proteins, which play a central role in the process in part by carrying the docked activities to designated membrane compartments within the cell. Insulin either via Shc or via IRS is a weak activator of the MAPK pathway. The phosphatidylinositol 3-kinase (PI3-K) − protein kinase B (PKB) pathway mediates most of the effects. PKB activates a vast number of response mechanisms, including the rapamycin-sensitive cell cycle regulatory processes, vasodilatation by increasing the activity of endothelial nitric oxide synthase (NOS), glucose uptake (via GLUT4 mobilization) and other metabolic activities. Refer to the text for additional explanation.

vary with the target cell of insulin. PI3-K phosphorylates membrane lipids to yield phosphatidylinositol-3,4,5-trisphosphate [PtdIns(3,4,5)P$_3$].

PI3-K activates PKB by a complex mechanism. PtdIns(3,4,5)P$_3$ located in the inner leaflet of the membrane binds the pleckstrin homology domain of PKB. This results in a conformational change that exposes a threonine residue of PKB to the constitutively active *PDK1* (3-phosphoinositide-dependent protein kinase 1). PtdIns(3,4,5)P$_3$ at the membrane activates *PDK2*, which phosphorylates a serine residue of PKB. After being phosphorylated at both sites, PKB detaches from the plasma membrane and phosphorylates its targets.

PKB (also known as *AKT* or *RAC*) serves as a focal point of several PI3-K-mediated metabolic and growth factor-like effects of insulin (see Fig. 9-13). The metabolic actions of PKB include:

- Translocation of *GLUT4* from the vesicular compartment to the cell surface plasma membrane. Although several mechanisms may activate PI3-K thereby recruiting PKB, only their activation via IRS will achieve mobilization of GLUT4 probably because IRS directs the signaling complex to the vesicular compartment instead of the plasma membrane per se. Increased levels of circulating FFA decrease the IRS-1-associated PI3-K activity and GLUT4 mobilization in skeletal muscle. In contrast, the *contraction pathway* of GLUT4 mobilization is not inhibited by FFA in skeletal muscle.
- Activation of *cyclic phosphodiesterase* (cyclic PDE). Because stimulation of glucagon- and β-adrenergic receptors achieve intracellular signaling by increasing cyclic AMP, insulin may directly antagonize these hormones via increasing the degradation of cyclic AMP. This mechanism might be important in the insulin-induced inhibition of hormone-sensitive lipase in adipose tissue, and the inhibition of glycogenolysis in liver and muscle. Note, however, that insulin does not inhibit glycogenolysis in human liver.
- Inactivation of *glycogen synthase kinase-3* results of decreased phosphorylation state of glycogen synthase, which equals with increased activity of glycogen synthase.
- PKB directly activates *acetyl-CoA carboxylase,* thereby stimulating fatty acid synthesis. This action is complemented by an activation of PDH phosphatase, which activates PDH. Note that activation of PDH is an IRS-mediated action that does not involve the PI3-K–PKB pathway.
- PKB induces *nitric oxide synthase* (NOS) in endothelial cells. The NO generated by the endothelium activates the soluble guanylyl cyclase in the adjacent vascular smooth muscle cells, thereby causing vasorelaxation. NIDDM and *syndrome X* (see later) are often associated with hypertension, and the decreased endothelial NOS activity secondary to insulin resistance has been implicated in its pathomechanism.

The growth factor function mediated by the PI3-K–PKB pathway involves the activation of *FKBP-rapamycin associated protein* (FRAP). FRAP is a member of the *phosphatidylinositol kinase (PIK-) related kinases* and is closely related to *ataxia telangiectasia mutated* (ATM). The PIK-related kinases function in signal transduction pathways involved in surveillance, cell-cycle checkpoints, DNA repair and recombination. The *FRAP* gene maps to chromosome 1p36.2, a region deleted in neuroblastomas. FRAP is the target of the rapamycin-induced inhibition of progression through G_1 of the cell cycle. *Rapamycin* (a potent immunosuppressive drug) and *FK506* (another immunosuppressive drug similar to *cyclosporin A*) bind to the same intracellular receptor, *FK-binding protein 12* (FKBP12), yet the resulting complexes are involved in distinct signaling pathways. The FKBP12-rapamycin complex inhibits the mitogen-stimulated signaling pathway that leads to activation of *p70 S6 kinase* (p70S6k), *cyclin-dependent kinases* (CDKs) and progression through the G_1 checkpoint of the cell cycle at least in osteosarcoma cells, hepatocytes and T lymphocytes. This pathway has also been implicated in the induction of glucose-6-phosphate dehydrogenase (G6PDH) expression and upregulation of the pentose monophosphate shunt.

The Activated Insulin Receptor Recruits the Mitogen-Associated Protein Kinase Pathway Via the SH2/SH3 Domain Adapter Proteins Grb-2, Crk, and Nck or the Tyrosine Kinase Fyn   We have discussed the mitogen-associated protein (MAP) kinase pathway in Chap. 5. The activation of this pathway results in early gene expression and stimulation of DNA replication. The activated insulin receptor recruits the MAP kinase pathway via a small SH2/SH3 domain adapter protein known as *Grb-2*. Depending on the cell type, Grb-2 may engage a number of insulin receptor-activated proteins such as IRS-1 (the preferred pathway in skeletal muscle), IRS-2, or Shc. The activated Grb-2 forms a complex with the guanine nucleotide exchange factor *SOS ("son of sevenless"),* which in turn facilitates the exchange of GDP for GTP in $p21^{ras}$. The activated $p21^{ras}$ then recruits the MAP kinase pathway. Activation of the MAP-kinase pathway increases the expression of GLUT1 and stimulates glucose uptake. Although activation of the MAP-kinase pathway by insulin is well-documented, it is relatively insensitive to insulin, and results in only a modest increase in GLUT1-mediated glucose uptake.

IRS molecules also serve as Grb-2-independent docking sites for other SH2/SH3 adapter proteins such as crk and nck, which may also activate the MAP-kinase pathway via SOS. Fyn, a tyrosine kinase, also may bind to IRS and activate the MAP-kinase pathway via activating raf (see Fig. 9-13).

The Regulation of Insulin Secretion

Plasma Glucose Concentration Is the Main Regulator of Insulin Secretion Via a Complex Metabolic Coupling Mechanism   The regulatory mechanism of insulin secretion monitors the *changes* of intracellular glucose concentration in the pancreatic β cell. This equals with monitoring *plasma* concentrations, but not the intracellular concentrations of glucose in peripheral tissues. The most important stimulus of insulin secretion is hyperglycemia (Fig. 9-14). The β cells take up glucose by a low-affinity glucose transporter protein GLUT2 (see details of GLUTs above). Thus, β cells are relatively starved under euglycemic conditions. Upon hyperglycemia, glucose may enter the β cells, where it joins the glycolytic pathway upon being phosphorylated by the low-affinity glucokinase enzyme. *Glucokinase* is normally the rate limiting step in the process, and thus regarded as the *glucose sensor*. The subcellular localization of glucokinase appears to be important in its regulatory role: it is associated with *porin* in the outer mitochondrial membrane. The glycolytic pathway produces acetyl-CoA, which is used for the generation of ATP by the Krebs cycle, terminal oxidation and oxidative phosphorylation in *mitochondria*. The low affinity steps of GLUT2 and glucokinase assure that cytoplasmic ATP levels will reach signaling concentrations only upon hyperglycemia. The increased concentrations of cytoplasmic ATP or the increased ATP/ADP ratio inhibits the function of a specific type of potassium channel (*ATP-sensitive K^+-channel, inward rectifying K^+-channel 6.2* [$K_{ir}6.2$]). The reduced efflux of K^+ results in depolarization of the cell membrane, which in turn activates *voltage-gated Ca^{++}-channels*. The increase in cytoplasmic Ca^{++} activates the microtubules and results in exocytosis of the secretory granules containing insulin crystals.

ATP regulates the K^+-channel via the *sulfonylurea receptor* (SUR). SUR is a member of the *ATP-binding cassette superfamily,* and serves as a subunit of the potassium channel. SUR has 12 transmembrane segments, two putative sites for binding ATP and sulfonylurea drugs, and is homologous with *cystic fibrosis transmembrane regulator* (CFTR, a chloride channel) and *multidrug resistance protein* (MDR, which pumps organic anions out of the cytoplasm). Sufonylurea drugs exert the same effect on β cells as the increased intracellular levels of ATP. Rare mutations of SUR result in *familial hyperinsulinemic hypoglycemia of infancy* (FHHI). In FHHI, the second nucleotide-binding fold of SUR is missing, which results in the inhibition of the K^+-channel without an increased ATP/ADP ratio. Mutations of $K_{ir}6.2$ may also lead to FHHI.

As noted above, BIRKO mice (mice lacking insulin receptors in their pancreatic β cells) do not respond with insulin release to an acute glucose challenge. The β cells do not require insulin for glucose uptake, and BIRKO mice have normal levels of GLUT2. The mechanism of insulin receptor signaling in the glucose-induced release of insulin is currently unknown.

Loss-of-function mutation of certain components of the signaling pathway of *regulated* insulin secretion results in early onset types of diabetes known as MODY and mitochondrial diabetes.

MODY has the characteristics of NIDDM except that it starts early in life (at an age younger than 25 years), in most cases follows an autosomal

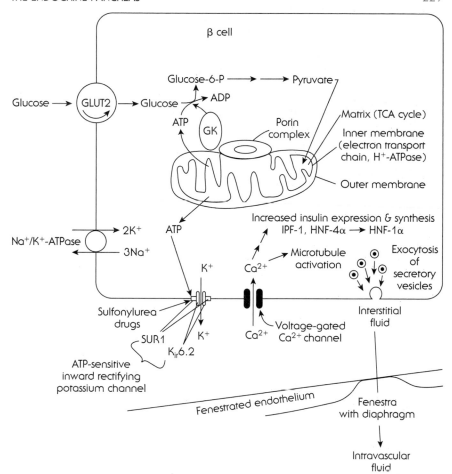

Figure 9-14. The regulatory mechanisms of glucose-induced insulin-release in the pancreatic β cell. The components are not drawn to scale. The ATP-sensitive potassium channel is a multiunit cylindrical structure assembled as $(SUR1/K_{ir}6.2)_4$. SUR1, sulfonylurea receptor-1; $K_{ir}6.2$, inward rectifying potassium channel. The flux of K^+ ions is inhibited either by an increased ATP/ADP ratio in the cytosol or by sulfonylurea drugs (oral hypoglycemic agents). The retained K^+ ions increase the intracellular positive charge leading to depolarization and opening of voltage-gated Ca^{2+} channels. The increase in intracellular Ca^{2+} is the signal for exocytosis of stored insulin and the increased hormone synthesis. Adequate insulin secretion is achieved by metabolic coupling, which involves the low-affinity glucose transporter (GLUT2), glucokinase (GK), and mitochondrial activity. GK is strategically positioned at the porin complex, where the outer and inner mitochondrial membranes form a button-like attachment.

dominant pattern, and is usually associated with a nonobese phenotype. MODY is a primary defect of the function of the β cells. Measurements of antibodies and C-peptide are very useful in differentiating MODY from IDDM:

- Antibodies against insulin and GAD65 are absent in MODY but present in IDDM patients.
- Levels of C-peptide are much more severely diminished in IDDM partly because the *constitutive* secretion of insulin continues in MODY.

Several MODY genes have been identified (Table 9-6). Most cases are related to mutations of glucokinase/MODY2 (the glucose sensor). The MODY1 gene encodes the *hepatocyte nuclear factor-4α* (HNF-4α), which is a member of the orphan nuclear receptor/steroid hormone receptor superfamily and a regulator of HNF-1α expression. HNF-1α/MODY3 is encoded by the *TCF1* gene; it is a weak activator of the insulin gene. These three MODY genes are all expressed both in the liver and the pancreatic β cells. Note that glucokinase in the liver is expressed via a different promoter. The MODY4 gene was identified as *insulin promoter factor-1 (IPF-1)*. Like all other MODYs, the MODY4 manifests in the heterozygous state. As mentioned, IPF-1 is identical to IDX-1, and its total absence (homozygous mutation) causes pancreatic agenesis. There is little if any support for a causative role of GLUT2 mutations in MODY.

Mitochondrial diabetes is due to mutations of mitochondrial DNA, most often involving an A-to-G transition in the tRNA$^{Leu(UUR)}$ at nucleotide 3243. The mutation results in a reduced capacity of the mitochondrion to increase ATP synthesis upon availability of glucose, which in turn hampers insulin release. In addition, patients may develop hearing impairment, cataract and a syndrome consisting of myopathy, encephalopathy, lactic acidosis, and stroke-like episodes *(MELAS syndrome)*. Mitochondrial diabetes is inherited from the mother. Note that mitochondrial aging (a process related to cumulative damage of mitochondrial DNA inflicted by free radicals) in itself may yield a condition similar to mitochondrial diabetes; this may explain the deteriorating glycemic control (hyperglycemia) in elderly patients.

Table 9-6   MODY Genes

Designation	Gene	Location
MODY1	HNF-4α or TCF14	20q
MODY2	Glucokinase	7p13
MODY3	HNF-1α or TCF1	12q
MODY4	IPF-1 or IDX-1	13q12.1
MODY5	HNF-1β or TCF2	17cen-q

ABBREVIATIONS: HNF, hepatocyte nuclear factor; IPF1, insulin promoter factor-1.

Table 9-7   Regulators of Insulin Secretion

Direct stimulators	Amplifiers	Inhibitors
Acute hyperglycemia (requires normal insulin receptor signaling)	Incretins: Secretin-family: GLP-1[7-37], secretin, GIP, VIP Gastrin-family: gastrin, CCK	Hypoglycemia Sustained hyperglycemia (glucose toxicity)
Leucine	Arginine, lysine	SRIF
	β_2 adrenergic receptor agonists	α_2 adrenergic receptor agonists
	Parasympathetic stimulus (M_3 muscarinic receptor stimulation)	Increased plasma levels of free fatty acids TNF-α

ABBREVIATIONS: GLP-1, glucagon-like peptide-1; GIP, gastric inhibitory peptide; VIP, vasoactive intestinal polypeptide; SRIF, somatostatin; CCK, cholecystokinin; TNF-α, tumor necrosis factor α.

Amino Acids, Hormones, and Autonomic Nerves also Directly Modulate Insulin Secretion   These additional regulators of insulin secretion may function either as direct stimulants, amplifiers of glucose-induced insulin secretion, or inhibitors (Table 9-7). *Amplifiers* differ from direct stimulants in that they do not stimulate insulin secretion without concomitant hyperglycemia. *Incretins* such as GLP-1[7-37] (see above) function mainly as amplifiers of insulin secretion in response to *oral* glucose. Other amplifiers include *β_2 adrenergic receptor agonists* (mainly adrenaline). The incretins and β-adrenergic stimulation activate the adenylyl cyclase enzyme and increase cyclic AMP. Another important amplifier is increased *parasympathetic (vagal) tone*, i.e., stimulation of muscarinic (mainly M_3) cholinergic receptors, which acts by the mobilization of Ca^{2+} via IP_3.

Amino acids may serve either as direct stimulators (leucine) or amplifiers (arginine, lysine). Note that leucine is a ketogenic amino acid: its increase signals a potential for increased ketone body production, which is antagonized by insulin. Therefore, leucine-induced insulin secretion may be viewed as a negative feedback regulation of ketone body production. This action is supported by leucin's inability to stimulate glucagon, a potent ketogenic hormone. Arginine and lysine appear to amplify insulin secretion related to the effect of their positive charge on the membrane potential of β cells.

The *inhibitors* of insulin release exert their action mainly by blunting hyperglycemia-induced release of insulin. The most important inhibitors are *α_2-adrenergic receptor agonists* (mainly noradrenaline), *somatostatin* (SRIF), increased levels of circulating FFA, and TNF-α. The stimulation of α_2- and β_2-adrenergic receptors exerts opposite effects on insulin secretion. During stress, the net effect of their stimulation is an inhibition of insulin secretion (and stimulation of glucagon secretion, see above).

Free fatty acids are taken up by the β cells and delivered into the mitochondrial matrix by the carnitine shuttle, where they undergo β-oxida-

A

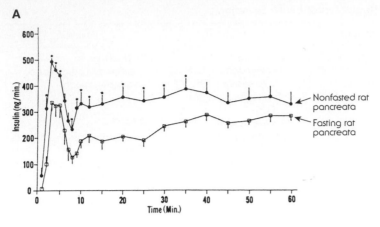

B

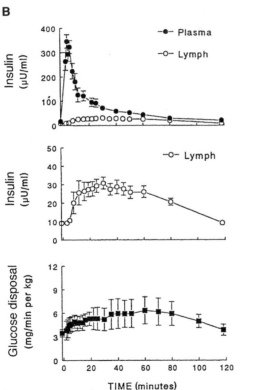

TIME (minutes)

Figure 9-15. The biphasic response of insulin secretion and its conversion into a monophasic response in the interstitial fluid. A. The insulin secretion of rat pancreata perfused with a medium containing 200 mg/dL glucose. Note that the rapid high-amplitude first phase (secretion of stored insulin) is followed by a decline (depletion of insulin stores), then a slow, lower amplitude second phase occurs (newly synthesized insulin). B. Although present, the second phase of insulin increase as observed in plasma is less prominent in comparison with the first phase increment (top panel). In the same in vivo experiment, the profile of insulin in lymph (which represents the concentration of insulin in the interstitial fluid) is clearly

tion that generates acetyl-CoA. Another mitochondrial enzyme, the PDH complex generates acetyl-CoA from pyruvate in the process of oxidative metabolization of glucose. *The activity of PDH complex is inhibited by the accumulation of acetyl-CoA. The inhibition of PDH by FFA-derived acetyl-CoA explains in part why elevated plasma FFA levels blunt insulin responses to changes in circulating glucose.* An additional mechanism of blunting insulin responses by elevated plasma FFA is the direct inhibition of insulin receptor signaling in the β cells. TNF-α, a lipolytic agent that increases plasma FFA levels, is a potent inhibitor of glucose-induced release of insulin. A local production of TNF-α by unspecified cells in the pancreatic islets has been demonstrated, and might contribute to the pathomechanism of NIDDM.

A Prolonged Hyperglycemic Stimulus Results in a Biphasic Insulin-Release Response   When glucose infusion is initiated in a fasting patient, the insulin stored in secretory vesicles of β cells is rapidly released. In spite of maintaining the hyperglycemic stimulus by continued glucose infusion, insulin release rapidly decreases, which is indicated by returning to near-basal plasma insulin concentrations. This is the *fast, early, or first phase of insulin release,* which is completed about 10 to 15 min after the onset of glucose infusion. If glucose infusion continues, plasma insulin levels increase again reflecting increased rate of secretion. This second peak, which is attained more slowly and has a longer duration is referred to as the *slow, late, or second phase of insulin release.* The slow phase is attributed to the secretion of newly synthesized insulin. After 1.5 to 3 h of continued glucose exposure, insulin secretion returns to 15 to 25% of peak values. This still represents a higher than basal rate of insulin release, which can be maintained for more than 48 h (Fig. 9-15). The first-phase insulin response during intravenous glucose infusion is markedly blunted or absent in NIDDM and MODY patients.

Due to a Slow Transendothelial Transport, Biphasic Insulin Response in Plasma Is Transformed into a Monophasic Insulin Response in Interstitial Fluid, Resulting in Monophasic Responses in Peripheral Glucose Disposal, Inhibition of Lipolysis, and Hepatic Glucose Output   Of the three traditionally recognized main targets of insulin, only the liver is readily reached by plasma insulin because the liver has a discontinuous endothe-

---

Figure 9-15. (*Continued*) monophasic and follows a different time course than insulin in plasma (middle panel). The difference is due to the endothelial barrier in muscle and adipose tissue. Glucose disposal (bottom panel) follows a time course that is identical with that of insulin in the interstitial fluid, and different from the time course of insulin in plasma. (*Source:* A. Fig. 1 in Curry DL: Insulin content and insulinogenesis by perfused rat pancreas: Effects of long term glucose stimulation. Endocrinology 118:170–175, 1986; B. Fig. 5 in Bergman RN: New concepts in extracellular signaling for insulin action: The single gateway hypothesis. Recent Progress Hormone Res 52:359–366, 1997.)

lium. In contrast, the capillary endothelium of muscle and adipose tissue is of the continuous type, and insulin penetrates this barrier by a relatively slow non-receptor-mediated transcytosis. The delivery of insulin into the interstitial fluid is a diffusion-limited process, and under normal conditions the concentration ratio of insulin between plasma and the interstitial fluid is 3:2. Because the effect of insulin requires reaching the skeletal muscle fiber or the adipocyte, transcytosis becomes the dynamic determinant of glucose disposal. Due to the kinetics of transcytosis, the biphasic pattern of insulin seen in plasma is transformed into a monophasic increase of insulin in the interstitial fluid, which in turn correlates well with the time course of glucose disposal (see Fig. 9-15B).

Due to the difference in their endothelial barriers and the first passage phenomenon, the kinetics of the response to insulin by the liver is expected to be faster than the response by muscle or adipose tissue. However, the response by the liver (decreased hepatic glucose output) follows the same kinetics as the response by the peripheral tissues (glucose uptake by muscle and adipose tissue, inhibition of lipolysis in adipose tissue). This observation has led to the conclusion that insulin's effect to inhibit hepatic glucose output is mediated *indirectly* by a signal emanating from the periphery. The signal was identified as the insulin-induced decrease in FFA output by adipose tissue (i.e., the inhibition of hormone-sensitive lipase). This concept is known as the *single gateway hypothesis*. Indeed, the ED_{50} plasma level of insulin to suppress lipolysis as well as hepatic glucose output are equal (<200 pM), whereas stimulation of peripheral glucose disposal has a much higher ED_{50} (>500 pM).

Ingestion of carbohydrates triggers a rapid insulin secretory response, which practically immediately exposes the liver to high levels of insulin. If direct inhibition were the dominant mechanism of hepatic glucose output, the response could be too rapid and yield hypoglycemia. Because the transcytosis in adipose and muscle tissues follows the same timecourse, the single gateway mechanism guarantees that hepatic glucose production does not decrease until peripheral glucose utilization increases.

Glucagon stimulates hepatic glucose output mainly by direct hepatic actions (increased glycogenolysis and gluconeogenesis), and in part by increasing lipolysis in adipose tissue, which in turn supports gluconeogenesis. The *relative importance* of the indirect (FFA-mediated) and the direct hepatic action of insulin to inhibit hepatic glucose output depends on the plasma level of glucagon: with increasing plasma levels of glucagon, the relative contribution of insulin's direct hepatic action also increases (Fig. 9-16). Glucagon levels are high during fasting, yet even under these circumstances approximately 80% of insulin's action is mediated via inhibition of lipolysis. These observations put the concept of *insulin:glucagon ratio* (see above) into a new perspective.

The single gateway hypothesis places FFA in the center of the pathomechanism of NIDDM. This notion is supported by several findings:

• Hepatic insulin resistance (increased hepatic glucose output) in

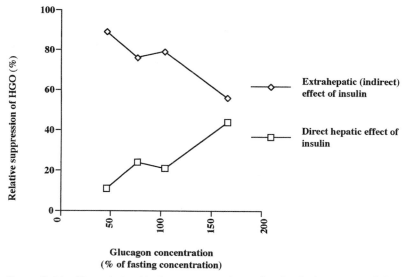

Figure 9-16. The relationship between circulating levels of glucagon and the relative importance of insulin's direct hepatic and indirect (extrahepatic) site of action in suppressing hepatic glucose output (HGO). Insulin was infused at a constant rate. Although the relative importance of the hepatic site of action increased with increasing concentrations of glucagon, the extrahepatic site was at least as important as the direct action even when plasma glucagon was very high.

NIDDM can be explained mainly by insulin resistance of the adipocyte, i.e., the inability of insulin to suppress lipolysis.

- As discussed above, increased levels of plasma FFA are responsible for

    - decreased insulin response of the β cell to hyperglycemia and

    - decreased insulin-induced GLUT4 mobilization in skeletal muscle.

- The insulin-sensitizer drugs *thiazolidinediones* (such as troglitazone and rosiglitazone) activate the peroxisome proliferator-activated receptor γ (PPARγ; see Chap. 5) predominantly acting on adipocytes. Although skeletal muscle expresses only low levels of PPARγ mRNA (up to 5% that of white adipocytes), its PPARγ *protein* levels are unexpectedly high (about 70% that of white adipocytes). It is noteworthy that the expression of PPARγ is regulated differently in muscle and adipose tissue. PPARγ levels are similar in skeletal muscles of lean nondiabetic and insulin-resistant obese diabetic subjects.

Ultradian Oscillations of Insulin Secretion Can Be Entrained by Oscillations of Glucose Infusion Rate Only if the Pancreatic β Cells Function Normally   When glucose is intravenously infused at a *constant rate* (e.g., 5 mg/kg/min), plasma glucose and insulin levels display regular oscillations with a periodicity of 90 to 120 min, termed *ultradian oscillations*. The oscillations of insulin temporally lag behind the oscillations of glucose, indicating that insulin secretion is driven by endogenous oscillations of glucose. If the glucose is infused at a variable rate with regular oscillations having a periodicity shorter or longer than the endogenous rhythm, insulin secretion follows this exogenously enforced new rhythm. This phenomenon is termed *entrainment. Insulin secretion by normally functioning β cells can be completely entrained by exogenous glucose oscillations.* In contrast, entrainment of insulin secretion is lost in patients who have either mildly impaired glucose tolerance or overt NIDDM. In these patients, insulin secretion at first glance fluctuates similarly as in healthy patients; however, the fluctuations are temporally unrelated to the oscillations of exogenous glucose infusion (Fig. 9-17). The loss of entrainment might be explained by the elevated plasma levels of FFA; PPARγ-activator drugs may at least in part restore entrainment in NIDDM.

Glycemic Control Is Determined by the Relationship between Insulin Secretion and the Insulin Sensitivity of Target Tissues   Among individuals displaying normal glucose control, *body mass index* (BMI, an index of the degree of adiposity, see Box 10-4) is positively associated with plasma insulin levels. This observation indicates that obesity, especially *central obesity,* decreases insulin sensitivity (i.e., obesity causes insulin resistance), and euglycemia may be achieved only at the expense of hyperinsulinemia. The relationship between insulin sensitivity and fasting insulin levels is hyperpolic in healthy young adult human subjects (Fig. 9-18). Another important determinant of insulin sensitivity is the contribution of *skeletal muscle fiber types* to lean body mass. The contribution of type I (areobic, red) skeletal muscle fibers (see Chap. 11) is increased by regular exercise. These muscle fibers primarily rely on FFA as their fuel, and improve insulin sensitivity probably by decreasing plasma FFA levels. In contrast, a preponderance of type II (anaerobic, white) muscle fibers, which is typically observed in subjects with a sedentary lifestyle, contributes to insulin resistance. Individuals with impaired glucose tolerance and diabetes mellitus have a combination of insulin sensitivity and plasma insulin concentration that places them below and to the left of the normal hyperbolic function.

The hyperbolic relationship in euglycemic subjects means that the product of insulin sensitivity and insulin secretion is constant, which suggests a negative feedback loop between these two parameters. Such a feedback loop is essential in the long-term regulation of body weight, and probably involves *leptin* (see also Chaps. 12 and 15). Leptin is a helix-bundle peptide hormone that is secreted by adipose tissue. Increasing plasma levels of leptin indicate increased degree of adiposity. Leptin's main target is the hypothalamus, where it suppresses appetite and increases sympathetic activity. This in part explains why obese subjects have a higher lipolytic activity, elevated plasma FFA levels, and decreased insulin sensitivity. Elevated plasma FFA levels in obese subjects is in part explained by the autocrine action of increased TNF-α activity in adipose tissue. Mutations of the *obese* (leptin) gene in *ob/ob* mice lead to leptin deficiency and obesity. Loss-of-

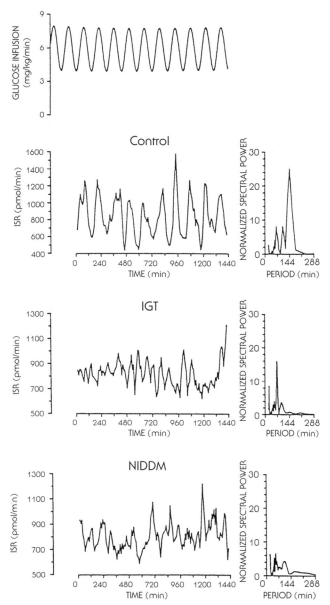

Figure 9-17. The entrainment of the insulin secretory response (ISR) by oscillating infusions of glucose in a clinical setting. The periodicity of glucose infusion was 144 minutes. The ISR was evaluated by measurements of the C peptide and computer-aided deconvolution analysis. The normalized spectral power of control patients yielded a peak periodicity of 144 minutes, indicating that their ultradian insulin secretion was entrained by the oscillating glucose input. In patients with impaired glucose tolerance (IGT) a shorter period time with a lower amplitude was observed. Entrainment was totally lost in patients with non insulin-dependent diabetes mellitus (NIDDM). Without deconvolution, the loss of entrainment is not obvious because insulin secretion fluctuates in all three groups. The loss of entrainment means that the temporal relationship reflecting a causal link between the fluctuations of glucose and insulin is absent. (Source: Fig. 10 in Polonsky KS: Lilly Lecture 1994. The β-cell in diabetes: From molecular genetics to clinical research. *Diabetes* 44:705–717, 1995.)

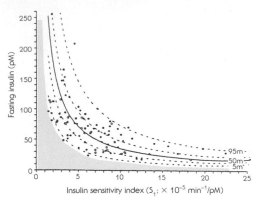

Figure 9-18.   The relationship between the insulin sensitivity index and fasting plasma insulin levels in young euglycemic patients. The solid line indicates the best fit (50th percentile), dashed lines display the 5th and 95th percentiles. The hyperbolic relationship reflects the feed-back relationship between these parameters. The variations in insulin sensitivity are mainly attributed to the degree of adiposity as determined by body mass index. Patients with impaired glucose tolerance and diabetes mellitus fall in the region left and below the hyperbolic function (highlighted in color). (*Source:* Fig. 2 in Kahn SE et al: Quantification of the relationship between insulin sensitivity and β-cell function in human subjects. Diabetes 42:1663–1672, 1993.)

function mutations of the leptin receptor are responsible for NIDDM in the *db/db* mouse. Hyperphagia in these mutant animals is a direct cause of elevated plasma FFA. Leptin improves insulin sensitivity, at least in part, independent of its hypothalamic action, probably by regulating the expression of fatty acid translocase (FAT; see below).

As a consequence of the hyperbolic function, basal plasma insulin may be a better indicator of insulin sensitivity in obese, insulin-resistant subjects, whereas direct determination of insulin sensitivity would be more reliable in lean, insulin-sensitive individuals.

Administration of PPARγ-activator drugs to insulin resistant diabetic patients *decreases* plasma insulin levels as well as plasma glucose, indicating that the mechanism of action is enhancement of insulin sensitivity. This is in contrast with the action of sulfonylureas, which decrease plasma glucose mainly by increasing pancreatic insulin secretion. The most effective therapy in diabetic patients with marked insulin resistance are the insulin sensitizers, such as the PPARγ-activators troglitazone and rosiglitazone. In contrast, in diabetic patients whose insulin sensitivity is close to normal, insulin or insulin inducers (such as sulfonylureas) are the most effective therapeutic agents. A combination of insulin sensitizers and insulin inducers may be required to normalize glycemic control.

Fatty Acid Translocase Deficiency Underlies Insulin Resistance, Defective Fatty Acid Metabolism, and Hypertriglyceridemia in Spontaneously Hypertensive Rats and May Be Important in the Pathogenesis of Human Syndrome X The uptake of FFA across the plasma membrane may be mediated by at least three distinct proteins:

- *Fatty acid translocase* (FAT). The normal function of FAT is transporting fatty acids to the cytosol *for re-esterification.*
- *Plasma membrane fatty acid binding protein* (FABP$_{pm}$).
- *Fatty acid transport protein* (FATP). FATP may transport FA toward mitochondria *for oxidation.*

Syndrome X refers to insulin resistance syndrome, which may include the association of several conditions such as NIDDM, obesity, combined hyperlipidemia, and hypertension. The defective *SHR gene* of spontaneously hypertensive rats (a model of syndrome X) is the equivalent of *FAT* also known as *CD36* (encoded by human chromosome 7), the protein product of which was originally identified in human platelets and in lactating mammary epithelium. Transgenic mice overexpressing FAT have decreased blood lipids. In contrast, the FAT protein is undetectable in the plasma membrane of spontaneously hypertensive rats. In differentiated adipocytes, levels of the FAT mRNA are downregulated by increased cytoplasmic concentration of cyclic AMP independent of the activation of hormone-sensitive lipase.

Lipopolysaccharide (LPS, endotoxin), TNF-α, or IL-1 are lipolytic agents, which induce insulin resistance. These compounds:

- decrease FAT and FATP gene expression in tissues where FFA uptake and/or oxidation is decreased during sepsis, such as in adipose tissue, skeletal muscle and heart.
- decrease FATP mRNA expression but increase FAT mRNA levels in the liver, where FFA oxidation is decreased during sepsis but the uptake of peripherally derived FFA is increased to support re-esterification.

In the leptin-deficient *ob/ob* mice FAT mRNA levels are disproportionately induced in the liver and white adipose tissue compared to control heterozygous, nonobese littermates (fifteenfold higher in liver but only 60 to 80% higher in adipose tissue), whereas FATP mRNA levels are unaffected. Similar to the effect of TNF-α, this arrangement would favor movement of FFA from white adipose tissue to the liver for re-esterification (VLDL production) and cause hyperlipidemia. Thus, the normal action of leptin favors movement of FFA to adipose tissue and away from the liver, and decreases plasma lipids, thereby improving insulin sensitivity. Because leptin decreases appetite, the shift of FFA to adipose tissue does not result in obesity.

Peroxisome proliferators improve plasma lipid profile by influencing both the metabolism and the cellular uptake of fatty acids. FAT mRNA is induced in the liver and intestine of mice by PPARα-activating drugs, such as clofibrate. In white adipose tissue of obese mice, the insulin-sensitizing PPARγ activators (such as troglitazone and rosiglitazone), which are known to antagonize the action of TNF-α in this target tissue, induce FAT and FATP even more efficiently than clofibrate.

Diabetic Complications

Diabetic complications may present as

- acute conditions, such as
  - the life-threatening events of hyperosmolar or ketoacidotic coma
  - the Somogyi effect
- slowly developing consequences of
  - chronic hyperglycemia, such as diabetic microangiopathy,
macroangiopathy, neuropathy, nephropathy, ophthalmopathy, and
compromised defenses against infections
  - insulin resistance, such as hypertension related to decreased
NOS activity in endothelial cells.

***Hyperglycemia May Result in Coma Secondary to Hyperosmo-
lality*** *Hyperosmolar coma* typically presents with plasma glucose levels
exceeding 700 mg/dL. The main determinant of plasma osmolality is sodium: sodium (together with its counterions) accounts for about 270 to 290
mOsm/kg of the total plasma osmolality of 275 to 295 mOsm/kg. Normally
glucose adds only about 5 mOsm/kg to plasma osmolality (glucose level of
90 mg/dL). However, diabetic patients may experience extreme hyperglycemia. Using the empirical formula to estimate plasma osmolality (see Chap.
1), a plasma glucose of about 700 mg/dL could yield a plasma osmolality
close to 340 mOsm/kg, i.e., sufficiently high to cause coma.

Diabetic ketoacidosis (DKA) usually develops in type I diabetic
(IDDM) patients and if untreated may *acutely* proceed to *DKA coma*. In
contrast, type II diabetic patients are more prone to develop *hyperosmolar
coma* without ketoacidosis; the onset of this hyperosmolar coma tends to
be *gradual*. It is not widely recognized that the cause of coma and death
in the DKA coma patient is primarily due more to the hyperosmotic condition than to the acidosis.

As noted earlier, glucosuria serves as an emergency overflow safety
valve in the regulation of plasma glucose levels. The kidney starts to spill
glucose into urine if the plasma levels of glucose exceed the renal threshold
of about 160 to 240 mg/dL. However, together with the glucose, water and
electrolytes are lost in urine because the osmotic activity of glucose is
generating *solvent drag*. The condition is termed *osmotic diuresis*. At this
stage, the plasma (blood) volume is maintained; that is, water is essentially
lost from the interstitial fluid compartment.

The continued hepatic glucose output and diminished cellular glucose
uptake maintains osmotic diuresis, the volume of the ECF becomes reduced
and its osmolality is further increased. The decreased volume of ECF
activates the sympathoadrenal system in an attempt to maintain blood
pressure (see Chap. 12). This has several deleterious consequences:

- Sympathoadrenal activation increases glucagon secretion.
- Adrenaline directly increases hepatic glucose output.

• Noradrenaline stimulates lipolysis. The increased FFA supports hepatic ketogenesis and gluconeogenesis.

• Noradrenaline causes peripheral (mainly cutaneous) vasoconstriction that results in decreased heat dissipation and consequent fever. Fever induces glucocorticoids, which promote gluconeogenesis and exert a permissive action on lipolysis.

The increasing hyperglycemic hyperosmolality of ECF initiates movement of water from the intracellular fluid (ICF) into the ECF. This autotransfusion of water decreases cell volume and increases intracellular osmolality. Such a cellular dehydration in the brain is a direct cause of impaired central nervous system (CNS) function. The cellular dehydration and the reduced ECF volume result in coma and *hypovolemic shock*, respectively. The condition, if untreated, will inevitably result in death through these two mechanisms.

Osmotic diuresis may lead to severe volume depletion/dehydration (usually 5 to 10% of body weight), which results in decreased GFR, increased levels of aldosterone, and antidiuretic hormone (Chaps. 10 and 12), and prerenal azotemia (see also Chap. 7). *Prerenal azotemia* is characterized by the disproportionate accumulation of blood urea nitrogen (BUN) and creatinine in plasma. Both compounds increase in plasma because of the decreased GFR. Unlike creatinine, urea is reabsorbed from the renal tubules (see Chap. 10). As long as there is no renal damage (which, however, may be present in long-standing diabetes), the tubular function of the kidney is unimpaired, leading to more accumulation of BUN than creatinine (their mass ratio rises above the normal range of 10 to 12). Note, however, that the ketone bodies interfere with the chemical determination of creatinine. Thus, ketoacidosis may present with a falsely elevated creatinine, and mask the prerenal azotemia. In clinical practice, hydration status is often assessed from urine output. In poorly controlled diabetic patients with osmotic diuresis the "normal" urine output does not indicate proper hydration, but further volume loss in spite of dehydration.

Osmotic diuresis results in the loss of several electrolytes, which must be replenished during the therapeutic intervention.

• In diabetic ketoacidosis, the H^+ ions are exchanged with intracellular K^+. This mechanism is important in attenuating the degree of acidosis because the intracellular proteins represent the largest buffering capacity. The K^+ entering the ECF is lost because of the osmotic diuresis. Depending on the actual stage in these fluxes, a patient may have hyperkalemia, hypokalemia, or normal potassium levels. In any case, *total body potassium is depleted*. The treatment of diabetic ketoacidosis involves volume replacement with saline and the administration of exogenous insulin. Insulin corrects the metabolic problem that led to acidosis in part by inhibiting ketone body production. Thus, the fluxes of H^+ and K^+ become reversed. In addition, insulin stimulates cellular uptake of potassium. Without adding potassium to the infusion, the patient could shift into life-threatening *hypoka-*

lemia. Before administering potassium, however, one must confirm that the patient is not hyperkalemic.

- *To correct the acidosis,* insulin must deliver sufficient quantities of glucose to the intracellular compartment. This glucose replenishes the pool of oxaloacetate, the acceptor molecule of acetyl-CoA in the TCA cycle. Thus, glucose allows a greater metabolization rate of ketone bodies. To achieve normal pH, *glucose often needs to be added to the infusion,* when plasma glucose decreases to about 250 mg/dL.

- The patient loses both phosphate and calcium with the osmotic diuresis. The hypocalcemia leads to increased secretion of PTH, which normalizes calcium but worsens the *hypophosphatemia.* Thus, part of the potassium replacement is often administered in the form of potassium phosphate.

- Insulin therapy is aimed at decreasing plasma glucose concentration at a slow rate (75 to 100 mg/dL/h). This allows time for the movement of glucose from the brain interstitial and cerebrospinal fluids into brain cells (to be utilized) and to the general ECF. Fast decrease of plasma glucose would induce the movement of water from the ECF to the brain and cause *cerebral edema.*

DKA is often precipitated in IDDM patients by stressful events, such as infections, surgery, or emotional upheavals. Stress mobilizes several insulin-antagonist hormones, including cortisol, adrenaline, glucagon, and GH. In the absence of functional β cells, the hyperglycemic action of these hormones can be antagonized only if the dose of insulin is increased. During the early stages of IDDM, the functional β cell mass may be sufficient to support glucose homeostasis under normal circumstances, but a stressful event may cause decompensation and result in DKA. Upon cessation of stress (such as the healing of an infection), the patient may be able to maintain euglycemia without exogenous insulin, until the β cell mass decreases below a critical threshold. At this point, exogenous insulin is needed even in the absence of stress. The phase in which exogenous insulin is needed only during stressful events is referred to as the *honeymoon period.*

Lactic acidosis may develop as a consequence of hypoxia related to poor perfusion of tissues. Severe lactic acidosis, however, is usually associated with the use of certain *biguanide* oral antidiabetic drugs.

The Somogyi Effect Is the Consequence of a Too-High Evening Dose of Insulin   Insulin-dependent diabetic patients usually receive several doses of insulin daily, which precede meals. If the evening dose of insulin is too high, after correcting the postprandial hyperglycemia, insulin will shift the patient into hypoglycemia, which occurs during sleep. This hypoglycemia activates counterregulatory mechanisms, such as glucagon, GH, adrenaline, and cortisol. In the absence of both endogenous and further exogenous insulin, these hormones cause significant hyperglycemia which occurs during the early morning hours, and worsens the overall glycemic control of the patient. This phenomenon is known as the *Somogyi effect*. This type of morning hyperglycemia can be corrected by decreasing the evening dose of insulin, thereby avoiding the activation of counterregulatory hormones.

The mechanism of the Somogyi effect is distinct from two other prebreakfast hyperglycemias: the dawn phenomenon and the waning of circulating insulin levels.

- The *dawn phenomenon* is caused by sleep-associated GH secretion that results in decreased insulin sensitivity with a few hours of lag time. Whereas, in the Somogyi effect the circulating levels of insulin are too high, they are normal in the dawn phenomenon, yet insufficient because of the decreased insulin sensitivity.
- The *waning of circulating insulin levels* is characterized by the decrease of plasma insulin to subnormal concentrations irrespective of the insulin sensitivity of tissues.

Prebreakfast hyperglycemia may be caused by these mechanisms alone or in combination.

Nonenzymatic Glycosylation of Proteins Can Be Exploited to Monitor Glycemic Control   Glucose is a reducing aldohexose, and as such carries a highly reactive hydroxyl group on its first carbonic atom known as the glycosidic hydroxyl group. When proteins are exposed to glucose, they become glycosylated in a non-enzymatic manner. The reaction is directly proportionate with the concentration glucose, and targets the primary amino groups carried by proteins. The targeted primary amino group is most often an ε-amino group of lysine or the α-amino group of the N-terminal amino acid. The reaction involves two steps:

- *Schiff base production* and
- *Amadori rearrangement*

The *Amadori products* are also known as *early glycosylation products*. At this stage the glycosylation is *very slowly reversible*.

This process affects mainly the extracellular matrix proteins, including collagens. The extracellular matrix proteins have a long half-life; this allows for the slow rearrangements of the early glycosylation products to form *irreversibly* glycosylated cross-linked proteins known as *advanced glycosylation end products* (AGE). AGEs are resistant to proteolytic degradation and have a prolonged lifespan. Formation of AGEs may occur between two collagen molecules; however, the process may result in the *trapping* of circulating proteins by collagen. This mechanism may account for trapping of LDL in the wall of blood vessels and development of atherosclerosis (see below). The glycosylation of collagen in the glomerular basement membrane alters its filter characteristics, and albumin becomes able to penetrate, which leads to proteinuria. The resulting glumerulosclerosis ultimately leads to the most severe form of *diabetic nephropathy*—chronic renal failure. Altered structure of the capillary basement membrane is a component of diabetic microangiopathy, which leads to leakiness of the capillaries and formation of edema. The microangiopathy is usually assessed by fundoscopy because the retinal vessels are readily visible. Their impairment, which is accentuated by long-term hypertension, may cause *diabetic retinopathy,* a leading cause of blindness in developed countries.

Measurement of the Amadori products of certain proteins in blood is suitable for monitoring *long-term* glucose control. The nonenzymatic glycosylation at any point in time is a function of glucose concentration, and compared to the lifespan of these circulating proteins the Amadori glycosylation can be considered irreversible. This means that glycosylation of these proteins functions as an integrator and reflects the "area under the curve": the duration and extent of hyperglycemia. Two proteins are used for this purpose in practice:

- *Glycosylated* (or glycated) *hemoglobins* (HbA_1 and HbA_{1c}). The lifespan of the RBC is 120 days, during which no new protein synthesis occurs. Glucose concentration within RBCs is identical with plasma glucose. The levels of glycosylated hemoglobins reflect blood glucose concentrations over the 4- to 8-week period prior to sampling. An empirical formula can be used for estimating the *average* blood glucose:

$$\text{glucose (mg/dL)} = 33.3\ HbA_{1c} - 86.$$

HbA_{1c} is normally 4 to 5.2% of total Hb.

- *Fructosamine test.* Fructosamine is generated from glycosylated proteins in a test tube; the test actually measures glycosylated serum proteins. Its normal value is 1 to 2% of the total serum protein. Due to the shorter half-life of serum proteins, the fructosamine test reflects blood glucose concentrations over the 2- to 3-week period prior to sampling. Thus, the effect of therapy adjustment on glucose control can be assessed earlier with the fructosamine test than with glycosylated hemoglobins, which is essential in the close monitoring of gestational diabetes.

Activation of the Polyol Pathway Is a Leading Cause of Diabetic Neuropathy and Contributes to Impaired Resistance to Infections   Many cells contain the enzyme *aldose reductase,* which reduces the aldehyde group of aldohexoses into an alcohol; the resulting molecules are termed polyalcholos or *polyols*. Glucose is reduced to *sorbitol,* galactose is reduced to *dulcitol.* Sorbitol can be further processed by a dehydrogenase to fructose. There are three requisites for overproduction of the polyols:

- Increased substrate level in plasma (hyperglycemia).
- Insulin-independent uptake of the substrate.
- Presence of aldose reductase in the cell.

Although the CNS takes up glucose in an insulin-independent fashion, it is largely unaffected by the polyol pathway because of the lack of aldose reductase. Axons of peripheral nerves, Schwann cells, endothelial cells, the cells in the lens of the eye, and white blood cells (especially neutrophil granulocytes) on the other hand are very sensitive to this mechanism.

- *Sorbitol accumulation means* the accumulation of an osmotically active substance, which in turn results in water influx and swelling of the cells (i.e., *osmotic cell injury*). Sorbitol accumulation is associated with a decrease of intracellular myoinositol content, which leads to decreased activities of the DAG-PKC and the IP_3-Ca^{2+}-pathways. This mechanism explains:
  - diabetic neuropathy, which primarily affects sensory and autonomic nerves. Involvement of pudendal autonomic nerves is a leading cause of erectile dysfunction. Diabetic neuropathy plays an essential role in the development of poorly healing *ulcus cruris* (ulceration affecting the skin of the leg and the foot), and cartilage degeneration in the foot *(Charcot's joint)*.
  - endothelial dysfunction and microangiopathy.
  - cataract formation.

Experimental *galactose* overfeeding of rats is suitable to activate the polyol pathway and induce a condition indistinguishable from diabetic neuropathy.

- The activation of the polyol pathway consumes intracellular NADPH, which is generated by the hexose monophosphate shunt. Because NADPH is crucial for the *neutrophil respiratory burst activity* (NRBA), NRBA is decreased and so is the efficiency of bacterium-killing by neutrophil granulocytes. In line with this, NRBA is negatively correlated with levels of HbA_1. This mechanism is in part responsible for decreased defenses against infections in diabetic patients. Diabetic patients often develop skin infections (such as staphylococcal *carbuncles* or corynebacterium-induced *erythrasma*) and fungal lesions such as vaginal yeast infections.

Tolrestat, an inhibitor of aldose reductase, has been effective in prevention of several diabetic complications both experimentally and in clinical trials.

Diabetic Macroangiopathy Is Caused by Derangement of Lipoprotein Metabolism and Hypertension   FFA are transported in blood bound to albumin. The plasma transport of other hydrophobic lipids is accomplished by macromolecular complexes known as *lipoproteins*. The highly hydrophobic triglycerides and cholesteryl esters found in the core of lipoproteins are enveloped by a *monolayer* of typical membrane components such as the amphipathic phospholipids, free cholesterol, and proteins. These proteins are known as *apolipoproteins,* which regulate the transport, processing, and cellular uptake of lipoproteins. The metabolism of lipoproteins is classified as the exogenous and endogenous pathways (Fig. 9-19).

Figure 9-19. Lipoprotein metabolism. Solid arrows indicate either movement or stimulation/increase. Touching curved arrows: lipoprotein interaction and material transfer. Dashed arrows indicate decrease/inhibition. Abbreviations: VLDL, very low density lipoprotein; IDL, intermediate density lipoprotein; LDL, low density lipoprotein; HDL$_2$, HDL$_3$ (two main subtypes), high density lipoprotein; surface (exchangeable) apolipoproteins, A-I, A-II, A-IV, C-I, C-II, C-III, E; core (nonexchangeable) apolipoproteins, B-48, B-100; apobec-1, apolipoprotein B mRNA-editing catalytic polypeptide-1; lipoprotein core lipids: TG, triglyceride; CE, cholesteryl ester; lipoprotein surface lipids: FC, free cholesterol; PL, phospholipid; LPL, lipoprotein lipase; HTGL, hepatic triglyceride lipase; LCAT, lecithin cholesterol acyltransferase; FFA, free fatty acid; FAT, fatty acid translocase; LRP, LDL-receptor-related protein. The left side

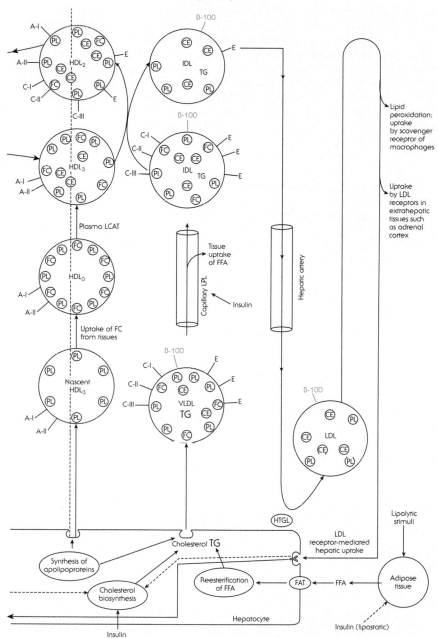

Figure 9-19. (*Continued*) of the diagram displays the exogenous pathway (chylomicron processing), the right side shows the endogenous pathway (VLDL/IDL processing) of lipoprotein metabolism. HDLs are shown in the midline: the apolipoproteins of nascent HDLs are produced by both the enterocytes and hepatocytes, and HDL interactions are crucial in the processing of both chylomicrons and IDL. HDL thus removes cholesterol from peripheral tissues (reverse transport) and enhances the clearance of lipoproteins via cycles of interaction involving transfer of both lipids and surface apolipoproteins.

• The *exogenous pathway* starts with the intestinal absorption of dietary lipids from the intestines. The absorptive enterocyte assembles *chylomicrons,* which in their nascent form contain apolipoproteins (apo) A-I, A-II, A-IV, and B-48. *ApoB-48* in humans is a unique product of enterocytes. The enterocytes and the liver express the same *apoB* gene, but only the enterocytes express the *apoB mRNA-editing catalytic polypeptide-1 (apobec-1),* which is responsible for the alternative splicing of apoB mRNA. This results in the appearance of an early STOP codon and a truncated protein product (apoB-48), as opposed to the hepatic form (apoB-100). Chylomicrons are approximately 1-μm diameter lipoproteins, which enter the intestinal lymphatic system that carries the milky-appearing *chylus* (hence the name of chylomicrons). Through the *thoracic duct,* lymph joins a low-pressure point of the venous system (the junction of the internal jugular and subclavian veins). Chylomicrons are normally cleared *rapidly* from blood involving several steps and mechanisms:

   • *High density lipoproteins* (HDL), whose apolipoproteins are made by the intestines and the liver, take up some cholesterol from chylomicrons, and directly transfer apolipoproteins C-I, C-II, C-III, and E to chylomicrons.

   • *Lipoprotein lipase* (LPL) is an enzyme associated with the glycocalyx of capillary endothelium in muscle and adipose tissue. This enzyme can be liberated from its endothelial binding by *heparin.* LPL liberates FFA from chylomicrons, which may be taken up by muscle fibers or adipocytes and used as an energy source or stored after re-esterification, respectively. *ApoC-II acquired from interaction with HDL is a mandatory component of LPL activation.* After being acted on by LPL, the *chylomicron remnant* returns the borrowed apoC proteins to HDL.

   • The mainly hepatic uptake of the triglyceride-deprived/cholesterol-rich chylomicron remnant is a process probably mediated by the interaction between the *apolipoprotein E* component of the remnant and apoE receptors, such as *LDL receptor-related protein* (LRP).

• The *endogenous pathway* starts with hepatic VLDL secretion. VLDL has an apolipoprotein composition similar to that of mature chylomicrons (i.e., contains apoC-I, -II, -III, and -E), except that it contains apoB-100. The production rate of VLDL is mainly determined by the availability of substrate. Thus, large amounts of VLDL are produced when plasma FFA levels are high, such as in diabetes mellitus. VLDL is processed by LPL in a manner similar to that of chylomicrons. The resulting lipoprotein is known as *intermediate density lipoprotein* (IDL), which is subject to further cleavage by *hepatic lipase* (an LPL-related ectoenzyme) yielding LDL. LDL is cleared from the circulation by the *LDL receptor* mainly in the liver, but also in peripheral tissues (see also Chap. 5). The LDL receptor-mediated clearance of LDL (a cholesterol-rich VLDL remnant) is significantly slower than that of the chylomicron remnant. The difference is due to the type of apoB present (Box 9-5). The high production rate of VLDL increases LDL production, which results in downregulation of LDL receptors and further accumulation of LDL in plasma. LDL may undergo peroxi-

BOX 9-5   Involvement of LDL-Receptor and Apo-B Subtypes in Hypercholesterolemia and Atherosclerosis

Patients with heterozygous familial hypercholesterolemia have 50% less LDL receptors than normal, and suffer from severe atherosclerosis especially of the large arteries (aorta, renal artery). In contrast, even homozygous LDL-receptor knockout mice are resistant to the condition. This is a direct cause of hepatic expression of apobec-1 in rodents, and the different clearance of lipoproteins containing apoB-48 and apoB-100. Apobec-1/LDL-receptor double knockout mice develop every facet of the human familial hypercholesterolemia, including the accentuated presentation in males.

dation, which makes it a ligand for the *scavenger LDL-receptor* expressed by several cell types, including macrophages. These macrophages may take up large quantities of cholesterol-rich LDL and turn into *foam cells,* which may become deposited in the subendothelial layer of the intima of large arteries and cause the development of *atherosclerotic plaques.*

Vitamin E, acting in concert with the selenoprotein *glutathion peroxidase,* effectively antagonizes peroxidation of lipids and the development of atherosclerosis. Dietary supplementation of vitamin E (400 IU/d) and selenium (50 to 100 μg/d) has been recommended for the prevention of atherosclerosis and certain malignancies, such as prostate cancer.

In diabetes, the accumulation of VLDL (known as *type IV hyperlipidemia*) is the cause of atherosclerosis and coronary heart disease. In type II diabetes (NIDDM), due to the upregulation of HMG-CoA reductase, the cholesterol content of VLDL is increased and more severe atherosclerosis develops. Hypertension hastens the development of atherosclerosis. As seen, insulin resistance may directly contribute to hypertension by decreasing endothelial nitric oxide synthase activity. Atherosclerotic plaques often develop in the renal arteries, and cause *renovascular hypertension* (see Chap. 12).

Other Pancreatic Hormones

Somatostatin Is an Inhibitor of Insulin Secretion But Has Uncertain Physiologic Relevance   SRIF is discussed in detail in relation with GH (Chap. 10). SRIF is produced by pancreatic δ cells, which are located mainly at the periphery of the islets. Thus, due to the preferentially central to peripheral perfusion of the islets, SRIF probably has minimal action on insulin secretion, and might inhibit glucagon secretion in a paracrine manner. Exogenously administered SRIF or its analogs, such as *octreotide,* used in the treatment of acromegaly may suppress insulin secretion and cause *hypoinsulinemic hyperglycemia. Somatostatinomas* of the pancreas may manifest in hypochlorhydria (decreased gastric acid secretion) and poor gallbladder motility leading to *steatorrhea* (undigested lipids in stool) and *cholelithiasis* (gallstones).

Amylin Is a Calcitonin-Related Peptide Product of β Cells, Which May Form Amyloid Deposits   *Amylin* (also known as *islet amyloid polypeptide* [IAPP]) is a minor product of the β cells and is cosecreted with insulin. In hyperinsulinemic NIDDM patients, the hypersecretion of amylin results in amyloid deposits surrounding the β cells. These deposits resemble those observed in Alzheimer's disease in the brain, and may contribute to the dysfunction of the β cells.

Pancreatic Polypeptide, the Product of F Cells, Is an Inhibitor of Digestive Functions   Pancreatic polypeptide is a 36 amino acid peptide, which is homologous with *neuropeptide Y* (NPY) and peptide YY (PYY). Pancreatic polypeptide is produced by the F cells in response to a mixed meal or duodenal acidification. The response is mediated by vagal parasympathetic fibers. Pancreatic polypeptide inhibits bicarbonate and enzyme secretion by the exocrine pancreas, and causes gallbladder relaxation.

Pancreatic Tumors May Be Manifestations of Multiple Endocrine Neoplasia Type I Syndrome and Produce Various Polypeptide Hormones   Type I multiple endocrine neoplasia (MEN) syndrome includes tumors of the pancreas, pituitary and the parathyroid glands. It is further discussed in Chap. 10 (see Box 10-3). Pancreatic tumors may secrete hormones that are normal products of islet cells (insulinoma, glucagonoma, somatostatinoma). However, they may produce other hormones such as

- *gastrin*, which induces overt gastric acid production and peptic ulcer disease of the duodenum. This condition is known as *Zollinger-Ellison syndrome.*
- VIP, which causes watery diarrhea, hypokalemia, achlorhydria (WDHA) syndrome.
- GHRH, which causes *ectopic acromegaly* via its action on pituitary somatotrophs.

10

THE HYPOTHALAMOHYPOPHYSEAL SYSTEM

OBJECTIVES

1. Discuss the anatomy and the development of the pituitary gland. Describe the neural and vascular connections between the hypothalamus and the pituitary gland. Describe the blood supply and the venous drainage of the pituitary gland.

2. Identify *parvocellular* hypothalamic neuronal groups that project to the median eminence, *magnocellular* hypothalamic neuronal groups that project to the posterior lobe of the pituitary gland, neurons that project to other areas of the brain, or function as intrahypothalamic connections.

3. Identify the normal and typical ectopic sources of *antidiuretic hormone* (ADH). Describe the transcription and translation of the ADH gene, the processing of pre-proADH, and the storage and release of ADH.

4. Discuss the ADH receptors and the biologic actions of ADH. Discuss the renal actions of ADH in detail. Describe the quantitative relationship between ADH-dependent and ADH-independent types of water reabsortion.

5. Discuss *aquaporins* (AQPs) and *urea transporters* (UTs). Identify ADH-dependent and other types of AQPs and UTs. Describe their role in the osmotic concentration of urine.

6. Discuss the quantitative aspects of water intake and water losses. Describe the assessment of water balance.

7. Discuss the regulation of ADH secretion and thirst. Identify overlapping and distinctive features, and the potential for dissociation of ADH and thirst regulation.

8. Discuss deranged regulatory processes: the types of *diabetes insipidus, syndrome of inappropriate ADH* secretion (SIADH), *primary polydipsia*, and *adipsic conditions*.

9. Describe the cell types and hormones of the *adenohypophysis*. Discuss general causes of pituitary hypofunction and hyperfunction, including pituitary adenomas and the *multiple endocrine neoplasia* (MEN) type I syndrome.

10. Describe the relationship between *growth hormone* (GH) and *insulin-like growth factor-1* (IGF-1). Discuss the structure, the receptors and the binding proteins of GH and IGFs.

11. Identify the direct and indirect (IGF-1-mediated) biologic actions of GH. Discuss effects of GH and IGFs on growth in utero and postpartum. Discuss the metabolic actions of GH and IGFs. Identify "other" actions of GH and IGF-1.

12. Discuss the *Pit-1* transcription factor and the regulation of gene expression and biosynthesis of GH. Discuss *GH-releasing hormone* (GHRH), *somatostatin* (SRIF), *GH secretagogues*, and their relationships with each other in the regulation of GH secretion. Discuss the regulation of episodic GH secretion. Discuss SRIF receptors, and describe their actions on secretion, cell proliferation, and neuronal electrical activity.

13. Identify the types of feedback loops used by pituitary hormones and discuss the feedback regulation of GH. Identify nutritional, physiologic, and endocrine factors, and neurotransmitter-specific drugs that either stimulate or inhibit GH secretion. Discuss the use of these factors in the clinical assessment of GH regulation.

14. Discuss states of GH deficiency and GH excess, identify the major features of clinical presentation, etiologies, and distinctive laboratory diagnostic features.

ANATOMIC CONSIDERATIONS

Anatomy and Development of the Pituitary Gland

The pituitary gland *(hypophysis)*, an endocrine organ weighing 0.5 to 0.9 g in nonpregnant adults, occupies the *sella turcica* (Turkish saddle) of the sphenoid bone (Fig. 10-1). The sella turcica is bordered on each side by the *cavernous sinus,* a venous sinus through which pass the internal carotid artery and cranial nerves III, IV, V/1, and VI. Doublings of the dura mater housing the cavernous sinuses hang from two pairs of bony structures known as the *anterior and posterior clinoid processes*. The doublings of the dura mater actually form the ceiling of the sella turcica known as the *diaphragma sellae,* leaving only a narrow opening for the passage of the *pituitary stalk* that connects the hypophysis with the hypothalamus. Although the arachnoid membrane follows the surface of the dura mater, the *basilar cisterns* containing cerebrospinal fluid (CSF) normally remain superior to the diaphragma sellae. The *optic chiasm* is found in the suprasellar space between the two anterior clinoid processes.

These anatomic relationships are important in understanding certain clinical situations:

• Tumors of the pituitary gland with suprasellar growth may compress the optic chiasm, compromise its blood supply, and impair vision. This usually presents as *bilateral (bitemporal) hemianopsia* (Fig. 10-2) because the compressed nerves that cross in the midline are derived from the medial portion of the retina (i.e., the portion receiving optical input from the lateral visual field). The compression is sometimes severe and may cause blindness.

   • The venous blood carrying the pituitary hormones enters the cavernous sinus, which is subsequently drained by the *superior and inferior petrosal sinuses,* and eventually by the *internal jugular vein.* In clinical practice, the blood of the inferior petrosal sinus is sometimes directly sampled by catheterization via the jugular vein to ascertain whether an overproduced hormone is derived from the pituitary gland or an ectopic site.

   • Whiplash type head/neck injuries may sever the pituitary stalk at the site where it passes through the diaphragma sellae. The injury results in the characteristic triad of diabetes insipidus, hypopituitarism and hyperprolactinemia (see Dysregulation of Water Balance and The Hormones of the Adenohypophysis).

   • When the subarachnoid space protrudes through the diaphragma sellae, the CSF may expand the sella turcica and flatten the pituitary gland. This condition, known as the *empty sella syndrome,* is usually associated with normal pituitary function, but may be mistaken for an adenoma on regular X-ray images of the skull.

The pituitary gland develops from two sources:

   • A protrusion of the nerve tissue of the hypothalamus together with a funnel-like extension of the third cerebral ventricle *(infundibular recess)* gives rise to the *neurohypophysis (posterior lobe).*

   • The developing neurohypophysis induces the development of the *adenohypophysis* (glandular hypophysis) that is derived from the evaginating placodial ectoderm of the primitive pharynx. The evagination yields a flattened, ball-like structure known as *Rathke's pouch.* The posterior wall of Rathke's pouch that is in direct contact with the neurohypophysis becomes the *intermediate lobe,* which is rudimentary in humans. The anterior wall of Rathke's pouch develops into the *pars distalis* (or *anterior lobe*), which contains the functionally most relevant and largest part of the adenohypophysis, and a thin mantle-like *pars tuberalis* (or *pars infundibularis*), which grows around the pituitary stalk. Remnants of the lumen of Rathke's pouch are present as cystic structures at the intermediate lobe.

Important clinical implications of the pituitary development include the following:

   • Because the development of Rathke's pouch requires the prior development of the neurohypophyseal process, *anencephaly* (lack of brain development, a neural tube defect) is usually associated with impaired pituitary development and function.

   • *Craniopharyngioma* is typically a slow-growing tumor derived from remnants of Rathke's pouch, which presents in children and young adults with hypothalamic and/or pituitary dysfunction.

A

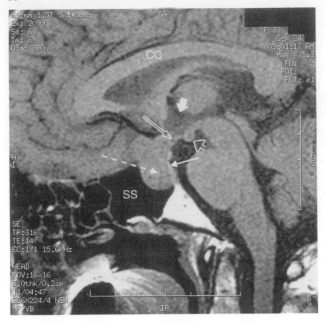

B

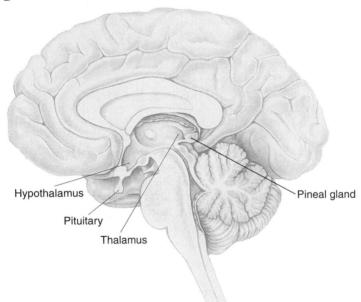

Hypothalamus

Pituitary

Thalamus

Pineal gland

Figure 10-1. The hypothalamus and the sella turcica. A and C are magnetic resonance imaging (MRI) scans of a patient having a pituitary macroadenoma; B and D are schematic representations of the normal anatomic conditions. A. Sagittal MRI of the brain at the hypothalamus and the pituitary gland. The adenomatous pituitary is shown by the dashed arrow; the posterior pituitary can be recognized by its high intensity (longer solid arrow). The wide solid arrow indicates the third cerebral ventricle; the long open arrow points at the *infundibular recess.* The wide open arrow indicates the *mamillary body,* which is the posterior border of the hypothalamus. CC, *corpus callosum;* SS, *sphenoid sinus.* B. Schematic representation of the brain comparable with the view seen in A.

C

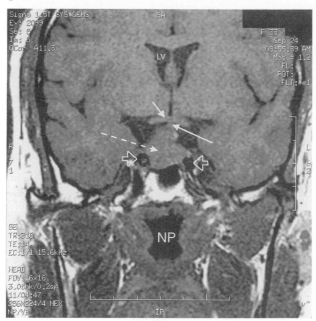

D

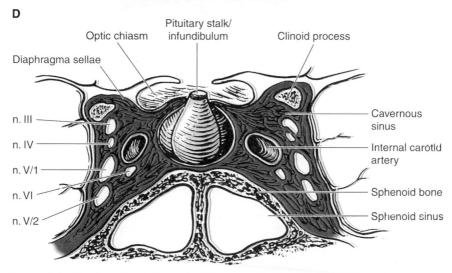

Optic chiasm

Pituitary stalk/
infundibulum

Clinoid process

Diaphragma sellae

n. III

n. IV

n. V/1

n. VI

n. V/2

Cavernous
sinus

Internal carotid
artery

Sphenoid bone

Sphenoid sinus

Figure 10-1. (*Continued*) C. Coronal MRI image of the brain in the plane of the pituitary adenoma (dashed arrow). On either side of the pituitary gland, the internal carotid arteries are seen as they pass through the cavernous sinus (open arrows). Short solid arrow: optic chiasm; long solid arrow: pituitary stalk/infundibulum. LV, lateral ventricle; NP, nasopharynx. D. Schematic representation of the pituitary in a plane similar to that seen in C. The cavernous sinus within the doubling of the dura mater contains the internal carotid artery and several cranial nerves. The *diaphragma sellae* spans between the clinoid processes and allows passage of the stalk. The arachnoidea follows the dura into the *hypophyseal fossa,* but the subarachnoideal space is normally negligible. Note the anatomical relationship between the sphenoid sinus and the hypophyseal fossa, which provides the basis of transsphenoidal operations of the pituitary. [*Source:* B: Kupferman I: Hypothalamus and Limbic System I: Peptidergic Neurons, Homeostasis, and Emotional Behavior. In: Kandel ER, Schwartz JH (eds): *Principles of Neural Science,* 2nd ed., p. 615: Fig. 46-3. A; Elsevier, 1985.)

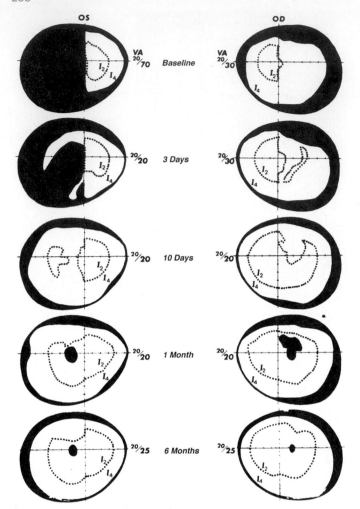

Figure 10-2. Asymmetrical bilateral hemianopsia. The visual field of this patient was narrowed due to compression of the optic chiasm by a prolactin-secreting pituitary adenoma. Therapy with the dopamine agonist drug bromocriptine resulted in a rapid involution of the tumor and recovery of the visual field and visual acuity. (*Source:* Rapid regression of pituitary prolectinomas during bromocriptine treatment. Thorner MO et al: J Clin Endocrinol Metab 51:438–445, 1980).

Neural and Vascular Connections Between the Hypothalamus and the Pituitary Gland

The pituitary gland is often referred to as a master gland because it regulates the function of several major endocrine glands. In turn, the function of the pituitary gland is regulated by the hypothalamus and feedback information from the "peripheral" endocrine organs acting either directly on the pituitary or indirectly via the hypothalamus. The coordinated function is achieved by neural and vascular connections between the hypothalamus and the pituitary gland.

The Anterograde Flow in the Hypophyseal Portal Vessels Delivers Hypothalamic Neurohormones from the Median Eminence to the Adenohypophysis   The arterial blood supply of the pituitary is provided by three pairs of direct branches of the internal carotid artery:

• The *superior hypophyseal arteries* supply the *median eminence* (the floor of the third ventricle, from which the pituitary stalk originates), where they form the *primary capillary plexus*. The blood of this plexus is drained by the *long hypophyseal portal veins* into the *secondary plexus,* which is the network of sinusoid (i.e., large diameter) capillaries of the adenohypophysis (Fig. 10-3). Both plexuses are formed by fenestrated capillaries. The hypothalamic neurohormones are liberated from the nerves into the extracellular fluid (ECF) of the median eminence near the capillaries, and are delivered by the *anterograde flow* of portal blood plasma to the anterior pituitary at high concentrations. They regulate the secretion of adenohypophyseal hormones. Note that a *retrograde flow* in the *subependymal plexus* (which forms anastomoses with the primary plexus) has also been demonstrated. The function of the retrograde flow is probably an immediate feedback from the pituitary to the median eminence.
• The *middle and inferior hypophyseal arteries* supply the pituitary stalk and the posterior pituitary. The *short portal vessels* connect the capillary plexus of the posterior lobe with that of the pars distalis.

Neural Tracts Originating from Magnocellular Hypothalamic Neurons and Projecting to the Neurohypophysis Liberate Their Neurohormones Near the Capillaries of the Posterior Lobe   The anatomic and functional connection between the hypothalamus and the neurohypophysis is primarily neural. The hormones of the neurohypophysis (*oxytocin* [OT] and *vasopressin* also known as ADH) are synthesized in the *paraventricular* and *supraoptic nuclei* of the hypothalamus. Both hormones are produced in both nuclei, but by separate sets of neurons. Unlike the small (parvocellular) neurons that produce the regulators of adenohypophyseal function, OT and ADH are produced by *magnocellular* neurons. The unmyelinated axons of these neurons form the *hypothalamohypophyseal tract,* which terminates in the posterior lobe. OT and ADH are structurally related nonapeptides synthesized as larger preprohormones in the perikarya (see "The Structure and Functions of Antidiuretic Hormone"). The cleavage of the prohormones occurs within the secretory granules during their *fast axonal transport,* an ATP-driven, colchicine-sensitive microtubular transport that proceeds at a rate of 2 to 8 mm/h. The axons pass through the median eminence and terminate in the posterior lobe. There the secretory vesicles accumulate and the hormones are stored in the *Herring's bodies* (varicosities of the axons). The hormones (and the associated cleavage products known as

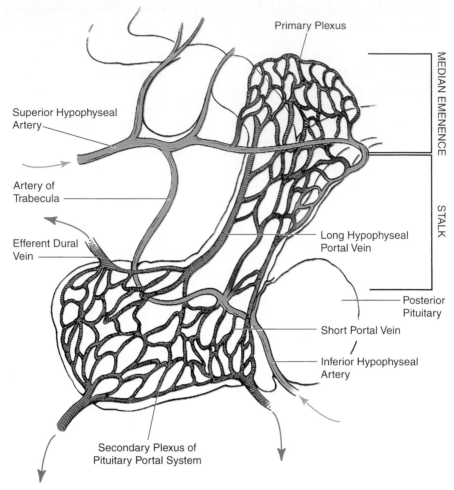

Figure 10-3. Pituitary portal circulation. The anterior pituitary is supplied by blood that first passed through the capillary bed of either the median eminence (long portal vessels) or the posterior pituitary (short portal vessels). (*Source:* Krieger DT: The hypothalamus and neuroendocrinology. In: Krieger DT, Hughes JC (eds): *Neuroendocrinology,* Sinauer Associates, Inc., Sunderland, MA, HP Publishing Co., Inc., New York, 1980.)

neurophysins) are liberated by exocytosis if action potentials travel down the same axon. The hormones are liberated near the fenestrated capillaries of the neurohypophysis, which is mainly drained directly by the cavernous sinus into the systemic circulation. The *pituicytes* of the posterior lobe are modified glial cells that are apparently not involved in hormone secretion.

Hypothalamic Structure

The hypothalamus is the inferior portion of the diencephalon located between the *lamina terminalis* and the *mamillary bodies* (Fig. 10-4). The hypothalamus is separated in the midline by the *third cerebral ventricle*. At the bottom of the third ventricle, the two sides of the hypothalamus are connected by the *median eminence*. The median eminence contains the nerve terminals that discharge the hypothalamic neurohormones into the primary capillary plexus, and the nerves in transit destined to terminate in the posterior pituitary. Thus, the pituitary stalk is a direct extension of the median eminence.

Clusters of perikarya (gray matter) form the *hypothalamic nuclei,* which are surrounded by nerve tracts (white matter). Some of the perikarya project to other parts of the central nervous system (CNS) or other hypothalamic nuclei, while others are neurohormonal in nature. These include the parvocellular and magnocellular neurosecretory systems. The names reflect a difference in neuronal size, which is related to the quantity of the neurohormones produced. The same nucleus may contain perikarya belonging to both systems.

- The hypophyseotrophic *parvocellular neurons* secrete minute quantities of *releasing hormones* and *release inhibiting hormones* near the capillaries of the median eminence. These factors reach high local concentrations and regulate the function of the adenohypophysis.
- The *magnocellular neurons* release their neurohormones near the capillaries of the neurohypophysis. These neurohormones reach their targets via the systemic circulation; thus, they are released in larger quantities.

Most of the nonhypophyseotrophic functions of the hypothalamus are related to the immediate regulatory mechanisms of reproduction and survival (such as thirst, hunger/satiety, energy expenditure, and thermoregulation). The regulatory systems of emotions, sexual behavior, and sex hormones are closely associated with one another. The morphologic basis of the association is the intimate connection between the hypothalamus and the limbic system. The arrangement of the hypothalamic nuclei is shown in Fig. 10-4. The nuclei can be localized in the topographical areas or zones of the hypothalamus:

- in the rostrocaudal orientation:
    - preoptic area

A

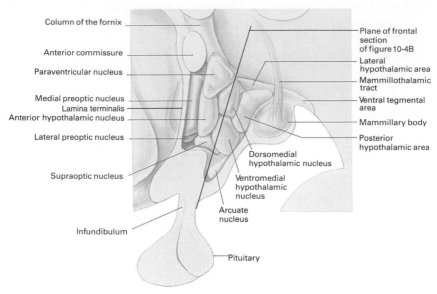

Column of the fornix

Anterior commissure

Paraventricular nucleus

Medial preoptic nucleus
Lamina terminalis
Anterior hypothalamic nucleus

Lateral preoptic nucleus

Supraoptic nucleus

Infundibulum

Plane of frontal
section
of figure 10-4B

Lateral
hypothalamic area

Mammillothalamic
tract

Ventral tegmental
area

Mammillary body

Posterior
hypothalamic area

Dorsomedial
hypothalamic nucleus

Ventromedial
hypothalamic
nucleus

Arcuate
nucleus

Pituitary

B

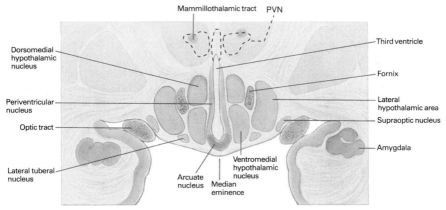

Mammillothalamic tract   PVN

Dorsomedial
hypothalamic
nucleus

Periventricular
nucleus

Optic tract

Lateral tuberal
nucleus

Arcuate   Median
nucleus   eminence

Ventromedial
hypothalamic
nucleus

Third ventricle

Fornix

Lateral
hypothalamic area

Supraoptic nucleus

Amygdala

Figure 10-4. Anatomic arrangement of hypothalamic nuclei. The dotted lines indicate structures that are anterior to the plane of this section: the contour of the third ventricle and the paraventricular nucleus (PVN). (*Source:* Fig. 46-3, p 615 and Fig. 46-4, p 616 in Kupferman I, Hypothalamus and limbic system I: Peptidergic neurons, homeostasis, and emotional behavior, in Kandel ER, Schwartz JH: *Principles of Neural Science*, 2nd ed., New York, Elsevier, 1985.)

- tuberoinfundibular area
- mamillary area (posterior hypothalamus)
- in the transverse orientation:
  - medial hypothalamus, which consists of the periventricular and the more lateral intermediate zones
  - lateral hypothalamus

- in the axial orientation:
  - dorsal and ventral hypothalamus.

Some of the prominent hypothalamic nuclei are listed in Table 10-1.

THE NEUROHYPOPHYSIS

As mentioned, the two major neurohypophyseal hormones are ADH and OT. In this section, we shall discuss only ADH in detail, and we defer discussion of OT to Chap. 13.

The Structure and Functions of Antidiuretic Hormone

ADH, Also Known as Arginine Vasopressin, Is a Nonapeptide Acting on Various G-Protein Coupled Heptahelical Receptors   The genes encoding ADH and OT are found on chromosome 20. They probably evolved by duplication and inversion of the ancestral gene as reflected by their homologous structures and opposite orientation on the opposite strands of DNA. After the cleavage of the signal peptide, the prohormones are cleaved to yield the nonapeptides ADH and OT, their neurophysins (neurophysin II and I, respectively) and, in case of the proADH, a glycopeptide (Fig. 10-5). The neurohypophyseal system is the psysiologic source of ADH and OT. However, circulating ADH maybe derived from ectopic sources: *small cell bronchial cancers* (derived from the amine precursor uptake and decar-

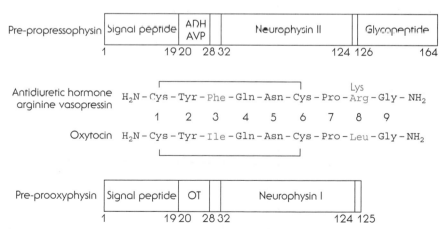

Figure 10-5.   The structures of the precursors of human antidiuretic hormone (ADH; also known as arginine vasopressin [AVP]) and oxytocin (OT). The OT precursor (preprooxyphysin) lacks the glycopeptide moiety. OT per se differs from AVP only in two residues of the nonapeptide sequence. The difference between AVP and lysine vasopressin (porcine ADH) at position 8 is also displayed.

Table 10-1   The Hypothalamic Nuclei and Their Main Functions

Nucleus	Location	Major neurohormones and/or functions
Supraoptic (SON)	Anterolateral, above the optic tract	ADH: osmoregulation, regulation of ECF volume; OT: regulation of uterine contractions and milk ejection

Paraventricular (PVN)	Dorsal anterior periventricular	Magnocellular PVN
		  ADH, OT: same functions as above
		Parvocellular PVN
		   TRH: regulation of thyroid function
		   CRH: regulation of adrenocortical function, regulation of the sympathetic nervous system and adrenal medulla, regulation of appetite
		   ADH: coexpressed with CRH, regulation of adrenocortical function
		   VIP: Prolactin-releasing factor (?)

Suprachiasmatic (SCN)	Above the optic chiasm, anteroventral periventricular zone	Regulator of circadian rhythms and pineal function ("Zeitgeber" [pacemaker]): VIP, ADH neurons project mainly to the PVN
Arcuate (ARCN)	Medial basal hypothalamus close to the third ventricle	GHRH: Stimulation of growth hormone GnRH: Regulation of pituitary gonadotropins (FSH and LH) Dopamine: functions as PIH SRIF: inhibition of GHRH release Regulation of appetite (NPY, ART, α-MSH, CART)
Periventricular	Anteroventral	SRIF: inhibition of growth hormone secretion by direct pituitary action; most abundant SRIF location
Ventromedial (VMN)		GHRH (as above) SRIF: inhibition of GHRH release Functions as a satiety center
Dorsomedial (DMN)		Focal point of information processing: receives input from VMN and lateral hypothalamus and projects to the PVN
Lateral hypothalamus		Functions as a hunger center (MCH, orexins)
Preoptic area (POA)		Main regulator of ovulation in *rodents*. Only a few GnRH neurons in primates
Anterior hypothalamus		Thermoregulation: "cooling center" AV3V region: regulation of thirst
Posterior hypothalamus		Thermoregulation: "heating center"

ABBREVIATIONS: ADH, antidiuretic hormone; ECF, extracellular fluid; OT, oxytocin; TRH, thyrotropin-releasing hormone; CRH, corticotrophin-releasing hormone; VIP, vasoactive intestinal polypeptide; GHRH, growth hormone releasing hormone; GnRH, gonadotropin-releasing hormone; FSH, follicle stimulating hormone; LH, luteinizing hormone; PIH, prolactin inhibiting hormone; SRIF, somatostatin; NPY, neuropeptide Y; ART, agouti-related transcript; α-MSH, α-melanocyte-stimulating hormone; CART, cocain and amphetamine-regulated transcript; MCH, melanin concentrating hormone.

boxylation [APUD] cells of the bronchi known as *Kulchitsky's cells*) often cause paraneoplastic syndromes. Their secretory product is most often ADH, leading to SIADH (see below). Their second most prevalent product is ACTH that may lead to ectopic Cushing's syndrome (see Chap. 12).

The name ADH refers to the renal action of the hormone (*antidiuresis* due to increased water reabsorption). It is also known as vasopressin because it may raise blood pressure by causing vasoconstriction, i.e., increasing peripheral resistance. Human ADH contains an arginine in position 8, whereas porcine ADH contains a lysine residue at the same position. For this reason, human and porcine ADHs are also referred to as *arginine vasopressin* (AVP) and *lysine vasopressin* (LVP), respectively.

ADH stimulates ACTH secretion from the corticotroph cells of the anterior pituitary gland; this action is in part due to potentiation of the action of corticotrophin releasing hormone (CRH). Because ADH has a direct ACTH-releasing action, researchers erroneously thought that ADH was the main physiologic hypothalamic releasing factor that regulated ACTH secretion. The ADH fulfilling CRH-like function does not necessarily originate from the magnocellular neurons and the posterior lobe: ADH is coexpressed with CRH in parvocellular paraventricular neurons, which project to the median eminence.

ADH is expressed by various sets of neurons and functions as a neurotransmitter. ADH along with neuronal α-MSH are *"physiologic antipyretics,"* which lower core body temperature. ADH improves memory by a hippocampal action. The latter action maybe rationalized as the need for remembering the site where water is available.

Circulating ADH acts on the *area postrema* (a circumventricular organ outside the blood brain barrier [BBB]) thereby modulating baroreceptor-mediated regulation of blood pressure.

ADH and OT circulate in plasma unbound to carrier proteins. They are rapidly cleared from the circulation mainly by the kidneys, but also by the liver and to a lesser extent by the brain. The placenta may also be a significant site of degradation. Both hormones have very short half-lives, which have been reported to be between 5 to 15 min. The action of ADH is mediated by various trimeric G-protein coupled heptahelical receptors (Table 10-2).

Accumulation of Solutes in the Renal Medulla Contributes to the Corticopapillary Gradient, the Driving Force of Water Reabsorption About 65% of the filtered NaCl is reabsorbed in the *proximal convoluted tubules* (PCT). The *thick ascending limb* (TAL) and the *distal convoluted tubule* (DCT) reabsorb 10 to 15% and 5 to 7% of the filtered NaCl, respectively. Unlike in the proximal tubules where water movement follows the reabsorption of NaCl, water reabsorption is minimal in these segments (and also in the thin ascending limb) because of the absence of aquaporins (see ADH Increases Water Reabsorption in the Collecting Ducts of the Kidney by

Table 10-2 ADH Receptors in Humans

Receptor subtype	Second messenger system	Tissue distribution	Function
V_1 (V_{1a})	PLC/PLA$_2$: DAG, IP$_3$, Ca^{2+}, arachidonate metabolites	Smooth muscle in the mesenteric artery	Vasoconstriction
V_3 (V_{1b})	Same as V_1	Pituitary gland	Release of ACTH, partly by potentiating the action of CRH
V_2	Adenylyl cyclase	Kidney	Antidiuresis by mobilization of AQP2 in the collecting ducts, stimulation of NaCl reabsorption in the thick ascending limb, stimulation of UT1-mediated urea reabsorption in the terminal inner medullary collecting ducts

ABBREVIATIONS: PLC, phospholipase C; DAG, diacylglycerol; PLA$_2$, phospholipase A$_2$; IP$_3$, inositol trisphosphate; ACTH, adrenocorticoph hormone; CRH, corticotrophin releasing hormone; AQP2, aquaporin-2; UT1, urea transporter 1.

Mobilizing Aquaporin 2). Due to the location and orientation of the thick ascending limbs and the distal convoluted tubules, reabsorption of NaCl generates a *corticopapillary osmolality gradient* (i.e., the osmolality is the lowest in the renal cortex and increases towards the renal papillae; see Fig. 10-6). Stimulation of the V_2 receptors in the thick ascending limb of the loop of Henle results in increased NaCl transport from the lumen into the interstitial space. In addition to NaCl reabsorption, ADH-regulated urea recycling is a significant contributor to the corticopapillary gradient (see ADH Stimulates the Reabsorption of Urea in the Inner Medullary Collecting Ducts Via Urea Transporter 1). Thus, ADH contributes to the development of the osmotic gradient in the renal medulla. Note that this action of ADH is antagonized in hypercalcemic states by stimulation of the calcium sensing receptors in the thick ascending limb (see Chap. 8).

The terminal segments of the renal tubules known as the *medullary collecting ducts* (MCD) run antiparallel with the thick ascending limb. The high osmolality of the medullary interstitial fluid would drive the reabsorption of water from the lumen of the medullary collecting ducts. This movement is regulated by ADH, which regulates water permeability of the collecting ducts.

ADH Increases Water Reabsorption in the Collecting Ducts of the Kidney by Mobilizing Aquaporin 2   As discussed (Chap. 1), the phospholipid bilayer of membranes is permeable to water. However, the water *permeability coefficient* of certain membranes (such as those in the thin descending loop of Henle, 1500 to 2000 μm/s) exceeds that of most other plasma membranes (50 μm/s) by thirty- to fortyfold. The increased water permeability found in certain tissues is related to the presence of water-selective channels called AQPs, a subfamily of the *membrane integral proteins* (MIPs). To date, nine aquaporins have been identified (Table 10-3).

AQP2, a water-channel exclusively expressed in the *collecting ducts* of the kidney (Fig. 10-6), is the only aquaporin directly regulated by ADH via V_2-receptor-mediated mechanisms:

- ADH induces the *biosynthesis* of AQP2 via a CREB-mediated transcriptional control mechanism (slow, long-term control).
- ADH *mobilizes* AQP2. Under resting conditions, the AQP2 protein is confined to intracellular membranes. The cyclic adenosine monophosphate (cyclic AMP)-activated PKA phosphorylates the Ser^{256} residue of preexisting AQP2 molecules. The phosphorylation results in the translocation of the vesicles and insertion of AQP2 into the apical (luminal) membranes of collecting duct cells. The vesicular movement involves *actin* filaments and colchicine-sensitive mechanisms, including *dynein*. This mechanism, which is the most important and rapid renal action of ADH, is reminiscent of that of insulin-induced translocation of GLUT4 (see Chap. 9).

The analogy is similar also in the sense that *renal water-handling includes ADH-dependent water-reabsorption via AQP2* (similar to insulin-dependent glucose disposal via GLUT4) *and ADH-independent water-reabsorption via AQP1, AQP3, AQP4 and AQP6* (similar to insulin-independent glucose disposal via GLUT1 and GLUT3).

As stated above, water moves across the cells of the collecting ducts toward the high concentration of solutes found in the interstitial space of the renal medulla. This movement is enabled if water channels are present both in the apical and the basolateral membranes of the collecting duct cells. Thus, the function of AQP2 in the apical membrane is complemented by AQP3 and AQP4 in the basolateral membrane of the same tubules. Note that similar to AQP2, AQP3 is also induced by dehydration. However, induction of AQP3 does not involve ADH. The transported water eventually enters the peritubular capillaries and joins the systemic circulation.

ADH Stimulates the Reabsorption of Urea in the Inner Medullary Collecting Ducts Via Urea Transporter 1 Urea, the major end product of nitrogen metabolism, is excreted by the kidney (see also *blood urea nitrogen* [BUN] in Chap. 7). An important element of the urinary concentrating process is the accumulation of urea in the interstitial compartment of the inner medulla. The accumulation of urea is a facilitated diffusion mediated by UTs (Fig. 10-6).

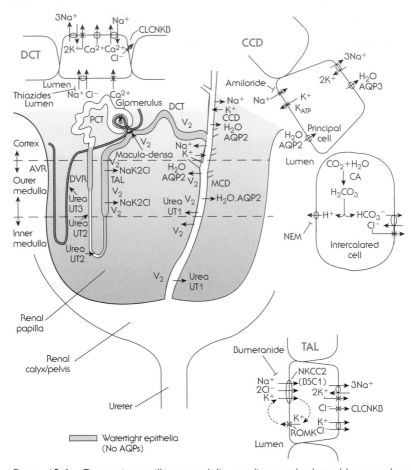

Figure 10-6. The corticopapillary osmolality gradient and selected hormonal regulatory mechanisms of renal function. The corticopapillary osmolality gradient (indicated by color gradient) is generated by sodium reabsorption in the thick ascending limb (TAL) of the loop of Henle and by UT1-mediated urea reabsorption in the medullary collecting duct (MCD). Both processes are stimulated by antidiuretic hormone (ADH). The renal actions of ADH are mediated by V_2 receptors. The action of ADH on TAL is antagonized by stimulation of calcium-sensing receptors (CaR) in states of hypercalcemia. Watertight epithelia lacking aquaporins (AQPs) are shown in color; in these segments, the movement of water following the transport of solutes is minimal. The proximal convoluted tubule (PCT) and the descending thin limb mainly express AQP1. AQP2 is mobilized by ADH in the cortical collecting duct (CCD) and the MCD; water reabsorption is driven by the accumulated osmolality. The CCD is the main site of action of mineralocorticoids. The handling of Na^+, K^+, H^+, Cl^-, and bicarbonate by the TAL, DCT and CCD are shown in the inserts. *Urea recycling* is achieved by the combined actions of UT1 in the MCD and UT2 in the descending thin limb. Urea may be washed out from the renal papilla by increased circulation and UT3-mediated uptake

- UT1 found in the apical membrane of terminal inner medullary collecting ducts mediates ADH-regulated urea reabsorption. The underlying mechanism is similar to the mobilization of preexisting AQP2 and does not appear to involve enhanced biosynthesis of UT1.
- The role of UT2 and UT3 is to minimize the escape of urea from the inner medulla.
  - UT2 enables urea reentry from the intersitial compartment into the descending thin limb thereby facilitating the process of *urea recycling.*
  - UT3 is constitutively expressed in the descending but not the ascending *vasa recta.*

The biosynthesis of UT2 (but not UT1) is upregulated by dehydration in an ADH-independent manner. In contrast, the biosynthesis of UT1 (but not UT2) is upregulated by a long-term low-protein diet. This mechansim helps to maintain the concentrating ability of the kidney by increasing urea reabsorption that compensates for the decreased hepatic urea production.

UT3 is also expressed in astrocytes and ependymal cells of the brain and in the Sertoli cells of the testis. At these sites significant quantities of urea are produced in the process of polyamine biosynthesis. Polyamines are important regulators of cell proliferation, which are mainly produced from orinithine by a decarboxylase enzyme (ODC; see also Chap. 5). UT3 allows for a rapid exit of the byproduct urea from the intracellular fluid (ICF).

Healthy Adults on a Normal Diet Must Excrete 800 to 1000 mOsm Solute Daily   As seen (Chap. 1), the normal range of plasma osmolality is between 275 and 295 mOsm/kg, and the ability of the kidney to modify the concentration of solutes in urine ranges between 50 and 1200 mOsm/kg. Healthy adults on a normal diet must excrete 800 to 1000 mOsm of solute daily. To excrete 1000 mOsm solute, the *obligate urinary water excretion* is 1000 mOsm per 1200 mOsm/kg water = 0.8 kg (0.8 L) water per day. This urine is maximally concentrated, which is indicated by a dark yellow/orange color (Box 10-1). If the requirement of obligate water excretion is not met, solutes accumulate in the ECF leading to the condition of *uremia.*

Conversely, due to the limits of renal dilution capacity, the maximum volume of urine is calculated as 1000 mOsm per 50mOsm/kg water = 20 kg (20 L) water per day. The maximally dilute urine is almost colorless.

Figure 10-6. (*Continued*)   in the descending vasa recta (DVR). AVR: ascending vasa recta. (*Source:* Modified from Fig. 1 in Dibas Al et al: Aquaporins (water channels): Role in vasopressin-activated water transport. Proc Soc Exp Biol Med 219:183–199, 1998; Fig. 1 in Hebert SC: Roles of Na-K-2Cl and Na-Cl cotransporters and ROMK potassium channels in urinary concentrating mechanisms. Am J Physiol 275:F325–F327, 1998; Fig. 3 in Tsukaguchi H et al: Urea transporters in kidney: Molecular analysis and contribution to the urinary concentration process. Am J Physiol 275:F319–F324, 1998.)

Table 10-3 Aquaporins

AQP subtype	Transport specificity	Tissue distribution and function
AQP0 (MIP26, a connexin [gap junction protein])	Water, sucrose, ascorbate, KCl, cyclic AMP, IP_3, Ca^{2+}, polyethylene glycol	Lens: AQP0 dysfunction may lead to cataract and presbyopia
AQP1 (CHIP28)	Water (glycerol?)	Proximal renal tubules, thin descending loop of Henle: 80–90% of the total renal water reabsorption Ciliary body: aqueous humor formation Choroid plexus: CSF formation Lungs: airway hydration and respiratory water loss, reabsorption of alveolar fluid RBC membranes: a determinant of osmotic resistance of RBCs Gallbladder: water reabsorption
AQP2	Water, H^+	Apical (luminal) membrane of collecting ducts of the kidney: ADH-mediated water reabsorption (responsible for concentrating urine)
AQP3	Water, urea, glycerol	Basolateral membrane of collecting ducts of the kidney (facing the interstitial space): allows the movement of water from the cell to the interstitial space; dehydration induces renal expression of AQP3. Cornea: assuring corneal transparency by removing glycerol phosphate and other small metabolites
AQP4	Water	Basolateral membrane of collecting ducts of the kidney (facing the interstitial space): allows the movement of water from the cell to the interstitial space Ciliary body: aqueous humor formation Choroid plexus: CSF formation
AQP5	Water	Salivary glands, lacrimal glands Lungs: fluid secretion
AQP6	Water	Kidney-specific expression. Probably involved in renal water handling
AQP7	Water, urea, glycerol	Spermatozoa: physiologic role unknown; responsible for the properties of sperm during cryopreservation
AQP8	The most water-selective channel	Salivary glands (including exocrine pancreas): secretion of saliva and pancreatic juice Colon: reabsorption of water

ABBREVIATIONS: AQP, aquaporin; AMP, adenosine monophosphate; CSF, cerebrospinal fluid; RBC, red blood cells; ADH, antidiuretic hormone; MIP, membrane integral protein; CHIP, channel-forming integral protein.

BOX 10-1 Urochrome

Urochrome, also known as *uroerythrin* a tripyrrole red pigment structurally related to the bile pigment *biliverdin.* In urine samples, it is adsorbed by the amorphous urate sediments. The daily excretion of urochrome is constant. Thus, urine color can be used for the quantitive assessment of hydration status.

If water intake exceeds the maximum urinary output, plasma osmolality decreases and *water intoxication* occurs.

Note that during starvation the amount of excreted solutes may decrease to as little as 300 mOsm/d. In this case, the obligate urinary water excretion becomes 0.25 L/d. Conversely, the maximum volume of urine becomes 6 L. Thus, during starvation, otherwise healthy individuals are more susceptible to water intoxication, and uremia will not occur in spite of subnormal urinary volume.

Because the volume of the isoosmotic glomerular filtrate is about 180 L/d, the *maximal ADH-dependent water-reabsorption* is calculated as $(20 - 0.8) = 19.2$ L, or $19.2/180 = 0.106$ (i.e. 10 to 11% of the filtered volume). The *minimal ADH-independent water-reabsorption* is $180 - 19.2 = 160.8$ L, or 89 to 90% of the filtered volume.

Water Balance Is Achieved by Regulated Water Intake and Water Losses The average adult loses approximately 2.5 L of water per day. To achieve water balance, this must be matched by the sum of water intake and metabolic production of water (Table 10-4). (Metabolic production of water is due to the oxidation of hydrogen derived from carbohydrates or lipids.)

Assuming a daily excretion of 1000 mOsm solutes in 1.5 L urine (the average daily values) the average osmolality of urine is 1000 mOsm/1.5 kg $= 667$ mOsm/kg (i.e. about 2.3-fold higher than that of plasma). This indicates that under normal circumstances, significant ADH-dependent water reabsorption occurs.

Table 10-4 Components of Water Balance

Input	Output
Water as liquids: 1600 mL	Urine: 1500 mL
Water in foods: 700 mL	"Insensible perspiration":
	• Cutaneous evaporation: 400 mL
	• Lung/respiratory water loss: 300 mL
Metabolic water production: 200 mL	Perspiration (sweating): 100 mL
	Stool: 200 mL
Total: 2500 mL	Total: 2500 mL

Obviously, the volumes shown in Table 10-4 are influenced by several environmental factors, such as the ambient temperature and humidity. For example, in a hot and dry environment such as the Arizona desert, to prevent hyperthermia, the body evaporates significant volumes of water, and the volume is replenished by drinking. Thus, temperature regulation has a significant impact on water homeostasis.

Disturbances of the gastrointestinal (GI) function may also have a significant impact on water balance. For example, choleriform diarrhea may result in a life-threatening loss of water via the GI tract.

The loss of water is accompanied by a loss of solutes, such as Na^+, Cl^-, HCO_3^-, K^+, and H^+. Depending on the relative losses of water and solutes, hyperosmolar or hypoosmolar conditions, acidosis or alkalosis, hyperkalemia or hypokalemia may develop, which provoke appropriate homeostatic responses. Thus, the homeostatic responses must restore both the volume and the composition of bodily fluids. The discussion here is focused on the regulation of "free water" by modulation of water intake and urinary loss of water.

Free Water Clearance Is the Volume of Solute-Free Water Excreted Per Day   To assess free water clearance, we calculate what would be the volume of urine if it were isosmotic with plasma ("osmolar clearance"), and we subtract this volume from the measured volume of the 24-h urine specimen:

$$C_{fw} = U_{vol} - (U_{osm} * U_{vol})/P_{osm} \tag{10-1}$$

This equation can be rearranged as

$$C_{fw} = U_{vol} * (1 - U_{osm}/P_{osm}) \tag{10-2}$$

where C_{fw} is the clearance of free water, U_{vol} is the volume of urine, U_{osm} is the osmolality of urine, and P_{osm} is the osmolality of plasma. $(U_{osm} * U_{vol})/P_{osm}$ found in the first equation is the osmolar clearance.

For example, the U_{osm} and U_{vol} of a 24-h specimen are 100 mOsm/kg water and 10 L, respectively. This represents approximately 1000 mOsm solutes per 24 h. The patient's plasma osmolality is 280 mOsm/kg water. Thus, the 1000 mOsm solute would be isosmotic if it were distributed in 1000/280 = 3.6 kg water (approximately 3.6 L urine).

As we can see, the free water clearance is a positive virtual volume when urinary osmolality is below that of plasma, and a negative virtual volume when urinary osmolality exceeds that of plasma. The free water clearance is useful in the quantitative assessment of water balance.

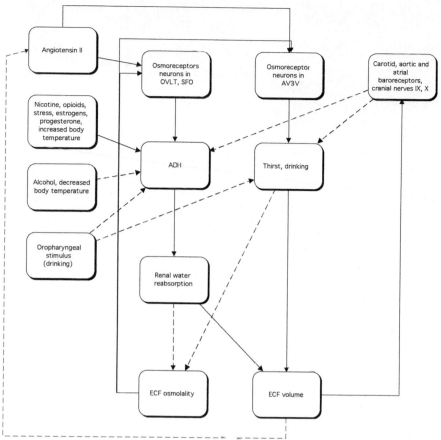

Figure 10-7. Feedback regulatory loops involved in the regulation of antidiuretic hormone (ADH) and thirst. The solid arrows indicate stimulation/increase; the dashed arrows indicate inhibition/decrease. Compare with Fig. 12-11 depicting the regulatory mechanisms of the renin–angiotensin–aldosterone axis.

The Regulation of Antidiuretic Hormone and Thirst

The Main Regulators of ADH Secretion Are Plasma Osmolality and Intravascular Pressure The regulatory mechanisms of ADH secretion and thirst are summarized in Fig. 10-7. As discussed, the main effect of ADH is water retention. Water retention may have two nonexclusive outcomes:

- decreasing the osmolality of ECF.
- increasing the volume of ECF.

These outcomes may also be achieved by drinking, a behavior prompted by thirst. *Thirst* is defined as a conscious sensation of a need for water and a desire to drink. There is an obvious need to limit expansion of ECF and

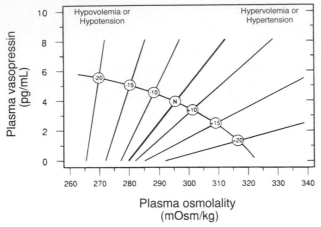

Figure 10-8. The impact of blood volume and/or pressure on the osmolality-induced secretion of ADH (vasopressin). The line labeled N indicates normovolemic (normotensive) conditions. The lines labeled with negative numbers indicate percent decrease in blood volume/pressure (hypovolemia, hypotension), those with positive numbers indicate percent increase in blood volume/pressure (fluid retention, hypertension). (*Source:* Robertson GL: Regulation of vasopressin secretion, in Seldin DW, Giebisch G (eds): *The Kidney: Physiology and Pathophysiology*, New York, Raven, 1985.)

to confine its osmolality within narrow limits. Not surprisingly, both ADH secretion and thirst are regulated by two main feedback mechanisms:

• Osmoreceptor control, the primary regulator of ADH, responds to a 1 to 2% increase in osmolality with a practically immediate hormone release. In healthy adults, the *osmotic threshold* at which the secretion of ADH begins is 280 to 284 mOsm/kg water.
• Baroreceptor control, which responds to a larger than 10% drop in the volume of ECF.

These two controls act in a coordinated fashion. At any given ECF volume, ADH secretion is proportionately increased with increasing plasma osmolality. A decrease in the volume of ECF enhances the ADH-response to any given increase in osmolality (Fig. 10-8). Note that other factors are also involved in the regulation of ADH.

• Stimuli of ADH secretion include
    • *Stress, via endogenous opioids.*
    • *Postural change.* Upon standing up after being in a recumbent position, the baroreceptor reflex stimulates ADH secretion (see below).
    • *Angiotensin II* (A-II, the regulator of aldosterone secretion) acts on the osmoreceptors of the circumventricular organs, which are unprotected by the BBB. A-II synergizes with the osmotic stimuli to induce ADH secretion and to increase thirst.

- *Nicotine.*
- *Estrogens* and *progesterone.* These hormones cause water retention during the luteal phase of the menstrual cycle.
- *Increased body temperature.*
- *Alcohol* induces diuresis by directly inhibiting ADH secretion. A *decrease in body temperature* also inhibits hypothalamic ADH; this action may reflect a negative feedback mechanism because ADH is a hypothermic agent.

Decreases in the Volume of ECF Elicit Concurrent Responses Leading to Sodium Retention via Aldosterone, Water Retention via ADH, and Water Intake via Increased Sensation of Thirst Changes in the volume of ECF often include concurrent loss of water and sodium under common conditions such as diarrhea, vomiting, or hemorrhage. To preserve and/or restore volume, the baroreceptor-mediated mechanisms typically exert a similar impact on ADH and thirst (regulation of water) and aldosterone (regulation of sodium). In contrast, osmoreceptor-mediated mechanisms selectively activate ADH and thirst, but not aldosterone. The control of sodium by aldosterone is further discussed in Chap. 12.

The *baroreceptors* involved in the regulation of ADH include the stretch receptors of the atria and the aortic and carotid sinuses. The signals from these receptors are communicated to the brain stem by cranial nerves IX and X. When blood pressure and the volume of ECF are normal, baroreceptors exert a tonic inhibitory influence over ADH secretion (compare to Chap. 12).

On occasion, the osmoreceptor and baroreceptor controls may be in conflict with each other. Severe volume depletion and the resultant hypotension override the hyposmotic inhibition of ADH secretion. This phenomenon is sometimes referred to as *the law of circulating volume.* Under these circumstances the baroreceptor mechanism may provoke high rates of ADH secretion that exceed even those seen during maximal hyperosmotic stimuli. These very high levels of plasma ADH cause hyposmotic volume retention and vasoconstriction that helps to increase blood pressure. In healthy individuals, the pressor response induced by exogenous ADH is short-lived mainly because of the baroreceptor feedback control of blood pressure.

The baroreceptor mechanism is also involved in the regulation of thirst: *hypotension and hypovolemia are dipsogenic stimuli.* Patients shifting toward hypovolemic shock complain about thirst.

A Distinct Set of Osmoreceptors Regulate ADH Secretion and Thirst The osmoreceptors responsible for regulating ADH secretion from the neurohypophysis are neurons found in certain circumventricular organs, mainly the *organum vasculosum laminae terminalis* (OVLT) and the *subfornical organ* (SFO). These neurons communicate with the ADH-producing hypothalamic neurons by *glutamate* receptors. The ADH responses to increased osmolality are not mediated by cholinergic mechanisms. Thus, the long-recognized antidiuretic effect of tobacco smoking which is mediated by the nicotinic receptors of ADH-producing neurons is not part of the physiologic osmoregulatory pathway. The high level of expression of AQP4 in the paraventricular and supraoptic nuclei suggest that ADH-producing neurons may directly respond to osmotic stimuli. However, the physiologic significance of this direct osmotic control of ADH is unestablished.

The osmoreceptors controlling thirst are probably located in a distinct area near the OVLT in the anteroventral region of the third ventricle termed the *AV3V region*. These osmoreceptors eventually communicate their signal to the cerebral cortex, but the neural pathway is largely unknown. Note, however, that the OVLT and mainly the SFO are the mediators of angiotensin II-induced drinking. The osmotic threshold of thirst coincides with that of ADH secretion. The osmoreceptors for thirst are *solute specific,* and respond preferentially to increased levels of *sodium* in the ECF. In contrast, acute elevations of *glucose* either in healthy volunteers or in patients with diabetes mellitus are not dipsogenic. Thirst in poorly controlled diabetes mellitus is related to hypovolemia secondary to polyuria.

Due to the selective damage to one or the other distinct set of osmoreceptors, osmoregulation of thirst and ADH seretion may become dissociated.

Oropharyngeal Inhibition: ADH and Thirst Are Acutely Regulated by the Act of Drinking   The act of drinking promptly inhibits ADH secretion and decreases thirst. The purpose of this mechanism, which involves *oropharyngeal receptors,* is to prevent overhydration. If drinking were stopped only when plasma osmolality returned to normal, hyperhydration would occur due to the delay between ingestion of water and its intestinal absorption.

The baroreceptor-mediated and oropharyngeal inhibition of ADH secretion are decreased in the elderly. In contrast, oropharyngeal inhibition of *thirst* is normal, whereas osmoreceptor-mediated thirst is decreased in this population. Taken together, these factors may contribute to the high incidence of *hypernatremia* among nursing home patients.

Dysregulation of Water Balance

Disturbances in ADH-Regulated Water Balance   The two main types of disturbances in ADH-regulated water balance are diabetes insipidus and SIADH. As pointed out (Chap. 7), conditions such as these may be suspected by the association of laboratory findings:

- Less than concentrated urine in face of high-normal plasma sodium (i.e., high plasma osmolality) may suggest diabetes insipidus.

Table 10-5 Normal Values
of ADH in Normotensive Individuals

Plasma osmolality (mOsm/kg)	ADH (pg/mL [pM])
270–280	<1.5 [<1.4]
280–285	<2.5 [<2.3]
285–290	1–5 [0.9–4.6]
290–295	2–7 [1.9–6.5]
295–300	4–12 [3.7–11.1]

• The laboratory hallmark of SIADH is the association of low plasma osmolality with less than maximally dilute (i.e., inappropriately concentrated) urine.

Accordingly, the normal plasma values of ADH must be interpreted in comparison with plasma osmolality and blood pressure. Table 10-5 shows the normal values of ADH in normotensive individuals (compare with Fig. 10-8).

Diabetes insipidus ("tasteless polyuria") develops when ADH-dependent water reabsorption is impaired. The water losses are replenished by increased water consumption *(secondary polydipsia)*. Secondary polydipsia is maintained by relatively high plasma osmolality (above the osmotic threshold of 284 mOsm/kg), which indicates that the regulation of thirst is normal. Diabetes insipidus causes an initial depletion of the ECF volume. The resulting hyperreninemia (see Chap. 12) causes increased plasma levels of angiotensin II, which contributes to the secondary polydipsia.

The relatively high plasma osmolality helps in the differential diagnosis of diabetes insipidus from *primary polydipsia* (a disorder of thirst, see below). In primary polydipsia, plasma osmolality is decreased by excessive water intake below the osmotic threshold, which leads to suppressed ADH secretion and consequent polyuria.

Diabetes insipidus may have central and peripheral etiologies.

• *Central diabetes insipidus* is usually related to the lack of ADH secretion.
• *Nephrogenic diabetes insipidus* is due to the resistance to the action of ADH.

Both types of diabetes insipidus may be either acquired or congenital. The central and nephrogenic types may be distinguished by the effectiveness of exogenously administered *desmopressin* (ddAVP), a long-acting agonist peptide analog of ADH. Desmopressin is well absorbed from the nasal mucosa. This route of administration is used in the therapy of central diabetes insipidus.

Acquired diabetes insipidus has various etiologies, including

- *Head trauma.* As noted earlier, whiplash injuries may disrupt the pituitary stalk. The subsequent *diabetes insipidus develops in three phases.* First, the disruption of axon continuity prevents action potentials of hypothalamic neurons from reaching the posterior pituitary, which leads to a prompt inhibition of ADH secretion. Second, after a few days, the axons degenerate, and the stored ADH is liberated in an unregulated manner. Thus, if ddAVP therapy was instituted during the first phase, the patient is in danger of water intoxication during the second phase. Finally, with the depletion of posterior pituitary ADH stores, permanent diabetes insipidus commences.

- *Craniopharyngiomas* may have the same impact on ADH as a head trauma, but due to the slowly progressing lesion, the above phases are not observed.

- *Lithium* therapy. Lithium is often used in the treatment of manic depression. Lithium decreases V_2 receptors in the kidney, which also leads to reduced expression of AQP2. Thus, lithium decreases renal responsiveness to ADH.

- *Colchicine* therapy of gout or antineoplastic therapy by *vinblastine* decreases renal responsiveness to ADH by inhibiting the mobilization of AQP2.

- *Electrolyte disturbances* including hypercalcemia (see Chap. 8) and hypokalemia.

- *Chronic renal diseases.*

Congenital diabetes insipidus also has multiple etiologies, including mutations of

- the ADH gene, which is inherited in an autosomal dominant manner;
- the V_2 receptor gene, which is inherited in an X-linked manner; and
- the AQP2, which is inherited in an autosomal recessive manner.

SIADH is characterized by continued ADH secretion in spite of plasma osmolality below the osmotic threshold. As mentioned, one of the leading causes of SIADH is ectopic production of ADH, which is not subject to the normal feedback control. The patients are *euvolemic* because the fluid retention is attenuated by an increase of glomerular filtration rate (GFR), which is maintained by hypertension. Another factor contributing to euvolemia and ameliorating the degree of hyponatremia is that, by an unknown mechanism, long-term exposure to ADH downregulates AQP2 synthesis. The treatment of SIADH includes fluid restriction and *demeclocycline.* The latter interferes with the action of ADH by blocking postreceptor mechanisms.

Other causes of SIADH include severe untreated cases of hypothyroidism *(myxedema)* and adrenal insufficiency (Addison's disease). A major difference in the presentation of SIADH between these and ectopic ADH-producing patients is blood pressure, which is characteristically low in patients with myxedema and Addison's disease. These patients tend to be hypovolemic and have decreased GRF. The hypovolemia may activate ADH secretion via disinhibition of baroreceptor feedback. The decreased GFR increases the fractional reabsorption of water in the renal proximal tubules. Both components predispose the patients to hyponatremia, which is exaggerated by the lost aldosterone function (sodium reabsorption) in Addison's disease patients.

Disturbances in the Regulation of Thirst   The two main types of dysregulation of thirst are primary polydipsia and adipsic conditions. *Primary polydipsia* is a pathologically increased desire for water intake. As discussed above, most cases of diabetes insipidus are accompanied by secondary polydipsia indicating that regulation of thirst is normal. The sensation of thirst in secondary polydipsia persists throughout the night, whereas *thirst dissipates at night in patients with primary polydipsia.* The laboratory analysis of randomly collected samples is sometimes insufficient for distinguishing secondary polydipsia from primary polydipsia, and a *water deprivation test* may be required. Water deprivation is done under supervision because primary polydipsia patients cannot resist obtaining water even if instructed otherwise. The patient's weight and urine output are monitored. Water deprivation results in a decrease in urine output (<0.5 mL/min) and an increase in specific gravity in primary polydipsia, but not in diabetes insipidus.

The causes of primary polydipsia are varied. One etiology is a selective dysfunction of the osmoreceptors mediating thirst sensation: the osmotic threshold of these receptors is lowered such that the patient feels thirsty at plasma osmolalities that completely suppress ADH secretion. Primary polydipsia may be a manifestation of schizophrenia or organic brain damage.

Adipsic (hypodipsic) disorders are characterized by the inappropriate lack of thirst and failure to correct hyperosmolality by drinking. In most cases the baroregulation of thirst and ADH are retained indicating that the condition is a dysfunction of osmoreceptors (Box 10-2).

BOX 10-2   Adipsic Disorders

Type A adipsia, also known as *essential hypernatremia,* is due to the increased osmotic threshold of the osmoreceptors. The osmoreceptors regulating both thirst and ADH secretion function at an elevated setpoint, *but the slope of the osmolality-ADH relationship is normal.* This condition may be misdiagnosed as central diabetes insipidus if thirst is not formally assessed. *Type B adipsia* involves a normal setpoint of thirst associated with abnormally shallow slopes of the osmolality-ADH and osmolality-thirst relationships. Complete destruction of the osmoreceptors results in *type C adipsia,* which may develop after surgical repair of an aneurysm of the *anterior communicating artery* of the circle of Willis. This artery supplies the OVLT and the AV3V region.

THE ADENOHYPOPHYSIS

In this section, an overview of the adenohypohyseal hormones is presented. Most of the adenohypophyseal hormones regulate classical endocrine glands, and are best discussed in detail together with their targets. In humans, growth hormone (GH, somatotropin) and prolactin (PRL, lactotrope, or mammotrope hormone) do not target classical endocrine glands. In this section, we shall discuss the growth hormone–insulin-like growth factor 1 (GH–IGF-1) axis, which serves as a prototype for the regulation of anterior pituitary function. Because the main functions of PRL are related to reproduction, the discussion of PRL is deferred to Chap. 13.

The Hormones of the Adenohypophysis

Similar to those of the neurohypophysis, all adenohypophyseal hormones are peptides. The adenohypophysis contains various hormone-producing cell types (Table 10-6).

The classical adenohypophyseal hormones belong to three hormone *families:*

- Derivatives of *proopiomelanocortin* (POMC), mainly *adrenocorticoph hormone* (ACTH).
- *Glycoprotein hormones. Thyroid stimulating hormone* (TSH), *follicle-stimulating hormone* (FSH), *luteinizing hormone* (LH), and the *placentally expressed* LH-like *human chorionic gonadotropin* (hCG) share a common subunit structure involving the same α subunit. The specificity of hormone-receptor interaction is assured by the β subunit, which is unique to each hormone. Note that the β subunits of LH and hCG are distinct,

Table 10-6   Adenohypophyseal Hormones and Their Cellular Sources

Cellular source and histological staining	Main hormone product(s)	Structure of hormone	Main functions
Somatotroph (acidophil)	GH also known as STH or somatotropin	191 amino acids, 22-kDa protein, mainly nonglycosylated	Stimulates the production of IGF-1 (the mediator of the indirect actions of GH). Also exerts direct actions on growth and metabolism. Modulator of immune function and hemostasis.
Lactotroph or mammotroph (acidophil)	PRL	198 amino acids, 23-kDa protein, mainly nonglycosylated (note: most of the decidually produced PRL is glycosylated.)	Stimulation of milk production (protein and lactose synthesis, water excretion, and sodium retention). Inhibits gonadotropin secretion. Immunomodulator.

Table 10-6 (*Continued*)

Cellular source and histological staining	Main hormone product(s)	Structure of hormone	Main functions
Corticotroph (small cells with "basophil" granules with strong PAS positivity indicating the presence of glycoproteins)	Derivatives of POMC, mainly ACTH and β-LPH	POMC: glycosylated polypeptide of 134 amino acid residues. ACTH: simple peptide of 39 amino acid residues, 4.5-kDa. β-LPH: simple peptide of 91 amino acid residues, 11.2-kDa.	ACTH: stimulation of glucocorticoids and sex steroids in the zona fasciculata and zona reticularis of the adrenal cortex, inducing hyperplasia and hypertrophy of the adrenal cortex. β-LPH: weak lipolytic and opioid actions
Thyrotroph (large cells with "basophil" granules with PAS positivity)	TSH	Glycoprotein hormone consisting of a shared α (89 amino acid) and a TSH-specific β (112 amino acid) subunit. Total size: 28 kDa.	Stimulation of all aspects of thyroid gland function: hormone synthesis, secretion, hyperplasia, hypertrophy, and vascularization.
Gonadotroph (small cells with "basophil" granules with PAS positivity)	LH: named after its effect in females. It is identical with the ICSH originally described in males.	Glycoprotein hormone consisting of a shared α and an LH-specific β (115 amino acid) subunit. Total size: 29 kDa	Females: stimulates steroid hormone synthesis in theca interna cells, lutein cells, and hilar cells; promotes luteinization and maintains the corpus luteum. Males: stimulates steroid hormone production in Leydig cells.
	FSH	Glycoprotein hormone consisting of a shared α and an FSH-specific β (115 amino acid) subunit. Total size: 29 kDa.	Females: targets the granulosa cells to promote follicular development. Stimulates aromatase expression and inhibin secretion by granulosa cells. Males: targets the Sertoli cells to promote spermatogenesis, and to stimulate inhibin secretion
Folliculostellate (glia-like) cells (part of the chromophobe cell population)	bFGF (FGF-2)	155 amino acids	Paracrine actions in the pituitary gland

ABBREVIATIONS: GH, growth hormone; STH, somatotroph hormone; IGF, insulin-like growth factor; PRL, prolactin; POMC, proopiomelanocortin; ACTH, adrenocorticotroph hormone; β-LPH, β-lipotropin; TSH, thyroid stimulating hormone; LH, luteinizing hormone; ICSH, interstitial (Leydig) cell stimulating hormone; FSH, follicle-stimulating hormone; bFGF, basic fibroblast growth factor. PAS, periodic acid Schiff (histochemical staining reaction).

yet recognize the same receptor. The selective immunologic detection of β-hCG in urine is utilized as a pregnancy test.

  • *Lactogenic* (somatomammotropic) hormones, including *growth hormone* (GH; also known as *somatotroph hormone* [STH] or *somatotropin*), *prolactin* (PRL), the *placentally expressed human chorionic somatomammotropins* (hCSs) also known as *human placental lactogens* (hPLs), and the molecular variants of these hormones. Similar to hCG, the pituitary glycoprotein hormones and all somatomammotropic hormones appear in urine.

In experimental animals, the main secretory product of the intermediate lobe is *α-melanocyte stimulating hormone* (α-MSH), a peptide identical with the N-terminal 13 amino acid residues of ACTH. In humans, the intermediate lobe is rudimentary and produces significant amounts of α-MSH only during fetal life. In adults, α-MSH is produced by neurons as a transmitter, whereas circulating α-MSH is derived from extrapituitary sources such as the skin (see Chap. 12).

Note that with the exception of GH and PRL, all classic adenohypophyseal hormones act on G-protein linked receptors, and their actions are at least in part mediated by cyclic AMP.

All hormone-producing adenohypophyseal cells store relatively large amounts of the preformed hormone(s) in secretory granules, whose staining is used for the classification of the adenohypophyseal cell types. The adenohypophysis is classified into *chromophobic* (nonstaining) and *chromophilic* (easily stained) cell populations. The classical adenohypophyseal hormones are produced by the chromophilic cells, which are subdivided into *acidophilic* and *basophilic* cells. The term "basophilic" refers to the blue staining of the secretory granules. This is actually a misnomer because the blue staining of the granules is achieved with anilin dyes and does not reflect true basophilic but *mucoid* (highly glycosylated) chemical character. In the adult human adenohypophysis, the chromophobic, acidophilic, and basophilic cells account for about 50, 40, and 10% of the cells, respectively. This percentage of chromophobic cells includes folliculostellate and unidentified cell populations. Today, the cell types are identified by immunocytochemistry, which utilizes hormone-specific antibodies. Hormone secretion by individual cells in vitro can be quantitatively assessed by methods such as the *reverse hemolytic plaque assay*. These studies have revealed functional heterogeneity among the producers of a given hormone, such as the amount of PRL released by lactotroph populations and their responsiveness to stimulatory and inhibitory factors.

The distribution of various cell types within the pituitary gland is nonrandom.

  • *Gonadotrophs* (FSH/LH-producing cells) and *somatotrophs* are most numerous in the *posterolateral region* of the pars distalis. This location apparently makes them the most vulnerable: gonadotroph function is the first to be impaired in most diseases that inflict mechanical damage on the pituitary gland.

• The *anteromedial region* of the pars distalis is the predominant location of *corticotrophs* and an almost exclusive location of the *thyrotrophs*. These cell populations, especially the thyrotrophs, are resiliant to locally damaging maladies such as tumors and granulomatous diseases.

• The lactotrophs are found throughout the pituitary gland. Some of the lactotrophs are associated with gonadotroph cells, which may provide the basis of paracrine interaction between these cells in the regulation of reproductive function. Others form a cluster close to the intermediate lobe, which may reflect the function of α-MSH in lactotroph development. The lactotroph is a relatively resilient cell population.

During pregnancy, the acidophilic lactotroph cells respond to the high levels of estrogens by hyperplasia. As a consequence, the pituitary almost doubles in size, which is only partially reversed after the cessation of lactation. Prolonged exposure to estrogens (such as contraceptive pills) is associated with the development of PRL-secreting adenomas *(prolactinomas)* in a dose-dependent manner. It is unclear whether estrogens cause the adenomas, or serve only as growth factors for the preexisting adenomas.

Pituitary adenomas are common in adults but rare in children. Pituitary tumors are usually monoclonal and are most often *microadenomas* (the largest diameter of the tumor is <10 mm). Larger diameter tumors are called *macroadenomas*. Bitemporal hemianopsia is usually due to macroadenomas exceeding 15 mm in diameter and having a *suprasellar extension* (Fig. 10-2). A common feature of these tumors that their hormone secretion is no longer subject to normal feedback suppression, and they function independent of hypothalamic input. Most adenohypophyseal tumors hypersecrete their specific hormone(s), a condition sometimes called *hyperpituitarism*. *Pituitary apoplexy* is the sudden hemorrhage of pituitary adenomas, a life-threatening event that may destroy the entire hypophyseal tissue.

Pituitary adenomas may occur as solo tumors or may be manifestations of MEN *syndrome* (Box 10-3). Among solo pituitary tumors, *prolactinomas* are the most common (26%), followed by the GH cell adenoma (13%). About one third of GH-secreting adenomas (4 to 5%) also secrete PRL and typically have two separate populations of cells (GH and PRL producers). These are distinct from the *acidophil stem cell adenomas,* which secrete both hormones from a single cell population reflecting the ontogeny of somatotrophs and lactotrophs (see later). Among basophil adenomas, corticotroph (8% of all anterior pituitary tumors) and gonadotroph (6%) adenomas are more common, and the incidence of TSH-producing adenomas is the lowest (<1%).

All adenohypophyseal hormones are secreted in a pulsatile (or episodic) manner (see Chap. 7). The episodic pattern is dictated by the synchronized secretory pattern of the hypothalamic neurohormones. The synchronization indicates that the neurons are organized into networks referred

BOX 10-3 Type I MEN Syndrome

Multiple endocrine neoplasia (MEN) syndromes are dominantly inherited familial disorders. MEN type I, also known as *Wermer's syndrome,* can be remembered as the "PPP" syndrome because it involves tumors of the pituitary, parathyroid, and the pancreas. These organs are involved in 65, 80, and 75% of MEN type I cases, respectively. In 20% of the cases, other organs may be involved, usually *carcinoid tumors* derived from gut and bronchial APUD cells. Cutaneous nonendocrine malignancies *(angiofibroma, collagenoma,* and *lipoma)* are also common. It is a prudent clinical practice to exclude MEN type I syndrome whenever a tumor of any of these glands is discovered. Thus, in case of a pituitary adenoma, plasma calcium should be evaluated to exclude primary hyperparathyroidism. Pancreatic tumors may secrete a number of bioactive peptides, such as GHRH, VIP, gastrin, and the peptides, which are also produced by normal islet cells. Some of these hormones do not cause overt symptoms and the tumor is localized by radiologic imaging. Gastrin-producing tumors, however, manifest in peptic ulcers due to the hypersecretion of hydrochloric acid by gastric parietal cells. This condition is known as *Zollinger–Ellison syndrome.*

The cause of MEN type I is the mutation of the *MEN1* gene on chromosome 11q13. The normal *MEN1* gene encodes *menin,* a 610-amino acid nuclear putative tumor suppressor protein that contains two nuclear localization signals. Menin inhibits the tumorigenicity of Ras as demonstrated with Ras-overexpressing transgenic cells that were injected into mice. The tumor suppressor function of menin involves direct binding with the JunD transcription factor and inhibition of JunD/Fos-activated transcription. Mutational analysis of the *MEN1* gene indicates its involvement in both familial and sporadic tumors of the glands involved in Wermer's syndrome. The mutation causes tumor development only in homozygous (or compact heterozygous) states supporting Knudson's *two-hit model of tumorigenesis.* The requirement for the second hit explains the delayed (usually 2nd or 3rd decade) manifestation of Wermer's syndrome.

Although the etiology of MEN type I is distinct from that of MEN type II (see Box 12-2), mixed forms of MEN types I and II have also been described.

to as *pulse generators.* The best characterized is the *gonadotropin-releasing hormone* (GnRH) *pulse generator,* which regulates gonadotropin secretion (see Chap. 13).

Most adenohypophyseal hormones are under a primarily stimulatory hypothalamic control. However, PRL is mainly under a tonic inhibitory control by the *PRL-inhibiting factor* (PIF), which has been identified as dopamine. This explains why, after an injury to the pituitary stalk that disrupts the hypophyseal portal vessels, the secretion of all pituitary hormones (including ADH and OT of the posterior pituitary) become diminished *(hypopituitarism)* except that of PRL, which is increased due to disinhibition.

If the hypophyseal tissue per se is destroyed, the secretion of all pituitary hormones becomes diminished, including PRL. This condition, known as *panhypopituitarism,* may develop after the infarction of the pituitary gland such as *Sheehan's syndrome,* which is usually due to sudden postpartum hypovolemia and reflex vasospasm leading to ischemia of the hyperplastic pituitary.

The Growth Hormone–Insulin-Like Growth Factor-1 Axis

In addition to being a major regulator of skeletal and "soft" tissue growth, GH functions as an important regulator of metabolism, mineral homeostasis, hematologic parameters and other physiologic functions. IGF-1 is produced in the liver (the main source of *circulating* IGF-1) and in most "peripheral" tissues (such as fibroblasts and chondroblasts) in response to *stimulation by GH*. The IGF-1 produced in the peripheral tissues may act in a paracrine/autocrine fashion. Thus, the biologic actions of GH are categorized as

- direct actions of GH and
- indirect actions of exerted by IGF-1 (also known as *somatomedin-C* [*somato*tropin's *medi*ator of action]).

Due to the local production and paracrine actions of IGF-1, the identification of direct and indirect actions has often been difficult. The biologic effects of GH and IGF-1 are usually classified as *growth promoting, metabolic,* and *other* actions. GH has direct growth-promoting actions that can be demonstrated by in vitro experiments. However, IGF-1 can mimic all the in vivo growth-promoting actions of GH. Thus, it is uncertain whether in vivo GH exerts a significant direct growth-promoting action. GH has direct *diabetogenic* metabolic actions, which antagonize those of IGF (see details later).

The clinical picture of GH overproduction presents either as *gigantism* (when the onset of GH overproduction is before epiphyseal closure) or as *acromegaly* (overproduction of GH after the epiphyseal closure is complete). Pituitary giants develop acromegalic features. Congenital selective *GH deficiency* results in *dwarfism* with normal bodily proportions. Taken together, these conditions help us in understanding the physiologic role of the GH–IGF-1 axis as a whole.

The lack of functional GH receptors results in a phenocopy of GH deficiency. This condition is known as *Laron-type dwarfism* or *congenital GH resistance syndrome*. These patients are treated with recombinant

Table 10-7   Selected Members and groups of Helix Bundle Peptides (HBPs)[a]

Group	Members	Group	Members
I: Lactogenic (somatomammotropic) hormones	**GH** (and its variants), **PRL**, hCSs (also known as [hPLs])	V	**LIF** oncostatin–M, IL–12, CNTF
II	EPO	VI	**GM–CSF**, IL–3, IL–4, IL–5
III	IL–2	VII	IL–7, IL–9
IV	IL–6, IL–11, M–SCF	VIII	Leptin

[a]The hormones in **bold** typeface are discussed in this book.

ABBREVIATIONS: GH, growth hormone; PRL, prolactin; hCS, human chorionic somatomammotropin; hPL, placental lactogen; LIF, leukemia inhibiting factor; IL, interleukin; CNTF, ciliary neurotrophic factor; GM-CSF, granulocyte macrophage colony stimulating factor; M-SCF, macrophage colony stimulating factor; EPO, erythropoietin.

IGF-1. This clinical setting helps us to understand the isolated biologic effects of IGF-1 and to decipher some of the direct actions of GH.

First, we shall discuss the structure, transport and actions of these hormones. Then we turn our attention to the regulation of their synthesis and secretion.

The Structure, Plasma Transport, and Receptors of Growth Hormone and Insulin-Like Growth Factor-1

GH Is a Member of the Helix Bundle Peptide Superfamily   The hormones of the *helix bundle peptide* (HBP) superfamily share the same overall 3-dimensional structure consisting of four antiparallel α-helices connected by random coil segments. The HBP superfamily consists of several groups of proteins, including the family of lactogenic hormones (Table 10-7). The amino acid sequences *within* each group are homologous, but dissimilar *among* the groups. HBP hormones act on members of *cytokine receptor superfamily* (see Table 5-1) and often display broad, partially overlapping biologic activities.

GH Belongs to the Family of Lactogenic (Somatomammotropic) Hormones   The genes of *GH* and *PRL*, which are phylogenetically derived from a common GH-like ancestral gene, are found on chromosomes 17 and 6, respectively. The *GH* locus on human chromosome 17q22-24 contains *hGH-N* (hGH-normal), a hCS-like pseudogene, *hCS-A*, *hGH-V* (hGH-variant), and *hCS-B*. The *hGH(-N)* gene is expressed in the pituitary gland, whereas the other four genes are expressed in the placenta. Due to alternative splicing, the *hGH* gene encodes for two polypeptides: the main 22-kDa GH and a minor 20-kDa variant. GH and hCS have two and PRL has three intrachain disulfide bridges, which stabilize their 3-dimensional structures.

The relationship between GH and PRL is also reflected by the following observations:

• Due to their structural homology, GH may crossreact on PRL receptors (see below).

- The GH and PRL receptor genes are closely associated on chromosome 5.

- PRL-producing cells develop from postmitotic GH-producing cells during ontogeny. The cell population reflecting this stage of development is referred to as the *somatomammotroph*. Pituitary adenomas secreting GH and PRL from a single population of cells (*acidophil stem cell adenomas,* see above) may arise from these cells.

- The gene expression of GH, PRL, and the β-subunit of TSH is directly regulated by a pituitary specific transcription factor known as *Pit-1*. Mutations of Pit-1 result in a simultaneous deficiency of these three hormones; the mutation was originally discovered in *Snell dwarf mice. Prophet of Pit-1 (PROP-1)*, a paired-like homeodomain transcription factor, serves as an early enhancer of Pit-1 gene expression. Its mutation, originally described in *Ames dwarf mice,* is probably the leading cause of *combined pituitary hormone deficiency (CPHD)* in humans, a condition that includes deficiency in all pituitary hormones, except ACTH. PROP-1 regulates the development and hormone expression of GH-, PRL-, and TSH-producing pituitary cells via Pit-1, and those of gonadotropin-producing pituitary cells via a Pit-1-independent mechanism.

Growth Hormone Is Transported in Plasma Either as a Free Hormone or Associated with GH-Binding Protein Derived from the Extracellular Domain of the GH Receptor   GH is circulating in plasma with an initial half-life of approximately 20 min. The initial half-life is related to the elimination of *unbound* GH from the circulation mainly by the liver (a major target organ of GH) and by renal filtration. Immunoreactive GH is present in urine.

Some of the circulating GH is associated with *GH-binding protein* (GHBP). GHBP is the extracellular domain of the GH receptor, which is probably liberated by proteolytic cleavage. The GH binding capacity of normal adult plasma is low and easily saturated by GH during the peaks of episodic secretion. However, between episodes of GH bursts when plasma GH levels are low, a significant proportion of GH is bound to GHBP. The eliminated free GH is continuously replenished from this pool. This explains that after the initial rapid elimination, the half-life of GH is about 50 min.

As noted, Laron-type dwarfism is a dysfunction of the GH receptors. In most cases, the GH receptors and thus GHBP are absent. Heterozygous individuals can be identified by their decreased plasma GHBP levels (about 50% of normal).

GH Activates the JAK–STAT Pathway by Dimerization of the Receptors by a Single Ligand   Human GH acts on its cognate receptor, but at high concentrations it crossreacts with the human PRL receptor. This explains why acromegalic patients may experience breast discharge (*galactorrhea;* see also Chap. 13). Note that the crossreactivity between GH and PRL is not mutual: even exterme hyperprolactinemia will not cause acromegaly without increased levels of plasma GH. Human placental lactogen (hPL or hCS), unlike its rodent counterpart, is structurally closer to GH than to PRL. Thus, hCS exerts more GH-like than PRL-like biologic activities.

Unlike the insulin receptor, the human GH receptor is highly species specific for its ligand. The mandatory need for human GH in the treatment of GH deficiency was initially resolved with hormone purified from human cadaver pituitary glands. Some of these GH preparations were contaminated with human *prion protein,* which caused *Creutzfeldt–Jakob disease.* This ultimately fatal "slow virus" *spongiform encephalopathy* (which is similar to *kuru, mad cow disease,* and *scrapie*) became avoidable with the introduction of human recombinant GH.

A single GH molecule can bind with two GH receptors (see Fig. 5-4). Dimerization of the GH receptor activates the Jak–STAT pathway (see Chap. 5). The receptor binding sites of GH are referred to as site-1 and site-2. Human GH receptor antagonists have been developed (such as Trovert®, B2036-PEG), in which site-2 is modified at a single amino acid thereby enabling GH-binding with only a single receptor. Dimers of GH found in the circulation ("big GH") are stabilized by the rearrangement of disulfide bonds to form interchain bridges. Big GH has a reduced biologic activity that is explained by steric hindrance of a receptor binding site.

The Type 1 Insulin-Like Growth Factor Receptor Mediates the Action of Both IGF-1 and IGF-2   We have already discussed some of the basic aspects of IGFs (*somatomedins* [Sm-s]) and their receptors (Chap. 9). Somatomedins were originally discovered as *"sulfation factors,"* which stimulated incorporation of sulfate into glycosaminoglycans synthesized by chondroblasts. A separate line of research led to the discovery of *nonsuppressible insulin-like activity* (NSILA) in serum (see Box 9-3). Sequencing of the purified polypeptides revealed that the sulfation factor Sm-C was identical with IGF-1, a major component of NSILA.

IGF-1 (Sm-C) and IGF-2 (Sm-A) are single-chain polypeptides of 70 and 67 amino acids, respectively. Together with insulin and the more distantly related *relaxin* (see Chap. 13) they comprise the *insulin-IGF family.* At least in mice, both *IGF-2* and the *type 2 insulin-like growth factor receptor* (IGF-2R) genes are imprinted: in most tissues *IGF-2* is expressed only from the paternally derived chromosome, and *IGF-2R* is expressed from the maternally derived chromosome. Neither the *IGF-1* nor the *IGF-1R* gene is imprinted. Unlike that of IGF-1, the secretion of IGF-2 is not GH-dependent.

The 3-dimensional structure of IGFs is similar to that of insulin (Fig. 9-11). Not surprisingly, the IGF-1 receptor (IGF-1R or type 1 IGF receptor) is a heterotetramer tyrosine kinase receptor, which is highly homologous with the insulin receptor (IR). In tissues expressing both IGF-1R and IR, hemireceptors may form hybrid tetramers. These *hybrid IGF-1R/IR receptors* are found at increased numbers in muscle and adipose tissues of NIMDD patients and may contribute to insulin resistance because they recognize IGFs but have a diminished avidity (affinity) for insulin. *The IGF-1R mediates the action of both IGF-1 and IGF-2.* The IGF-1R displays a hierarchy of binding affinities: IGF-1 > IGF-2 ≫ insulin. This binding hierarchy is essentially reversed for the insulin receptor: insulin ≫ IGF-2 > IGF-1. Hyperinsulinemia in the fetus of diabetic mothers results in *macrosomia* at least in part by activating type 1 IGF receptors.

The signal transduction pathway of the IGF-1R is also similar to that of the IR and involves *IRS-1* as a docking molecule.

The main function of the IGF-2 receptor (IGF-2R, also known as type 2 IGF receptor or *cation-independent mannose-6-phosphate receptor*) *is the clearance of IGF-2 from the ECF* (see also in Chap. 5). The IGF-2R does not bind either IGF-1 or insulin.

IGFs Are Mostly Confined to an Approximately 150-kDa GH-Dependent Protein Complex, Which Consists of IGF, IGFBP-3, and an Acid-Labile Subunit

Unlike insulin, IGFs circulate mainly in a carrier protein-bound form, which leads to a half-life of about 24 h. Six structurally homologous high affinity *IGF-binding proteins* (IGFBPs) with distinct tissue expression, regulation, and functions have been characterized. None of these proteins binds insulin. Less than 1% of the total plasma concentration of IGFs is unbound. At least 95% of the total concentration of IGF-1 and IGF-2 is confined to an approximately *150-kDa GH-dependent protein complex,* which consist of a molecule of *IGF-1* or IGF-2 (7.5 kDa), *IGFBP-3* (50 kDa), and an *acid-labile subunit* (ALS; 86-kD dimer). On the average, less than 4% of plasma IGF is bound to IGFBP-1, -2, and -4.

The name ALS refers to the observation that upon acidification-induced dissociation of the 150-kDa complex (pH 4.0), this subunit was irreversibly denatured. ALS functions as a binding protein of the preformed IGFBP-3/IGF complex by interacting with IGFBP-3. ALS, a member of the *"leucine-rich repeat" family of proteins,* is a glycoprotein.

All components of the 150-kDa complex are produced by the liver. It is important that *the biosynthesis of all components of the 150-kDa complex is regulated in a similar fashion: it is stimulated by GH and suppressed by catabolic conditions* such as caloric restriction, malnutrition, IDDM, or severe burns. A major difference in the regulation is that IGFBP-3 is stimulated by both GH and IGF-1, whereas ALS is stimulated only by GH and not by IGF-1.

Caloric restriction suppresses IGF-1 via a decrease of GH receptors. In case of protein restriction (with normal caloric input), the IGF-1 decrease appears to involve a mechanism distal to the GH receptor.

IGF-2, which is not regulated by GH, is most often the causative agent of non-islet-cell tumor-induced hypoglycemia (see also Chap. 9). The tumor-derived IGF-2 displays a higher than normal molecular size ("big IGF-2") and an impaired ability to bind to the IGFBP-3 150 kDa complex. These tumors may coexpress IGF-2 and IGFBP-6, which explains the shorter plasma half-life and greater bioavailability of tumor-derived IGF-2.

The Functions of GH and IGF-1   As mentioned, the effects of GH and IGF-1 can be categorized as growth factor-like, metabolic and diverse "other" effects. Both the growth factor-like and the metabolic actions contribute to the *promotion of skeletal and soft tissue growth*. The growth factor-like activities include direct stimulation of cell proliferation, promotion of differentiation and prevention of apoptosis.

Bone and Cartilage Are Major Direct and Indirect Targets of GH

A well-recognized effect of GH is the stimulation of bone growth and advancement of bone age (see also Chapter 8). These effects are in part direct actions of GH and in part mediated by IGF-1 produced mainly in skeletal tissue in response to GH. The skeletal growth effects include the stimulation of cell proliferation of *cartilage* (including the epiphyseal *growth plate*), fibroblasts, and mesenchymal cells, such as those of the periosteum and perichondrium. Thus, the GH–IGF-1 axis stimulates both endochondral and periosteal growth of bones. After epiphyseal closure, only appositional (both periosteal and perichondrial) growth is stimulated. This, as an exaggerated effect, accounts for certain *acromegalic features* (Figs. 10-9 and 10-10); that is, enlargement (*megaly*) of the *acra* (tips, edges, extremities) of the body, such as

- thickening of the skull bones;
    - growing of the jaw
    - because the teeth are unable to grow, the space between teeth widens
        - the chin becomes prominent
        - the more pronounced growth of the mandible than that of the maxilla results in a pronounced underbite *(prognathism)*;
- enlargement of the ears and nose;
- broadening of the hands and feet.

It must be emphasized that GH promotes soft tissue growth, and (mainly through IGF-1) may cause *organomegaly* in acromegalic patients. Organomegaly may include the liver, spleen, thymus, thyroid, tongue, and heart. The broadening of the hand is in part due to soft tissue overgrowth, which may cause *carpal tunnel syndrome.* Acromegalic patients typically have a "bulky" and moist handshake.

GH stimulates bone turnover (BMU activity) leading to an increase in the laboratory indicators of bone formation as well as bone resorption, such as plasma *alkaline phosphatase* activity. The long-term effect of physiologic levels of GH is the increase of bone mass and *bone mineral density* (BMD). Osteoporosis seen in the axial skeleton of acromegalic patients is the consequence of the PRL-like biologic activity of supranormal GH, which suppresses pituitary gonadotroph function and results in hypogonadism.

GH, IGF-1 and IGF-2 Play Different Physiologic Roles in Prenatal and Postnatal Growth

The role of GH in prenatal and early postnatal

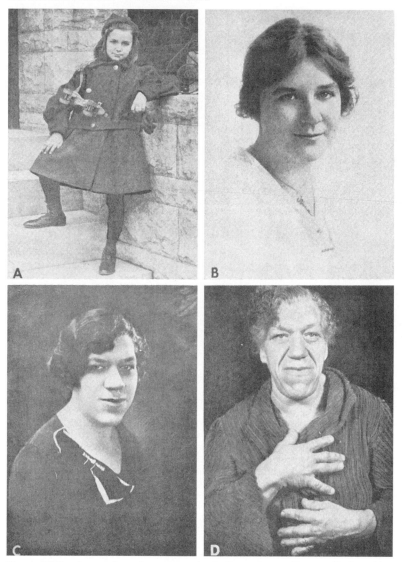

Figure 10-9. Progression of acromegaly. A. Normal, age 9 years; B. Age 16 years with possible signs of early coarsening features; C and D. Ages 33 and 52, respectively: well-established acromegaly. (*Source*: Mendeloff AI, Smith DE (eds): Acromegaly, diabetes, hypermetabolism, proteinuria and heart failure. Clinical Pathological Conference. Am J Med 20:133, 1956.)

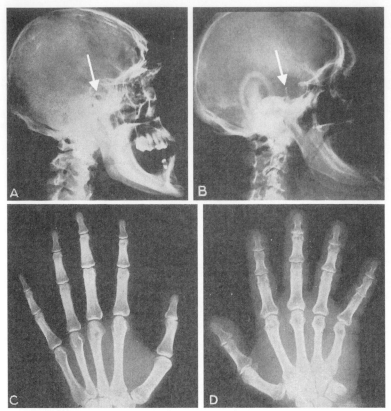

Figure 10-10. Radiologic manifestations of acromegaly. A, B: Lateral x-ray of the skull of acromegalic patients. The enlargement of the sella is due to macroadenoma (arrow). The mandible is elongated (prognathism). The calvaria is thick and the paranasal sinuses are enlarged, which contributes to the nasal quality of voice. C. Normal hand of a "big-boned" Swedish man. D. The hand of an acromegalic patient of about the same size. The acromegalic hand shows marked thickening of soft tissues, broadened bones with small osteophytes, and tufting of the distal phalanges. (*Source:* Fig. 18-40, p. 604 in Daughaday WH: The anterior pituitary. In Wilson, JD, Foster DW (eds): Williams Textbook of Endocrinology, 7th ed, Philadelphia, W.B. Saunders Company, 1985.)

growth has been a matter of controversy. Recent developments, however, have allowed a more accurate assessment:

• *While GH itself is not required, the stimulation of GH receptors is needed for normal prenatal somatic growth.* GH deficient infants are born with normal length and weight. However, Laron-type dwarf infants are born short and below normal weight. In addition, experiments with IGF-1 knockout mice indicate that IGF-1 is involved in normal intrauterine growth and maturation of bone, muscle and skin. These observations suggest that the GH receptor-IGF-1 axis is a regulator of intrauterine growth, and the activation of GH recetors maybe carried out by alternative ligands, such as hCS or placental GH-variant.

- *Whereas IGF-1 regulates somatic growth both in utero and postpartum, IGF-2 is important only in prenatal somatic growth.* Experimental evidence obtained with knockout mice indicate that IGF-1 and IGF-2 equally contribute to prenatal stimulation of growth. Knockout mice deficient in the IGF-1R are born with severe growth retardation and die because their hypoplastic breathing muscles are unable to expand their lungs. This finding illustrates the essential function of IGFs in the normal development and growth of skeletal muscle. Unlike IGF-1 knockout mice, IGF-2-deficient mice grow at a normal rate *after* birth.

Note that plasma IGF-1 levels increase from birth (11 to 206 ng/mL) and reach peak values in preadolescent or early adolescent years (134 to 836 ng/mL). Thereafter, plasma IGF-1 slowly but progressively decreases. The preadolescent peak value indicates the involvement of IGF-1 in the pubertal growth spurt. Indeed, increased rate of statural growth is the first (albeit easily overlooked) sign of puberty. The peak of plasma IGF-1 is accompanied by increased urinary GH output, indicating that GH secretion is enhanced during the pubertal growth spurt. The increased pubertal GH secretion is difficult to ascertain in plasma because of the episodic secretory pattern. Note that the episodic pattern of GH secretion is a more effective stimulus of growth than the constantly elevated plasma concentration of GH. The pulse amplitude of GH bursts is higher in males than in females. Accordingly, the *average* plasma IGF-1 is higher in males than in females, albeit the normal values show a very similar range.

As discussed below, GH secretion is under a negative feedback influence by IGF-1. Thus, under normal circumstances, hypersecretion of GH is prevented by the rise in circulating IGF-1. The concomitant increase of both IGF-1 and GH during puberty implies that the set point of negative feedback becomes elevated. Stimulation of hypothalamic estrogen receptors by circulating estrogens in females, or local hypothalamic conversion of circulating testosterone into estradiol in males, has been implicated in resetting the threshold of feedback. However, it is unresolved why both GH and IGF-1 begin their age-dependent decline at a time when no change in sexual steroid production is evident.

Thyroid Hormones Acting at Multiple Sites Are Essential for the Normal Growth-Promoting Function of the GH–IGF-1 Axis Hypothyroidism in infancy and childhood results in severe retardation of growth and mental development. The effects of thyroid hormones on growth include

- maintenance of GH production;
- permissive action for the IGF-1-stimulating effect of GH;
- permissive action for the growth-promoting effects of IGF-1.

Thus, upon correction of hypothyroidism, circulating levels of GH increase and the GH-induced increase of plasma IGF-1 is augmented. The thyroid hormone-enhanced growth promoting action of IGF-1 is more prominent in bones than in soft tissues. Thyroid hormones are important determinants of bone age.

The maintenance of GH production by thyroid hormones involves species-specific differences. In rodents, GH gene expression in the pituitary gland is directly augmented by thyroid hormones. In humans, thyroid hormones (T_4, T_3) suppress GH gene expression if they are present in supraphysiologic concentrations. Although the mechanism is uncertain, euthyroid concentrations of thyroid hormones are nevertheless mandatory for normal GH production.

GH Is Primarily a Diabetogenic Hormone, Which Opposes the Actions of Insulin and IGFs on Carbohydrate and Lipid Homeostasis   The metabolic effects of GH and IGF-1 are summarized in Table 10-8. GH is directly lipolytic and (mainly indirectly) promotes protein synthesis, thereby increasing *lean* body mass. For these effects, GH has been abused by professional athletes. In contrast, GH deficiency results in decreased muscle mass, increased lipid stores and may lead to obesity indicating that GH is a physiologic regulator of both muscle mass and adiposity (Box 10-4).

GH exerts several direct effects on adipose tissue:

• In vivo, GH inhibits the differentiation of committed preadipocytes into adipocytes and stimulates IGF-1 production of preadipocytes. IGF-1 may result in clonal expansion of preadipocytes by an autocrine/paracrine mechanism (see Chap. 15).

Table 10-8   Metabolic Effects of GH and IGF–1 in vivo

Function/parameter group	Function/parameter subgroup	GH	IGF-1
Carbohydrate metabolism	Glucose uptake in extra-hepatic tissues	Decrease[a]	Increase
	Hepatic glucose output	Increase	Decrease
	Hepatic glycogen stores	Increase (jointly with gluco-corticoids and insulin)	
	Plasma glucose	Increase	Decrease
	Insulin sensitivity	Decrease	Increase
Lipid metabolism	Lipolysis in adipocytes, plasma FFA levels	Increase	Decrease
	Plasma ketone bodies	Increase	Decrease
Protein metabolism (muscle, connective tissue)	Amino acid uptake	Increase (?)	Increase
	Protein synthesis	Increase (?)	Increase
	Nitrogen excretion	Decrease (?)	Decrease

[a]In GH-deficient patients, administration of GH results in a short-lived insulin-like action. During this time, glucose uptake by "peripheral" (extrahepatic) tissues increases.

ABBREVIATION: FFA, free fatty acid.

BOX 10-4   Body Mass Index

Body mass index (BMI) is used as an indicator of adiposity. BMI is calculated as the body weight (in kg) divided by the square of height/length (in meters). The BMI is an age-dependent parameter. The BMI in children decreases until the age of 6 years, followed by a gradual increase toward adult BMI. In lean adults, the BMI ranges between 20 and 24 kg/m² in women, and between 21 and 25 kg/m² in men. The sexual difference of BMI is mainly due to the larger muscle and bone mass in males. Obesity is usually diagnosed when the BMI exceeds 28 to 30 kg/m². The BMI, however, underestimates the degree of adiposity in GH deficiency and Laron syndrome because the increased adiposity is masked by the diminished bone and muscle (lean body) mass. Under these conditions, *skin fold thickness* is a more reliable measure of adiposity than BMI.

• *GH induces lipolysis,* an effect requiring the *permissive action of glucocorticoids*. Thus, whereas GH promotes adipose tissue growth via IGF-1, it directly depletes the triglyceride stores of adipocytes.

The breakdown of triglycerides increases plasma levels of FFA. As we have seen (Chap. 9), increased plasma FFA increases hepatic glucose output by providing the energy source for increased ATP generation, and the increased intracellular ATP shuttles the metabolic pathway toward gluconeogenesis. The increased FFA is probably the main cause of the *insulin resistance* observed in acromegalic patients.

In adults, GH is one of the defenses protecting against hypoglycemia below plasma glucose levels of 65 mg/dL (the average physiologic threshold of GH response). GH deficient adults compensate by using other hyperglycemic hormones such as glucagon, adrenaline, and cortisol. In neonates, however, GH is a preeminent antihypoglycemic hormone: GH-deficient and Laron syndrome infants often experience hypoglycemic episodes.

As their name implies, IGFs are insulin-like not only in structure but also in their metabolic actions. Due to the regulation of IGF-1 and because of the differences between IGF-1 and insulin, the impact of IGF-1 on metabolic regulation is complex.

• In acromegaly, when both GH and IGF-1 are elevated, the insulin-antagonist actions of GH prevail over the insulin-like effects of IGF-1 in terms of carbohydrate and lipid metabolism. Thus, the lipolytic and hyperglycemic actions of GH override the lipostatic and hypoglycemic actions of IGF-1. This is in part due to the GH-dependent increase of plasma IGFBP-3 and ALS, which in turn decreases the concentration of free IGF-1 thereby limiting the availability of IGF-1 for the interstitial compartment. In spite of the increased hepatic glucose output, acromegalic patients have increased hepatic glycogen stores. In terms of protein metabo-

lism, if GH exerts any effect directly, it is synergistic with that of IGF-1. Thus, IGF-1 and GH together yield a positive nitrogen balance and increase lean body mass.
  • As pointed out, GH deficiency may lead to obesity. This is also the case in Laron-type dwarfism (GH resistance), a condition treated with recombinant IGF-1. Insulin (in conjunction with glucocorticoids) is known to increase adiposity, and this effect is also expected from IGF-1. High doses of IGF-1 are indeed capable of increasing adiposity. However, when physiologic (replacement) doses of IGF-1 are administered, Laron syndrome patients typically react with growth accompanied by a *decrease* in adiposity. This is best explained by the relative effectiveness of IGF-1 in muscle and adipose tissues: *Unlike insulin, which (due to different numbers of spare receptors) is more effective in adipose tissue than in muscle, IGF-1 is more effective in muscle than in adipose tissue.* Indeed, IGF-1R expression is very low in adipose tissue. Thus, IGF-1 preferentially increases glucose uptake and utilization in muscle, and in the absence of overt caloric intake it results in a decrease of lipid stores.

  IGFs stimulate amino acid uptake and protein synthesis by muscle and fibroblasts, thereby promoting a positive nitrogen balance. The action of GH in this regard is unsettled. GH certainly does not oppose the effects of IGFs on amino acid/protein homeostasis. Some authorities argue that the effects of GH on nitrogen balance are all mediated by IGFs. Others argue that during protein deprivation, when a GH postreceptor defect leads to reduced production of IGF-1 (and a consequent increase in GH secretion), the metabolic actions of GH are retained, and its action on amino acid/protein homeostasis attenuates the degree of negative nitrogen balance.

  The GH–IGF-1 Axis Targets the Liver, Heart, Bone Marrow, Kidney, Brain, and Skin   Selected biologic effects of increased activity of the GH-IGF-1 axis are listed in Table 10-9. In most cases, it is uncertain whether GH or IGF-1 is the physiologic mediator of the effect.
  Acromegalic patients have a decreased life expectancy due to an increased risk for cardiovascular events, especially stroke and myocardial infarction. Acromegalic patients are usually hypertensive, which is in part due to the direct cardiovascular trophic action of GH. Cardiomegaly, however, is in part also the consequence of hypertension ("work hypertrophy"). GH stimulates the hepatic production of the clotting factor *fibrinogen*. The combination of these factors with altered metabolic parameters (such as hyperglycemia, hypertriglyceridemia) promote atherosclerosis and thromboembolism.
  GH affects both the connective tissue of the *skin* and epidermal skin appendages. Acromegalic patients have a thick dermis and hyperactive sweat glands, which accounts for a "wet bulky handshake." Laron syndrome patients often have sparse hair and a decreased ability of sweating. Hair

Table 10-9   Main Biologic Effects of GH–IGF-1 Axis[a]

Target/source	Parameter	Effect
Blood and Plasma (liver, bone and bone marrow actions)	IGF-1, ALS	Increased by GH only
	IGFBP-3	Increased by both GH and IGF-1
	Alkaline phosphatase (bone-specific)	Increase (mainly IGF-1)
	Fibrinogen	Increase
	Hemoglobin, hematocrit	Increase (mainly IGF-1 action on bone marrow)
Cartilage, bone	Length (before epiphyseal closure), width (periosteal and perichrondrial growth)	Stimulation (mainly IGF-1)
Visceral organs (liver, spleen, thymus, thyroid), tongue and heart	Growth	Stimulation/organomegaly (both GH and IGF-1)
Renal 25(OH) vitamin D 1α-hydroxylase activity	Plasma calcitriol	Increase (mainly GH), promotes positive calcium balance
Kidney	GFR	Increase (IGF-1)
Skin	Hair growth	Stimulation (IGF-1?)
	Sweat glands	Hyperplasia, hypertrophy, hyperfunction (GH?)
	Dermis	Thickening (both GH and IGF-1)

[a]For metabolic effects, see Table 10-8.

ABBREVIATIONS: IGF, insulin-like growth factor; GH growth hormone; IGFBP, IGF binding protein; GFR, glomerular filtration rate.

growth is promoted by IGF-1 in vitro and the distribution IGF-1 receptors in hair follicles suggest an involvement in the morphogenesis of hair. These findings indicate a physiologic regulation of hair follicles and sweat glands either by GH and/or by IGF-1.

GH is transported across the choroid plexus and reaches the brain via the CSF. The effects of pareneterally administered GH on neurotransmitter metabolism have been demonstrated in GH deficient adults. Moreover, in animal experiments parenteral GH has been demonstrated to induce ornithine decarboxylase (ODC) activity in several tissues including the brain suggesting a growth factor-like function of GH in the CNS. Because GH resistant patients are not mentally retarded, the CNS actions of GH and/or IGF-1 do not appear to be essential.

The Regulation of Growth Hormone

The Main Hypothalamic Neurohormones Regulating GH Secretion Are GHRH and SRIF   The main regulatory mechanisms of GH secretion are summarized in Fig. 10-11. The neurohormones GHRH and SRIF are liberated at the median eminence. They act directly on pituitary soma-totrophs and represent the *final common pathway* of most other GH-regulating mechanisms. Historically the hypothalamic neurohormones were referred to as "releasing (or inhibiting) factors" before their chemical identities were established, and the term releasing (or inhibiting) *hormone* is properly used for substances with defined chemical structures. However, not every authority subscribes to this terminology, and GHRH is still re-ferred to by some authors as *GH-releasing factor* (GRF). The term GRF, however, may refer to substances other than GHRH. Depending on the species, the age of the individual and the physiologic conditions, substances other than GHRH may fulfill the role of GRFs. To avoid confusion, in this text we shall use the term GRF in a broad sense as a "GH-stimulating sub-stance."

In addition to the dual (GHRH/SRIF) hypothalamic control, a novel regulatory system has been discovered. We shall discuss this system briefly under the heading of *GH secretagogue* (GHS).

GH Synthesis Requires Normal Levels of Glucocorticoids, Thyroid Hormone, GHRH, and a Functional Pit-1 Transcription Factor The prerequisite of GH release is prior synthesis, which requires expression of the GH gene. As mentioned above, the tissue-specific transcription factor Pit-1 plays a crucial role in the transcriptional control of GH. Expression of Pit-1 is enhanced by

- prophet of Pit-1 (PROP-1)
- IP_3 and Ca^{2+} in thyrotrophs (see Chap. 11);
- cyclic AMP in somatotrophs and lactotrophs. In these cells cyclic AMP is stimulated by GHRH and VIP (or unidentified *PRL-releasing factors* [PRFs]), respectively.

The shared cyclic AMP mechanism of somatotrophs and lactotrophs indicates that the Pit-1 response elements of GH and PRL genes rely on different co-activators. These coactivators include activated steroid hor-mone receptors: The expression of the GH gene requires normal levels of cortisol and thyroid hormones, whereas that of PRL requires estrogens. As mentioned above, the requirement for thyroid hormones for GH production involves different mechanisms in humans and rodents.

SRIF inhibits GH synthesis by several mechanisms (see SRIF Is a Functional Antagonist of GHRH and of Thyrotropin-Releasing Hor-mone [TRH]).

GHRH Stimulates the Synthesis and Release of GH, and Is Trophic for the Somatotroph Cells GHRH was originally isolated from an ectopic source: a benign pancreatic adenoma, which caused acromegaly. Due to the trophic action of GHRH, the patient had an enlarged pituitary gland,

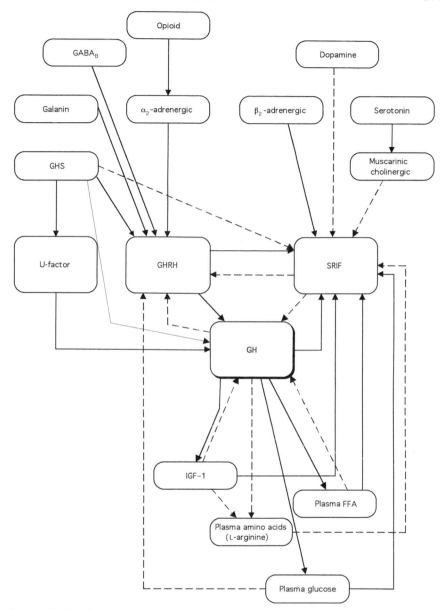

Figure 10-11. Regulation of the GH–IGF-1 axis. The figure neglects the impact of IGF-binding proteins, which are also regulated in part by GH and/or IGF-1R stimulation. The solid arrows indicate stimulation/increase, the dashed arrows indicate inhibition decrease. Note that two consecutive inhibitory mechanisms indicate an overall stimulatory influence due to disinhibition. GH, growth hormone; IGF-1, insulin-like growth factor-1; GHRH, GH-releasing hormone; SRIF, somatostatin-14; GHS, GH secretagogue; U-factor, unidentified GH-releasing factor; GABA, gamma aminobutyric acid. The putative U-factor requires normal GHRH-signaling for its action.

which led to the original (mistaken) diagnosis of pituitary adenoma and hypophysectomy. The otherwise silent pancreatic adenoma was sought only after histologic analysis revealed that instead of a cluster of monoclonal somatotrophs (as expected in a tumor), the entire pituitary displayed a hyperplasia of somatotrophs intermingled with other types of normal pituitary cells.

GHRH is normally expressed in neurons found in the arcuate and ventromedial nuclei of the hypothalamus. GHRH produced in other parts of the brain, the testis, or other tissues is not related to the regulation of GH. The most abundant isoform of GHRH is a 44-amino-acid long simple peptide. GHRH belongs to the secretin-glucagon family. Not surprisingly, its receptor is a heptahelical G-protein-coupled receptor (see also McCune–Albright syndrome, Chap. 8), whose action is primarily mediated by stimulation of adenylyl cyclase and PLC. PKA, by activating plasma membrane Ca^{2+} channels, and PLC, by IP_3, increase cytoplasmic levels of Ca^{2+} from extracellular sources and the endoplasmic reticulum, respectively.

In addition to its trophic action on somatotrophs, GHRH is a positive regulator of both the synthesis and the release of GH. An acute challange with intravenous GHRH results in a sudden discharge of stored GH secretory granules leading to a burst of plasma GH levels. The amplitude of the burst, however, is dependent upon several factors including

- the dose of the acute GHRH
- the GHRH receptor status of the somatotrophs
- the amount of stored GH.

In cases of suspected GHRH deficiency, the clinical evaluation may require *"priming"* with GHRH prior to the acute GHRH challenge test. The priming induces the synthesis of GH and enables the subsequent stimulus to release the stored hormone.

The episodic secretion of GH is directly coupled with the *episodic release of GHRH* (see Both GHRH and SRIF Contribute to the Episodic Pattern of GH Secretion). This pattern of GHRH secretion is important in the maintenance of GHRH responsiveness: continuous exposure to GHRH results in a significant *downregulation of GHRH receptors* and a blunted (submaximal) GH response to GHRH. Note that the continuous exposure to GHRH (such as in ectopic GHRH-induced acromegaly) maintains elevated GH secretion. Thus, the degree of GHRH receptor downregulation is not as severe as that seen in the case of the GnRH receptor (see Chap. 13).

Glucocorticoids exert a major influence over the GHRH system. Normal levels of cortisol induce not only GH expression but also that of the GHRH receptor. An acute challenge with glucocorticoids induces GH release. In Cushing's syndrome (*chronic* hypersecretion of, or exposure to, glucocorticoids) GH secretion is diminished. This is probably due to suppression of hypothalamic GHRH expression. Although normal concentrations of glucocorticoids are essential for certain actions of GH (such as lipolysis), excess glucocorticoids directly inhibit somatic growth by promoting a catabolic state involving increased muscle breakdown and decreased collagen synthesis.

SRIF Is a Functional Antagonist of GHRH and of Thyrotropin-Releasing Hormone (TRH)   The highly conserved *SRIF* gene on chromosome 3 encodes a 116 amino acid pre-proSRIF. ProSRIF is processed by tissue specific proprotein convertases predominantly yielding a 14 amino acid form (SRIF-14) in the brain and the pancreas, and a 28 amino acid form (SRIF-28) in the GI tract. SRIF-14 contains a single disulfide bond.

SRIF is produced by several neuronal groups in the brain and also in other tissues such as the placenta, immune system and APUD cells. The SRIF neurons involved in the direct inhibition of pituitary GH secretion are located in the anterior periventricular nucleus. An additional group of SRIF neurons is found within the arcuate and ventromedial nuclei. These SRIF neurons inhibit the release of GHRH, thereby depriving the somatotroph cells from a stimulatory signal.

The SRIF receptors (SSTRs, often designated as *sst*-s) are members of the G-protein coupled heptahelical receptor family. The effector coupling of these SSTRs is partially overlapping and heterogenous (Table 10-10). Note, however, that *all SSTRs inhibit adenylyl cyclase activity* (and thus antagonize GHRH) and, except for SSTR-4, all SSTRs are expressed in the pituitary gland. *SRIF is utilized as a general "turn-off" signal.* As such, *SRIF inhibits neuronal electrical activity, secretory processes and cell proliferation.* The inhibition of adenylyl cyclase and calcium channels explains the inhibition of secretion and, in certain tissues such as the pituitary, cell proliferation. The activation of K^+-channels leads to hyperpolarization, which in turn inhibits the voltage-gated Ca^{2+}-channels. The antiproliferative effects are in part mediated by the inhibition of MAPK and by stimulation of tyrosine phosphatase activities. This latter action antagonizes tyrosine kinase activity, which is typically increased upon activation of growth factor receptors. Stimulation of SSTR-3 may induce apoptosis in proliferating cells.

All SSTRs bind both SRIF-14 and SRIF-28. SSTRs-1 through -4 display preference for SRIF-14, SSTR-5 is weakly selective for SRIF-28. SSTRs can be categorized as two subfamilies:

• The first subfamily includes SSTR-2, -3, and -5, which react well with octapeptide and hexapeptide agonist SRIF analogs such as *octreotide* or *lanreotide*.
• The second subfamily includes SSTR-1 and -4, which react poorly with the same analogs.

The pituitary action of SRIF is not specific for the somatotroph cell, but include all Pit-1-expressing cell types. SRIF is a potent inhibitor of

Table 10-10 Effector Coupling and Tissue Distribution of Somatostatin Receptors[a]

	SSTR-1	SSTR-2[b]	SSTR-3	SSTR-4	SSTR-5
Adenyl cyclase activity	Decrease	Decrease	Decrease	Decrease	Decrease
Tyrosine phosphatase activity	Increase	Increase	Increase	Increase	—
MAPK activity	—	—	Decrease	Increase	Decrease
K$^+$ channels	Increase (hyperpolarization)	Increase (hyperpolarization)	Increase (hyperpolarization)	Increase (hyperpolarization)	Increase (hyperpolarization)
Chromosomal localization	14q13	17q24	22q13.1	20p11.2	16p13.3
Tissue distribution	Stomach Brain Pituitary Pancreas Kidney Liver —	Stomach Brain Pituitary Pancreas Kidney — Lung: carcinoids, small cell cancers, some non-small cell cancers	Stomach Brain Pituitary — — — —	Stomach Brain — Pancreas Kidney — Lung	Stomach Brain Pituitary — — — —

[a]Modified from Patel YC, Srikant CB. Trends Endocrinol Metab 8:398–405, 1997.
[b]Due to alternative splicing, SSTR-2 exists as two isoforms (SSTR-2A and SSTR-2B).

TSH secretion and thus acts as a functional TRH antagonist. SRIF is a modulator of lactotroph function: it only inhibits stimulated but not basal secretion of PRL. Proliferation of adenomas derived from all Pit-1-expressing cell types is typically inhibited by octreotide. In spite of the wide range of SRIF targets, long-term administration of octreotide in acromegalic patients is relatively free of side effects. In acromegalic patients, the GH-inhibiting action of octreotide is *more* pronounced than its inhibitory effect on insulin or TSH secretion. Nevertheless normalization of GH by octreotide may result in relative insulin-deficiency and hyperglycemia. The main (albeit preventable) side effect of octreotide therapy is the development of gallstones due to decreased emptying of the gallbladder.

Tumor cells often overexpress SSTRs, which can be exploited for diagnostic imaging. Scintigraphy after the administration of [111]Indium-labeled octreotide is especially useful in the localization of carcinoid tumors and small cell bronchial cancers. In addition, the growth of some of these tumors can be inhibited by octreotide therapy. Tumor cells are usually more sensitive to octreotide than normal tissues because they are less susceptible to receptor downregulation.

Both GHRH and SRIF Contribute to the Episodic Pattern of GH Secretion

As mentioned, GHRH is released in an episodic fashion. During a burst of GH, the increased GHRH secretion is accompanied by a decrease in SRIF secretion. It appears that the two subsets of SRIF neurons act in a coordinated manner: When the activity of GHRH release-inhibitors decreases (which permits increased GHRH output), the activity of those SRIF neurons, which inhibit GH directly at the pituitary level also decreases. Note that this latter is a disinhibition of GH secretion, which in itself stimulates GH release by a rebound effect. However, the rebound effect is accentuated by the concomitant release of GHRH, leading to an enhanced amplitude of the GH burst.

Whereas SRIF inhibits GHRH, the primary effect of GHRH on SRIF is stimulation. This, at least in part, explains the experimental finding that small doses of intracerebroventricularly administered GHRH inhibit GH secretion. GHRH may also inhibit its own secretion independent of its effect on SRIF (ultrashort-loop feedback). These mechanisms appear to be involved in the termination of the GH burst. *The main contributing factor to the termination of GH burst is the negative feedback provided by GH (short-loop feedback), which stimulates the biosynthesis and release of SRIF.* The long-loop feedback by IGF-1 shares these effects of GH. However, feedback through IGF-1 is probably too slow to account for the termination of bursts. Instead, feedback through IGF-1 regulates the overall daily GH output.

The feedback by GH can be experimentally demonstrated by a periodic infusion of GH that imitates episodic secretion. By using an appropriate time period, the endogenous episodic pattern becomes *entrained*.

GH Secretagogue Acts on the Pituitary, but Mainly Stimulates GH Secretion by a Complex Hypothalamic Action Enhancing the Episodic Secretory Pattern When testing various analogs of the endogenous opioid metenkephalin, it was discovered that some of these peptides were very potent inducers of GH secretion, albeit incapable of binding to opioid receptors. This led to the development of *GH-releasing peptides* (GHRPs) such as *GHRP-6* and *hexarelin*. Today the term *GH secretagogue* is used for GHRPs and nonpeptide drugs such as *MK-0677* stimulating the same receptors. All subtypes of the *GH secretagogue receptors* (GHSRs) belong to the G-protein coupled heptahelical receptor family. Unlike the GHRH receptor, GHSRs do not activate adenylyl cyclase but utilize signaling mechanisms similar to those of TRH. Thus, the effector of GHSRs is the PLCβ pathway, which increases cytoplasmic Ca^{2+} via IP_3. The GHSRs are currently orphan receptors: their endogenous ligand is unknown. Experimental and clinical pharmacologic data, however, provide an insight into the physiologic role of the (not necessarily peptide) "endogenous GHRPs."

Although GH secretagogues stimulate GH secretion by a direct pituitary action, their dominant GH-releasing action is mediated by the hypothalamus. The hypothalamic action involves

- actions on the arcuate and ventromedial nuclei
    - a direct stimulation of GHRH neurons projecting to the median eminence
    - an inhibition of those SRIF neurons, which project to GHRH neurons within the arcuate nucleus (the inhibition of SRIF neurons is probably mediated by local NPY neurons)
    - probable stimulation of an unknown alternative GRF ("U-factor"), which in turn acts on the pituitary.

The net effect of these actions is an *enhancement of episodic GH secretion by amplifying the amplitude of GH bursts*. Because GH is more effective when secreted in an episodic (rather than a continuous) manner, GH secretagogues may become the preferred therapy of certain types of GH deficiencies. An increasingly recognized GH deficiency is due to aging: above the age of 60 years, most individuals are GH deficient if the levels of young adulthood are used as a normal reference range. Restoration of GH in the elderly is still controversial: its benefits are variable and there is a potentially increased risk for development of tumors, especially colon cancer. However, GH secretagogues are promising drugs. An advantage of GH secretagogues over recombinant GH is that GH must be injected (similar to insulin or IGF-1), whereas GHRPs can be effectively delivered as nasal sprays, and nonpeptide GH secretagogues are active orally.

Endogenous GH secretion as well as the GH responses to various stimuli (including GHRH) are blunted in obese individuals mainly because of the inhibitory impact of free fatty acids (FFA). Although the response to GHS is also decreased, it appears to be the most potent GH-stimulus in obesity. GHRP has been used in assessing the pituitary GH reserve. Combined administration of GHS and GHRH induces an enhanced GH response, which exceeds those induced either by GHS or by GHRH alone. The enhanced GH response is in part explained by the SRIF-inhibiting action of GHS.

The Regulation of GH Involves Long-Loop, Short-Loop, and Ultrashort-Loop Feedback Mechanisms In the regulation of pituitary hormones, three types of feedback are distinguished (see Fig. 7-5). We have already discussed some of these feedback mechanisms above. IGF-1 exerts its action at two sites. In the pituitary, IGF-1 suppresses the transcription and synthesis of GH. In the hypothalamus, IGF-1 inhibits GHRH, which (at least in part) may be mediated by stimulation of SRIF. The hypothalamic action of IGF-1 is a more rapid mediator of feedback than its pituitary action. The long-loop feedback inhibition of GH is exerted not only by IGF-1, but also by metabolic parameters regulated by GH:

• *Decrease in circulating amino acids.* The decrease of amino acids (mainly arginine) is more along the lines of the withdrawal of a stimulus: postprandial hyperaminoacidemia stimulates GH, whereas the GH–IGF-1 axis decreases plasma amino acid levels by increasing the amino acid uptake and incorporation into proteins. Arginine infusion (0.5 g/kg arginine HCl over 30 min) is used as a GH-provocation test in clinical practice.

• *Hyperglycemia and elevated FFA. The inhibitory feedback by these metabolic parameters is operational only if at least normal levels of IGF-1 are present.* This is evidenced in poorly controlled type I diabetic patients, whose IGF-1 levels are low due to relative cellular starvation, and their elevated plasma glucose and FFA are unable to suppress GH secretion.

   • GH promotes hyperglycemia. Hyperglycemia stimulates the SRIF neurons thereby inhibiting GH. Conversely, hypoglycemia is among the strongest stimuli of GH secretion. Hypoglycemia not only inhibits SRIF (which is its main target) but also stimulates GHRH. The released GH attempts to restore euglycemia. Glucose-mediated suppression of GH (in conjunction with an oral glucose tolerance test) is used in the diagnosis of acromegaly: in case of an adenoma, glucose is unable to inhibit GH secretion. As a clinical test, insulin-induced hypoglycemia (<40 mg/dL plasma glucose) is used in the diagnosis of GH insufficiency.

   • GH increases plasma FFA by its lipolytic action. The elevated FFA in turn suppresses GH secretion. This is a strong inhibitory input that may override the stimulatory action of arginine. The target of FFA action is at least in part the stimulation of SRIF neurons, although a direct pituitary inhibition of GH has also been suggested.

GHRH and SRIF Are Influenced by Several Physiologic and Pharmacologic Factors As mentioned, GHRH and SRIF (and perhaps the

Table 10-11   Selected Physiologic and Pharmacologic Regulators
of GH Secretion

Category	Stimulators of GH	Inhibitors of GH
Nutrition	Hypoglycemia (absolute and relative)	Hyperglycemia
	Postprandial hyperaminoacidemia (primarily arginine)	Supranormal plasma FFA
	Prolonged fasting and/or protein deprivation	Obesity
Stress	Acute stress: Exercise, psychological stress, pain, physical stress (such as high environmental temperature)	Chronic stress
Hormones	GHRH	Hypothyroidism
	Sex steroids (via estrogen receptors)	Glucocorticoid excess (Cushing's disease) or deficiency (Addison's disease)
	VIP, TRH (only if a GH secreting adenoma is present)	Progesterone (cortisol-like action)
Neurotransmitters and drugs	Dopamine agonists penetrating the blood brain barrier (central action, healthy subjects): bromocriptine, levodopa	Dopamine agonists (in *acromegalic* subjects, pituitary action dominates): bromocriptine
	—	Dopamine antagonists (in nonacromegalic subjects): phenotiazines, pimozide
	α_2 adrenergic agonists: clonidine	α_1 adrenergic agonists: prazosin, nonselective α-adrenergic agonists (action uncertain in humans)
	β_2 adrenergic antagonists: propranolol	β_2 adrenergic agonists: isoproterenol
	Serotonin precursor: 5-HTP	Serotonin antagonists: methysergide, LSD
	Opioids: morphin, endogenous opioids (β-endorphin)	Opioid antagonists: naloxone
	Cholinergic tone: physostigmine	Muscarinic cholinergic antagonists: atropine

ABBREVIATIONS: GH, growth hormone; FFA, free fatty acids; GHRH, GH-releasing hormone; LSD, lysergic acid diethylamide; VIP, vasoactive intestinal peptide; TRH, thyrotropin releasing hormone; 5-HTP, 5-hydroxy-L-tryptophan.

"U-factor") are the final common pathways of the neural inputs modulating GH secretion. The precise mechanisms underlying the regulation of GH by physiologic stimuli are still incompletely understood. Table 10-11 lists selected physiologic and pharmacologic regulators of GH secretion.

The secretory activity of GHRH neurons is at least in part regulated by a stimulatory pathway that involves endogenous opioids and α_2-adrenergic receptor stimulation. This explains the well-established GH-stimulating effects of morphine and clonidine. The dopamine precursor L-DOPA (levodopa) may exert its GH-stimulating action after being converted into dopa-

mine acting on dopamine receptors or when further processed into adrenaline acting on α_2-adrenergic receptors. Although the mechanisms are
different (Fig. 10-11), the outcome in terms of GH stimulation is similar.
Serotonin apparently regulates both GHRH and SRIF mechanisms. Muscarinic cholinergic stimulation inhibits SRIF, thereby stimulating GH. This
cholinergic pathway is part of the negative feedback regulation by GH.

The daily secretory pattern of GH is significantly influenced by meals
and sleep. The increased GH secretion occurring during deep NREM sleep
(non-rapid eye movement or delta sleep) is not a direct stimulatory effect
of sleep. It appears that increased GHRH activity is responsible for inducing
both NREM sleep (an effect within the brain) and increased GH secretion
as a direct effect on the pituitary gland.

Major Disorders of the GH–IGF-1 System   The disorders of the GH–
IGF-1 system can be categorized as states of hyperfunction and hypofunction.

The hyperfunctional state is represented by *gigantism* and *acromegaly,*
which have been discussed at some detail throughout this chapter. As noted,
hyperfunction is usually due to a hormone-secreting pituitary adenoma,
and rarely to ectopic production of GHRH or as a part of McCune–Albright
syndrome. Pituitary adenomas typically escape from the normal hypothalamic and feedback regulatory processes. Thus, GH secretion is permanently
elevated, does not follow the normal episodic pattern, and is not suppressible by hyperglycemia. The tumor cells display certain characteristic responses distinct from the physiologic regulation. These responses include
suppression of GH secretion by dopamine agonists (such as the D_2 receptor
agonist bromocriptine), and stimulation of GH secretion by TRH or VIP.
It appears that normal somatotrophs express TRH receptors, but the action
of TRH is prevented by a TRH-degrading membrane-anchored ectoenzyme
expressed by normal somatotrophs (see also Chap. 11). The protection
from TRH action by the ectoenzyme is lost in somatotroph tumor cells. The
treatment of GH hypersecretion may involve surgery and/or conservative
therapy with octreotide or bromocriptine.

GH-deficient states, which result in growth retardation or dwarfism in
children, have several etiologies. Indeed, just about any checkpoint of the
regulatory pathway (Fig. 10-11) has been implicated. Except for IGF-1
resistance, the sine qua non of GH deficiencies is that plasma levels IGF-
1 (and not necessarily GH) are decreased. The differential diagnosis is then
focused on GH per se:

- A decrease of plasma GH indicates a pituitary and/or hypothalamic
defect, which may include
    - Mechanical damage (such as craniopharyngioma, injury).
    - GH deficiency with or without "midline" defects of devel-
    opment (such as optic hypoplasia, cleft palate, absent *septum pel-
    licidum*).

- Neurosecretory GH deficiency, a common disorder in which spontaneous GHRH secretion is diminished, but can be stimulated by several mechanisms, such as clonidine, GH secretagogues, or stress. *Psychosocial dwarfism* (also known as *maternal deprivation syndrome*) may be a subset of this condition.
- GHRH resistance due to the congenital defect of the GHRH receptor. This condition, which is the human homologue of the *lit/lit* little mouse, is an autosomal recessive disorder involving chromosome 7p14. It is known as the *dwarfism of Sindh,* named after a province in Pakistan, where the first affected individuals were identified. The condition is characterized by somatotroph hypoplasia. It is noteworthy that in addition to GHRH, GHS compounds (such as hexarelin) are also ineffective in stimulating GH secretion, which may reflect a mandatory role of GHRH signaling in the normal GH response evoked by GHS.
- Congenital absence of GH due to mutations of the GH gene.
- Congenital absence of GH, PRL and TSH due to a Pit-1 defect; congenital absence of GH, PRL, TSH and pituitary gonadotropins due to a PROP-1 defect.
- Acquired panhypopituitarism (Sheehan's syndrome).
- Pituitary agenesis.
- Other endocrine diseases such as hypothyroidism, Cushing's disease or Addison's disease.
- An elevated (or sometimes normal) plasma GH is consistent with a GH-resistant state, which may include
    - Laron syndrome (defective GH receptor).
    - Biologically inactive GH syndrome (the mutant GH is immunoreactive but does not bind to the GH receptor).
    - Pygmies (lack of pubertal increase of IGF-1 production leading to the absence of pubertal growth spurt; the etiology is unknown).
    - Catabolic states, such as poorly controlled diabetes mellitus, caloric deprivation, protein deprivation, burn injuries.
    - IGF-1 resistance. This extremely rare condition is accompanied by elevated levels of GH *and* IGF-1.

Because GH is normally low and secreted in bursts, the verification of subnormal GH secretion requires various provocations tests and/or measurement of GH in 24-h urine samples. The GHRH test is designed to distinguish between hypothalamic and pituitary defects. Other tests, such as hypoglycemia, arginine infusion, levodopa, clonidine, and exercise depend on a combined hypothalamic and pituitary function.

The differential diagnosis is intended to select the most appropriate therapy. Current choices include recombinant hGH (pituitary GH deficiencies), recombinant hIGF-1 (Laron syndrome) and GH secretagogues (certain GH deficiencies of hypothalamic origin). GHRH is not used as a treatment because of its very short half-life.

11

THE THYROID GLAND

OBJECTIVES

1. Discuss the anatomy, embryology, and histology of the thyroid gland.
2. Discuss the *thyroid-stimulating hormone receptor* (TSH-R) as a major regulator of thyroid function.
3. Discuss the biosynthesis of thyroid hormones. Discuss the physiology of iodide including its sources, distribution, clearance, membrane-transport, and organification. Discuss the uses of radioactive iodine isotopes.
4. Discuss the metabolism of thyroid hormones. Distinguish between processes leading to hormone degradation and hormone activation.
5. Discuss the transport of thyroid hormones in the circulation and the various types of binding proteins. Discuss the laboratory evaluation of total and free thyroid hormones.
6. Discuss the thyroid hormone receptors and their mechanism of action. Discuss the nongenomic actions of thyroid hormones.
7. Discuss the biologic actions of thyroid hormones. Compare and contrast the consequences of hypothyroidism versus hyperthyroidism in adults and in infants.
8. Discuss the regulation of temperature and metabolic rate. Identify the mechanisms responsible for the calorigenic effect of thyroid hormones. Discuss *uncoupling proteins* (UCPs).
9. Discuss the regulation of thyroid function in the context of the hypothalamic-pituitary-thyroid axis. Discuss the ontogeny of thyroid function and its regulation.
10. Discuss the major derangements of thyroid function. Explain their clinical and laboratory presentation based on their roles in, and/or impact on, the hypothalamic-pituitary-thyroid axis and other target sites.

OVERVIEW OF THE ANATOMY, EMBRYOLOGY, AND HISTOLOGY OF THE THYROID GLAND

The thyroid gland is a highly vascular ductless gland normally weighing 10 to 25 g. Enlargement of the thyroid gland is referred to as *goiter* or *struma*, which may present either with a *diffuse* or a *nodular* (focal) morphology. Note that goiter may be present in any state of thyroid function, i.e., in euthyroidism, hypothyroidism, or hyperthyroidism.

The inferior parts of the two *lateral lobes* of the thyroid gland are connected by the *isthmus* just anterior to the 2nd to 4th cartilaginous rings of the trachea (Figs. 11-1). The entire gland is ensheathed by the *pretracheal fascia*. The superior extension of the thyroid gland is limited by the insertion of the *sternothyroid muscle* in the *oblique line* of the thyroid cartilage. The

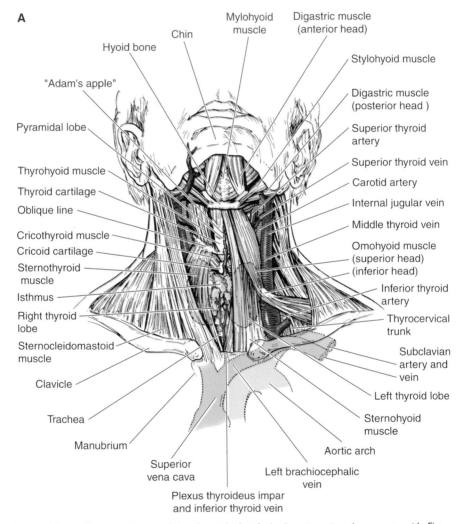

A

Mylohyoid muscle
Digastric muscle (anterior head)
Chin
Hyoid bone
Stylohyoid muscle
"Adam's apple"
Digastric muscle (posterior head)
Pyramidal lobe
Superior thyroid artery
Thyrohyoid muscle
Superior thyroid vein
Thyroid cartilage
Carotid artery
Oblique line
Internal jugular vein
Middle thyroid vein
Cricothyroid muscle
Cricoid cartilage
Omohyoid muscle (superior head) (inferior head)
Sternothyroid muscle
Inferior thyroid artery
Isthmus
Right thyroid lobe
Thyrocervical trunk
Sternocleidomastoid muscle
Subclavian artery and vein
Clavicle
Left thyroid lobe
Trachea
Sternohyoid muscle
Manubrium
Aortic arch
Superior vena cava
Left brachiocephalic vein
Plexus thyroideus impar and inferior thyroid vein

Figure 11-1. Gross anatomy of the thyroid gland. A. Anterior view (compare with Fig. 11-8). The thyroid gland is shown in color. Note the position of the lateral lobes and the pyramidal lobe. The arterial supply and venous drainage are shown in lighter and darker shades of blue, respectively. Note the palpable landmarks: hyoid bone, thyroid cartilage, cricoid cartilage, manubrium sterni, clavicular head, sternocleidomastoid muscle.

B

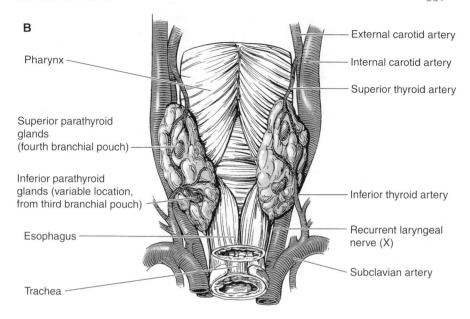

Pharynx

Superior parathyroid glands (fourth branchial pouch)

Inferior parathyroid glands (variable location, from third branchial pouch)

Esophagus

Trachea

External carotid artery

Internal carotid artery

Superior thyroid artery

Inferior thyroid artery

Recurrent laryngeal nerve (X)

Subclavian artery

C

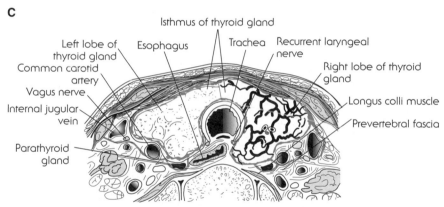

Isthmus of thyroid gland

Left lobe of thyroid gland
Common carotid artery
Vagus nerve
Internal jugular vein

Parathyroid gland

Esophagus

Trachea   Recurrent laryngeal nerve

Right lobe of thyroid gland

Longus colli muscle

Prevertebral fascia

Figure 11-1. (*Continued*) B. Posterior view. Note the position of the parathyroid glands and the recurrent laryngeal nerve. C. Cross-sectional view. Note the relative position of the thyroid and parathyroid glands, and the recurrent laryngeal nerve. The thyroid gland, the strap muscles and the great cervical vessels are all invested in the pretrachial fascia (shown in color). (*Sources:* B: modified from Fig. 21-9, p. 359 in Ganong WF: *Review of Medical Physiology*, 17th ed, Appleton & Lange 1995. C: modified from Fig. 7-2, p. 193 in Greenspan FS: The Thyroid Gland, in Greenspan FS & Strewler GJ (eds): *Basic and Clinical Endocrinology*, 5th ed, Stamford, CT, Appleton & Lange, 1997.)

sternothyroid and the *sternohyoid* muscles, which belong to the infrahyoid "strap" muscles, take their origins on the inner surface of the sternum. Thus, these muscles create a preformed space for the expansion of the thyroid gland, which may actually extend to the anterior mediastinum *(substernal struma)*. When enlarged, the thyroid gland usually becomes distinctly palpable, and protrudes posterolaterally.

Medially the lateral lobes are in touch with the cricoid and thyroid cartilages of the larynx. The anatomical relationship between the thyroid gland, the laryngeal and tracheal cartilages explains *laryngomalacia,* the softening and destruction of the cartilages by the mechanical pressure sometimes exerted by the enlarged thyroid gland. The posterior edge of each lateral lobe touches the ipsilateral *recurrent laryngeal nerve,* a branch of cranial nerve X. This nerve innervates the *posterior cricoarytenoid muscle,* the only muscle that opens the glottis by diverting the vocal cords. The *parathyroid glands* are found at the posterolateral edges of the lobes. Accidental injuries to the recurrent nerve and removal of the parathyroid glands are potential complications of surgical thyroidectomy.

The thyroid gland is supplied by two pairs of arteries, the *superior thyroid artery* from the external carotid artery, and the larger *inferior thyroid artery,* which is derived from the thyrocervical trunk of the subclavian artery. The venous blood is first gathered by a venous plexus, which is primarily drained by a single *inferior thyroid vein* into the *left brachiocephalic vein.* The lymphatic vessels of the thyroid lead to the deep cervical and anterior mediastinal lymph nodes. These lymph nodes are preferred sites of early metastases of thyroid malignancies.

Among all endocrine glands, the thyroid gland develops first, starting about 24 days after fertilization. The *follicular epithelium* of the thyroid gland develops from the *thyroglossal duct,* an endodermal outgrowth of the primitive pharynx. The *parafollicular* cells develop from the neural crest and migrate to the thyroid gland through the last pharyngeal pouch (see details in Chap. 8). The *foramen cecum* of the tongue is the remnant of the embryonic evagination site of the thyroglossal duct. During its descent, the thyroglossal duct penetrates the root of the tongue, then turns ventrally and passes between the cartilages of the second and third branchial arches. After the passage of the duct, these cartilages fuse to form the corpus of the hyoid bone. The thyroglossal duct bifurcates at the site of the future isthmus. After the development of the permanent thyroid structures, the thyroglossal duct degenerates. When the degeneration and/or the descent is incomplete, thyroid tissue may be present at any location along the course of the thyroglossal duct. This accessory thyroid tissue may form either cysts or solid masses. A frequently encountered developmental variation is the *pyramidal lobe* extending from the isthmus toward the hyoid bone. Rarely, the thyroglossal duct fails to descend, and presents as a *lingual thyroid gland*. Functional ectopic thyroid tissue may be present in ovarian teratomas: this rare condition is known as *struma ovarii* (ovarian goiter).

In the beginning, the thyroglossal duct is a hollow tube. Its development is comparable with that of exocrine glands: after repeated bifurcations, a compound alveolar (acinar) gland is formed, where the secretory acini communicate their products to the surface by the branching (thyroglossal) duct system. However, the involution of the duct system results in a ductless acinar lumen (a transcellular fluid compartment) for each secretory unit. These ball-shaped secretory units are the *thyroid follicles,* which are lined by the *simple cuboidal follicular epithelium* and filled with *colloid* (Fig. 11-2). The colloid contains *thyroglobulin* (Tg), which serves as a precursor and storage form of thyroid hormones. Approximately 30% of the thyroid

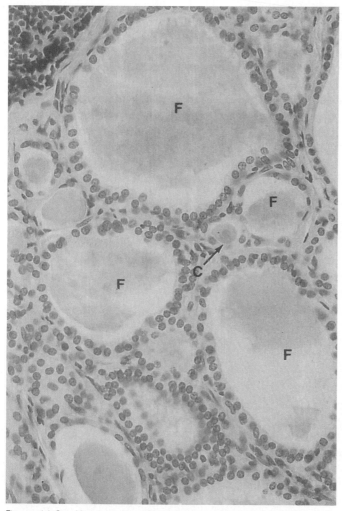

Figure 11-2. Histologic image of the thyroid gland. F, follicles; C, C cells (clear, calcitonin cells) also known as parafollicular cells. The follicular lumen is filled with thyroglobulin ("colloid"). Active reabsorption of the colloid leads to vacuolization (empty spaces) near the simple cuboidal follicular epithelium. (*Source:* Fig. 17-15, p 267 in Berman I: *Color Atlas of Histology,* Stamford, CT, Appleton & Lange, 1993.)

mass is colloid. Tight junctions joining the follicular epithelial cells prevent the paracellular transport of most compounds, including iodide and thyroglobulin. The parafollicular (C) cells are found in the stroma, which fills the space between the follicles.

The height of the follicular epithelial cells is determined by the activity of their *thyroid stimulating hormone receptors* (TSH-R) and the consequent increase in cytoplasmic levels of cyclic AMP. In the absence of a stimulus, the follicular epithelium is described as low cuboidal (essentially squamous). Upon intense stimulation, the epithelium becomes tall cuboidal or even columnar. The increased epithelial height reflects hyperfunction of the cells, including an increased production of Tg. The follicular cells display *dual polarity:* their secretory activity is bidirectional. They secrete Tg *apically* into the follicular lumen. On demand (also signaled by TSH), they endocytose Tg, and liberate thyroid hormones from it by proteolytic cleavage. The thyroid hormones leave the cells at their *basolateral* surface to enter the bloodstream.

The stimulation of TSH-Rs therefore has two seemingly opposite actions: increased synthesis/secretion and increased reabsorption of Tg. However, both actions support increased secretion of thyroid hormones into the circulation. If the intense TSH-R stimulation is prolonged, the reabsorption of Tg dominates, and the morphology is a characterized by the association of tall cuboidal/columnar epithelium with depleted and highly vacuolar colloid stores.

The thyroid hormones liberated from Tg by its lysosomal degradation do not need to be exocytosed: they are lipophilic and penetrate the cell membrane toward the basal surface. This diffusion is enhanced by a steep gradient which is in part maintained by thyroid binding globulin (TBG), a plasma protein that keeps the concentration of free thyroid hormones very low (see also Chap. 4).

THE THYROID STIMULATING HORMONE RECEPTOR (TSH-R) AND THE BIOSYNTHESIS OF THYROID HORMONES

The Main Regulator of Thyroid Function Is the Activity of the TSH-Receptor

Although the physiologic regulator of the TSH-receptor (TSH-R) activity is TSH (Fig. 11-3) under varied and common pathologic conditions TSH-R is activated in a TSH-independent fashion.

As mentioned (see Chapter 10) all pituitary glycoprotein hormones (TSH, luteinizing hormone [LH], follicle-stimulating hormone [FSH]) act on G-protein-coupled seven transmembrane-segment receptors. The receptors of these glycoprotein hormones are closely related to each other, mainly in their intracellular domains indicating shared postreceptor mechanisms, which mainly involve the activation of adenylyl cyclase.

Stimulation of the TSH-Rs

- enhances every aspect of thyroid hormone synthesis and secretion, which is accompanied by morphologic changes of the follicular epithelium and colloid (see above);
- stimulates the secretion of *vascular endothelial growth factor* (VEGF) by follicular epithelial cells. VEGF is secreted toward the *basal* surface (i.e., toward the interstitial connective tissue). VEGF targets the pericytes to increase vascularization of the thyroid gland. Autoantibody-induced hypervascularization (together with the increased cardiac output) is responsible for the *bruit* audible over the thyroid gland of Graves' disease patients (see below).
- promotes proliferation of the follicular epithelium, which may result in hyperplasia and goiter.

The similarity in the extracellular domains of the pituitary glycoprotein hormones is sufficient to yield cross-reactivities among these hormones, provided the hormones are present in very high concentrations. Such a cross-reactivity is seen in *choriocarcinoma* (a tumor of syncytiotrophoblast cells invading the mother's tissues), which produces excessive quantities of human chorionic gonadotropin (hCG, an LH-like hormone) potentially resulting in hyperthyroidism.

Unique features of the TSH-R are that

- its polypeptide chain is cleaved by a protease in the extracellular domain (Fig. 11-4), and
- the TSH-R is "noisy," meaning that it normally has a detectable ligand-independent activity.

It is uncertain whether the cleavage of the extracellular domain is responsible for the noisy nature of the TSH-R. The cleavage of the TSH-R results in two chains designated as the *A* and *B subunits* of the TSH-R, which are held together by disulfide bonds. The A subunit (which contains the N-glycosidic groups of the TSH-R) can be detached from the membrane-anchored B subunit by the cooperative action of a matrix metalloproteinase and disulfide isomerase. This is known as the *shedding of the A subunit*, which explains the presence of the A subunit in the circulation. Unlike the cleaved extracellular domain of the GH receptor, the A subunit does not appear to function as a TSH-binding carrier protein.

The TSH-R is a common target of *autoantibodies* (Fig. 11-5). The two main types of TSH-R autoantibodies bind to *different regions of the TSH-binding site* of the TSH-R:

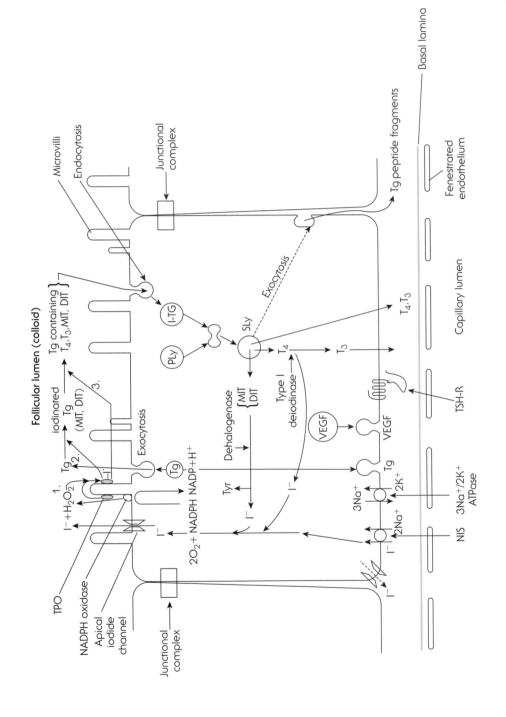

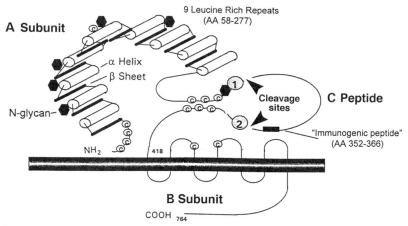

Figure 11-4. Schematic representation of the thyroid stimulating hormone receptor (TSH-R). An unusual feature of the TSH-R is its cleavage at two sites. The "C peptide" is not homologous with that of insulin. The name, however, refers to an analogous process: upon removal of the C peptide segment, two chains are generated which are held together by disulfide bonds. The A subunit may become shed. The residues labeled with "C" indicate cysteines. Note the location of immunogenic peptide (compare with Fig. 11-5). (*Source:* Fig. 2 in Rapoport B et al: The thyrotropin (TSH) receptor: Interaction with TSH and autoantibodies. Endocrine Rev 19:673–716, 1998.)

- *Anti-TSH-R [stim]* (also known as thyroid-stimulating immuno-globulin [TSI] or antibody [TSAb]), which is the causative agent of hyper-thyroidism in *Graves' disease* (also known as *Basedow's disease*). This population of antibodies was formerly called *long-acting thyroid stimulator (LATS).* In the laboratory diagnosis of Graves' disease, these antibodies are demonstrated in the patient's serum by an in vitro cell culture adenylyl cyclase stimulation assay. Stimulation of adenylyl cyclase 130 to 200% above the basal activity indicates the presence of the antibodies in conditions usually different from Graves' disease. The simulation of adenylyl cyclase above 280% is characteristic in Graves' disease.
- *Anti-TSH-R [block]* (also known as thyroid stimulation-blocking antibody [TSBAb]) binds to a distinct region of the TSH-R without activating it. However, the binding of TSBAb prevents the binding of TSH, thereby inhibiting the stimulatory action of TSH on adenylyl cyclase activity. These antibodies are causally involved in the hypothyroidism seen in *idiopathic*

Figure 11-3. The biosynthesis and secretion of thyroid hormones in the follicular epithelium. The thyroid stimulating hormone receptor (TSH-R) in the basolateral membrane and the intracellular concentration of iodide (I^-) regulate the process. NIS, $2Na^+/I^-$symporter; Tg, thyroglobulin; I-Tg, iodinated Tg; TPO, thyroid peroxidase; MIT, monoiodotyrosine; DIT, diiodotyrosine; T_4, thyroxine; T_3, triiodothyronine; PLy, primary lysosome containing cathepsins; SLy, secondary lysosome (PLy merged with endocytosed I-Tg). The reactions catalyzed by TPO are peroxidation (1), organification (2) and coupling (3); all occur at the follicular aspect of the apical membrane. Note the recycling of I^- by *dehalogenase*, and the cytoplasmic conversion of T_4 into T_3 by type I *deiodinase*. The junctional complexes (if intact) prevent leakage of colloidal thyroglobulin and access of antibodies to TPO. The mechanism of iodide leakage through the basolateral membrane is uncertain. Vascular endothelial growth factor (VEGF) is secreted upon stimulation of TSH-R and increases vascularity of the thyroid gland.

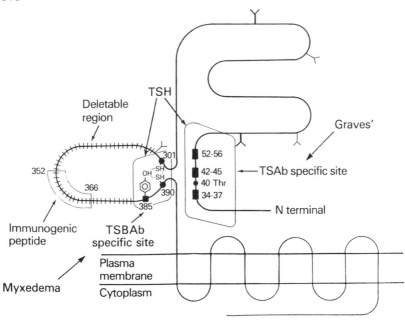

Figure 11-5. Model of the thyroid stimulating hormone receptor (TSH-R) displaying the putative binding sites of TSH, blocking TSH-R antibodies (TSBAb) and Graves' disease-specific stimulatory antibodies (TSAb). Note the locations of the "deletable region" (C peptide in Fig. 11-4) and the immunogenic peptide. The "Y"-s indicate sites of glycosylation. (*Source:* Fig. 12 in Kosugi et al.: Identification of thyroid-stimulating antibody-specific interaction sites in the N-terminal region of the thyrotropin receptor. Molecular Endocrinol 7:114–130, 1993.)

myxedema and *Hashimoto's disease*. Both TSAb and TSBAb prevent the binding of TSH to TSH-R. Thus, the routine clinical test based on the inhibition of TSH-binding does not prove the epitope specificity of the antibody, and the test is positive in Graves' disease.

Because these antibodies belong to the immunoglobulin G (IgG) class, they cross the placental barrier. Therefore, maternal autoantibodies may interfere with fetal and, due to the long half-life of IgGs, neonatal thyroid function, resulting either in congenital hyperthyroidism or hypothyroidism.

The TSH-R gene is found on chromosome 14. The main regulator of its expression in the thyroid gland is *thyroid transcription factor 1* (TTF-1). Overexposure of the thyroid gland to TSH significantly down-regulates TSH-Rs. However, normal levels of TSH are apparently required for normal expression of TSH-R in follicular epithelial cells. Thyroid hormones (especially T_3) stimulate TSH-R expression. Clonally expanded somatic gain-of-function mutations of the TSH-R gene manifest in a dominant manner, and are responsible for the development of *toxic multinodular goiter* and *toxic adenoma (Plummer's disease)* of the thyroid gland. (Note that the term *toxic* refers to *thyrotoxicosis,* the exaggerated and deleterious effects of overt thyroid hormone levels.) Inherited germline gain-of-function mutation of the TSH-R may cause a rare form of congenital hyperthyroidism presenting with symptoms at birth. Gain-of-function mutations of $G_{\alpha s}$ (McCune–Albright syndrome) may involve follicular epithelial cells and imitate TSH-R activation (see also Chap. 8).

In contrast with the traditional view, the expression of the TSH-R is not restricted to the follicular epithelium: transcripts and receptor protein have been detected in *in the adipocytes and perimysial fibroblasts of the orbital connective tissue*. Increased expression of orbital connective tissue TSH-R has been observed in Graves' disease patients. The autoantibodies of Graves' disease target not only the thyroid gland but also orbital (and possibly other extrathyroidal) TSH-Rs, which explains certain manifestations of Graves' disease, such as *exophthalmos* and *pretibial myxedema*. Note that the pretibial myxedema is a direct action of anti-TSH-R antibodies and is seen in Graves' disease, as opposed to the generalized myxedema of hypothyroidism.

Thyroid Hormones Are Heavily Iodinated Amino Acid Derivatives

The thyroid hormones are *iodothyronines* synthesized by coupling specific iodinated tyrosyl residues of Tg via an ether linkage (Fig. 11-6). A unique feature of the thyroid gland that *crucial steps of the hormone synthesis occur in the extracellular space*, in the follicular lumen. The thyroid gland mainly secretes *thyroxine* (3,5,3',5'-tetraiodothyronine, T_4), and smaller amounts of the three to eight times more potent *triiodothyronine* (3,5,3'-triiodothyronine, T_3). Thyroid hormones are lipophilic molecules that could not be contained by membranes. To keep them in a hydrophilic and therefore containable phase, their synthesis and storage are performed while they exist as residues of the polypeptide chain in Tg. The biosynthesis of these heavily iodinated compounds includes the following steps:

- Accumulation of iodide (iodide transport or *iodide trap*).
- Biosynthesis and secretion of the glycoprotein *thyroglobulin* (Tg) into the follicular lumen.
- Extracellular posttranslational modification of Tg:
    - *Organification* of iodide by the iodination of tyrosine residues in Tg. This reaction requires prior *peroxidation* of iodide.
    - *Coupling* of specific iodotyrosyl residues of Tg to form iodothyronines residing within the peptide chain.
- *Storage* of iodinated Tg as colloid in the follicular lumen.
- *Endocytosis* of iodinated Tg and merging with primary lysosomes.
- *Secretion:* Proteolytic cleavage of Tg into peptides and amino acids, including the diffusible thyroid hormones.
- *Metabolization* of thyroid hormones by *deiodinase* enzymes: Metabolization is involved both in the potentiation of T_4 (by *conversion* to T_3) and in the *degradation* of thyroid hormones.

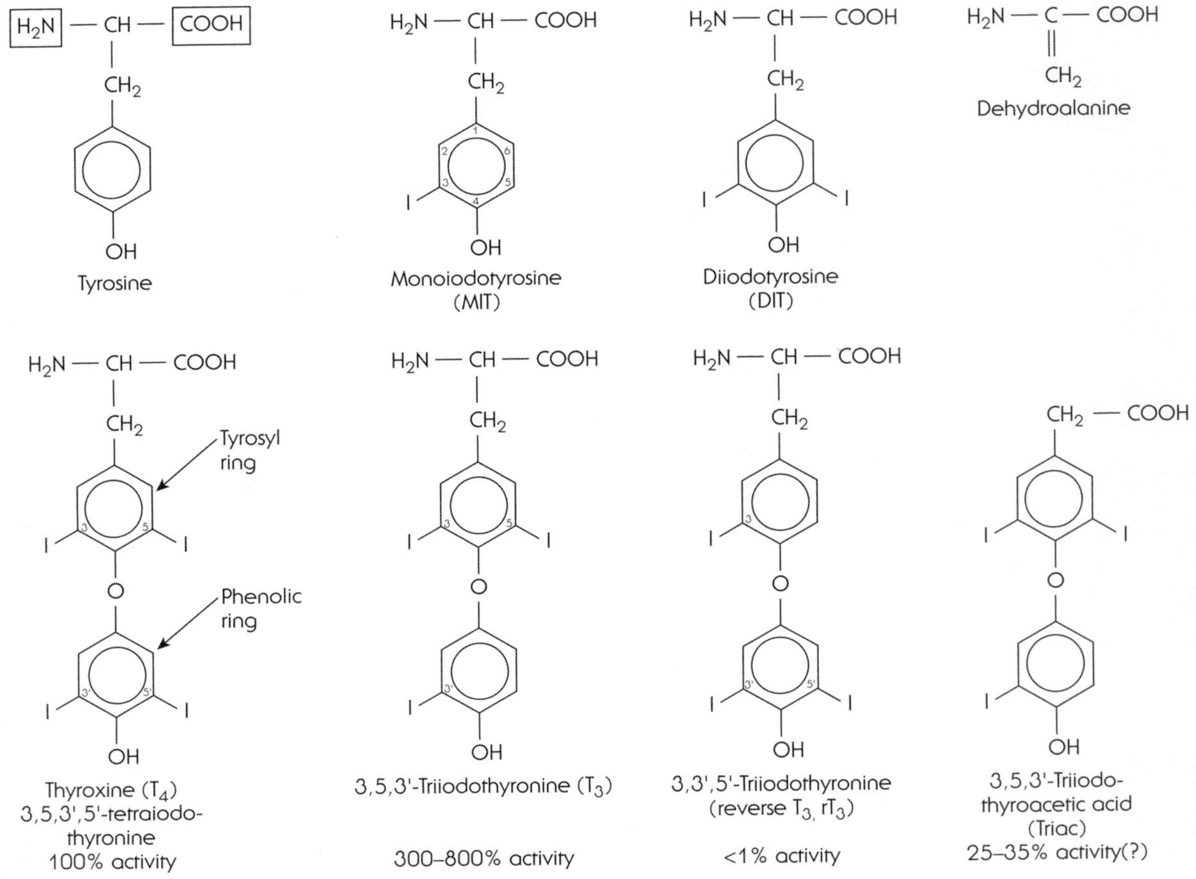

H_2N — CH — COOH
|
CH_2
|
(benzene ring)
|
OH

Tyrosine

H_2N — CH — COOH
|
CH_2
|
(benzene ring with I)
|
OH

Monoiodotyrosine
(MIT)

H_2N — CH — COOH
|
CH_2
|
(benzene ring with 2 I)
|
OH

Diiodotyrosine
(DIT)

H_2N — C — COOH
‖
CH_2

Dehydroalanine

H_2N — CH — COOH
|
CH_2
|
(ring)—O—(ring)
|
OH

Thyroxine (T_4)
3,5,3',5'-tetraiodo-
thyronine
100% activity

Tyrosyl ring
Phenolic ring

H_2N — CH — COOH
|
CH_2
|
(ring)—O—(ring)
|
OH

3,5,3'-Triiodothyronine (T_3)

300–800% activity

H_2N — CH — COOH
|
CH_2
|
(ring)—O—(ring)
|
OH

3,3',5'-Triiodothyronine
(reverse T_3, rT_3)

<1% activity

CH_2 — COOH
|
(ring)—O—(ring)
|
OH

3,5,3'-Triiodo-
thyroacetic acid
(Triac)
25–35% activity(?)

We next discuss the most important details of the biosynthetic process. *Note that with the exception of storage, all aspects of thyroid hormone production are stimulated by TSH.*

Iodide is Delivered to the Follicular Lumen by the Combination of a Secondary Active Transport Process Involving the Sodium Iodide (Na^+/I^-) Symporter in the Basolateral Membrane and a Passive Transport Through the Apical Iodide Channel

Plasma levels of iodide are very low (15 to 30 nM [0.2 to 0.4 μg/dL]). Iodide, similar to other ionic compounds, does not penetrate the phospholipid bilayer of the cell membrane. Iodide is concentrated by an active transport process in the thyroid gland usually twenty- to fortyfold relative to plasma iodide concentrations. Under intense stimulation by TSH, the concentration of iodide in the thyroid may exceed that in plasma over a hundredfold. The plasma concentrations of iodide are directly proportional to its dietary intake. In case of dietary iodine deficiency (<50 μg iodide/d), the concentrating ability of the thyroid may become insufficient to supply normal quantities of iodide for the production of thyroid hormones.

To reach the follicular lumen, iodide must penetrate two cell membranes:

- the basolateral membrane is penetrated by a secondary (indirect) active transport mechanism involving the *sodium iodide (Na^+/I^-) symporter* (NIS),
- the apical membrane is penetrated by diffusion along the electrochemical gradient of iodide through an *iodide channel*.

Iodide enters the cytoplasm of the follicular epithelial cells via the NIS, an integral membrane protein with 12 transmembrane segments, found in the basolateral membrane of the follicular epithelial cells. Iodide is transported against both electrical and chemical gradients. The driving force of iodide uptake is the concurrent transport of sodium, which is driven by the high electrochemical gradient of Na^+. Two sodium ions are transported for each iodide. The Na^+ gradient is generated by the $3Na^+/2K^+$-ATPase, which constantly pumps Na^+ out of the cytoplasmic compartment. This mechanism is similar to that of the intestinal sodium glucose transporter (SGLT1, see

---

Figure 11-6. Chemical structures of thyroid hormones and related compounds. The framed amino and carboxyl groups indicate the linkage sites in the polypeptide chain of thyroglobulin. Dehydroalanine is generated as a byproduct during the coupling of two iodotyrosines. The biologic activity of thyronine compounds and TRIAC are displayed below the structures. TRIAC is a degradation product of T_3 generated by oxidative deamination. Note that the carbonic atoms of the outer ring are numbered as 1' through 6' (pronounced: prime).

Chap. 9). In cases of congenital defects of NIS, iodide may be delivered to the thyroid gland by passive diffusion (probably through iodide channels); however, the dietary intake of iodide needs to be increased by fifty- to a hundredfold.

The *NIS* gene is found on the short arm of chromosome 19. Its expression in the follicular cells is stimulated by TSH. *NIS is expressed* at several extrathyroid sites *in a TSH-independent manner,* resulting in iodide *secreting* capabilities of these tissues against a concentration gradient. These tissues include the *placenta* (delivering iodide for the fetal thyroid gland), *mammary gland* (delivering iodide for the thyroid gland of the breastfed infant), the choroid plexus, and certain parts of the alimentary system such as salivary glands, gastric mucosa, and the colon. In contrast, the small intestine is the site of *absorption* of iodide. The molecular mechanism of iodide absorption is poorly understood.

Because the organification of iodide (which is synonymous with the iodination of thyroglobulin) takes place at the luminal (extracellular) side of the apical membrane of the follicular cells, the iodide concentrated by the follicular epithelium must be leaked into the lumen. Opening of the *apical iodide channels,* thereby increasing the efflux of iodide into the follicular lumen, is among the earliest effects of TSH. Cyclic AMP activates these iodide channels, whereas DIDS (4,4'-Di-isothiocyanatostilbene-2,2'-disulfonic acid, an inhibitor of several anion channels) inhibits their function.

The iodine concentrating ability of the thyroid gland is the basis of several clinical procedures such as the diagnostic evaluation of thyroid function with radioactive iodine and radiothyroidectomy (Box 11-1).

Iodide Transport by NIS Can Be Inhibited by Lithium and by Several Anions

Lithium has multiple actions on the thyroid gland, and may be used as an inhibitor of thyroid function in thyrotoxicosis. Therapeutic doses of lithium carbonate (such as used in psychiatric practice) may inhibit the iodide-concentrating ability of the thyroid gland. This effect partly explains *lithium-induced hypothyroidism,* a common side effect of lithium therapy. The effect of lithium on iodide uptake by the thyroid is poorly understood. Because the affinity of lithium for NIS is much lower than that of sodium, the primary action of lithium may be on the second messengers activated by the TSH-R.

Certain anions can bind to the iodide site of NIS, which results in a competitive inhibition of the iodide transport:

- *Perchlorate* (ClO_4^-) is sometimes used in the diagnosis of organification defect (Box 11-2, Fig. 11-9). Unlike the other anions listed below,

BOX 11-1   Medical Uses of Radioactive Iodine Isotopes

The *radioactive iodine uptake* (RAIU) *test* follows the kinetics and extent of radioactive iodide accumulation. Orally administered ^{123}I sodium iodide (100 to 200 μCi) is used for this purpose, and the radioactivity is measured with a scintillation counter placed over the thyroid gland 6 and 24 h after the ingestion of the isotope (Fig. 11-7). ^{123}I has a physical half-life of 13.3 days. This isotope emits a 28-kEV x-ray and a 159-kEV gamma photon, but has no β emissions.

The purpose of *radioimaging (thyroid scan)* is to reveal the size and shape of the thyroid, and the distribution of iodine uptake within the gland. The scan is performed 8 to 24 h after oral administration of 200 to 300 μCi ^{123}I sodium iodide. (This technique is similar to the ^{99m}TcO$_4^-$ scintigraphy.) Focal lesions may present as

- *hot nodules*, which accumulate radioiodine more than the surrounding thyroid tissue. Hot nodules are rarely signs of malignancy.
- *cold nodules*, whose iodine uptake is lower than that of the surrounding thyroid tissue (Fig. 11-8). About 16% of cold nodules are due to malignant tumors of the thyroid because these tumors often have a decreased or absent expression of the *NIS* gene.

Radiothyroidectomy is the ablation of the entire thyroid gland (including the C cells) by loading the thyroid with 80 to 120 μCi/g ^{131}I. This technique is used as an alternative to surgical thyroidectomy. ^{131}I has a physical half life of 8 days, and emits both γ and β radiation. The latter delivers high *radiation absorbed dose* (in other words: penetrates the tissue only at very short distances), and is mainly responsible for the *localized* tissue damage. The total dose of ^{131}I is calculated from the estimated total weight of the thyroid and by the results of the 24-h ^{123}I sodium iodide RAIU test: Total dose = dose rate (μCi/g) * estimated thyroid weight * 100/RAIU$_{24}$(%). Without supplementation of T$_4$, radio-thyrectomy would cause *hypothyroidism commencing about 6 to 12 weeks after the exposure to radioiodine.*

perchlorate binds with NIS, but it is not transported into the cytoplasmic compartment.

- *Pertechnetate* (TcO$_4^-$) is used as ^{99m}TcO$_4^-$ for radioimaging evaluation of the thyroid gland. The usual dose of ^{99m}TcO$_4^-$ is 1 to 10 mCi, administered intravenously 30 to 60 minutes before the scan is performed. ^{99m}Tc emits a 140-kEV γ radiation and has a physical half-life of 6 hours.
- *Nitrate* (NO$_3^-$) and *thiocyanate* (SCN$^-$) are environmental iodide transport inhibitors. Consumption of water with a high nitrate concentration (>50 mg/L, most often seen in well water) may cause primary hypothyroidism. Dietary intake of thyocyanate precursors (such as those found in

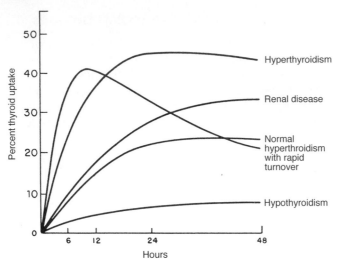

Figure 11-7. Typical thyroidal radioiodine uptake (RAIU) curves in health and disease. The various pathologic conditions are indicated in the figure. (*Source:* Fig. 39-2, p 620 in Sarne DH, Refetoff S: Thyroid function tests, in DeGroot LJ (ed): *Endocrinology,* vol I, Philadelphia, Saunders, 1995. Figure originally appeared in DeGroot LJ et al: *The Thyroid and Its Diseases.* New York, Wiley, 1984.)

cabbages) may contribute to hypothyroidism and aggravate hypothyroidism related to low dietary iodide intake. Note that large doses of *thiocyonates also inhibit organification of iodine.*

• Large doses (30 to 100 mg/d) of stable (nonradioactive) idodide are useful in preventing thyroid uptake of radioactive iodine isotopes following nuclear accidents. The mechanism involves competition between "cold" and radioactive idodide for NIS and the inhibition of the *overall* iodide uptake by exposure to massive doses of iodide (see also at thyroid autoregulation).

Tg, an Immunogenic Molecule, Is Mainly Secreted into the Immunologically Sequestered Follicular Lumen, but Small Amounts Are Directly Secreted into the Circulation

The expression of the human *Tg* gene (found on chromosome 8q) is stimulated by TSH. Tg is a glycoprotein dimer of 660 kDa; its carbohydrate content is approximately 10% by weight. The bulk of Tg is secreted into the follicular lumen, a sequestered transcellular space. However, small amounts of Tg are secreted directly at the basal surface. Because this Tg never entered the follicular lumen, it is devoid of iodine. Its normal concentration in plasma is 3 to 42 ng/mL. Its plasma levels increase upon stimulation of the TSH-R (e.g., in Graves' disease), in thyroiditis, and in follicular and papillary cancers of the thyroid.

The polypeptide chain of the monomeric Tg consists of 2748 amino acid residues. About two thirds of the sequence at the N-terminal side

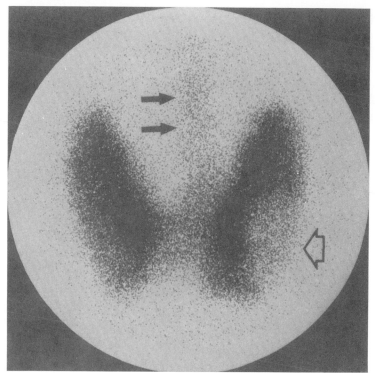

Figure 11-8. Thyroid scan with $^{99m}TcO_4^-$ demonstrating a cold nodule in the left lobe and a diffuse toxic goiter. This hyperthyroid patient had a 24-h ^{123}I uptake of 70%. The cold nodule (open arrow) was proved to be a papillary carcinoma. The solid arrows indicate the radiological evidence of a functioning pyramidal lobe (compare with Fig. 11-1A). (*Source:* Fig. 19-19, p 467 in Khafagi FA et al.: Nuclear medicine, in: Moore WT, Eastman RE (eds): *Diagnostic Endocrinology*, St. Louis, Mosby, 1996.)

consists of tandem repeats of four motifs (types 1, 2, 3a, and 3b). The type 1 motif, which is repeated 10 times, is homologous with a cystein-rich motif of the invariant chain of the *class II major histocompatibility antigen.* The C-terminal 570-amino acid sequence of Tg is homologous with *serum cholinesterase.* Low titers of anti-Tg antibodies are detected in 10% of healthy individuals. In autoimmune diseases of the thyroid gland the anti-Tg autoantibodies are usually present in high titers and recognize epitopes distinct from those recognized by the antibodies of healthy individuals. The antigenicity of Tg is enhanced by iodination.

Tg is iodinated after its secretion into the follicular lumen. At the apical membrane, four constituents of the thyroid hormone synthesis apparatus meet (Fig. 11-3):

- iodide
- hydrogen peroxide generating system
- thyroid peroxidase (TPO)
- thyroglobulin.

Reactive Iodide Is Generated by Thyroid Peroxidase (TPO) Utilizing Hydrogen Peroxide as an Electron Acceptor

NADPH oxidase generates hydrogen peroxide (H_2O_2) by transferring electrons from NADPH to molecular oxygen. NADPH itself is generated by the pentose monophosphate shunt. The production of hydrogen peroxide is stimulated by TSH. Unlike most actions of TSH, the stimulation of NDPH oxidase activity is not mediated by cyclic AMP, but by *the IP_3-Ca^{2+} pathway*. The Ca^{2+}-dependent NADPH oxidase is associated with the apical plasma membrane of the follicular cells. *The concentration of hydrogen peroxide controls the rate of iodination and coupling.* Hydrogen peroxide functions as an electron acceptor in the generation of reactive iodide, a reaction catalyzed by TPO:

$$I^- + H_2O_2 = 2\ OH^- + TPO\text{-}I^{\textbf{·}} \tag{11-1}$$

TPO-I˙ is also known as *compound I*. TPO is encoded by a gene on chromosome 2p; its expression is stimulated by TSH. Two protein products of 933 and 876 amino acids arise because of alternative splicing of the primary transcript. TPO is anchored in the plasma membrane by a C-terminal 25-amino-acid hydrophobic tail; TPO itself is on the luminal side of the membrane. Similar to the closely related but soluble *myeloperoxidase* (MPO), TPO is a heme-containing enzyme. TPO has multiple catalytic activities:

- *Peroxidation* of I^- (see equation 11-1).
- *Iodination* of tyrosyl residues in Tg, where TPO functions as compound I.
- *Coupling* of iodotyrosyl residues, where TPO functions as *compound II*. Compound II can be demonstrated experimentally: in the absence of I^- and in presence of equimolar hydrogen peroxide, compound I is spontaneously converted to compound II. Compound II does not catalyze the iodination reaction. In the presence of excess hydrogen peroxide, compound II is converted into the inactive compound III. Inactivation of compound II is prevented by iodide.

Thiocyanate (see above) and carbamide drugs such as *methimazole* and *propylthiouracil* (PTU) inhibit the activities of TPO, and are clinically used as inhibitors of organification in hyperthyroid states (see Box 11-2). Unlike methimazole, PTU also inhibits the conversion of T_4 into T_3 by 5′-deiodinase (see The Metabolization of Thyroid Hormones).

In autoimmune diseases of the thyroid, especially in Hashimoto's disease, autoantibodies specific for TPO are typically present in the circulation in high titers. *TPO autoantibodies* are identical with those referred to as *thyroid microsomal antibodies*. The immunometric assay used for the detection of TPO antibodies is more sensitive and specific than the typical

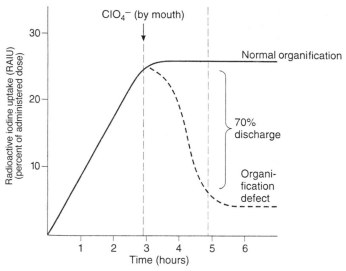

Figure 11-9. Perchlorate discharge of thyroidal inorganic iodine. Three hours after a tracer dose of ^{123}I, perchlorate is administered. In case of organification defect, iodide leaks out of the thyroid gland. Compare with Figs. 11-3 and 11-7. (*Source:* Fig. 7-12, p 199, in Greenspan FS, The thyroid gland, in Greenspan FS, Strewler GJ (eds): *Basic and Clinical Endocrinology,* 5th ed. Stamford, CT, Appleton & Lange, 1997.)

hemagglutination-based assays of microsomal antibodies. In vivo, the TPO autoantibodies inhibit the organification process and are involved in the pathogenesis of primary hypothyroidism. TPO antibodies may activate the complement cascade, thereby causing cellular damage in the thyroid follicles. The ability to form TPO autoantibodies is inherited as an autosomal dominant trait with a penetrance that is markedly higher in women than in men. *Lymphocytic thyroiditis,* a usually self-resolving condition often

BOX 11-2   Perchlorate Discharge Test of Radioiodide

Organification defects can be demonstrated by the discharge of trapped radioiodide upon the administration of perchlorate. As discussed above, perchlorate is a competitive inhibitor of NIS. During a RAIU test, about 3 h after the administration of ^{123}I sodium iodide, an oral dose of potassium perchlorate is given, which prevents further accumulation of ^{123}I in the thyroid gland. If the organification of iodine is normal, there is a negligible change in the radioactivity detected in the thyroid gland. In contrast, there is a rapid decline of thyroidal radioactivity if the organification is defective (Fig. 11-9) because in the absence of active accumulation, the efflux of *inorganic* iodide becomes evident. Defects of organification may be induced by several factors such as drugs (methimazole, PTU), dietary goitrogens (thyocyanate precursors), or autoantibodies to TPO.

seen in the postpartum period, may be associated with a transient appearance of TPO autoantibodies. In this condition, the damage to the thyroid gland causes a transient increase of plasma thyroid hormone levels followed by an also transient hypothyroid state.

Only 6 to 8 of the 134 Tyrosyl Residues in Thyroglobulin Dimers Are Hormonogenic

Tg is a protein not especially rich in tyrosyl residues. Moreover, only 5 to 52 (on the average 25 to 30) of the 134 tyrosyl residues of the dimeric human Tg become iodinated, and only 6 to 8 tyrosyl residues are hormonogenic. This reflects that the tyrosyl residues of Tg are not equally accessible for iodination. Those tyrosyl residues which are the most accessible for iodination are also more available for coupling. Depending on the degree of iodination, *3-monoiodotyrosyl* (MIT) and *3,5-diiodotyrosyl* (DIT) residues are formed.

In the *coupling reaction* (catalyzed by the compound II activity of TPO), specific iodotyrosyl residues function as *donors* of an *iodophenoxyl group*, whereas others function as acceptors. The donors and acceptors provide the outer *(phenolic)* and inner *(tyrosyl)* rings of *thyronines*, respectively (Fig. 11-6). The coupling of two DITs yields a T_4, whereas that of a MIT and a DIT usually yields a T_3, and rarely a hormonally inactive rT_3. The coupling of two MITs produces trace quantities of the inactive 3,3'-diiodothyronine. Concomitant with the transfer of the iodophenoxyl group, the donor tyrosyl is converted into a *dehydroalanine*, which also remains in the polypeptide chain.

The decreased availability of iodide increases the *MIT/DIT ratio* upon the iodination of Tg. As a consequence, the production of T_3 by direct coupling of MIT and DIT increases. Because T_3 is more potent than T_4, this mechanism may be viewed as a compensation for iodine deficiency.

The Degradation of Thyroglobulin Liberates Iodothyronines and Iodotyrosines, Which Are Secreted and Recycled, Respectively

TSH stimulates the endocytosis of Tg from the colloid. After the fusion of the endocytotic vesicles with primary lysosomes, the lysosomal enzymes (mainly *cathepsins* B, D, and L) cleave Tg into small peptides and amino acids. The liberated MIT and DIT are rapidly transported from the secondary lysosome into the cytoplasmic compartment, where they become deiodinated by the enzyme *iodotyrosine dehalogenase*. Most of the regenerated iodide is recycled for organification; minor amounts are leaked back to the extracellular fluid (ECF). In fact, *dehalogenase provides twice as much iodine or organification than does the sodium iodide symporter*. The congenital defect of dehalogenase results in *symptoms* of iodine deficiency (the deficiency is effectively present only in within the thyroid) because MIT and DIT enter the ECF and are eventually lost with urine.

The lysosomally liberated T_4 and T_3 reach the circulation by diffusion across the membranes. There is evidence that their transport is enhanced by integral membrane protein transporters. While within the cytoplasm of the follicular cell, T_4 may become converted into T_3 by *type I 5'-deiodinase*. The activity of this enzyme in the thyroid gland is increased upon stimulation by TSH. In euthyroid individuals, the daily secretion of T_4 is about 80 to 90 μg (105 to 115 nmoles); the ratio of secreted $T_4 : T_3$ is usually about 20:1 to 10:1. In hyperthyroidism, especially in Graves' disease, the activity of thyroid T_4 conversion into T_3 may become exaggerated due to the stimulation of TSH-R. In this case, plasma T_4 levels may be close to normal in spite of an overt hyperthyroid clinical picture. This is known as *T_3 toxicosis,* which can be verified by direct measurement of plasma T_3.

Iodine is Not Only a Component of Thyroid Hormones but Also a Regulator of Their Synthesis and Secretion

The supply of iodide regulates thyroid hormone synthesis and secretion, and alters the TSH sensitivity of the thyroid gland. These effects are independent of TSH secretion and are therefore collectively referred to as *thyroidal autoregulation*. Excess iodine exerts generally inhibitory effects, which are probably mediated by *iodolipid compounds*. These effects allow the thyroid to secrete normal amounts of thyroid hormones in spite of increased dietary intake of iodide. Thyroidal autoregulation includes the following effects:

• *The responses of both* TSH-receptor-activated *second messenger pathways* (cyclic AMP and the PLC/IP$_3$/DAG) *become blunted* in the thyroid gland.
• The *Wolff-Chaikoff effect,* which is an inhibition of organification by an *acute* excess of iodine, is mediated by decreased hydrogen peroxide production.
• The decreased hydrogen peroxide production may also be responsible for the *decreased coupling reaction,* which leads to an increase in the iodotyrosine:iodothyronine ratio in Tg.
• *Downregulation of iodide transport.*
• *Inhibition of colloid reabsorption,* an effect also exerted by lithium.
• *Decreased production of VEGF,* which results in decreased vascularity.

These processes are activated with a daily oral iodide dose of >2 mg (usually > 6 mg). The outcome of acute iodine surplus is more predictable if it joins a previously instituted treatment with PTU or methimazole. The susceptibility for thyroid autoregulation is enhanced in patients whose TSH receptors are supranormally activated. Graves' disease patients are hyper-thyroid because of the production of an autoantibody that binds to the TSH receptor and mimics the actions of TSH. In preparation for surgical thyroidectomy of Graves' disease patients, high oral doses of iodide are administered, which transiently (lasting about 10 to 14 days) inhibit thyroid function and reduce vascularization. The transient nature of the effect, known as the *escape phenomenon*, is explained by the substantial downregu-lation of iodide transport (an effect mediated by the blunted second messenger responses of the TSH receptor), indicating that the intracellular (rather than the extracellular) supply of iodide is the key element in thyroid auto-regulation.

For reasons unknown, in some patients an iodide load will induce hyperthyroidism instead of an inhibition of thyroid hormone production. This condition is called the *jodbasedow effect*, referring to an iodide-induced Basedow's (Graves') disease-like condition.

Insufficient Dietary Intake of Iodine, a Trace Element, Is the Leading Cause of Endemic Goiter

The recommended daily allowance (RDA) of iodine intake is 150 μg. The average daily iodine intake in the United States is 240 to 740 μg, mainly in the form of iodized salt, iodide added to bakery products, and iodide naturally present in seafood. Iodine is ingested in the form of iodide (I^-) or iodate (IO_3^-), the latter being converted into iodide in the stomach. Iodide is rapidly absorbed from the small intestine. The compartmentaliza-tion and fluxes of inorganic iodide are shown in Fig. 11-10. The thyroid gland normally organifies about 75 μg iodide/d. The rest of the trapped *net* inorganic iodide is leaked back from the gland into the ECF. During the degradation of thyroid hormones, some of the organified iodide is liberated by deiodinase enzymes and joins the inorganic pool. Most of the iodide leaving the body (usually greater than 90 to 95%) is excreted by the kidneys. The fecal loss is primarily related to active secretion by the colon; the iodide secreted by the salivary glands and the gastric mucosa is absorbed by the small intestine. The iodide losses by sweating are variable. During pregnancy and lactation, significant quantities of iodide are transferred to the fetus and the infant. Therefore, the RDA of iodine during pregnancy and lactation are 175 and 200 μg, respectively.

When the dietary intake of iodine is below 150 μg/d, the thyroid secretes more thyroid hormone than it synthesizes. The difference is derived from thyroid hormones stored as Tg in the colloid. If the low iodine intake persists for more than 3 months, the thyroid hormone stores become de-pleted. The consequence is an initial decrease of thyroid hormone secretion. Due to the negative feedback regulation of thyroid function (see below and in Chap. 7), this leads to an increase of TSH secretion. In turn, the

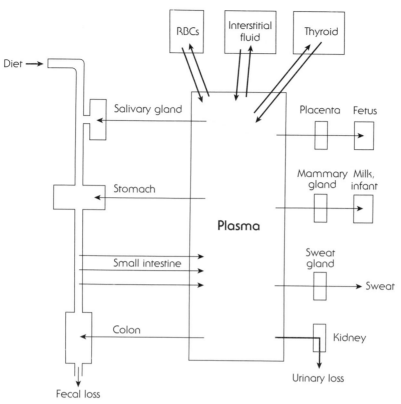

Figure 11-10. The distribution and fluxes of iodide among fluid compartments. The thick arrows indicate the highest fluxes. In an individual in iodine balance, the dietary intake and total losses are equal. Most of the iodide (>90 to 95%) is lost via urine. During pregnancy and lactation, significant amounts of iodide are lost via the placenta and the mammary gland, respectively.

elevated TSH causes thyroid hyperplasia and hypertrophy. Due to the increased concentrating ability and the increased functional tissue mass (goiter), the thyroid gland meets the daily requirement in the *amount* of thyroid hormone production in spite of low plasma iodide *concentration*. The plasma levels of T_4 reach the normal range. This *compensated iodine deficiency* is a euthyroid state achieved at the expense of increased plasma TSH and increased thyroid tissue mass. When the dietary intake of iodine drops below 50 μg/d, this compensatory mechanism becomes insufficient and the goiter is associated with hypothyroidism.

Because dietary iodine deficiency follows the geographical distribution of iodine in earth's crust, this type of condition presents as an *endemic goiter*. If the iodine deficiency is severe, the adult population suffers from hypothyroidism, whereas the condition may present in infants as *endemic cretinism* (see later). Iodine is relatively abundant and evenly distributed in the oceans, and is available in sufficient quantities along the seashores. In contrast, mountainous and inland areas have very limited supplies of iodine. Especially in these areas, prophylaxis of endemic goiter by using iodized salt is utterly important.

THE METABOLIZATION OF THYROID HORMONES

The metabolization of thyroid hormones includes deiodination, conjugation (mainly sulfation), deamination and decarboxylation reactions. These reactions are not mutually exclusive.

Deiodination is the predominant pathway of thyroid hormone metabolization. The reaction is performed by three types of *deiodinase enzymes* (Table 11-1), which are distinct from the thyroidal monotyrosine dehalogenase. All deiodinases are selenoproteins, which (similar to glutathione peroxidases) contain a selenocysteine residue at their active site. This explains their dysfunction in selenium deficient states, and the need for thiol cofactors in maintaining their normal activity. The thiol cofactors vary with the tissues and probably also with the type of deiodinases. Reduced glutathione (GSH) is an important cofactor of type I deiodinase. Deiodinase activities are regulated by the thyroid status. In general, the changes in deiodinase activities can be seen as attempts to normalize plasma and tissue levels of T_3.

Type III deiodinase is a purely hormone degrading enzyme. Its function is to limit the effect of thyroid hormones. Because it is a tyrosyl ring

Table 11-1   Iodothyronine Deiodinase Enzymes

Type	Main sites of expression	Main functions	Substrate preference	Activity in hypothyroidism	Activity in hyperthyroidism
Type I (5'-deiodinase) PTU-sensitive deiodinase	Liver, kidney	Activation of thyroid hormone, the main source of circulating T_3 Degradation of thyroid hormones, conservation of iodine	Sulfoconjugated $T_4/T_3 > rT_3 \gg$ $T_4 > T_3$	Decreased	Increased
	Thyroid gland	Intrathyroidal activation of thyroid hormone providing T_3 for plasma		Increased* (certain forms of primary hypothyroidism)	Increased*
Type II (5'-deiodinase) PTU-resistant deiodinase	Brain, pituitary gland, brown adipose tissue, cardiac and skeletal muscle	Provides intracellular T_3; conserves iodine by deiodination of the inactive rT_3	$T_4 = rT_3$	Increased	Decreased
Type III (5-deiodinase or tyrosyl ring deiodinase) PTU-resistant deiodinase	Brain, skin, placenta, fetal liver	Protection against overexposure to T_3 by inactivation of thyroid hormones.	$T_3 > T_4$	Decreased	Increased

*Enzyme activity is increased by stimulation of the TSH receptor.

deiodinase, it converts T_4 into rT_3, and T_3 into $3,3'T_2$. The placental expression of type III deiodinase explains the relative (although not absolute) inability of thyroid hormones to penetrate the placental barrier.

Type I 5'-deiodinase is a mixed function enzyme, which contributes to both degradation and activation of thyroid hormones.

- The hormone-degrading activity of type I deiodinase depends on the substrate. *Type I deiodinase primarily degrades already biologically inactive thyronine compounds thereby conserving iodide.* Sulfoconjugation of T_4 and T_3 by the liver diminishes their biologic activity. These compounds are excreted with bile, but join the enterohepatic circulation. Sulfoconjugated T_4 and T_3 are the most preferred substrates for deionination by type I deiodinase. Reverse T_3 is also rapidly metabolized by type I deiodinase. The conversion of T_4 into T_3 is an activating function of type I deiodinase (see below). The resultant T_3 is a poor substrate of type I deiodinase, which prevents its degradation before it can reenter the circulation.

- As noted, the function of the type I 5'-deiodinase *in the thyroid gland* is to increase the relative secretion of T_3. Because T_3 is 3 to 8 times more potent than T_4, this is an activating function of deiodinase. About 80% of the T_4 secreted by the thyroid gland is deioninated by peripheral tissues to yield approximately equimolar amounts of T_3 and rT_3. Thus, the secreted T_4 functions as a prohormone. Peripheral conversion of T_4 into T_3 mainly by the liver and the kidney is the source of about 75% of the *circulating* T_3. More T_3 is generated by peripheral conversion than the amount that appears in the circulation. The difference is related to the T_3 produced by the tissues and degraded before it can enter the circulation. Although in humans (but not in laboratory rodents) cardiac and skeletal muscle tissues express the type II deiodinase gene, most of the T_4 to T_3 conversion is performed by hepatic and renal type I deiodinase: PTU, which inhibits type I but not type II or type III deiodinase, effectively decreases the circulating levels of T_3. This feature of PTU is utilized in the treatment of thyrotoxicosis.

Type II deiodinase is crucial in achieving high intracellular concentration of T_3 in specific target tissues of thyroid hormones. Such an action in the pituitary gland and the hypothalamus is essential in the feedback regulation of TSH secretion by thyroid hormones. Note that deiodinase activity is conspicuously absent from the paraventricular nucleus, the site of thyrotropin-releasing hormone (TRH) neurons involved in the regulation of TSH, a finding that implicates other hypothalamic areas in the local conversion of T_4 into T_3 (see also Regulation of Thyroid Function: The TRH-TSH-Thyroid Axis). Because type II deiodinase is resistant to therapeutic levels of PTU, PTU does not impair the negative feedback action of plasma T_4. Note that type II deiodinase is widely distributed in the brain, where it contributes to normal brain development and function. In *brown adipose tissue* (BAT), type II deiodinase activity is increased upon cold adaptation.

The elevated intracellular levels of T_3 increase heat production via *uncoupling protein 1* (UCP-1; see The Action of Thyroid Hormones).

Several factors decrease the conversion of T_4 into T_3:

- Hepatic disease, selenium deficiency, fetal life, or caloric restriction. Note that thyroid hormones increase the metabolic rate, and the reduced conversion rate of T_4 into T_3 during starvation may be viewed as an adaptive response to conserve the limited energy supply.
- Glucocorticoid excess.
- Certain iodine-containing drugs, such as *amiodarone* and lipid-soluble x-ray contrast materials used in cholecystography (*iopanoic acid*, tyropaonate, etc.). The radiographic contrast agents (which inhibit all three types of deiodinases) are useful in the *acute* treatment of thyrotoxicosis. Amiodarone, which is used for the *long-term* treatment of arrhythmia, significantly alters thyroid hormone metabolism. By inhibiting the conversion of T_4 into T_3, it results in elevated total and free (non-protein-bound) plasma T_4, a decrease in plasma T_3, which taken together, result in a euthyroid state. Because of the oversupply of T_4 to pituitary type II deiodinase (see below), TSH may become suppressed. This effect strengthens the point that the increased levels of plasma T_4 are derived not from increased production but by decreased conversion of T_4.

TRANSPORT OF THYROID HORMONES

The Free (Biologically Active) Fractions of T_4 and T_3 Are About 0.04% and 0.4% of Their Total Concentrations, Respectively

The characteristics of plasma proteins that serve as carriers of thyroid hormones and the relative proportions of thyroid hormones bound to them are shown in Tables 4-1 and 4-2. As lipophilic substances, thyroid hormones primarily circulate as protein-bound hormones. The half-life of T_3 is shorter than that of T_4 (1 versus 7 days), which is explained by the higher proportion of free T_3 in the circulation. It is important to emphasize that *the free fraction of the thyroid hormones is responsible for the biologic effects*, and that *the concentration of free thyroid hormones is regulated by the hypothalamohypophyseal system*.

The quantitatively most important thyroid hormone carrier in plasma is *thyroxine-binding globulin* (TBG). TBG binds 68% of total T_4 and 80% of total T_3. As is the case with most hormone-binding globulins, estrogens increase the plasma levels of TBG, which explains the sexual difference observed in *total* T_4 and T_3 concentrations in adult plasma samples during the reproductive years. Due to the very high levels of estrogens, total (but not free) T_4 and T_3 levels dramatically increase in pregnancy. About 9 to 11% of plasma T_4 is bound to *transthyretin* (TTR, also known as *thyroxine-binding prealbumin* [TBPA]). The affinity of T_3 to TTR is tenfold lower

Table 11-2 Normal Values of Thyroid Hormones and TSH

Test	Normal value
Total T$_4$	Males: 4.6–10.5 μg/dL (59–135 nM)
	Females: 5.5–11.0 μg/dL (71–142 nM)
	Gestation (wk 15–40): 9.1–14.0 μg/dL (117–181 nM)
Total T$_3$	70–204 ng/dL (1.08–3.14 nM)
	Gestation (wk 15–40): 116–247 ng/dL (1.79–3.80 nM)
Free T$_4$ (direct equilibrium dialysis or equilibrium tracer dialysis)	Adults: 0.8–2.7 ng/dL (10–35 pM)
	Gestation (wk 15–40): 0.5–1.6 ng/dL (6–21 pM)
Free T$_3$ (equilibrium tracer dialysis)	Children and adults: 0.26–0.48 pg/dL (4.0–7.4 pM)
	Gestation (wk 15–40): 0.20–0.34 pg/dL (3.0–5.2 pM)
Thyroid hormone binding ratio (THBR)	Adults: 0.85–1.14
	Gestation (wk 15–40): 0.68–0.87
Free thyroxine index (FT$_4$I)	Pubertal children and adults: 4.2–13.0
Thyroid-stimulating hormone (TSH)	Adults: 0.4–4.2 μU/mL
	Whole blood (3–7 days postpartum): <20 μU/mL

than that of T$_4$. *Albumin* is a low-affinity but high-capacity carrier that binds approximately 20% T$_4$ and T$_3$. None of the three major thyroid hormone-binding proteins is essential for life; however, they have a substantial impact on most aspects of thyroid hormone homeostasis. Certain drugs such as aspirin may compete for T$_4$-binding sites of carrier proteins and cause a transient increase in free thyroid hormone levels.

The *total* and *free serum concentrations* of thyroid hormones are shown in Table 11-2. To screen for congenital hypothyroidism, total T$_4$ is measured in *whole blood* samples collected 48 hours after birth. Congenital hypothyroidism is highly unlikely if this value is >7.5 μg/dL (>97 nM). The routine screening procedure calls for the measurement of TSH from the same blood sample in those infants, whose T$_4$ values are in the bottom 10 to 12% of the population. Unfortunately, most laboratories only report TSH levels, which are elevated in primary hypothyroidism. Thus, the laboratory screening may miss the rare cases of TSH deficiency (secondary hypothyroidism).

The Concentration of Free Thyroid Hormones Can Be Either Directly Measured or Estimated

Free T$_4$ can be directly measured by radioimmunoassay (RIA) either after *equilibrium dialysis* or after *ultrafiltration* of the serum sample. These methods separate the protein-bound and free hormones before the measurement. All other methods are indirect measurements yielding estimates of free thyroid hormones.

Equilibrium tracer dialysis is used for estimating free T_4 and free T_3 concentrations. In this assay, trace quantities of radioactive T_4 or T_3 are added to the dialysis system and the radioactivity in the protein-free fraction at equilibrium is measured.

The traditional estimate of free thyroid hormones is the *free T_4 (or free T_3) index* (FTI). In the United States, this is gradually replaced by the direct measurements discussed above. Unlike the other methods, which provide either measures or estimates of concentration in units such as ng/dL, FTI is a unitless estimate of the free hormone concentration, which is calculated by multiplying the T_3 *resin uptake test* (T_3RU) with the total concentration of T_4 (μg/dL) or T_3 (ng/dL). The T_3RU test estimates the *available* thyroid hormone-binding sites in serum (mainly in TBG). Trace quantities of radiolabeled T_3 (or sometimes T_4) are added to the patient's serum sample. When reaching an equilibrium according to the law of mass action, the ratio of (free T_3)/(bound T_3) is the same for radioactive and cold hormones. A resin is added to the sample, which binds *free* (radioactive and cold) T_3. The sample is centrifuged, and the radioactivity in the pellet (i.e., the resin) is measured. The ratio of the total/pelleted radioactivity is calculated. A high T_3RU indicates high binding of the radioactive T_3 to the resin because little radioactive T_3 bound to carrier proteins. This means that overwhelming concentrations of endogenous free thyroid hormones occupied the binding sites of serum proteins. In clinical medicine, FTI is not directly calculated from the results of the T_3RU test. Instead, the result of T_3RU (%) with the patient's serum is first normalized by dividing it with the T_3RU (%) of a reference serum. This is known as the *thyroid hormone-binding ratio* (THBR). The normal value of the THBR is centered around 1.0 (see Table 11-2). The *FT_4I* calculated with the THBR ranges between 4.2 and 13.0 with an average of 8.0.

Normal values of either the FT_4I or of the direct measures of free T_4 (and/or T_3) can be used as indicators of euthyroidism. These values are usually supranormal in hyperthyroidism and subnormal in hypothyroidism. The exposure of the thyroid hormone receptor to thyroid hormones may be different from the values estimated from serum measurements because of the intracellular conversion of T_4 into T_3. Thus, the laboratory findings must be interpreted together with plasma levels of TSH (reflecting feedback) and the clinical picture which is based on the biologic effects of thyroid hormones.

Thyroid Hormone-Binding Proteins Aid the Uniform Distribution and Delivery of Thyroid Hormones to Tissues, and Enhance the Reentry of Thyroid Hormones From Tissues into Plasma

It has been demonstrated in a liver perfusion system that in the absence of binding proteins, T_4 and T_3 are taken up rapidly and retained by the first cells encountered. This depletes T_4 and T_3 in the perfusion medium, and deprives the hepatocytes located more distally in the perfused liver. In the presence of binding proteins, thyroid hormone uptake becomes uniform throughout the perfused organ.

To limit the exposure of thyroid hormone receptors to thyroid hormones, several mechanisms are utilized:

- intracellular degradation of thyroid hormones mainly by deiodinases;
- active elimination of intracellular thyroid hormones by plasma membrane transport proteins;
- enhancement of the reentry of thyroid hormones from the interstitial fluid into plasma by the presence of available binding sites of binding proteins.

This latter mechanism has been experimentally demonstrated by preloading the tissues with radioactive thyroid hormones; their reentry into the circulation was enhanced by including binding proteins in the perfusion medium.

TTR is synthesized not only by the liver but also by the choroid plexus and the retinal pigment cells. Whereas TTR production by the liver decreases in starvation, it is maintained at high levels in the choroid plexus. Thus, plasma levels of TTR decrease as a component of the mechanisms leading to a decreased metabolic rate. At the same time, TTR in the cerebrospinal fluid (CSF) does not decrease, contributing to maintaining the normal delivery of T_4 needed for CNS activity. Experiments with TTR knockout mice, however, suggest that TTR is not essential for T_4 transport from plasma into the brain: although T_4 levels in brain tissue are lower in these mice, the T_3 levels (reflecting local conversion from T_4) are normal. It has been proposed that the distribution of T_4 within the CNS is influenced by TTR. Mutations of TTR may lead to various types of *amyloidoses* affecting the peripheral nerves *(familial amyloidotic polyneuropathy)* and the CNS *(familial oculoleptomeningeal amyloidosis)*.

THE ACTION OF THYROID HORMONES

Most actions of the thyroid hormones are mediated by their intracelullar receptors (TRs) as discussed in Chap. 5. Here we discuss specific aspects of the molecular mechanisms involved, and the biologic functions of thyroid hormones.

The Thyroid Hormone Receptors (TRs) Are Encoded by Two Genes (TRα and TRβ), and Each Gene Encodes at Least Two TR Isoforms

The TRα and TRβ genes are localized on chromosomes 17 and 3, respectively. Both genes are protooncogenes: they are the cellular homologs of the viral oncogene v-*erb*A carried by the avian erythroblastosis virus. The TR isoforms are generated from the human genes by distinct mechanisms:

- The TRβ gene utilizes two different promoters and first exons. This has two consequences:
    - The *isoforms of TRβ* (TRβ1 and TRβ2) are expressed differentially in a temporal and tissue-specific manner.
    - The amino terminals of TRβ1 and TRβ2, which serve as their transactivation domains (TAF-1), are different and display different specificities. The DNA-binding (DBD) and the hormone-binding domains (HBD) of TRβ1 and TRβ2 are identical.
- The TRα gene is transcribed from a single promoter. Due to alternative splicing of the primary transcript, the C-terminal HBD is different: unlike TRα1, TRα2 does not bind T$_3$. As a consequence, *TRα2 functions as a suppressor, which antagonizes the actions of T$_3$.*

The expression of TRβ2 is the most restricted: it is expressed at high levels only in the pituitary gland, mainly in the thyrotrophs, lactotrophs, and somatotrophs. The coexpression of TRβ2 and type II deiodinase is the basis for the long-loop negative feedback action of T$_4$ on TSH in the pituitary gland. In addition to the hypophysis, TRβ2 is expressed at lower levels in the adult brain, retina, liver, kidney, and the heart.

All other TR isoforms are coexpressed at varying proportions in every tissue. The practically ubiquitous expression of TRs explains the characteristic actions of thyroid hormones:

- the normal function of every organ system requires exposure to physiologic levels of thyroid hormones;
- thyroid hormones primarily function as quantitative modulators of physiologic processes rather than an "all-or-none" type of signal.

This notion is further substantiated by the involvement of nuclear cofactors (coactivators and co-repressors) in determining the specific action of the TRs.

Experiments with knockout mice indicate that the presence of the TRα gene encoding both TRα1 and TRα2 isoforms is needed for survival: TRα knockout mice die within 5 weeks after birth and display severe consequences of hypothyroidism. Surprisingly, the selective loss of either the TRα1 isoform or the TRβ gene is compatible with life, and these animals display mild to moderate hypothyroidism (see also at thyroid hormone resistance).

The Effects of TRs Are Influenced by the Dimerization Partner and the Presence of T$_3$

Mainly due to their different affinities for TRs, T$_3$ occupies about 90% of the binding sites of TRs, and T$_4$ occupies only about 10%.

Although monomeric TRs can bind to thyroid hormone-response elements (TREs), they typically function as dimers. TRs can form

- *homodimers,* which includes *any combination of TR isoforms,* and
- *heterodimers,* usually with RXR. Similar to the arrangement seen in the case of the vitamin D receptor, RXR occupies the upstream hexameric half-site of the TRE. Heterodimers bind to TREs with higher affinity than homodimers do.

The heterogenous nature of the TR isoform-homodimers and the presence of the heterodimers results in a complex regulation of T_3-regulated gene expression. Major aspects of the regulation include the following.

- The unliganded TR usually functions as a repressor of the same gene, which is induced by T_3.
- Involvement of TRα2 in the dimer results in suppression.
- T_3 disrupts TR homodimers, but not heterodimers.

Thyroid Hormones May Exert Nongenomic Actions

The nongenomic actions of thyroid hormones are poorly understood. These rapid responses include stimulation of glucose and amino acid transport and the prompt decrease of type II deiodinase activity in the pituitary gland.

Whereas the Physiologic Actions of Thyroid Hormones Are Well Defined, Their Precise Molecular and Cellular Targets Are Poorly Understood

Several genes have been identified whose expression is either stimulated or suppressed by thyroid hormones. However, several of these genes do not contain TREs in their promoter region, indicating that thyroid hormones regulate their expression in an indirect manner. Selected examples of genes regulated by thyroid hormones are shown in Table 11-3. Irrespective of

Table 11-3   Selected Genes Regulated by Thyroid Hormones

Increased expression	Decreased expression
UCP-1 and UCP-3	TRH (in the paraventricular nucleus)
	α and β subunits of TSH in thyrotrophs
Ca^{2+}-ATPase	Gα_i subunit of trimeric G-proteins
α-MHC	β-MHC
Na$^+$/K$^+$-ATPase	
Myelin basic protein	
Myelin-associated glycoprotein	
HMG-CoA reductase	
LDL receptor	
β-adrenergic receptors	

ABBREVIATIONS: UCP, uncoupling protein; TRH, thyrotropin releasing hormone; TSH, thyroid-stimulating hormone; MHC, myosin heavy chain; LDL, low density lipoprotein; HMG-CoA, 3-hydroxy-3-methylglutaryl coenzyme A.

Table 11-4   Effects of Thyroid Hormones and the Consequences of Hyperthyroidism and Hypothyroidism

Target system	Physiologic function	Symptoms in hyperthyroidism	Symptoms in hypothyroidism
Sympathetic adrenergic system	Increased β adrenergic receptor activity: increased receptor numbers in heart, liver, muscle, adipocytes, increased $G\alpha_s$ and decreased $G\alpha_i$ expression	Tachycardia, arrhythmia, fine tremor in extended hands, increased glycogenolysis, gluconeogenesis, increased lipolysis; relaxation of vascular smooth muscle; eye-lid retraction and lid lag	Bradycardia, reduced energy mobilization: decreased glycogenolysis, gluconeogenesis, and lipolysis; partial ptosis
Energy expenditure	Increased Na^+/K^+-ATPase expression, increased expression of UCP: increased thermogenesis and heat dissipation, increased core body temperature; adaptation to cold climate.	Increased core and skin temperature; flush, moist, and warm skin; heat intolerance; weight loss in face of increased appetite	Decreased core and skin temperature; hypothermia is typical in myxedema coma; pale, dry skin; cold intolerance; moderate weight gain in adults Children: retardation in height exceeds retardation in weight
Oxygen consumption, free radical production	Increased oxygen consumption mainly secondary to effects on Na^+/K^+-ATPase and UPCs; increased numbers of mitochondria in most tissues; increased levels of free radicals (increased terminal oxidation and a decrease in superoxide dismutase activity)	Increased oxygen requirements; concurrent bronchial asthma may be worsened by excess levels of free radicals	Decreased oxygen requirements
Erythropoiesis	Indirect increase of RBC production via the EPO mechanism; increased RBC elimination	No major net change	May result in anemia: decreased EPO, decreased absorption of iron and folate; autoantibodies may attack gastric parietal cells (B_{12} deficiency)
Heart	See also above at β adrenergic receptors Preferential expression of α-MHC over the β-MHC leading to increased contractility (positive inotropic effect); increased sarcoplasmic Ca^{2+}-ATPase expression	Tachycardia, arrhythmia, increased cardiac output; tachycardia persists in sleep; decreased peripheral resistance; hyperkinetic syndrome without major hypertension	Bradycardia, decreased stroke volume and cardiac output; low voltage EKG; increased risk for coronary heart disease (see cholesterol)
Skeletal muscle	Increased protein catabolism and glycogenolysis; fiber type switching from slow to fast twitch muscle fibers	Thyrotoxic myopathy due to breakdown of contractile proteins and decreased glycogen stores; increased SERCA1 isoform expression; enhanced type II MHC isoform expression	Muscle weakness: reduced mobilization of glycogen stores, decreased type II MHC and increased type I MHC expression, decreased SERCA activity, preferential expression of SERCA2a
GI tract	Maintenance of normal gut motility and intestinal transit time (normal: adult 24–72 h, newborn 10–18 h); increased glucose absorption	Decreased intestinal transit time; usually causes loose stool, rarely diarrhea; increased glucose absorption rate may exaggerate postprandial hyperglycemia	Increased intestinal transit time, constipation
Cholesterol	Increased cholesterol synthesis by inducing HMG-CoA-reductase; increased elimination of LDL from the circulation by inducing hepatic LDL receptors	Decreased total and LDL cholesterol	Increased total and LDL cholesterol; increased risk for atherosclerosis

Table 11-4 (Continued)

Target system	Physiologic function	Symptoms in hyperthyroidism	Symptoms in hypothyroidism
Maturation of hepatic bilirubin UDP glucuronosyl-transferase activity	Promotion of maturation	No obvious clinical manifestation	Neonatal jaundice (yellow skin and sclera) due to increased indirect bilirubin in congenital hypothyroidism
β-carotene metabolism	Stimulation of conversion of β-carotene into two molecules of retinal in the intestinal epithelium	No obvious clinical manifestation	Accumulation of noncleaved β-carotene in LDL; results in yellow color of skin; sclera remains white
Skeletal effects	Promotes bone maturation, advances bone age; promotes bone growth by permissive action for IGF-1 and maintenance of normal GH gene expression. Adults: increases bone turnover	Children: bone age ahead of chronological age. Adults: osteoporosis by preferential stimulation of osteoclastic activity	Children: severe growth retardation, disproportionate dwarfism, delayed bone age
GAGs	Increased turnover	No clinical manifestation	Myxedema (nonpitting edema), hoarse voice, macroglossia
Plasma half-lives of hormones	Maintains normal half-lives of several hormones and drugs	Decreased half-life (e.g., cortisol's half-life decreases from 90 to 50 min)	Increased half-life (e.g., cortisol's half-life increases to >2 h)
ADH	Maintains normal secretion of ADH	No obvious clinical manifestation	SIADH, especially in myxedema coma
Skin appendages	Maintenance of normal function, structure, growth rate; and cycle of skin appendages.	Fine textured hair and increased (but replenshed) hair loss; onycholysis; wet, warm, "velvety," newborn-like skin.	Hair loss, brittle hair and nails, dry skin
Menstrual cycle	Euthyroidism is required for normal gonadotropin secretion	Oligo-amenorrhea (by increasing plasma levels of SHbG)	Galactorrhea-amenorrhea syndrome in primary hypothyroidism via TRH-induced hyperprolactinemia and inhibition of GnRH
Brain/nervous system	Terminal differentiation of the brain during ontogeny; maintenance of normal mental and emotional function; maintenance of normal hypoxic and hypercapnic drives of respiration; maintenance of normoreflexia in proprioceptive reflex arches	Decreased ability to concentrate; restlessness, irritability, frequent emotional outbursts; increased respiratory rate to match increased oxygen demand; hyperreflexia (e.g., patella reflex)	Cretinism in congenital hypothyroidism; slow mentation in adults; depression; hypoventilation even in hypercapnic states; hyporeflexia (e.g., patella reflex)

ABBREVIATIONS: UCP, uncoupling protein; RBC, red blood cells; EPO, erythropoietin; MHC, myosin heavy chain; EKG, electrocardiogram; SERCA, sarcoplasmic Ca^{2+}-ATPase; GI, gastrointestinal; HMG-CoA, 3-hydroxy-3-methylglutaryl coenzyme A; LDL, low density lipoprotein; IGF, insulin-like growth factor; GH, growth hormone; GAG, glycosaminoglycan; ADH, antidiuretic hormone; SIADH, syndrome of inappropriate ADH secretion; SHBG, sex hormone-binding globulin; TRH, thyrotropin-releasing hormone; GnRH, gonadotropin releasing hormone.

the precise mechanism of action, the physiologic effects of thyroid hormones can be deciphered from the clinical presentation of hyperthyroid and hypothyroid patients. These effects are summarized in Table 11-4.

In Hyperthyroidism, the Activities of Both Anabolic and Catabolic Pathways of Metabolism Are Increased, and Their Balance Usually Shifts Toward Catabolism

In general, thyroid hormones stimulate turnover, i.e., both anabolic and catabolic pathways. The net effect of thyroid hormones is dose-dependent.

Euthyroidism supports the normal balance between anabolic and catabolic processes, and under these conditions thyroid hormones can be viewed as growth factors. Hyperthyroidism usually shifts the balance toward catabolism. The effects of thyroid hormones on metabolism include three main components:

- direct effects of thyroid hormones on protein (enzyme, receptor, ligand, etc.) expression and activity;
- increase of metabolism secondary to increased body temperature;
- catecholamine-dependent stimulation of metabolic pathways by upregulation of mainly β-adrenergic receptors (the plasma levels of catecholamines produced by the sympathoadrenal system remain normal). In addition to upregulating the receptors, the expression of G-proteins is also modulated by thyroid hormones. Thus, the increased expresssion of $G\alpha_s$, and the decreased expression of $G\alpha_i$ accentuate the cyclic AMP responses generated by the β-adrenergic receptors.

The increased activity of metabolic pathways also means *increased energy expenditure* (see below) and increased oxygen need of the tissues. The *increased oxygen supply* is ensured by the effects of thyroid hormones on

- the cardiovascular system to increase cardiac output (in part mediated by the upregulation of β-adrenergic receptors),
- the nervous system to enhance respiratory drive and
- via erythropoietin (EPO), red bone marrow to increase production of red blood cells.

To support the *increased energy (fuel) requirements*, thyroid hormones

- enhance appetite,
- increase the motility of the gastrointestinal (GI) tract and
- improve the efficiency intestinal absorption.

The clinically relevant effects of thyroid hormones on metabolic pathways are as follows:

- *Proteins*. Both hypothyroidism and hyperthyroidism may result in a negative nitrogen balance. In hypothyroidism, the negative nitrogen balance is caused by reduced protein synthesis. Correction of hypothyroidism by physiologic doses of T_4 stimulates cellular uptake of amino acids and protein synthesis, and decreases the excretion of nitrogen. Hyperthyroidism results in increased protein catabolism that may exceed the rate of protein synthesis.
  - *Lipids.*
    - *Triglycerides and free fatty acids* (FFA). Thyroid hormones increase hepatic lipid synthesis. Thyroid hormones stimulate low

density lipoprotein (LDL) receptor expression as well as the activity of lipoprotein lipase. The net effect in hyperthyroidism is a decrease in plasma lipoproteins. In adipocytes, hyperthyroidism primarily stimulates lipolysis by increasing the activity of hormone-sensitive lipase. This action, which is at least in part mediated by upregulation of β-adrenergic receptors of adipocytes, leads to increased plasma levels of FFA and glycerol. In hypothyroidism, both lipogenesis and lipolysis decrease with a net effect of increased levels of plasma LDL. The moderate weight gain is characterized with relative decrease in lean body mass.

- *Cholesterol.* Thyroid hormones increase the expression of *HMG-CoA-reductase* in the liver, the rate-limiting enzyme of cholesterol biosynthesis (HMG-CoA: β-hydroxy-β-methylglutaryl CoA; see Chap. 9). Cholesterol is secreted by the liver as a component of very low density lipoprotein (VLDL), which is converted to LDL (see Fig. 9-19). Thyroid hormones increase removal of LDL from the circulation by upregulating LDL receptors. The net effect in hyperthyroidism is a decreased plasma level of cholesterol. Hypothyroidism results in *hypercholesterolemia,* which predisposes the patients to atherosclerosis, particularly coronary heart disease.

- *Carbohydrates.*

  - Thyroid hormones are mildly diabetogenic: the net effect of hyperthyroidism on carbohydrate metabolism is mild hyperglycemia and decreased glucose tolerance. Due to the enhanced rate of glucose absorption from the GI tract and decreased glucose tolerance, glucose may reach very high postprandial plasma concentrations. The decreased glucose tolerance is in part due to insulin resistance mediated by the increased levels of FFA. Thyroid hormones stimulate hepatic gluconeogenesis and glycogenolysis; glycogenolysis is also enhanced in muscle. These effects on the liver may lead to hyperglycemia. However, the hyperglycemic actions are ameliorated by other actions of thyroid hormones, such as increased cellular uptake of glucose, increased glycolysis, and increased glycogen synthesis. *Myxedema coma* is usually associated with hypoglycemia.

  - Thyroid hormones increase both glycogen synthesis and glycogenolysis. The net effect of thyroid hormones on hepatic and muscle glycogen stores is a dose-dependent decrease: glycogen stores are increased in hypothyroidism and decreased in hyperthyroidism. The increased activity of hepatic glycogenolysis is in part mediated by the upregulated β- and possibly α_1-adrenergic receptors.

Skin and Eye Symptoms Are Useful in the Assessment of Thyroid Function

The structure and function of skin appendages and the dermis are strongly influenced by thyroid hormones. The term *myxedema* is often used as a synonym of hypothyroidism. To be precise, myxedema is a nonpitting type of edema, a characteristic symptom of hypothyroidism due to the accumulation of hydrated glycosaminoglycans (GAGs) in connective tissues. The cause of the accumulation is the *decreased breakdown of GAGs*, mainly hyaluronic acid. The condition is observed as puffiness of the skin, especially in areas of loose tissue, such as the periorbital connective tissue. The accumulation of GAGs in the vocal cords causes *hoarseness of the voice*. GAGs also accumulate in the connective tissue stroma of skeletal and cardiac muscles (i.e., in the endomysium and perimysium). This contributes to the enlargement of the heart and the tongue. Note that the mechanism of heart and tongue enlargement is different in acromegaly (see Chap. 10).

The skin of hypothyroid patients is often yellowish, which can be mistaken for jaundice. However, whereas in jaundice the color is related to bilirubin (a degradation product of heme), which impregnates both the skin and the sclera, in hypothyroidism the color is due to accumulation of β-carotene, which impregnates the skin *but not in the sclera*. The cause of *hypercarotenemia* is twofold:

• in the absence of thyroid hormones, the normal cleavage of β-carotene into two molecules of retinal in the enterocytes is decreased, which leads to increased absorption of intact β-carotene;
• the plasma concentration of LDL is increased in hypothyroidism (see Metabolic Actions of Thyroid Hormones), and the lipophilic β-carotene is dissolved in the circulating LDL.

Congenital hypothyroidism, however, may contribute to neonatal jaundice (see Thyroid Hormones Are Important Regulators of Development and Growth).

The perfusion of the skin by blood and the activity of *eccrine sweat glands* are stimulated by thyroid hormones. In hypothyroidism, the skin is cool and dry. In contrast, the skin of hyperthyroid patients is soft, moist, and velvety ("baby-like"). Graves' disease patients typically have a warm wet handshake, which is different from the cold wet (clammy) handshake of "nervous" (stressed) individuals. The clammy handshake is due to the direct activation of sympathetic nerves. The handshake of acromegalic patients is also wet but distinctively "bulky" (see also Chap. 10).

Increased hair loss occurs in both hypothyroidism and hyperthyroidism. In hyperthyroidism, the hair stems become fine and the turnover of hair is increased. Thus, the number of hair stems removed with regular combing is increased, but this is not accompanied by balding. In hypothyroidism, the replacement of lost hair is slowed, which may result in thinning of the hair. The hair loss of the lateral edges of supercilia is characteristic for hypothyroidism. The hair becomes brittle and looses its shine.

The nails separate from the nail bed in hyperthyroidism *(onycholysis)*. In hypothyroidism, the nails may become brittle.

The *superior tarsal muscle* of the eye (a smooth muscle) is innervated by sympathetic nerves from the superior cervical ganglion. Due to the upregulation of its β-adrenergic receptors, the tone of this muscle is increased by the hyperthyroid state. Hypothyroid patients may present with bilateral partial ptosis; this sleepy appearance is usually accompanied by a slow mentation. Hyperthyroid patients often present with *lid-retraction (Dalrymple's sign)*, which results in showing the sclera above iris (normally the superior eyelid covers part of the iris). This is typically accompanied with *rare blinking (Stellwag's sign)*, which results in accumulation of tears in the eyes. Sometimes the lid retraction is not spontaneous, but can be provoked if the patient follows a downward moving object with her or his eyes. The showing of the sclera above the iris during this test is known as *lid lag (Graefe's sign)*.

The *exophthalmos (proptosis,* bulging eyes) seen in Graves' disease is mainly the direct effect of autoantibodies (see above). The autoimmune ophthalmopathy may worsen even after thyroidectomy. However, the turgor of the retrobulbar tissues is regulated by sympathetic innervation: damage of the superior cervical ganglion results in *Horner's syndrome,* which includes *enophthalmos* (the opposite of exophthalmos). Because thyroid hormones influence the sympathetic input via modulating the expression of receptors, hyper- and hypothyroidism may be associated with mild exophtalmos and enophthalmos, respectively, in the absence of autoantibodies.

Thyroid Hormones Regulate the Isoform Expression of Myosin Heavy Chain and that of Sarcoplasmic Reticulum Ca²⁺-ATPase in Skeletal and Cardiac Muscles

Skeletal muscle fibers are classified as type I (aerobic, red, slow twitch) and type II (anaerobic, white, fast twitch) fibers. The skeletal muscle fiber types differ in their numbers of mitochondria, myoglobin content (hence the difference in their color), and amount of glycogen. Each myosin molecule consists of two heavy chains and two light chains. Myosin molecules are assembled into thick filaments, which slide along actin (thin) filaments in an ATP-powered process thereby generating muscle contraction. Type II muscle fibers primarily contain the fast-acting *myosin heavy chain* (MHC) II and *sarcoplasmic reticulum Ca^{2+}-ATPase* (SERCA1) isoforms. In contrast, type I muscles primarily contain the slow-acting MHC I and SERCA2a isoforms. *T_3 may induce partial or complete fiber type switching from type I (slow) to type II (fast) fibers by regulating the isoform expression of MHC and SERCA.* The increased activity of SERCA accumulates more Ca^{2+} in the sarcoplasmic reticulum, which leads to an enhanced influx of Ca^{2+} into the sarcoplasm upon stimulation. Note that under euthyroid conditions, nerve impulses to skeletal muscles and exercise are the main promoters of switching from white to red type of fiber. Hyperthyroidism antagonizes the exercise-induced fiber-type switching.

Cardiac muscle contains α and β isoforms of MHC. *Thyroid hormones increase the proportion of α-MHC*, the isoform that has more ATPase activity and can generate a faster and stronger contraction. The activity of α-MHC is supported by an increased expression of SERCA1. These effects of thyroid hormones increase the contractility of cardiac muscle *(positive inotropic action)*. The increased ATPase activity related to MHC isoform-switching in cardiac muscle is a significant component of the calorigenic action of thyroid hormones.

Thyroid hormones stimulate intestinal motility probably by a direct action on smooth muscle cells. Hypothyroidism prolongs intestinal transit time, results in increased water reabsorption from stool, and leads to consti-pation. The retention of stool causes abdominal distension that, in combina-tion with skeletal muscle weakness, often results in *umbilical hernia* in congenital hypothyroidism. Conversely, hyperthyroid patients have short-ened intestinal transit time and loose stool.

By Inducing the Expression of Uncoupling Protein-3 in Skeletal Muscle, Thyroid Hormones Increase Nonshivering Thermogenesis, and Raise Body Temperature and Basal Metabolic Rate

In homeothermic species, constant body temperature is maintained by a regulated balance between heat generation and heat dissipation (see Box 11-3). Heat is generated by muscles during voluntary physical activity and by various types of *involuntary forms of energy expenditure.*

• The *basal metabolic rate* (BMR) is defined as the metabolic rate in the thermoneutral zone 12 to 14 hours after the last meal in a nonsleeping, resting individual. (The *thermoneutral zone* is the temperature at which oxygen consumption is minimal.) The BMR is higher in males than in females. The average BMR is about 45 kcal/h/m^2 body surface area (approx-imately 200 kJ/h/m^2; 1 kcal = 4.187 kJ). Thus, the daily BMR in an average individual (1.8 m^2 body surface area) is 45×24 h $\times 1.8$ m$^2 \approx 2000$ kcal/d ($\approx$8600 kJ/d). Body surface area can be calculated with the following for-mula:

$$\text{Body surface area [m}^2] = 0.202 \times (\text{body weight [kg]})^{0.425}$$
$$\times (\text{height [m]})^{0.725}. \qquad (11\text{-}2)$$

• The *specific dynamic action* of foods is the obligatory energy expen-diture that occurs during the *assimilation* of the food. These are 30, 6, and 4% of the total caloric value of proteins, carbohydrates, and fat, respectively. This also means that the *net* energy in these foods after their assimilation is 70, 94, and 96% of their total caloric value for proteins, carbohydrates, and fat, respectively.

BOX 11-3   Hypothalamic Regulation of Temperature

The hypothalamus receives information about body temperature from the periphery (temperature receptors in skin and viscera) and from central temperature receptors located within the hypothalamus. The central temperature receptors are specialized neurons, whose firing rate is highly dependent on the temperature of blood (i.e., the core temperature of the body). Most cold receptors are found in the skin. In contrast, the central receptors are predominantly warm receptors. Both the cold- and warm-sensitive central *receptors* are confined to the anterior hypothalamus. These receptors determine the *set-point* of the thermostat mechanism. The set-point is in effect a set-range because the heat-generating and -dissipating mechanisms have different temperature thresholds. The *effector centers* of temperature regulation are the *anterior hypothalamic "cooling center"* and the *posterior hypothalamic "heating center."* Stimulation of warm receptors activates the anterior hypothalamus, which in turn induces cutaneous vasodilation (increased heat dissipation) and suppresses shivering. Stimulation of the cold receptors (in the anterior hypothalamus and in the skin) activates posterior hypothalamic mechanisms, and results in increased sympathetic activation, cutaneous vasoconstriction, increased shivering and nonshivering thermogenesis. *Fever* is the result of an elevated set-point of temperature regulation. The set-point is usually increased by *prostaglandin E_2 (PGE_2)* produced within the anterior hypothalamus upon increased exposure to *endogenous pyrogens*, such as interleukin-1 (IL-1), tumor necrosis factor-α (TNF-α) and other cytokines. This explains the antipyretic action of *nonsteroidal antiinflammatory drugs* (NSAIDs) such as aspirin, which are inhibitors of *prostaglandin synthase* enzymes (*cyclooxygenase-1* [COX-1] and COX-2). NSAIDs, which do not penetrate the blood-brain barrier (such as *diflunisal*), cannot reach the neurons of the anterior hypothalamus, and lack an antipyretic effect.

- *Shivering thermogenesis* is achieved by the involuntary (reflex) contractions of muscles.
- *Nonshivering thermogenesis* is traditionally defined as the heat generated by BAT. Unlike white adipose tissue (WAT), which is specialized for storing and mobilizing lipids to provide fuel for other tissues, BAT is specialized to burn lipids. The color of BAT is related to the large numbers of mitochondria containing cytochromes. BAT expresses UCP-1 (also known as thermogenin-1) from the *nuclear* DNA. UCP-1 is incorporated into the *inner* membrane of mitochondria in BAT. UCP-1 short-circuits the proton gradient generated by the electron transport chain: When the proton gradient is discharged through the H^+-ATPase, ATP is generated from ADP and P_i. In contrast, when the proton gradient is discharged through UCP-1, heat is generated instead of ATP. The activity of UCP-1 is primarily regulated by the stimulation of the β_3 adrenergic receptors of

brown adipocytes. Since the discovery of UCP-1, two additional UCPs have been cloned and characterized, which display different function, regulation and tissue distribution (Table 11-5).

In general, *UCPs serve as transport proteins of* free (nonesterified) fatty acids *(FFA) into mitochondria.* The FFA anions bind protons, and the transport of protonated fatty acids into the mitochondrial matrix (the site of β-oxidation of fatty acids) acts as an uncoupling mechanism. *Fatty acid-induced uncoupling probably regulates the efficiency of ATP-generation.* Note that the main mechanism of FFA transport into mitochondria is not the UCPs, but the *carnitine shuttle* (see details in biochemistry).

The relationship between fatty acid mobilization and UCPs indicates a potential role of UCP dysfunction in obesity. Leptin, a helix bundle peptide hormone produced by adipocytes, signals the degree of adiposity to the hypothalamus. Via this central action, leptin decreases food intake and increases energy expenditure. The latter action involves stimulation of β adrenergic receptors as well as upregulation of UCPs (see also in Chap. 15).

Thyroid hormones increase energy expenditure in most tissues with the notable exceptions of the adult brain, spleen, and testis. It seems that UCP-2 (the type of UCP expressed in some of these tissues) is not influenced by thyroid hormones. *In adults, the nonshivering thermogenesis induced by thyroid hormones is primarily mediated by UCP-3 in skeletal muscle.* The tissue mass of BAT is minimal in adult humans. Experiments with TRβ

Table 11-5   Uncoupling Proteins

	UCP-1	UCP-2	UCP-3 (short and long isoforms)
Function	Nonshivering thermogenesis in the newborn in response to cold ambient temperature	Regulation of body weight and energy balance, defense against the generation of reactive oxygen species (free radicals)	The main component of thyroid-dependent nonshivering thermogenesis in adults
Regulation by thyroid hormones	Increased transcription; increased sensitivity to sympathetic stimuli by upregulating β_3 adrenergic receptors Hyperthyroidism: paradoxic inhibition of thermogenesis in BAT	Mostly unresponsive to changes in thyroid state	Decreased transcription in hypothyroidism, increased transcription in hyperthyroidism; increased sensitivity to sympathetic stimuli by upregulating β_3 adrenergic receptors
Other known regulators	Cold via activation of the sympathoadrenal system	Leptin via activation of the sympathoadrenal system; caloric restriction increases mRNA	Leptin via activation of the sympathoadrenal system; caloric restriction increases mRNA
Tissue distribution	BAT	Most tissues, especially skeletal muscle, lung, spleen, thymus, leukocytes	High levels of expression in skeletal muscle, low expression in heart

ABBREVIATIONS: UCP, uncoupling protein; BAT, brown adipose tissue.

knockout mice indicate that the increased heart rate and the increased energy expenditure induced by thyroid hormones is solely mediated by TRα receptors.

In humans, BAT is an important component of temperature regulation in the newborn. The increased lipolysis and heat generation via the activation of UPC-1 is provoked by cold-activated sympathoadrenal activity and stimulation of the β_3 adrenergic receptors in BAT. While euthyroid levels of thyroid hormones are required for this mechanism, hyperthyroidism is associated with decreased heat production and increased accumulation of lipids in BAT. This paradoxical effect of hyperthyroidism may be secondary to increased heat production by other tissues.

Thyroid hormones increase the energy expenditure by several mechanisms:

- Increasing nonshivering thermogenesis in the muscles of adults by upregulating UCP-3 and the β adrenergic receptors.
- Increasing the BMR:
    - Thyroid hormones increase body temperature. The BMR increases 14% for each °C increase in core body temperature.
    - Thyroid hormones increase the activity of the Na$^+$/K$^+$-ATPase by inducing its expression. In euthyroid individuals, approximately 30% of the BMR is used by the Na$^+$/K$^+$-ATPase.

In vivo, the calorigenic action of thyroid hormones has a long latency period (1 to 2 weeks). Whereas hypothyroidism and hyperthyroidism cause hypothermia and hyperthermia, respectively, the role of thyroid hormones in cold adaptation in humans is less established than in rodents. In the newborn, TRH secretion by the hypothalamus is increased by cold, which leads to an acute secretion of TSH. In adults this acute mechanism is attenuated, and thyroid hormones are involved in the slow, long-term adaptation to cold climates.

Although the body temperature in hyperthyroidism is significantly increased, much of the generated heat is dissipated because thyroid hormones cause *cutaneous vasodilation*. The vasodilatory effect of thyroid hormones, which is mainly due to the local action of increased metabolism and accumulating metabolites, decreases the total peripheral resistance. This explains why hyperthyroid patients have only moderately increased blood pressure in spite of increased cardiac output.

Hyperthyroidism Causes a Hyperkinetic Syndrome with Increased Pulse Pressure but Only Moderate Hypertension

As mentioned, thyroid hormones exert several actions on the heart including preferential expression of the α isoform of MHC and SERCA1, which are responsible for the positive inotropic action. In addition, thyroid hormones upregulate the β_1-adrenergic receptors (thereby increasing the number of *spare receptors*) and their mediator G-proteins. The enhanced responses to adrenergic stimuli increase the heart rate (positive chronotropic effect) and often present with the sensation of *palpitations*. The net results are tachycardia and increased increased *cardiac output,* which are expected to increase blood pressure. Indeed, systolic pressure is typically elevated in hyperthyroid patients. However, due to the accumulation of metabolites in tissues (such as CO_2 and lactic acid), thyroid hormones cause significant vasorelaxation (see above). The resulting decrease in *total peripheral resistance* prevents the increase of diastolic blood pressure. Thus, *pulse pressure* (the difference between systolic and diastolic pressures) becomes increased in hyperthyroid patients.

The Life-Threatening Emergencies of Thyroid Dysfunction Are Often Related to the Effects of Thyroid State on the Cardiovascular System

The life-threatening complications of thyroid dysfunction are *thyrotoxic crisis* (thyroid storm) and *myxedema coma.*

Thyroid storm typically occurs in poorly controlled hyperthyroidism with a stressful "precipitating event" such as surgical or radiothyroidectomy, trauma, or acute infection. Total T_4 and T_3 levels are normal, the free T_4 and T_3 and the catecholamine binding sites are acutely elevated. The stressful event triggers the acute secretion of catecholamines by the sympathoadrenal system. The clinical presentation is dominated by hypermetabolism and excessive adrenergic response. The former manifests as high fever (or more precisely, hyperthermia); the latter is dominated by high pulse pressure, tachycardia, arrhythmia, and/or atrial fibrillation. The life-threatening complication is heart failure and cardiovascular shock. This mechanism is also indicated by the finding that the condition responds to cooling of the body combined with β-adrenergic blockers such as propranolol. The only acutely effective antithyroid drugs are the blockers of peripheral conversion of T_4 into T_3, such as PTU, iopanoic acid, and high doses of glucocorticoids.

Myxedema coma is characterized by unconsciousness, bradycardia with low voltage EKG, hypothermia, hypoventilation with hypoxia and hypercapnia (CO_2 retention), hypoglycemia, and SIADH. The condition has a very high rate of mortality, mainly due to cardiorespiratory failure. Because the condition is typically preceded by long-term hypothyroidism, there is a high incidence of coronary heart disease due to hypercholesterolemia. If the replacement of thyroid hormones is done rapidly, the increased oxygen demand of cardiac muscle cannot be met by the blood supply, which may lead either to *angina pectoris* or *myocardial infarction.*

The Menstrual Cycle Is Sensitive to Thyroid Dysfunction

The endocrine regulation of the menstrual cycle is discussed in detail in Chap. 13. Both hyperthyroidism and hypothyroidism may disrupt the normal menstrual cycle. This is especially important considering that most thyroid patients are women, who are of the reproductive age at the time of initial presentation.

Hyperthyroidism causes a characteristic increase in plasma levels of sex hormone binding globulin (SHBG). The increased binding protein decreases the concentration of free sex steroids, which interferes with the normal regulation of gonadotropin secretion.

Primary hypothyroidism upregulates hypothalamic secretion of TRH. TRH stimulates not only TSH secretion, but also prolactin (PRL; Fig. 11-11). As mentioned, related to acromegaly (see Chap. 10), the stimulation of PRL receptors inhibits gonadotropin-releasing hormone (GnRH) secretion of the hypothalamus, and leads to galactorrhea-amenorrhea syndrome.

It is understandable that dysfunction of the thyroid gland decreases fertility. Pregnancies often end in miscarriage or stillbirth. A surprising observation is that *thyroid hormones are not mandatory for lactation*. However, milk yield is improved by correction of the hypothyroid state.

Thyroid Hormones Are Important Regulators of Development and Growth

The classic example of the developmental effect of thyroid hormones is the thyroxine-dependent metamorphosis of amphibians. In humans, the developmental effects of thyroid hormones include skeletal maturation (advancement of bone age), terminal differentiation of the brain, and maturation of several biochemical processes. Accordingly, the consequences of *untreated congenital hypothyroidism* include:

- severe, obligatory mental retardation (cretinism, see below).
- severe, obligatory growth retardation which may present as *disproportionate dwarfism*. Dentition is delayed, the posterior fontanelle is enlarged, and the closure of both fontanelles occurs later than normal. These infants have subnormal levels of GH and IGF-1, reduced effectiveness of IGF-1, and a marked delay of bone age. The disproportionate nature of the dwarfism indicates that thyroid hormones exert significant actions on bone growth by GH-independent mechanisms.
- prolonged *neonatal jaundice* in most cases, which is due to the delay in the maturation of hepatic bilirubin uridine diphosphate (UDP) glucuronyltransferase activity.

Normal Levels of T₃ Are Required for Mental Development, but the Brain Is Strictly Protected from Overexposure to T₃ During Fetal Life

Thyroid hormones are required for *terminal* brain differentiation processes, such as dendritic and axonal growth, synaptogenesis, neuronal migration,

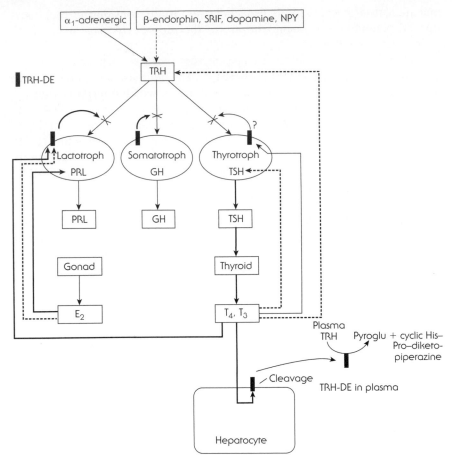

Figure 11-11. A model for the regulation of thyrotropin-releasing hormone degrading enzyme (TRH-DE) and its role in the feedback mechanisms of pituitary function. TRH receptors are expressed in all three cell types displayed, and all of them are exposed to high TRH concentrations in pituitary portal blood. The target cell-specificity of TRH is maintained by the expression of TRH-DE in lactotroph and somatotroph cells. Thyroid hormones upregulate TRH-DE in lactotroph and thyrotroph cells. Thyroid hormones suppress the expression of the TRH-receptor and both subunits of TSH in the thyrotroph cell. These actions together contribute to the negative feedback exerted by T_4/T_3 on the TRH-TSH axis. TRH-DE in lactotroph cells is suppressed by estradiol (E_2), thereby enhancing lactotroph sensitivity to TRH. Adenomatous lactotroph and somatotroph cells lose their ability to express TRH-DE; this is the basis of the TRH-induced growth hormone test in acromegaly. T_4/T_3 induces TRH-DE in the liver. Upon cleavage of the membrane-binding domain of the ectoenzyme, TRH-DE functions in plasma. Note that the figure neglects the involvement of deiodinases and plasma binding proteins in the regulatory circuit. PRL, prolactin; GH, growth hormone.

and myelination. The thyroid hormone-dependent development of the brain begins in utero and is completed by 2 to 3 years of age. Most of these processes in the brain are regulated by TRα isoforms. TRβ isoforms are the primary regulators of the development of the otic vesicle/cochlea. This role is supported by *deafness* observed in TRβ knockout mice and in human *thyroid hormone resistance syndrome* caused by mutations of the TRβ gene. This syndrome is often associated with mild mental retardation but not with the severe retardation seen in cretinism.

The expression of TRs in the developing brain precedes the endogenous production of thyroid hormones. Surprisingly, the first TR expressed in the brain is TRα2, a non-ligand-binding suppressor protein. The expression of TRα2 remains high in the developing brain. This suggests a mechanism protecting the brain from overexposure to thyroid hormones, which might cause terminal differentiation before the completion of the proliferative phase of brain development. Such protection is also supported by type III deiodinase expression by the placenta and the *fetal* liver. The TRα1 isoform is expressed later in brain development, especially in the differentiating cortical regions.

Although the thyroid gland develops very early (24 days after conception), it starts concentrating iodide only by the 11th gestational week and secreting significant amounts of thyroid hormones only during midgestation (18th to 20th weeks). Thus, during the first half of gestation, thyroid hormones in fetal plasma are derived from the mother. Preterm infants are born at an earlier stage of the development of thyroid regulation than term infants, and thus have subnormal total and free T_4 levels for newborns. Their TSH is also below normal, but their pituitary responds normally to exogenous TRH. This indicates that preterm infants have a *physiologic tertiary hypothyroidism,* a condition that usually resolves spontaneously and does not require treatment.

Untreated congenital hypothyroidism impairs terminal differentiation processes and leads to the severe mental (and growth) retardation known as *cretinism*. The term cretinism means "Christ-like"; these individuals are so retarded that they are incapable of committing sin. Today the mandatory screening for congenital hypothyroidism helps early diagnosis of the condition. With prompt treatment (orally administered L-thyroxine), most of these children have normal intellectual development. Any delay in therapy will lead to mental retardation, which (unlike the metabolic effects) cannot be corrected by later substitution of thyroid hormones. In contrast, the consequences of hypothyroidism on brain function in adults are reversible by T_4 substitution.

At birth, infants with thyroid agenesis or a complete absence of iodide organification have plasma T_4 levels 20 to 50% of the normal values. This indicates that in spite of the placental expression of type III deiodinase, significant amounts of T_4 are transferred from the maternal plasma into the fetal circulation. Because type II deiodinase activity in the brain increases in response to a decrease in circulating T_4, the intracellular levels of T_3 in the brain may be close to normal in these infants at birth. The placental transfer of T_4 may actually be increased in fetal hypothyroid states due to the increased concentration gradient of T_4. Due to these factors, the development of clinically evident hypothyroidism is delayed to 6 to 12 weeks postpartum.

REGULATION OF THYROID FUNCTION: THE THYROTROPIN-RELEASING HORMONE (TRH)-TSH-THYROID AXIS

The basic outline of thyroid hormone regulation by the hypothalamo-hypophyseal system was discussed in Chap. 7 (see Fig. 7-5, Table 7-1B).

The Main Hypothalamic Regulator of Thyroid Function Is the Tripeptide TRH

The tripeptide TRH (pyroGlu-His-Pro-NH$_2$) was the first hypothalamic releasing factor chemically identified. TRH is synthesized in perikarya located in the parvocellular portion of the paraventricular nucleus (PVN) and project to the median eminence. TRH expressed at other sites (see Box 11-4) is not involved in the regulation of TSH secretion. The product of the *TRH gene* (located on chromosome 3) is *pre-proTRH,* a 242-amino-acid polyprotein containing six copies of TRH in its sequence, which are liberated during proteolytic processing (see Chap. 3).

Under the influence of the suprachiasmatic nucleus, TRH is responsible for the circadian rhythm of TSH secretion. TRH is secreted in an episodic manner, which is reflected by the ultradian rhythm of TSH.

Whereas centrally acting α_1-adrenergic receptor agonists stimulate, bromocriptine (a dopamine agonist), endogenous opioids, and somatostatin

BOX 11-4   The Expression and Potential Functions of TRH Outside the Paraventricular Nucleus

TRH is widely expressed in the CNS, where it functions as a neurotransmitter and as a neurotrophic growth factor. As a neurotransmitter in the CNS, TRH raises body temperature via its action on the anterior hypothalamus, reverses the cognitive deficits by a hippocampal action, causes arousal, increases blood pressure and motor activity. As a neurotrophic factor, TRH improves the outcome of spinal cord and/or cerebellar injuries.

Pancreatic β-cells produce significant amounts of TRH, which might function as a stimulator of glucagon secretion. The function of TRH produced by the APUD cells of the gut is unknown.

(SRIF) inhibit the release of TRH. In vivo glucocorticoids inhibit TRH gene expression. The most important regulator of TRH is the thyroid hormone status, which represents a component of the long-loop negative feedback regulation. *Physiologic* plasma levels of both T_4 and T_3 are involved in the suppression of TRH in the PVN. Primary hyperthyroidism results in *further* suppression; primary hypothyroidism results in an increase of TRH synthesis and secretion by these cells. As mentioned, the PVN is devoid of deiodinase activity, which would suggest that circulating T_3 provides the feedback signal rather than T_4. However, the feedback would become effective only if free T_3 levels were in the supraphysiologic range. It has been suggested that T_4 contributes to the negative feedback by an indirect mechanism: T_4 is converted into T_3 outside the PVN (probably in the arcuate nucleus, where type II deiodinase activity is very high), from where the PVN receives neuronal input (see Fig. 15-5).

The action of TRH is mediated by its cognate receptor, a member of the G-protein-coupled heptahelical receptor family. The TRH-R gene is found on chromosome 8. The TRH receptor uses $G\alpha_q$ and increases the activity of PLC-β. The subsequent increase in PKC activity and activation of the IP_3 pathway result in increased synthesis and secretion of both subunits of TSH.

TRH is a relatively nonspecific hypothalamic releasing factor, which is often exploited in clinical practice. Exogenous TRH is used in provocation tests to evaluate secretory responses of TSH, prolactin (PRL), and growth hormone (GH). GH secretion in response to TRH is an abnormal response typically seen in acromegaly due to pituitary adenoma (see Chap. 10). Although exogenous TRH stimulates PRL, endogenous TRH does not function as the physiologic PRL-releasing factor (PRF) during lactation.

The Action of TRH Is Limited by a Hormonally Regulated and Highly Specific Peptidase

TRH is rapidly inactivated by the *TRH-degrading ectoenzyme* (TRH-DE; also known as *pyroglutamyl peptidase II*), a glycosylated, membrane-anchored zinc metallopeptidase. It appears that TRH is the only substrate of this enzyme, and that it is the only ectopeptidase capable of degrading TRH. TRH-DE converts TRH into pyroglutamic acid and *histidyl-proline diketopiperazine* (cyclo[His-Pro]).

TRH-DE has integrative functions in the control of TRH-stimulated secretion of TSH, GH, and PRL (see Fig. 11-11). After treatment with T_3, the mRNA levels of the TRH-DE markedly increase and those of TRH receptor decrease in the adenohypophysis. This effect is probably exerted on thyrotroph and lactotroph cells. Thus, in primary hypothyroidism not only TRH secretion is increased from the hypothalamus, but the TRH responsiveness of the pituitary gland is also enhanced by the decreased degradation of TRH and the increased numbers of TRH receptors. These effects all contribute to elevated levels of plasma TSH and PRL in primary hypothyroidism.

Estradiol (E_2) decreases adenohypophyseal expression of TRH-DE probably only in lactotrophs. Thus, in high estrogenic states (such as pregnancy) TRH might be a physiologic stimulator of PRL secretion. Testosterone, progesterone, aldosterone, and dexamethasone are ineffective. As mentioned (see Chap. 10), normal but not adenomatous somatotrophs are protected from TRH-stimulation by the expression of TRH-DE. In the brain, TRH-DE activity is unevenly distributed, which may indicate specific functions in TRH-mediated signaling. The expression of brain TRH-DE is not influenced by peripheral hormones.

T_3 increases the level of TRH-DE mRNA in the liver. The liver is probably the source of the active circulating form of TRH-DE: this membrane-anchored enzyme is apparently cleaved (similar to the mechanism seen in the generation of GHBP and angiotensin-converting enzyme [ACE]) and shed into plasma. Although significant amounts of orally administered TRH are absorbed from the GI tract, TRH is rapidly eliminated by the liver (first passage phenomenon).

TSH Synthesis and Secretion Is Regulated by TRH, T_4, and the Pit-1 Transcription Factor

As discussed earlier, TSH is one of the pituitary glycoprotein hormones, including FSH, LH, and the related placentally expressed hCG. The expression of the shared α subunit gene (found on chromosome 6) is regulated by different regions of the promoter in a cell-specific manner. This prevents inhibition of the α subunit expression in thyrotrophs by estrogen or progesterone or in gonadotrophs by thyroid hormones. The receptor-specificity is determined by the β subunit. The β subunit gene of TSH is located on chromosome 1.

Pit-1 is required for the expression of the TSH β subunit, but not for the TSH α subunit or the β subunit of the other glycoprotein hormones. Pit-1 is also expressed in somatotrophs and lactotrophs, where it increases the expression of GH and PRL, respectively (see Chap. 10).

T_4 is converted into T_3 within the pituitary gland by type II deiodinase. Thus, the primary feedback signal to the pituitary *in the circulation* is the concentration of T_4, rather than T_3. The T_3 generated in situ suppresses the expression of both α and β subunits of TSH. TRH antagonizes the action of T_3 by inducing the expression of both α and β subunits.

TSH circulates in plasma unbound to carrier proteins with a half-life of about 60 minutes. It is eliminated mainly by the kidneys in part by degradation, in part by excretion of the intact hormone. As mentioned above, TSH secretion follows a circadian rhythm. The peak values occur between 2:00 A.M. and 6:00 P.M., and the lowest values occur late afternoon between 5:00 and 6:00 P.M. The ultradian peaks of TSH-secretion occur at

2 to 4 h intervals and are superimposed on the circadian pattern The circadian rhythm is lost in secondary and tertiary hypothyroidism.

The normal plasma levels of TSH vary with age. The plasma TSH is lowest in adults (21 to 54 years of age: 0.4 to 4.2 μU/mL), and slightly higher in children and in the elderly. In term infants, a TRH-mediated TSH-surge is provoked by birth, which is related to the adaptation to a lower ambient temperature. This surge peaks about 30 min postpartum followed by a slow return to cord blood levels by the 3rd postpartum day. The physiologic tertiary hypothyroidism of preterm infants was discussed above.

Plasma TSH is perhaps the most sensitive indicator of thyroid state because of the tight control of its secretion by T_4 (mainly at the pituitary level) and T_3 mainly at the hypothalamic level. Measurement of plasma TSH is used as a gauge for adjusting the dose of drugs (such as L-thyroxine or PTU) in the treatment of thyroid diseases. The detection limit of currently used immunoradiometric IRMA type assays (0.01 μU/mL) is sufficient for demonstrating suppressed plasma levels of TSH.

Glucocorticoids Modulate the Function of the TRH-TSH-Thyroid Hormone Axis

Glucocorticoids inhibit the thyroid axis by several mechanisms:

- Inhibition of TRH gene expression and synthesis in the PVN;
- Decrease of TSH responsiveness to either endogenous or exogenous TRH leading to a decrease in plasma concentration of TSH and a consequent decrease in plasma T_4;
- Disproportionately large decrease in plasma T_3 secondary to inhibition of (mainly type I) deiodinase activity. This action of glucocorticoids is employed in the treatment of thyroid storm.

Although glucocorticoids decrease plasma levels of TBG, they increase those of transthyretin, thereby leaving the proportions of free and bound thyroid hormones approximately unaltered.

These effects of glucocorticoids are seen only if pharmacologic doses of glucocorticoids are administered. In Cushing's disease (which involves the overproduction of glucocorticoids), the suppression of thyroid function is typically mild and frank hypothyroidism is a relatively rare complication.

MAJOR PATHOLOGIC CONDITIONS OF THYROID FUNCTION

Disorders of thyroid function are common. Thus, primary care physicians routinely screen their patients for thyroid function. Selected disorders of thyroid function are summarized in Table 11-6.

Table 11-6   Selected Disorders of Thyroid Function°

Hypothyroidism		Hyperthyroidism	
Primary	Secondary/tertiary	Primary	Secondary/tertiary
Iodine deficiency, lithium therapy, dietary goitrogens	Premature birth	Graves' disease	TSH-secreting adenoma
Hashimoto's disease	Craniopharyngioma, pituitary apoplexy, Sheehan's syndrome, postablation state (hypophysectomy)	Gain-of-function mutations of TSH-R (toxic adenoma and toxic multinodular goiter)	Pituitary resistance to thyroid hormone action
Thyroid agenesis and ectopic thyroid gland	Mutations of Pit-1 and the β subunit of TSH	Thyrotoxicosis factitia (overdose of exogenous hormone)	Laboratory features of generalized resistance to thyroid hormone action with *hypothyroid* clinical presentation
Mutations of thyroglobulin, sodium iodide symporter, TPO		Struma ovarii	
Postablative condition (surgical or radiothyroidectomy)		Choriocarcinoma and hydatidiform mole (hCG production)	
Postpartum lymphocytic thyroiditis (2nd phase)		Postpartum lymphocytic thyroiditis (1st phase)	

° The assignment of disease entities reflects their laboratory diagnosis (plasma TSH and thyroid hormones).
ABBREVIATIONS: TSH, thyroid-stimulating hormone; TSH-R, TSH receptor; TPO, thyroid peroxidase; hCG, human chorionic gonadotropin.

Autoimmune Diseases Are the Most Common Pathologies Leading to Altered Thyroid Function

Most autoimmune diseases, including those of the thyroid gland, are more common in women than in men. The two prototypes of autoimmune thyroid diseases are Graves' and Hashimoto's diseases, which are the foremost causes of primary hyperthyroidism and hypothyroidism, respectively. Both diseases display association with certain HLA haplotypes, and both diseases usually present with diffuse goiter. It appears that the involvement of CD8$^+$ cytotoxic lymphocytes in the autoimmune reaction of Hashimoto's disease is responsible for their different pathomechanisms. However, mixed presentations may occur, which are referred to as *hashitoxicosis*.

The pathomechanism of *Hashimoto's disease* involves direct damage inflicted by cytotoxic (CD8$^+$) lymphocytes as well as antibody-mediated effects. The most characteristic and functionally important antibody is directed against thyroid peroxidase (TPO), which inhibits thyroid hormone synthesis. Because TPO is found at the apical membrane of the follicular epithelium (a sequestered space), the action of the anti-TPO immunoglobulins is puzzling. The cellular damage caused by the $CD8^+$ cells might make the TPO more accessible to the immunoglobulin.

Whereas the etiology of *Graves' disease* is still obscure, its pathomechanism is explained by effects of TSH-R-stimulating antibodies (TSAb). The production of TSAb is secondary to the aberrant expression of major histocompatibility complex class II antigens by thyroid follicular cells. These thyroid follicular cells acquire the capacity to present the TSH-R as an autoantigen to ($CD4^+$) helper T cells infiltrating the thyroid gland. The helper T cells direct B cells to produce TSAb-s. This mechanism is supported by experimental evidence: intraperitoneal immunization of inbred mice with syngeneic nonmitotic fibroblasts transfected with both the human TSH receptor and a major histocompatibility complex class II molecule, but not by either alone, results in the production of TSAb. These antibodies cause hyperthyroidism by acting on the murine TSH-R in the thyroid gland without the occurrence of lymphocytic infiltration of the gland per se. In thyroid follicular cells, aberrant expression of major histocompatibility complex class II antigens duplicating the autoimmune state can be induced by interferon-γ (IFN-γ). The IFN-γ-induced expression of major histocompatibility complex class II antigens is enhanced in the follicular cells of Graves' disease patients. Methimazole, a drug used for treating patients with Graves' disease, can suppress the interferon (IFN)-γ-induced increase in the expression of major histocompatibility complex class II antigens (HLA-DR α gene expression) and IFN-γ-induced endogenous antigen presentation by the cell. Graves' disease patients pretreated with iodide before surgery have lower levels of major histocompatibility complex class II RNA levels in their thyroid tissue than the patients who did not receive iodide pretreatment.

In some patients thyroid autoimmune disease (especially Hashimoto's disease) is associated with other autoimmune manifestations, including Addison's disease, type I diabetes mellitus, premature ovarian failure, hypophysitis, vitiligo (destruction of pigment cells in well-demarcated areas of the epidermis), and/or achlorhydria/pernicious anemia (destruction of gastric parietal cells). These combined autoimmune diseases are known as *type II multiple endocrine glandular failure* or *Schmidt's syndrome*.

Thyroid Hormone Resistance Syndrome (Refetoff Syndrome) Is a Rare Condition, Which Is Due to Mutations of the TRβ Gene

To date none of the thyroid resistance syndrome cases involved mutations of the TRα gene, which might indicate its lethal nature as evidenced in TRα-knockout mice. Apart from a few cases in which co-repressors of thyroid hormone receptors were mutated, all cases of thyroid hormone resistance have been mutations of the TRβ gene. Most mutations involve the C-terminal portion of the receptor, which eliminates its T_3 binding and converts the receptor into a functional repressor protein: the mutant receptor may form dimers with its regular partners and binds TRE segments of DNA, but prevents activation of transcription. This explains the autosomal dominant mode of inheritance of the condition.

Resistance to thyroid hormone is characterized by elevated free thyroid hormones in the serum and failure to suppress pituitary TSH secretion. This arrangement is also seen in secondary hyperthyroidism, which is usually due to TSH-producing basophil adenoma of the pituitary gland. Two major subtypes of the thyroid hormone resistance are recognized:

• *Generalized resistance,* which presents as a mild congenital hypothyroidism (attention-deficit/hyperactivity disorder, slight mental retardation, deafness, short stature).
• *Predominant pituitary resistance,* which presents with thyrotoxic features, especially tachyarrhythmia. In this condition, the TRβ2-mediated feedback appears to be affected, whereas the TRβ1-mediated functions are normal.

Both subtypes present with goiter and similar laboratory profile of increased TSH and thyroid hormones. The generalized resistance may be at least partially overcome by increasing the already high circulating levels of thyroid hormones with orally administered L-thyroxine. The thyrotoxic pituitary form often responds to treatment with 3,5,3′-triiodothyroacetic acid (TRIAC). TRIAC, a compound with little thyroid hormone activity, does not stimulate cardiac function. For reasons unknown, TRIAC may suppress pituitary TSH secretion thereby reducing goiter and the secretion of thyroid hormones.

Tumors of the Thyroid Gland May Be Caused by Mutations of TSH-R and the *RET* Protooncogene

As mentioned, gain-of-function mutations of the TSH-R may lead to development of toxic adenoma (Plummer's disease) or toxic multinodular goiter. Mutations of the *RET* protooncogene may cause cancer in two developmentally distinct populations of cells in the thyroid gland:

• *Familial medullary thyroid cancer* (FMTC) arises from the C-cells and is caused by gain-of-function mutations of the RET protooncogene, a single membrane spanning tyrosine-kinase receptor (discussed in more detail in Chap. 12). FMTC cells secrete calcitonin (see Chap. 8).
• The *RET/PTC* oncogenes are unique to *papillary thyroid cancer,* a derivative of the follicular epithelial cells. *RET/PTCs* are chimeric genes, which arise by the translocation and fusion between the *RET* protooncogene and three different fusion partners found on chromosome 10. The most common fusion partners are *H4 (PTC-1)* and *ELE1 (PTC-3).* The

rearrangement causes translocation of the protein from the membrane to the cytoplasm and constitutive activation of its tyrosine kinase activity. RET/PTC oncogene accounts for about 20% of human thyroid papillary carcinomas. Papillary thyroid cancers rarely cause thyrotoxicosis, but often secrete thyroglobulin. Most malignant tumors lack the sodium iodide symporter, and present as cold nodules on radioactive thyroid scan.

12

THE ADRENAL GLAND

OBJECTIVES

1. Identify the main components and/or layers of the adrenal gland, the main secretory products, and their physiologic functions.
2. Discuss the gross anatomy, histology, and embryology of the adrenal gland, the *paraganglia*, the *organ of Zuckerkandl*, and the ganglia of the autonomic nervous system.
3. Discuss the molecular basis of developmental derangements leading to *multiple endocrine neoplasia* (MEN) type II syndromes, *pheochromocytoma, medullary thyroid cancer*, and *Hirschprung's disease*.
4. Describe the biosynthesis, storage, and secretion of *catecholamines* in the adrenal medulla and sympathetic nerves. Discuss *vesicular monoamine transporters* and the molecular basis of the *uptake-1* and *uptake-2* systems (plasma membrane monoamine transporters).
5. Describe the plasma transport, half-life, and degradation of catecholamines.
6. Discuss adrenergic receptors, the tissue distribution, molecular action, and physiologic effects of catecholamines.
7. Discuss the regulation of sympathoadrenal activity and the stress response of Cannon. Describe catecholamine responses to postural changes.
8. Discuss the cardiovascular effects of catecholamines and *adrenomedullin*.
9. Describe the biosynthesis of steroid hormones and the cellular regulation of steroid hormone biosynthesis. Discuss the molecular basis of various enzyme defects related to steroid hormone biosynthesis. Identify the cell type-specific expression of steroidogenic enzymes and isoenzymes.
10. Discuss the plasma transport, degradation, action, and biologic effects of *mineralocorticoids*. Discuss the physiologic roles of *11β-hydroxysteroid dehydrogenase isoenzymes*.
11. Discuss the *renin-angiotensin system* and the regulation of mineralocorticoid homeostasis.
12. Discuss *natriuretic peptide* family and the *aldosterone escape phenomenon*.
13. Describe the transport, degradation, action and biologic effects of *glucocorticoids*.

14. Discuss the *CRH–ACTH–adrenocortical* axis, the regulation of glucocorticoid secretion, and the stress response of Selye.

15. Discuss the developmental changes in adrenocortical function and the molecular basis of *adrenarche*.

16. Be familiar with the main pathologic conditions of the adrenal gland. Identify the overlapping manifestations and interactions among diseases affecting various portions of the adrenal gland, such as the altered catecholamine synthesis in *Addison's disease*, the pathomechanism of *orthostatic hypotension* in Addison's disease, or the *apparent mineralocorticoid excess* in compensated glucocorticoid resistance.

INTRODUCTION

The adrenal gland is a multifunctional organ (Table 12-1). The medulla is a modified sympathetic ganglion. The cells of the adrenal medulla (the *pheochromocytes*) receive the same preganglionic synaptic innervation as the ganglionic cells. Unlike ganglionic cells, however, they do not send

Table 12-1 The Subdivision, Main Regulators, Hormones, and Functions of the Adrenal Gland

Division	Subdivision	Regulators	Hormone products	Functions
Cortex	Definitive zone, zona glomerulosa	Renin-angiotensin system and plasma K^+	Aldosterone	Stimulates Na-reabsorption leading to increased volume of ECF, decreases plasma K^+, increases plasma pH
	Definitive zone, zona fasciculata	CRH-ACTH axis	Mainly cortisol, some adrenal androgens (DHEA, DHEAS, androstenedione)	Stress response (of Selye); multiple actions on metabolism, blood pressure, and immune function
	Definitive zone, zona reticularis		Mainly adrenal androgens (DHEA, DHEAS androstenedione), some cortisol	Main source of androgens in females; serve also as precursors of estrogens generated by peripheral conversion; production increases at adrenarche
Cortex	Fetal zone	ACTH, CRH (both by direct action)	DHEA, DHEAS; minimal aldosterone and cortisol is produced from placentally derived progesterone	Provides estrogen precursors for the placenta
Medulla	N/A	Preganglionic sympathetic cholinergic fibers acting on nicotinic receptors	Adrenaline (epinephrine), noradrenaline (norepinephrine), adrenomedullin	Stress response (of Cannon), multiple actions on metabolism and blood pressure.

ABBREVIATIONS: ECF, extracellular fluid; CRH, corticotropin-releasing hormone; ACTH, adrenocorticotroph hormone; DHEA, dehydroepiandrosterone; DHEAS, DHEA sulfate.

axons to their targets. Instead, pheochromocytes release catecholamines into the extracellular fluid (ECF) to reach their targets via the bloodstream.

The cortex of the adrenal gland produces steroid hormones, including mineralocorticoids, glucocorticoids, and androgens. The adrenocortical, gonadal, and placental steroid hormone synthetic pathways represent variations of a basic theme. This results in cooperation between these steroid-producing organs and their regulatory systems in both health and disease.

In this Chap., we discuss the medulla, the general scheme of steroidogenesis, the mineralocorticoids, and the glucocorticoids. The adrenal androgens and the fetal zone of the adrenal cortex will be discussed in detail in Chap. 13.

OVERVIEW OF THE ANATOMY, HISTOLOGY, AND EMBRYOLOGY OF THE ADRENAL GLAND

Gross Anatomy

The *adrenal* or *suprarenal gland,* as its name indicates, is located near and superior to the kidneys. The Greek name of the gland *(epinephros),* which has the same meaning, is rarely used. However, *adrenaline,* the main secretory product of the gland's medulla, is often referred to as *epinephrine.*

The adrenal gland in adults consists of a medulla and a cortex, which have embryologically distinct origins (see Embryology). The two adrenal glands together weigh 8 to 10 g in adults. Ninety percent of the adrenal mass belongs to the cortex; 10% of the weight is the medulla. On gross examination, the cut surface of the gland reveals the cortex as a sulphur yellow layer surrounding a central brown-red medulla. Note that another steroid secreting organ, the corpus luteum of the ovary, also appears yellow on gross examination *(luteum* = yellow [Latin]).

The gland is embedded in the retroperitoneal adipose tissue, which also forms a capsule or padding around the kidneys. The blood supply of the gland is of major clinical importance (Fig. 12-1). The arterial supply is derived from three sources:

- *superior suprarenal artery* from the *inferior phrenic artery;*
- *middle suprarenal artery* directly from the *abdominal aorta;*
- *inferior suprarenal artery* from the *renal artery.*

The three arteries supply the gland by two means:

- They form a plexus in the connective tissue capsule of the adrenal gland and perfuse the gland from its periphery toward its center via a radially oriented sinusoidal system. This means that the medulla receives

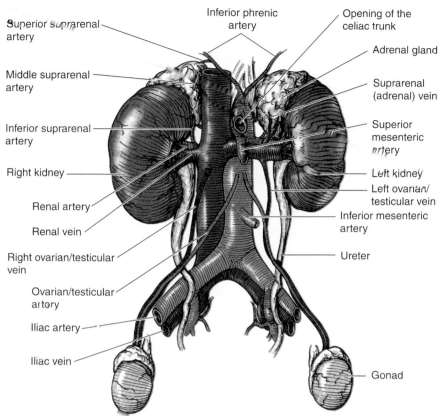

Superior suprarenal artery

Inferior phrenic artery

Opening of the celiac trunk

Middle suprarenal artery

Adrenal gland

Inferior suprarenal artery

Suprarenal (adrenal) vein

Right kidney

Superior mesenteric artery

Renal artery

Left kidney

Renal vein

Left ovarian/ testicular vein

Right ovarian/testicular vein

Inferior mesenteric artery

Ovarian/testicular artery

Ureter

Iliac artery

Iliac vein

Gonad

Figure 12-1. The anatomic arrangement and blood supply of the adrenal glands. The blood supply of the gonads are also displayed. Note the difference in the venous drainage between the left and right sides both for the adrenals and the gonads: Their veins on the left lead to the renal vein, those on the right open into the inferior vena cava. The suprarenal arteries are derived from three sources on each side. The lymphatics of the adrenals and the gonads follow the course of their arterial supply (not shown).

blood enriched with the secretory products of the cortex, but this blood has a decreased nutrient and oxygen content.

• The medulla receives nutrient-rich and oxygenated direct arterial supply. This blood, however, is not enriched by the secretory products of the cortex.

These two types of blood supply have a major impact on medullary hormone synthesis (see later).

The *venous drainage* is accomplished by a single adrenal vein on each side draining blood from the adrenal medulla. The arrangement is *similar to that of the venous drainage of the gonads:*

- the *right adrenal vein* (and the right *pampiniform plexus* from the testis or ovary) drains blood to the *inferior vena cava*;
- the *left adrenal vein* (and the left pampiniform plexus from the testis or ovary) drains blood to the *left renal vein*.

The lymphatic drainage of the adrenal gland (the preferred route of metastases of adrenal cancers) leads to the para-aortic lymph nodes.

Histology

The common histologic features of the adrenocortical zones are related to the steroidogenic nature of the tissue. Steroidogenesis is performed by cholesterol-processing enzymes found in the *smooth endoplasmic reticulum* (sER) and the *inner mitochondrial membrane*. Thus, steroid hormone-producing cells have a preponderance of sER in their cytoplasm, and *tubulovesicular* mitochondria (Fig. 12-2). The peculiar morphology of the mitochondrial cristae is related to the increased membrane surface, which is needed to house the rate-limiting enzyme of steroid hormone synthesis P450scc, which converts cholesterol into pregnenolone (see later). The only human pregnenolone-producing cell type, which has regular (lamellar) mitochondrial cristae, is the *zona glomerulosa* cell, which produces lower quantities of steroid hormones than the other cell types. For example, the zona glomerulosa cells produce aldosterone at the rate of 50 to 250 μg/d, whereas the zona fasciculata/reticularis cells produce cortisol at the rate of 15 to 20 mg/d.

The parenchymal cells of the adrenal cortex are capable of de novo synthesis of cholesterol. However, they mainly rely on uptake of cholesterol by receptor-mediated endocytosis of low density lipoproteins (LDL). The cells accumulate cholesterol-rich lipid droplets in the cytoplasm; thus, although they do not store steroid hormones, they store their precursor. LDL uptake by the cells is facilitated by the fenestrated endothelial lining of the adrenal gland. The fenestrations are of two sizes ($\approx$100 and 400 nm); the larger pore size is present in higher numbers towards the inner zones of the cortex.

The cytoarchitecture of the adrenal gland varies with the subdivisions of the gland and the arrangement of the cells is greatly influenced by the orientation of its blood vessels.

- The layers of the *permanent* or *definitive zone* of the cortex (Fig. 12-3) display the following characteristics:
  - The *zona glomerulosa* is found immediately beneath the connective tissue capsule. The vessels derived from the capsular plexus surround glomerulus-like spherical or elongated clusters of cortical epithelial cells. The mainly columnar cells contain scant lipid droplets, and the cytoplasm is dominated by sER resulting in an overall eosinophilic staining of the cytoplasm.

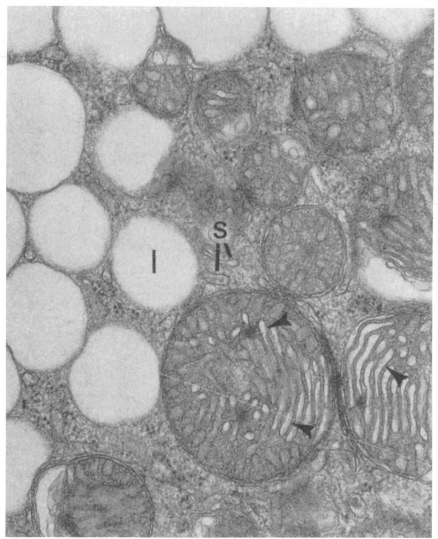

Figure 12-2. Electron micrograph of a steroid hormone producing cell from the zona fasciculata of the adrenal cortex. The cytoplasmic compartment is filled with lipid droplets (l), smooth endoplasmic reticulum (s) and mitochondria with tubulovesicular cristae (arrowheads). (*Source:* Inset of figure, p 235 in Cross PC, Mercer KL: *Cell and Tissue Ultrastructure. A Functional Perspective.* Freeman, 1993.)

• The *zona fasciculata* consists of large polyhedral cells arranged in one- to two-cell wide radial cords. The space between adjacent cords is occupied by the sinusoids. The plethora of lipid droplets in the parenchymal cells results in a foamy cytoplasmic appearance.

• In the *zona reticularis*, the radial parallel arrangement is replaced by an irregular, anastomosing network of cords. These

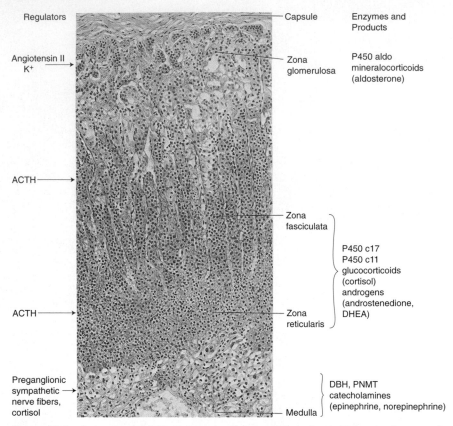

Figure 12-3. Low-power histologic image of the adrenal gland displaying the overall cytoarchitecture. Abbreviations: ACTH, adrenocorticotroph hormone; DHEA, dehydroepiandrosterone; DBH, dopamine β hydroxylase; PNMT, phenylethanolamine N-methyl transferase. (*Source:* Modified from Fig. 8.208, p 1380 in Warwick R, Williams PL (eds): *Gray's Anatomy*, 35th ed., Longman, 1973.)

cells are smaller, contain fewer lipid droplets, and often contain brown *lipofuscin* cytoplasmic inclusions, which are also known as *age pigments* (peroxidated membrane lipids of damaged mitochondria retained after their autophagocytosis). Note that the zona reticularis develops postnatally, and it is not recognizable until about 3 years of age.

• The *fetal zone* of the adrenal cortex is found *between the definitive cortex and the medulla.* The fetal zone gives the bulk of the adrenal gland during intrauterine life. The fetal adrenal gland is very large compared to the body or the adjacent kidney: its relative size is 10 times greater than in adults, and is about one third of the size of the kidney. The parenchymal cells in the fetal zone display an arrangement that is a mixture between those seen in the zona fasciculata and reticularis: anastomosing but in

principal radially arranged cords. The cytoplasm of the cells is more reminiscent of those in the zona reticularis.

The *adrenal medulla* contains few true sympathetic *ganglion cells*. The
pheochromocytes, which constitute the bulk of the parenchyma of the adrenal medulla, are axonless secretory cells that form an anastomosing network
of short cords and ovoid clusters. Unlike the cells of the adjacent zona
reticularis, the cytoplasmic staining of pheochromocytes is not eosinophilic
but either basophilic or pale. Pheochromocytes stain brown (*pheo* [Greek])
with potassium dichromate, which oxidizes their catecholamine content
into a polymerized melanin. For this reason, they are also referred to as
chromaffin cells. Chromaffin cells are found at other locations in the body,
such as the *paraganglia,* the *organ of Zuckerkandl* (see Embryology), and
the *carotid body*. The *pheochromocytes* have two subpopulations:

- *Noradrenaline-producing cells* display a strong chromaffin reaction.
They contain relatively large *dense core secretory granules* seen in electron
microscopic preparations.
- *Adrenaline-producing cells* are far more numerous and display a
weak chromaffin reaction. Their secretory granules are smaller, and contain
a homogenous, less electron dense material.

These cell types represent different physiologic states of the same
cell population. Thus, depending on exposure to different concentrations
of cortisol, adrenaline- and noradrenaline-producing cells may switch
phenotype (see The Biosynthesis, Storage, and Release of Catecholamines). The pheochromocytes also contain *chromogranin A,* a secretory
protein, in their granules. Measurements of chromogranin A in plasma
and its demonstration in tissues by immunocytochemistry are utilized in
the diagnosis of *pheochromocytoma* (a tumor derived from the adrenal
medulla) and other neuroendocrine tumors such as *carcinoids*. Chromogranin A is often secreted by "nonfunctional" tumors, which do not
secrete specific hormones.

The pheochromocytes secrete the contents of their granules by
exocytosis into the pericapillary ECF. The catecholamines secreted by
the adrenal medulla and the paraganglia reach their target cells via
the circulation. In contrast, postganglionic sympathetic adrenergic fibers
release their granules into the ECF near their target cells; thus, the
catecholamines from this source reach their primary targets without first
entering the bloodstream. Nevertheless, postganglionic sympathetic fibers
do not form true synapses with their target cells, and significant amounts
of the released catecholamines will reach the capillaries by diffusion
through the ECF.

Embryology

The adrenal gland develops from two primordial tissues:

•   The cortex develops from the mesothelial lining of the posterior abdominal wall between the *urogenital ridge* (the developing gonad) and the root of the *mesentery* (see Fig. 13-36).
•   The pheochromocytes develop from a subpopulation of neural crest cells known as *sympathogonia*. Thus, unlike the adrenal cortex, the medulla belongs to the *amine precursor uptake and decarboxylation* (APUD) system (see Box 9-1). Sympathogonia also give rise to *neuroblasts,* which form the sympathetic ganglia.

Steroidogenic factor-1 (SF-1) and *DAX-1* are nuclear orphan receptors, which are colocalized in developing tissues. Experiments with knockout mice indicate that SF-1 is required for the development of the adrenal glands, the gonads, and the ventromedial nucleus of the hypothalamus. Mutations of DAX-1 have similar consequences. Although SF-1 is expressed in the placenta (a major steroidogenic organ), it is not required for placental development.

The cortex develops in two waves: first the fetal zone develops starting with the 6th week. During the 7th week, sympathogonia migrate from the primitive sympathetic chain to the developing fetal zone, become encapsulated, and proliferate as *pheochromoblasts*. During the 8th week, the cells of the definitive cortex migrate and surround the primordial adrenal gland (second wave of cortical development). The absence of cortical development results in the *agenesis* of the entire adrenal gland.

In addition to the adrenal medulla, pheochromoblasts also form *paraganglia* on either side of the aorta and the *organ of Zuckerkandl,* which is found in the retroperitoneum anterior to the aorta between the *inferior mesenteric artery* and the bifurcation of the aorta. These organs function as "accessory adrenal medullae" not associated with adrenocortical cells. The organ of Zuckerkandl is a preferential site of extra-adrenal pheochromocytomas. It is the main source of circulating catecholamines in the fetus and during the first year of life, after which it normally involutes. Knockout mouse experiments suggest that *catecholamine production in the organ of Zuckerkandl is upregulated by the hypoxia-inducible transcription factor EPAS1* (see Box 12-1), and that the survival of the fetus mandates both EPAS1 and the enzymes involved in noradrenaline synthesis.

The migrating sympathogonia bring along their innervating preganglionic axons, which arise from perikarya located in the intermediolateral column of the *thoracolumbal spinal cord* (T1–L2). Other neural crest cells derived from the cranial and caudal portions of the developing nervous system develop into *parasympathetic ganglion cells,* which receive pregangli-

BOX 12-1   Regulation of Transcription by Hypoxia

Hypoxia is the subnormal concentration of oxygen (or Po_2) in tissues. Hypoxia caused by conditions such as high altitude, anemia, wound healing and developmental processes requires an adaptational response. The adaptation in part functions as a negative feedback system to ameliorate hypoxia by improving oxygen carrying capacity of blood, vascularization of the tissues, and by switching to anaerobic metabolism. Thus, hypoxia regulates genes involved in erythropoiesis, angiogenesis, energy metabolism, and apoptosis. Responsiveness to hypoxia is an ancestral mechanism: the oxygen sensor system in the nitrogen-fixing bacterium *Rhizobium meliloti* resembles that in mammalian cells. The putative main *oxygen sensors* are heme proteins, some of which are hemokinases, whereas others are flavohemoproteins (flavohemoglobins and NAD(P)H oxidases). Upon hypoxia, they phosphorylate the *hypoxia-inducible factor-1α* (HIF-1α, encoded by chromosome 14q21-q24), thereby preventing its degradation in the ubiquitin-proteasome pathway (see Box 12-9). Hypoxia increases protein, but not the mRNA, levels of HIF-1α. The stabilized HIF-1α forms a heterodimeric transcription factor with the *aryl hydrocarbon nuclear translocator* (ARNT; see Chap. 5). Both HIF-1α and ARNT are members of the PAS subfamily of basic-helix-loop-helix (bHLH) transcription factors (see Chap. 14). The HIF-1α/ARNT heterodimer enters the nucleus and upregulates the expression of genes involved in the adaptation of higher organisms to hypoxic conditions ("oxy-genes"). The enhancer DNA sequences of these oxy-genes are known as the *hypoxia response elements*. Examples of oxy-genes include *erythropoietin, vascular endothelial growth factor* (VEGF; see Chaps. 2 and 11), glucose transporters, and a number of glycolytic enzymes. Insulin also activates the HIF-1α/ARNT mechanism in part by inhibiting the proteasome pathway. The *von Hippel-Lindau* (VHL) tumor suppressor gene product *pVHL* plays a critical role in the regulation of HIF-1α. The direct interaction between HIF-1α and pVHL is iron dependent and necessary for the oxygen-dependent degradation of HIF-1α. In VHL-defective cells, HIF-1α is constitutively stabilized, which may explain the development of hemangiomas in von Hippel-Lindau disease.

In addition to hypoxia, transition metals (Co^{2+}, Ni^{2+} and Mn^{2+}) and iron chelation also stabilize HIF-1α. Induction of HIF-1α by hypoxia is blocked by the heme ligands carbon monoxide and nitric oxide. Homozygous HIF-1α knockout mouse embryos die during embryonic life due to neural tube defects, cardiovascular malformations, and marked cell death within the cephalic mesenchyme. Closely related, but differentially expressed, transcription factors have recently been cloned. At least one of these (*endothelial PAS-1* [EPAS1]) also forms heterodimers with ARNT and can be activated by hypoxia.

onic fibers either from the cranial nerves (III, VII, IX, X/XI) or from the sacral portion of the spinal cord. Most parasympathetic ganglion cells are not organized into compact ganglia, but become embedded in the wall of the innervated viscera, where they form plexuses.

The *migration* of intestinal parasympathetic ganglion cells and melanocytes from the neural crest is regulated by the *interaction between endothelin-3 (ET-3) and the endothelin B receptor*. Disruption of this signaling is the cause of the *multigenic* form of *Hirschprung's disease (congenital megacolon,* the consequence of agenesis of myenteric and submucosal plexuses in the gastrointestinal tract) and pigmentation deficits. This explains the association between Hirschprung's disease, white forelock of the hair, regional pigment deficits of the skin, and *heterochromia iridum* (bicolored irides).

The *proliferation* of certain neural crest-derived cells (such as the C-cells of the thyroid gland, autonomic ganglionic cells, and pheochromocytes but not the melanocytes) is regulated by *glial cell line-derived neurotrophic factor* (GDNF) acting on a receptor tyrosine kinase encoded by the *RET* protooncogene (Box 12-2).

BOX 12-2   Diseases Related to the *RET* Protooncogene

Mutations of the *RET* protooncogene, an unusual member of the transforming growth factor β (TGF-β) receptor family which maps to chromosome 10q11.1, are responsible for a variety of disease states.

- RET/PTC chimeric oncogenes are responsible for *papillary thyroid cancer* (see Chap. 11).
- Two types of gain-of-function mutations have been described, which are inherited in an autosomal dominant fashion:
    - a mutation that results in a ligand-independent dimerization of the RET receptor protein is the cause of both familial medullary thyroid cancer (*FMTC*) and type 2A multiple endocrine neoplasia (*MEN type 2A* or *Sipple's syndrome*). MEN type 2A may involve MTC, pheochromocytoma, and tumors of the parathyroid glands.
    - another mutation that activates the tyrosine kinase domain of the receptor in the absence of dimerization is the cause of *MEN type 2B* (also known as MEN type 3). MEN type 2B may involve MTC, pheochromocytoma, mucosal neuromas and is associated with marfanoid habitus.
- Loss-of-function mutations of RET are responsible for the autosomal dominant form of Hirschprung's disease, which has variable penetrance.

Neither sympathetic nor parasympathetic preganglionic fibers emerge from the cervical spine. The sympathetic ganglia in the cervical region, which supply the head and the neck, receive preganglionic fibers from upper thoracic spinal segments.

THE ADRENAL MEDULLA AND THE SYMPATHOADRENAL SYSTEM

The Biosynthesis, Storage, and Release of Catecholamines

Catecholamines Are Synthesized from L-Tyrosine in a Highly Regulated and Compartmentalized Process   The 3,4-dihydroxy derivatives of the aromatic ring are referred to as *catechol compounds*. In terms of chemical structure, the *catecholamines* are the 3,4-dihydroxy derivatives of phenylethylamine (i.e., the decarboxylation product of phenylalanine). The catecholamines include *dopamine, noradrenaline,* and *adrenaline,* compounds of the same biosynthetic pathway (Fig. 12-4). The substrate of the biosynthetic pathway, L-tyrosine, circulates in plasma at a concentration of 1 to 1.5 mg/dL, and its cellular uptake is mediated by an active transport mechanism. The processing of L-tyrosine to adrenaline involves four reactions; all but one reaction occurs in the cytosol:

- Ring hydroxylation by the Fe^{2+}-containing *tyrosine hydroxylase* is the rate-limiting step of catecholamine synthesis. This hydroxylation reaction requires *tetrahydrobiopterin* as a cofactor. The reaction product is L-*di*hydroxy-phenylalanine commonly known as *L-DOPA*. The activity of tyrosine hydroxylase is regulated by the preganglionic nerves and the intracellular levels of catechol compounds:
    - An acute increase of enzyme activity is achieved by activation of the preexisting enzyme. This mechanism involves phosphorylation by protein kinase A (PKA), protein kinase C (PKC), and calmodulin-dependent kinases.
    - Long-term stimulation upregulates the transcription and translation of tyrosine hydroxylase.
    - Catechol compounds inhibit tyrosine hydroxylase activity (product feedback).
    These mechanisms help to maintain catecholamine stores at times of increased demand and prevent overproduction, which is often referred to as the *synthesis-secretion coupling*. The reaction catalyzed by tyrosine hydroxylase should not be confused with that catalyzed by the copper-containing *tyrosinase,* which is involved in the biosynthesis of melanin.
- Decarboxylation by *DOPA-decarboxylase* yields *dopamine.* Like

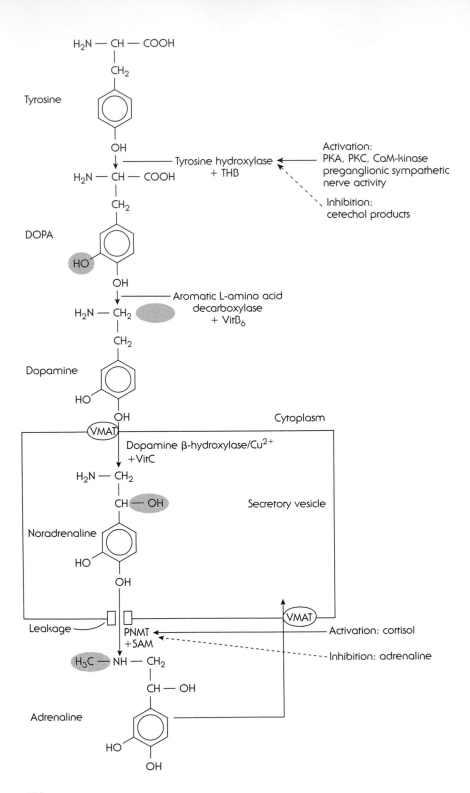

Tyrosine

Tyrosine hydroxylase
+ THB

DOPA

Aromatic L-amino acid
decarboxylase
+ VitB$_6$

Dopamine

VMAT

Cytoplasm

Dopamine β-hydroxylase/Cu^{2+}
+VitC

Secretory vesicle

Noradrenaline

Leakage

VMAT

PNMT
+SAM

Activation: cortisol

Inhibition: adrenaline

Adrenaline

the decarboxylation reactions in general, DOPA-decarboxylase requires *pyridoxal phosphate* as a cofactor. In dopaminergic neurons (found mainly in the central nervous system [CNS]) this is the end product, which is packaged into synaptic vesicles (secretory granules) by an active transport mechanism. Packaging of dopamine into secretory granules also takes place in noradrenergic and adrenergic neurons as well as the pheochromocytes. DOPA-decarboxylase is also known as *aromatic L-amino acid decarboxylase*. It is not specific for DOPA and generates serotonin from 5-hydroxy-L-tryptophane (5-HTP) in neurons, mast cells and certain APUD cells.

• The side-chain hydroxylation of dopamine is catalyzed by the copper-containing enzyme *dopamine β-hydroxylase* (DBH), which utilizes *ascorbic acid* (vitamin C) as a cofactor. *This reaction occurs within the synaptic vesicle/secretory granule*, and yields *noradrenaline*. DBH exists in the vesicles in two forms: membrane-anchored and soluble. Due to its location, soluble DBH is coreleased with both noradrenaline and adrenaline. Except for the cholinergic sympathetic nerves, noradrenaline is the end product in sympathetic nerves, the paraganglia, the organ of Zuckerkandl, and the vast majority of central catecholaminergic neural tracts.

• *Adrenaline* is derived from noradrenaline by N-methylation by *phenylethanolamine-N-methyltransferase* (PNMT). PNMT utilizes S-adenosylmethionine (SAM) as the methyl donor. Because this is a cytoplasmic reaction, *noradrenaline must leave the secretory granule*. This is a passive transport mechanism driven by concentration gradient. This also implies that *the adrenaline produced in the cytosol must reenter the secretory granule by active transport*. Few adrenergic neurons in the CNS and the vast majority of the pheochromocytes in the adrenal medulla express PNMT. *The expression and activity of PNMT in the adrenal medulla are dependent on the high local concentrations of cortisol* directly reaching the medulla from the cortex via the sinusoid system, and dynamically changes with the perfusion of the medulla by sinusoidal versus direct arterial blood supply (Box 12-3). The *transcriptional activation* of the *PNMT gene* involves the synergistic action between early growth response protein-1 (Egr 1 a zinc-finger transcription factor), APB2 (a transcription factor expressed in neural crest cells), and the ligand-activated glucocorticoid receptor. The glucocorticoid-stimulated PNMT *activity* involves poorly understood posttranscriptional events. Adrenaline is an allosteric inhibitor of PNMT (product feedback). PNMT is expressed in several extramedullary tissues, including the kidney, lung, and pancreas. The renal PNMT generates about half of the urinary adrenaline by converting circulating noradrenaline. A distinct, widely distributed *nonspecific NMT* also contributes to the peripheral conversion of noradren-

---

Figure 12-4. The biosynthetic pathway of catecholamines. Most reactions occur in the cytoplasmic compartment, except the conversion of dopamine into noradrenaline by dopamine β-hydroxylase (DBH) in the secretory vesicle. DBH exists in the vesicle both as a membrane-anchored and as a soluble enzyme. Dopamine and adrenaline enter the vesicle by active transport mechanism involving the vesicular monoamine transporters (VMATs). Noradrenaline leaves the vesicle by passive transport. The highlighted moieties in the structures show the change in the molecule in each reaction. The cofactors used by the enzymes include tetrahydrobiopterin (THB), S-adenosyl-methionine (SAM), vitamins B₆ (as pyridoxal phosphate) and C. The main regulators of the pathway are shown on the right.

BOX 12-3   Plasma Catecholamine Levels in Addison's Disease

The impact of locally high levels of cortsiol on PNMT activity is clinically relevant. In patients with autoimmune Addison's disease, the adrenal cortex is atrophied and cortisol production is diminished, yet the medulla is anatomically intact. Plasma levels of adrenaline in patients with Addison's disease are significantly reduced, and the *noradrenaline : adrenaline ratio* is elevated. Normally the molar ratio of noradrenaline : adrenaline in plasma is approximately 9 : 1 in both sexes. Probably due to a more intense autoimmune response, the decrease in plasma epinephrine is greater in females than in males, which results in a more increased ratio (approximately 45 : 1 in females versus 24 : 1 in males).

Noradrenaline-producing pheochromocytes are most often found in the vicinity of direct arterial supply of the medulla. In the case of paraganglia and the organ of Zuckerkandl, the physiologic absence of direct cortical influence explains that their secretory product is noradrenaline. In nonmammalian species, whose adrenal medulla and cortex remain anatomically separated during ontogeny, little if any adrenaline is produced by the medulla.

aline to adrenaline. Although 80% of the catecholamine output of the adrenal medulla is adrenaline and in spite of peripheral conversion by NMTs, the molar ratio of noradrenaline : adrenaline in plasma is approximately 9 : 1. This observation implies that circulating noradrenaline is dominantly derived from extra-adrenal sources (sympathetic nerves and paraganglia).

The Storage of Catecholamines Requires a Secondary Active Transport Involving the Adenosine Triphosphate-Driven Proton Pump and Reserpine-Sensitive Vesicular Monoamine Transporters   The storage of catecholamines in the secretory vesicles requires the continuous work of an active transport mechanism. The adenosine triphosphate (ATP)-driven proton pump embedded in the membrane of these vesicles generates a pH and electrical gradient. In turn, this gradient is utilized by electrogenic antiporter proteins known as *vesicular monoamine transporters* (VMATs). For every molecule of monoamine entering the vesicle, two protons are transported from the vesicle into the cytosol.

Two homologous but distinct *VMAT* genes have been cloned, which encode for the VMAT1 and VMAT2 transporters (Table 12-2). VMATs are characterized by 12 transmembrane helical segments and are structurally related to *plasma membrane monoamine transporters* (Box 12-4). VMAT1 is expressed exclusively in neuroendocrine, including chromaffin and enterochromaffin, cells. All pheochromocytes coexpress VMAT1 and VMAT2. Sympathomedullary tissues accumulate ^{131}*metaiodobenzylguanidine* (MIBG) by the action of VMATs; this is exploited in radioimaging for

Table 12-2   Characteristics of Human VMATs

Endogenous ligand	VMAT preference of the ligand	Inhibitor drug	VMAT preference of the ligand
Catecholamines	VMAT2 > VMAT1	Tetrabenazine	VMAT2
Histamine	VMAT2 ≫ VMAT1	Phenylethylamine, amphetamine	VMAT2 > VMAT1
		Reserpine, ketanserin	VMAT1 > VMAT2
		Fenfluramine	VMAT2 ≥ VMAT1

Tissue	VMAT type(s)
Central, peripheral, and enteric neurons; histamine-storing enterochromaffin-like cells of the oxyntic mucosa of the stomach	VMAT2
Pheochromocytes	VMAT1 and VMAT2

ABBREVIATION: VMAT, vesicular monoamine transporter.

the localization of pheochromocytomas and paragangliomas. The role of chromogranins in the storage of catecholamines is uncertain.

The Release of Secretory Granules from Pheochromocytes Involves Voltage-Gated Ca²⁺-Channels Acetylcholine released from the preganglionic fibers stimulates the nicotinic cholinergic receptors, thereby depolarizing the pheochromocytes. The depolarization activates voltage-gated Ca^{2+} channels, and the influx of Ca^{2+} results in the exocytosis of a *quantum* of secretory granules. During exocytosis, the entire vesicular content is released into the ECF. Thus, in addition to catecholamines, pheochromocytes and sympathetic nerves release chromogranins, DBH, ATP, and several biologically active peptides, including adrenomedullin (Box 12-5), cleavage products of proopiomelanocortin (POMC, including adrenocorticotropic hormone [ACTH], enkephalins), neuropeptide Y (NPY), and vasoactive intestinal peptide (VIP).

Although the classic fight or flight reaction involves simultaneous acti-

BOX 12-4   Plasma Membrane Monoamine Transporters

The *neuronal plasma membrane monoamine transporters* (termed *uptake-1*) found especially in nerve terminals are more specific and selective for neurotransmitters than VMATs. The plasma membrane transporters are inhibited by drugs such as *cocaine* (dopamine and noradrenaline transporters), *imipramine* (noradrenaline transporter), and *fluoxetine* (serotonin transporter). By inhibiting reuptake of neurotransmitters from the synaptic cleft, these drugs prolong the action of transmitters on their receptors found in the postsynaptic membranes.

The ubiquitous *extraneuronal amine transport system* (termed *uptake-2*) is not inhibited by cocaine. This system is involved in the removal of amines from the circulation and making them available to intracellular enzymes for degradation.

BOX 12-5   Adrenomedullin

Adrenomedullin (AM), a 52-amino acid peptide, belongs to the calcitonin gene peptide superfamily which also includes calcitonin (CT), calcitonin gene-related peptide (CGRP), and amylin. The posttranslational processing of the primary transcript of the adrenomedullin gene results in the translation of two biologically active peptides, AM and *proadrenomedullin N-20 terminal peptide* (PAMP). The two peptides display distinct mechanisms of action.

Although AM was initially isolated from human pheochromocytoma tissue and porcine adrenal medullae (hence its name), its mRNA is widely distributed among tissues. Both peptides are produced predominantly in the endothelial lining of the vasculature and act as very potent, long-lasting autocrine/paracrine vasodilatators. PAMP inhibits the release of neurotransmitters from vasoconstrictor nerves. AM stimulates cyclic AMP in both vascular and bronchial smooth muscle thereby resulting in vasodilatation and bronchodilatation, respectively. An AM receptor cloned from the lung is a typical heptahelical G-protein coupled receptor, but experimental evidence suggests the existence of additional AM receptors. By inhibiting the MAP kinase pathway, AM acts against proliferative changes of vascular and mesangial cells in hypertensive states.

AM is diuretic and natriuretic by a direct renal action. Both AM and PAMP inhibit aldosterone secretion from the adrenal cortex and suppress basal ACTH secretion from the pituitary gland. AM inhibits the secretion of ADH and suppresses water intake and salt appetite.

Taken together, *the hypotensive actions of AM and PAMP include decreasing total peripheral resistance as well as decreasing the volume of ECF.* Plasma AM and PAMP levels are increased in various cardiovascular diseases including hypertension, chronic renal failure, congestive heart failure, and septic shock. The direct cardiac effects (positive inotropism and chronotropism) and CNS actions (central sympathostimulation) of AM and PAMP may help to prevent vascular collapse during states of high AM secretion.

vation of both the sympathetic nerves and the adrenal medulla, under certain stimuli their activation may become dissociated. This is achieved by selective activation of preganglionic cells in the intermediolateral column of the spinal cord by descending pathways.

The Transport and Elimination of Catecholamines

Catecholamines Are Among the Shortest-Lived Signaling Molecules in Plasma   In spite of being hydrophilic molecules, 50 to 60% of catechola-

mines circulate in plasma in loose association with albumin, which is a low-affinity, high-capacity carrier protein. The initial biologic half-life of circulating catecholamines has been estimated between 10 seconds and 1.7 min. The extremely short plasma half-life of catecholamines contributes to their wide and rapid fluctuations in the circulation, which can present difficulty in the diagnosis of pheochromocytoma (see also Chap. 7). In addition, the duration of effect of parenterally administered adrenaline is also very short and may necessitate repeated administration.

Depending on their source, catecholamines are eliminated from the various fluid compartments by several mechanisms:

- In the synaptic cleft in the CNS and in the interstitial fluid near the axons of sympathetic autonomic nerves, catecholamines are primarily eliminated by *reuptake into nerve terminals by the uptake-1 mechanism.* After reuptake, catecholamines either reenter vesicles via VMAT or become degraded by monoamine oxidase (MAO).
- Catecholamines of either neuronal or glandular origin are degraded by catechol-O-methyltransferase (COMT; see below) in their target cells.
- After entering the circulation, catecholamines can be eliminated by
    - *rapid uptake by extraneuronal sites (uptake-2 mechanism) and subsequent degradation by COMT and/or MAO.* This mechanism is especially active in the liver. The high catecholamine-degrading activity of the liver explains why catecholamines are orally inactive (first passage phenomenon).
    - *direct filtration of the intact molecules into urine.* This mechanism is responsible for less than 5% of elimination of the total catecholamine output. Nevertheless, urinary catecholamine measurements are important in the diagnosis of pheochromocytoma.

Normal values of catecholamines in plasma and urine are shown in Table 12-3.

Monoamines Are Degraded by Intracellular Enzymes and Excreted in the Urine   The degradation of monoamines (including catecholamines) is typically a two-step enzymatic process occurring intracellularly in most tissues, which is followed by urinary excretion of the metabolites (Fig. 12-5 and Table 12-3).

A common enzyme involved in the degradation of monoamines is MAO, which is found in the *outer* mitochondrial membrane at several tissue locations such as nerve terminals and the liver. The substrates of MAO include catecholamines, serotonin, and histamine. MAO oxidizes the amino group of the monoamines to form aldehydes, which are further oxidized by the nonspecific *aldehyde dehydrogenase.* Thus, MAO ultimately converts either adrenaline or noradrenaline into *dihydroxymandelic acid*

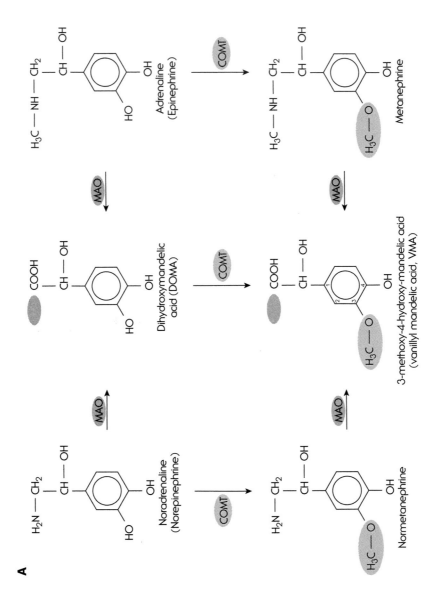

Figure 12-5.

378

B

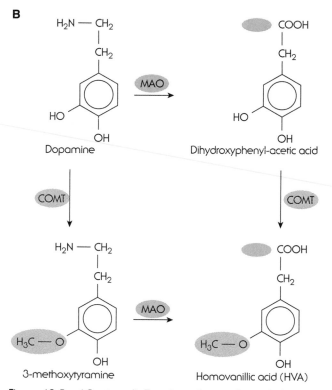

Figure 12-5. (*Continued*) The degradation of catecholamines by monoamino oxidase (MAO) and catechol-O-methyltransferase (COMT). The action of MAO is complemented by the *nonspecific aldehyde dehydrogenase* to yield the metabolites shown. The moieties affected by MAO are highlighted in gray, those affected by COMT are highlighted in color. A. The degradation of noradrenaline (norepinephrine) and adrenaline (epinephrine). B. The degradation of dopamine.

(DOMA). At least two types of the enzyme exist, which are encoded by two separate genes located on chromosome Xp11.4-p11.3. They display distinct substrate preferences and sensitivities to MAO-inhibitor drugs:

• *MAO-A* preferentially breaks down serotonin and noradrenaline, and is inhibited by *clorgyline;*
• *MAO-B* preferentially breaks down phenylethylamine (a synthetic substrate), and is inhibited by *selegiline* (deprenyl).

The extraneuronal catecholamine degradation involves COMT, which utilizes SAM as the methyl donor. COMT generates *metanephrine* from epinephrine (adrenaline) and *normetanephrine* from norepinephrine (noradrenaline). COMT is the most important enzyme that degrades *circulating* catecholamines.

Table 12-3   Normal Values of Catecholamines and Their Degradation Products in Adults

Laboratory parameter		Normal value
Urine (24 h)	Adrenaline	0–20 µg/d (0–109 nmol/d)
	Noradrenaline	15–80 µg/d (89–473 nmol/d)
	Dopamine	65–400 µg/d (424–2612 nmol/d)
	Metanephrine	74–297 µg/d (375–1506 nmol/d)
	Normetanephrine	105–354 µg/d (573–1933 nmol/d)
	Total (free plus conjugated)	<1 mg/d (<5 µmol/d)
	metanephrines	0.05–1.20 µg/mg (0.03–0.69 mmol/ mol) creatinine
	VMA	2.1–7.6 mg/d (11–38 µmol/d)
		1.8–4.8 µg/mg (1.0–2.7 mmol/mol) cre- atinine
	HVA	1.4–8.8 mg/d (8–48 µmol/d)
Plasma	Adrenaline	Supine (30 min): <50 pg/mL (<273 pM)
		Standing (30 min): <900 pg/mL (<4914 pM)
	Noradrenaline	Supine (30 min): 110–410 pg/mL (650– 2423 pM)
		Standing (30 min): 125–700 pg/mL (739–4137 pM)
	Dopamine (no postural change)	<87 pg/mL (<475 pM)

ABBREVIATIONS: VMA, vanillylmandelic acid; HVA, homovanillic acid.

The phenolic hydroxyl group of catecholamines and their metabolites may be *conjugated* either with sulfate or with glucuronate in the liver and the gut. The conjugated compounds are excreted with urine.

Either MAO or COMT may act first on their substrates. Their joint action produces *vanillyl mandelic acid* (VMA) either from adrenaline or from noradrenaline. All metabolites produced by either of these two enzymes separately, or produced by their joint action, appear in urine (see Table 12-3). The joint action of MAO and COMT converts dopamine into *homovanillic acid* (Fig. 12-5B).

In the degradation of serotonin, the action of MAO is followed by a nonspecific *aldehyde dehydrogenase,* which yields 5-hydroxyindoleacetic acid (5-HIAA).

The degradation of histamine involves the widely distributed *histamine-N-methyltransferase.* The metabolite N-methylhistamine is further metabolized either by MAO or by the nonspecific diamine oxidase (DAO).

The Actions and Regulation of Catecholamines

Circulating Catecholamines Have Limited Access to the Brain and the Fetus   Circulating catecholamines reach most tissues. However, catecholamines cannot penetrate the blood-brain barrier (BBB). For this reason, Parkinson's disease patients (whose nigrostriatal dopaminergic system is impaired) cannot be treated with dopamine. Instead, the dopamine precursor L-DOPA is administered, which can penetrate the BBB and be converted into dopamine in situ.

The fetus represents another protected compartment. As mentioned earlier, fetal production of (mainly) noradrenaline is essential for the survival of the fetus, which is primarily related to cardiovascular responses to hypoxia. To meet the minute-to-minute adaptational requirements of the fetus, the endogenously produced noradrenaline is rapidly cleared from the fetal circulation and the maternal transfer of cathecolamines is minimized by several mechanisms:

- The placenta expresses MAO-A, MAO-B, and COMT mainly in the syncytiotrophoblast cells. These enzymes may degrade both fetal and maternal catecholamines.
- The placenta expresses members of the *uptake-1 system,* the serotonin and mainly the norepinephrine transporters. The placental norepinephrine transporter is apparently essential for delivering the circulating fetal catecholamines into the syncytiotrophoblast for degradation. The inhibition of the norepinephrine transporter and the increase of fetal noradrenaline levels have been demonstrated in cocaine abusers, which may in part explain the deleterious effects of cocaine abuse on the fetus.

The Biologic Actions of Adrenaline and Noradrenaline Are Mediated by Several Subtypes of α- and β-Adrenergic G-Protein-Linked Receptors All adrenergic receptors are members of the G-protein-linked seven transmembrane segment receptor family. Based on their ligand preference, these receptors were originally classified as

- α-adrenergic receptors (adrenaline $\geq$ noradrenaline $\gg$ isoproterenol); and
- β-adrenergic receptors (isoproterenol $>$ adrenaline $>$ noradrenaline). Note that isoproterenol is an artificial ligand.

Each class of adrenergic receptors has several subtypes encoded by separate genes and performing different physiologic functions. The affinity of receptor-ligand interaction is modified by the subtype of the receptor:

- Due to a significantly higher affinity of adrenaline than noradrenaline for β_2-adrenergic receptors, physiologic levels of *circulating* noradrenaline are insufficient to stimulate β_2-adrenergic receptors. Thus, β_2-adrenergic receptors are either stimulated by circulating adrenaline or by the high concentrations of noradrenaline observed at the site of liberation near the sympathetic nerve terminals. The metabolic actions of catecholamines on the liver are therefore mediated exclusively by adrenaline.

- Noradrenaline has a higher affinity than adrenaline for β_3-adrenergic receptors. Thus, the main regulators of lipolysis are the sympathetic noradrenergic nerves rather than circulating adrenaline.
- The other adrenergic receptors bind these two ligands with approximately equal affinity.

The subtypes of the adrenergic receptors utilize various second messenger systems:

- All three known β-adrenergic receptor subtypes (β_1, β_2, β_3) utilize the $G\alpha_s$ G-protein and activate adenylyl cyclase.
- The α_1-adrenergic receptors (α_{1A}, α_{1B} and α_{1D}) mostly use $G\alpha_q$ G-proteins and usually activate PLCβ (thereby activating PKC via DAG and increasing intracellular Ca^{2+} via IP$_3$) and/or PLA$_2$.
- The coupling of α_2-adrenergic receptors (α_{2A}, α_{2B} and α_{2C}) is the most varied. $G\alpha_i$ and G_0 proteins couple the α_2-adrenergic receptors to effectors which may decrease the activity of adenylyl cyclase (an effect opposing the action of β-adrenergic receptors), activate K^+ channels, inhibit Ca^{2+} channels or activate PLCβ and/or PLA$_2$ (an effect similar to that of α_1-adrenergic receptors).

The physiologic effect of adrenergic receptor stimulation is influenced by other signaling systems present in the target cells. This is exemplified by the effect of adrenergic receptor activation in smooth muscle cells:

- Increasing intracellular cyclic adenosine monophosphate (cAMP) causes smooth muscle relaxation. This predictable outcome is seen in bronchial, vascular, and uterine smooth muscle upon stimulation by β-adrenergic receptors.
- Increasing intracellular Ca^{2+} upon stimulation by α_1-adrenergic receptors may either cause contraction or relaxation:
  - In vascular, bronchial, and uterine smooth muscle, contraction is achieved by calmodulin kinase-mediated phosphorylation of myosin light chain.
  - In intestinal smooth muscle, Ca^{2+}-dependent activation of K^+ channels causes hyperpolarization and relaxation.

In the peripheral nervous system, *α_2-adrenergic receptors are predominantly found in the "presynaptic" membrane of axons*. Their function is a local negative feedback: they are exposed to the catecholamines secreted into the ECF, and the *stimulation of α_2-receptors inhibits further release of noradrenaline*.

The Overall Actions of the Sympathoadrenal System Usually Either Antagonize or Complement Those of the Parasympathetic Autonomic Nerves Sympathetic and parasympathetic ganglion cells as well as pheochromocytes are innervated by cholinergic preganglionic nerves acting on *nicotinic* cholinergic receptors. The postganglionic parasympathetic nerves are cholinergic and activate atropine-sensitive *muscarinic* cholinergic receptors. Most postganglionic sympathetic nerves are noradrenergic, but some are cholinergic and (like the parasympathetic nerves) activate muscarinic receptors.

In general, the sympathoadrenal system activates mechanisms supporting fight or flight, which implies increased mobilization of energy and redistribution of blood supply to organs that are essential for the response. In contrast, the parasympathetic system promotes digestion of food and storage of energy. Table 12-4 compares and contrasts the actions of the sympathetic and parasympathetic systems. It must be emphasized that *the functional antagonistic nature of the sympathetic and parasympathetic systems often involves distinct target cell populations*. For example, although sympathetic stimulation causes *mydriasis* (pupillary dilatation) and parasympathetic stimulation causes *miosis* (pupillary constriction), the two actions are carried out by two different muscles. Accordingly, the muscarinic and adrenergic receptors are often expressed by different cell populations.

Although sympathetic and parasympathetic cholinergic fibers are activated under different *physiologic* conditions, *pharmacologic* manipulations of cholinergic transmission with drugs (such as atropine and cholinesterase inhibitors) are usually not selective for the origin of the innervation. For this reason, certain sympathetic cholinergic mechanisms are shown in Table 12-4 together with the effects of the parasympathetic system.

Similar to thyroid hormones and glucocorticoids, catecholamines have a vast array of targets. Nevertheless, most of the effects of sympathoadrenal activation can be conceptually integrated as follows:

- Increasing cardiac output and blood pressure;
- Causing bronchodilatation thereby matching increased perfusion of the lungs with increased ventilation;
- Diverting blood from the splanchnic region and the skin to muscle, while retaining blood perfusion of the brain;
- Mobilizing fuel from energy stores (hyperglycemic action, increasing plasma FFA).

Upon stress, the sympathoadrenergic and adrenocortical (ACTH-cortisol) systems are activated simultaneously. Their response and actions, however, follow a different timecourse. Catecholamines released from the adrenal medulla and the sympathetic nerves exert their actions instantaneously. The catecholamines and their actions are rapidly eliminated upon the termination of their release. In contrast, cortisol takes effect with a 20- to 30-min delay and its action is more prolonged. However, the two stress systems function in a similar and mutually supportive manner.

Table 12-4   Physiologic Effects of Sympathetic and Parasympathetic Activation[a]

| Effector organ | | Sympathoadrenal activation mediated by noradrenaline and/or adrenaline | | Parasympathetic (muscarinic cholinergic) activation |
Category	Target	Dominant receptor type	Response	Response
Heart	Sinoatrial node	β_1	Tachycardia	Bradycardia, vagal arrest
	Impulse conduction system		Increase in automacity and conduction velocity (may cause arrhythmia)	Decrease in automacity and conduction velocity
	Ventricles		Increase in contractility, automacity, and conduction velocity	Slight decrease in contractility
Arterioles	Coronary	α_1	Vasoconstriction[b]	—
	Skeletal muscle	α_1	Vasoconstriction[b]	Vasodilatation (*sympathetic* cholinergic; weak transitional effect)
		β_2	Vasodilatation[b] (response to low-dose exogenous adrenaline)	
	Cerebral	α_1	Weak vasoconstriction	Vasodilatation
	Splanchnic area (GI and renal)	α_1	Vasoconstriction	—
	Skin and mucosa	α_1	Vasoconstriction (pallor)	—
Veins		α_1	Vasoconstriction (leads to increased venous return of blood)	—
Lung	Bronchial muscle	β_2	Bronchodilatation	Bronchoconstriction
Metabolism	Muscle	β_2 (β_3?)	Stimulation of glycogenolysis; inhibition of glycogen synthesis	—
	Liver	β_2 (α_1)	Stimulation of glycogenolysis, gluconeogenesis; inhibition of glycogen synthesis	—
	Adipocytes	β_3	Lipolysis	—
Pancreatic islet	Insulin secretion	α_2	Inhibition	Stimulation
		β_2	Stimulation	
	Glucagon secretion	β_2	Stimulation	Stimulation
GI	Motility	α_1, α_2	Decrease	Increase
	Secretion of digestive juices	α_2	Inhibition	Stimulation
Salivary glands		β_1	Stimulation of mucous secretion making the teeth slippery	Stimulation of serous secretion (alkaline, watery secretion with α-amylase)
Skin	Sweat glands	α_1	Regional "adrenergic" sweating (e.g., underarm *apocrine* sweat glands and palm of the hand)	Generalized sweating by *eccrine* sweat glands (cholinergic sympathetic effect)
	Pilomotor muscle	α_1	Piloarrection (goosebumps)	—
Eye	Dilatator pupillae muscle	α_1	Mydriasis (pupillary dilatation)	—
	Sphincter pupillae muscle	—	—	Miosis (pupillary constriction)

Table 12-4   (*Continued*)

| Effector organ | | Sympathoadrenal activation mediated by noradrenaline and/or adreneraline | | Parasympathetic (muscarinic cholinergic) activation |
Category	Target	Dominant receptor type	Response	Response
	Ciliary muscle	β_2	Relaxation for far vision	Accommodation (contraction for near vision)
	Aqueous humor	β	Increased production acting on the ciliary body	Increased drainage by opening the canal of Schlemm via miotic action
Male sex organs (smooth muscles of glands, ducts, and penile vessels)		α_1	Ejaculation	Erection (noncholinergic mechanism involving neuronal nitric oxide synthase in parasympathetic nerves)
Uterus		β_2	Tocolytic (relaxation; pregnant and non-pregnant uterus)	Variable
		α_1	Contraction (pregnant uterus)	

[a] Modified from Table 6–1 in Goodman & Gilman's *The Pharmacological Basis of Therapeutics*, 9th ed, McGraw-Hill, 1996.

[b] The primary determinant of coronary vessel resistance in vivo is autoregulation. Whereas adrenaline causes vasoconstriction of isolated coronary arteries, its effect in situ is vasodilatation. This is due to the release of adenosine from cardiomyocytes on their increased work. Similarly, during a fight or flight reaction, the arterioles of only those skeletal muscles are *dilatated*, which perform active work, whereas in other skeletal muscles a weak vasoconstriction predominates. Thus, the effect of adrenaline on vascular smooth muscle is modulated by local metabolic activity. Due to the regional differences in the *relative* abundance of α_1- and β_2-adrenergic receptors of the arterioles, vasoconstriction in skeletal muscle is not as pronounced as in the skin or in the splanchnic area.

ABBREVIATION: GI, gastrointestinal.

The Sympathoadrenal System Is Activated by Threatening Changes in the Internal and/or External Environment   The adrenergic response to threatening changes is essentially homeostatic, i.e., it attempts to restore the original situation. Thus the sympathoadrenal response represents a negative feedback regulatory system (Table 12-5).

The responses are broad and not restricted to those associated with a particular stimulus in Table 12-5. For example, a diabetic ketoacidotic patient, who has lost significant volumes of fluid by osmotic diuresis responds to the hypovolemia by vasoconstriction and increased heart rate. This homeostatic response, however, occurs at the expense of increased body temperature because the vasoconstriction in the skin decreases heat dissipation. The febrile response increases the insulin requirement. In addition, the catecholamines are diabetogenic: they increase glucagon output from the pancreas and directly increase hepatic glucose output. Thus, whereas the sympathetic response is homeostatic in terms of antagonizing cardiovascular collapse, it worsens hyperglycemia (i.e., the underlying cause of hypovolemia) in a positive feedback loop, which would become fatal without intervention (insulin with fluid and electrolyte replacement).

Table 12-5   Stimuli Activating the Sympathoadrenal System and the Responses to Increased (Nor)adrenergic Activity

Stimulus	Response
Hypotension, hypovolemia, and postural changes by baroreceptor mechanism	Increased total peripheral resistance Increased cardiac output: tachycardia, increased venous return, increased stroke volume Increased renal renin secretion, consequent activation of the angiotensin-aldostesterone axis leading to volume retention
Hypoglycemia	Increased hepatic glycogenolysis and gluconeogenesis; decreased hepatic glycogen synthesis
Hypoxia and hypercapnia by direct action on CNS including the C1 area; hypoxia also by peripheral chemoreceptors (carotid and aortic bodies)	Increased cardiac output, increased tissue perfusion, bronchodilatation
Cold	Cutaneous vasoconstriction (reduced heat dissipation); increased metabolic rate (including nonshivering thermogenesis)
Anxiety, fright and pain stress by CRH-mediated activation of CNS and preganglionic sympathetic neurons	Fight or flight to eliminate the source of threat

ABBREVIATIONS: CNS, central nervous system; CRH, corticotropin-releasing hormone.

The Sympathetic Nerves Are Involved in the Regulation of Body Weight   *Leptin* secretion by adipocytes is proportional to the degree of adiposity of the body. Although leptin is helix bundle peptide hormone, it crosses the BBB by a receptor-mediated transport mechanism and acts on the hypothalamus. Leptin exerts two main effects: it decreases appetite and increases energy expenditure (see Chap. 15). The latter involves *activation of sympathetic nerve activity to adipose tissue without a concomitant activation of the adrenal medulla.* Adipocytes express β_3-adrenergic receptors, which (unlike other β-adrenergic receptors) are more responsive to noradrenaline than to adrenaline. Their increased stimulation results in enhanced lipolysis thereby reducing triglyceride stores. The decrease in triglycerides yields a decrease in leptin secretion. This feedback system involving leptin and increased sympathetic activity is part of the *lipostat mechanism.*

Modulation of Sympathetic Activity by Postural Changes and by Insulin-Induced Hypoglycemia Is Often Used in Clinical Practice   Healthy individuals maintain their blood pressure when standing up from a supine (reclining) position. The mechanism of adaptation to this postural change is shown in Fig. 12-6. Upon standing, gravity keeps blood in the lower half of the body leading to a reduced venous return. This results in an initial decrease in blood pressure. The *aortic arch* and the *carotid sinus* (found

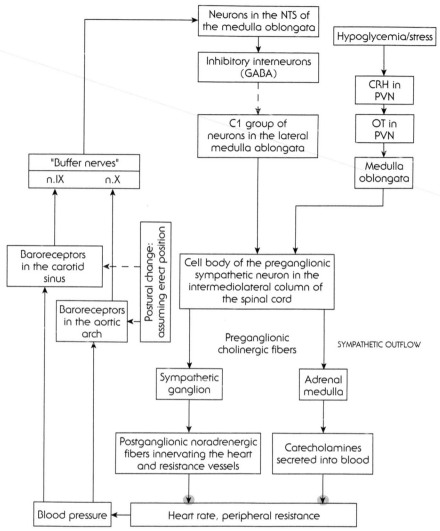

Figure 12-6. The sympathetic regulation of blood pressure and the baroreceptor control of sympathetic outflow. The solid arrows indicate stimulation/increase; the dashed arrows indicate inhibition/decrease. The firing rate of buffer nerves is proportional with the blood pressure as sensed by baroreceptors in the carotid sinus and the aortic arch. Buffer nerves stimulate neurons in the nucleus tractus solitarii (NTS), which (via GABAergic interneurons) inhibit the tonic activity of the C1 cells. An acute decrease in blood pressure in the vessels where the baroreceptors are located, such as the drop of blood pressure provoked by standing up, via this circuitry disinhibits the C1 neurons and returns blood pressure to normal by increased sympathetic outflow. If this mechanism is absent, orthostatic hypotension develops. The sympathetic outflow can be increased by stress via a pathway including cortico-trophin-releasing hormone (CRH) and oxytocin (OT) neurons located in the paraventricular nucleus (PVN). The circled areas are reminders of target cell responsiveness, which are maintained by thyroid hormones (β-adrenergic receptors) and glucocorticoids (α-adrenergic and angiotensin receptors). Compare this figure with Figs. 10-7 and 12-11.

in the *internal* carotid artery) contain stretch-sensitive receptors *(barorecep-tors)*. These baroreceptors generate signals that are proportional to blood pressure. The baroreceptor signal is conducted by the *"buffer nerves"* to the medulla oblongata in the brainstem. The buffer nerves are branches of cranial nerves X and IX, which supply the aortic arch and the carotid sinus, respectively, with sensory innervation. *The function of the buffer nerves is* to suppress the tonic activity of vasoconstrictor nerves (i.e., *to suppress the sympathetic outflow*). The initial decrease of buffer nerve activity upon standing results in increased sympathoadrenal activity. The resulting vasoconstriction increases total peripheral resistance indicated by a rise in diastolic pressure. In addition, heart rate and cardiac output also increase, which is indicated by an increase in systolic pressure.

If the efferent part of this reflex arch is dysfunctional, the blood pressure decreases, which is often associated with lightheadedness and may lead to fainting due to an acute drop of cerebral blood supply. If upon standing the systolic pressure decreases more than 20 to 25 mmHg and diastolic pressure decreases more than 10 to 15 mmHg, the patient might have a condition known as *orthostatic* or *postural hypotension*. As indicated in Table 12-3, noradrenaline and especially adrenaline increase in plasma upon standing. The increase in adrenaline clearly indicates that the postural regulation of blood pressure involves the adrenal medulla. Note, however, that in addition to sympathoadrenal activation, the response requires adequate circulating blood volume and normal venous return to the heart. Screening for orthostatic hypotension is an essential component of patient work-up.

The baroreceptor mechanism also protects against *acute hypertension.* However, during *sustained* hypertension, the baroreceptors undergo an adaptational process termed *baroreceptor resetting*. After resetting, the buffer nerve activity is normal at a supranormal value of blood pressure.

The increased vasoconstrictor tone upon standing has a disproportionately great effect on renal vessels. In part through this mechanism, in part through direct adrenergic stimulation of the *juxtaglomerular apparatus* (JGA), the kidneys secrete more renin which eventually leads to volume expansion. This mechanism explains that pheochromocytoma may be accompanied by secondary hyperaldosteronism (see also the aldosterone section).

Insulin-induced *hypoglycemia* is used as a clinical test for the assessment of growth hormone (GH) secretory capacity (see Chap. 10). During this test, patients become pale and are covered with cold sweat. The clinical signs of sympathoadrenal activation indicate a glucose value of about 50 to 55 mg/dL. In adults, *adrenaline* and glucagon are the first line of defense against hypoglycemia; these systems become activated at plasma glucose levels between 70 and 75 mg/dL, whereas the sympathetic *noradrenergic* nerves become activated only upon more severe hypoglycemia (45 to 55 mg/dL; see also Chap. 9).

Adrenergic Receptors Are Regulated by Thyroid Hormones, Cortisol, and Insulin   At increased numbers of spare receptors, a lower percentage of receptor occupancy (i.e., lower hormone concentration) is required for achieving the same biologic effect. As discussed in Chap. 5, adrenergic receptors are subject to homologous and heterologous downregulation. Thus, continued exposure of adrenergic receptors to adrenaline may reduce tissue responsiveness. For example, pheochromocytoma patients may present with normal blood pressure even if they have continuously elevated adrenaline secretion.

The receptor numbers are also regulated by other hormones. We have already discussed that *thyroid hormones* upregulate β-adrenergic receptors, thereby sensitizing most tissues more for adrenaline than for noradrenaline. In contrast, *cortisol* mainly upregulates α_1-adrenergic receptors and sensitizes the tissues for both catecholamines. This mechanism is important in maintaining *vascular reactivity*. Thus, in Addison's disease catecholamines are less effective in causing vasoconstriction, which contributes to the orthostatic hypotension seen in this condition. Another example is related to the treatment of hay fever and similar conditions. Stimulation of α_1-adrenergic receptors is the basis of most nasal decongestants. Prolonged (>5 to 7 days) use of these nasal sprays results in receptor downregulation and may lead to *rhinitis medicamentosa*. To wean these patients from the sympathomimetic treatment, glucocorticoid nasal sprays can be used, which upregulate the α_1-adrenergic receptors.

Lipolysis in adipocytes is stimulated by β_3-adrenergic receptors (see above). *Insulin suppresses the expression of β_3-adrenergic receptors in adipose tissue.* During fasting, insulin levels are low, and adipose tissue becomes more sensitive to sympathetic noradrenergic stimuli due to the disinhibition of β_3-receptor expression.

Dopamine Functions as a Third Peripheral Catecholaminergic System Mainly by an Autocrine/Paracrine Mechanism   Dopamine is the most abundant catecholamine in human urine (see Table 12-3). Dopamine exists in plasma and urine mainly as its sulfoconjugated derivative (dopamine sulfate), a biologically inactive metabolite. The sources and physiologic roles of dopamine outside the brain have been unsettled. The currently available data suggest the following conclusions:

- Dopamine acts as an autocrine/paracrine regulator of local organ function. The high levels of dopamine sulfate originate from the inactivation of dopamine within the tissues of origin.
- The main sources of circulating dopamine *sulfate* are non-neural elements in the gut and lungs, which are at least in part chromaffin APUD cells. Postprandial plasma levels of dopamine sulfate are twice as high as those during fasting. However, *free* dopamine remains unchanged in plasma.

• Generation of dopamine in non-noradrenergic, nonadrenergic cells explains why human urine contains higher concentrations of dopamine and its metabolites than the other catecholamines and their metabolites.

• Autonomic nerves significantly contribute to the plasma levels of *free* dopamine. Accordingly, plasma levels of free dopamine display postural changes, whereas dopamine sulfate (and for practical purposes: total dopamine) remains unchanged.

• Under physiologic conditions, the adrenal medulla is only a minor source of circulating and urinary dopamine sulfate. In pheochromocytoma, however, plasma free dopamine levels are elevated.

Dopamine exerts its biologic actions through at least five types of dopamine receptors, which (similar to other monoamine receptors) belong to the G-protein-coupled heptahelical receptor family. The D_1 receptor stimulates, whereas the D_2 receptor inhibits, the activity of adenylyl cyclase. Stimulation of D_1 receptors in the splanchnic area, especially in the renal vasculature, causes vasodilatation. Dopamine infusion is one of the most frequently used treatments of critically ill patients with low cardiac output states and/or acute oliguric renal failure.

The best established physiologic functions of dopamine are its antihypertensive and natriuretic actions. In vivo, L-DOPA is synthesized and secreted into the circulation in several tissues such as the muscles and the kidney. The proximal renal tubules also take up L-DOPA from plasma and convert it into dopamine. The locally produced dopamine acts upon dopaminergic receptors and decreases Na^+/K^+-ATPase activity thereby increasing natriuresis (see aldosterone). In primary hyperaldosteronism, plasma levels of free dopamine are elevated as a compensatory mechanism. This mechanism is also activated by volume expansion and/or by increased dietary sodium intake.

Impaired dopaminergic mechanisms have been implicated in *essential hypertension*. In patients suffering from essential hypertension, plasma levels and urinary excretion of *free* dopamine are suppressed, and the dopamine response to salt load is blunted. It has been suggested that the renal biosynthesis of dopamine is impaired. The natriuretic response to *exogenous* dopamine is enhanced in these patients. In genetically susceptible subjects, the decrease in renal dopaminergic activity precedes the development of hypertension, indicating that the decrease of dopamine is the cause rather than the consequence of this condition. In patients with orthostatic hypotension, plasma levels of dopamine are elevated.

The Main Pathologic Conditions of the Adrenal Medulla

The main pathologic conditions of the adrenal medulla include certain forms of orthostatic hypotension (hypofunction) and the tumors of the adrenal medulla, mostly pheochromocytoma (hyperfunction).

Orthostatic hypotension is not necessarily caused by diseases of the sympathoadrenal system. As discussed earlier, in *Addison's disease* the vascular reactivity to noradrenaline is diminished, which results in orthostatic hypotension even if the sympathetic outflow is increased by a postural change. Certain drugs acting at various points of the regulatory system may cause *drug-induced orthostatic* hypotension. *Primary orthostatic hypotension* (which is due to impaired sympathoadrenal activity) is classified as

- *peripheral type,* in which the sympathetic ganglionic cells, their axons and/or the pheochromocytes degenerate.
- *multiple system atrophy* (*Shy-Drager syndrome*), the degeneration of specific sets of neurons, including those in the basal ganglia and the preganglionic neurons of the intermediolateral column of the spinal cord. The condition is most common in middle-aged men.
- *familial dysautonomia* (*Riley-Day syndrome*) is a rare autosomal recessive condition affecting mostly children of Ashkenazi Jewish descent. The gene (*DYS*) maps to chromosome 9q31-q33.

Secondary orthostatic hypotension has varied etiologies such as diabetic neuropathy or Guillain-Barré syndrome.

Pheochromocytoma is a rare disease. The diagnosis is usually confirmed from the increased amounts of catecholamines and their degradation products in 24-hr urine. The clinical presentation is variable and may involve sustained hypertension, normal blood pressure with paroxysmal hypertensive attacks, headaches, and sometimes hypotension. The paroxysms may be mistaken for seizures or anxiety attacks. An attack may be provoked by palpation of the abdomen during physical examination or under conditions leading to elevated intraabdominal pressure. Although the symptomatology is mainly related to the cardiovascular system, laboratory findings indicate altered metabolism, which mainly presents as "endocrine diabetes."

The pheochromocytoma cells are not innervated by preganglionic nerves, and secrete catecholamines in an erratic, unregulated manner. Thus, in spite of the hypertension, the patients may experience an orthostatic drop in their blood pressure. Acute administration of the α_2-adrenergic receptor agonist clonidine normally imitates increased buffer nerve activity, and suppresses the activity of sympathetic preganglionic neurons. Unlike in other forms of hypertension, in pheochromocytoma patients acutely administered clonidine has no impact on catecholamine secretion and blood pressure. During a paroxysm, the catecholamine stores of the tumor may become severely depleted, and the patient experiences hypotension and orthostatic hypotension.

As discussed, pheochromocytoma may be a manifestation of MEN 2A or MEN 2B syndrome. The diagnosis of these MEN syndromes and the screening of family members relies on molecular genetic tests. Pheochromocytoma may be associated with other diseases, especially with *von Hippel-Lindau disease.*

The treatment of pheochromocytoma is surgical. In addition to computed tomography (CT) and magnetic resonance imaging (MRI), the VMAT-mediated accumulation of radiolabeled MIBG may be useful in the localization of the tumor.

THE ADRENAL CORTEX

Biosynthesis of Adrenocorticoids

Thorough Knowledge of the Chemical Structure and Nomenclature of Steroid Hormones Is Essential for Understanding Steroidogenesis and Steroid Hormone Degradation The precursor of all steroid hormones is *cholesterol* (Figs. 8-8 and 12-7). *Corticosteroid hormones* and their derivatives are produced by the adrenal cortex, the gonads, the placenta, the Schwann cells of peripheral nerves, and the brain. *Vitamin D derivatives* are also steroid hormones (see Chap. 8); however, unlike the steroid hormones discussed here, the sidechain of cholesterol during vitamin D biosynthesis

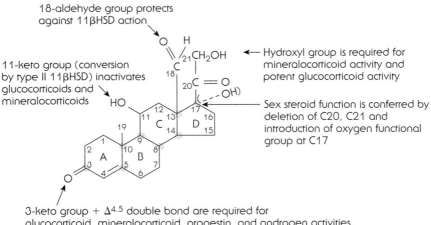

18-aldehyde group protects against 11βHSD action

11-keto group (conversion by type II 11βHSD) inactivates glucocorticoids and mineralocorticoids

← Hydroxyl group is required for mineralocorticoid activity and potent glucocorticoid activity

Sex steroid function is conferred by deletion of C20, C21 and introduction of oxygen functional group at C17

3-keto group + Δ4.5 double bond are required for glucocorticoid, mineralocorticoid, progestin, and androgen activities. Aromatization of the A-ring with deletion of C19 and introduction of 3-hydroxyl group are required for estrogenic activity.

Figure 12-7. The generic structure and structure-activity relationship of natural steroid hormones. The letters refer to the rings of the cyclopentanoperhydrophenanthrene core. The carbonic atoms are numbered by convention, and the asymmetric carbons are highlighted. Hydroxyl or other functional groups appended to the asymmetric carbonic atoms may be in either of two configurations: β-configuration (toward the reader, indicated by solid lines) or in the α-configuration (behind the page/away from the reader, indicated by dashed lines). (*Source:* Modified from Fig. 43-4, p 724 in Smith CM, Reynard AM (eds): *Textbook of Pharmacology.* Philadelphia, Saunders, 1992.)

is not cleaved. In contrast, the biosynthesis of corticosteroids and their derivatives does not involve opening of the B (or any other) ring.

Steroid hormones are often grouped based on their numbers of carbon atoms and named after their fully saturated core-molecules:

- *C-21 steroids,* also known as *pregnane-derivatives,* are the initially synthesized steroid hormones. They include progesterone (a characteristic product of the corpus luteum and the placenta), and the adrenal-specific mineralocorticoids and glucocorticoids.
- *C-19 steroids,* also known as *androstane-derivatives,* are androgens (male sex steroids) derived from certain C-21 steroids.
- *C-18 steroids,* also known as *estrane-derivatives,* are estrogens (female sex steroids) derived from androgens by oxidation of the C-19 methyl group, a reaction that leads to the aromatization of the A-ring.

The *chemical names* of steroid hormones are derived from these three ringed structures. Due to the presence of asymmetric carbon atoms, steroid hormones may have *stereoisomers.* These are referred to with the *iso-* or *epi-* prefix in the chemical name of the structures. The α and β designation refers to the steric position of the hydroxyl (or methyl) groups, whereby α is behind the plane of the rings and β is in the front. The hydroxyl (–OH) groups are referred to as *-ol* (as in alcoh*ol* and phen*ol*), the oxo (=O) groups are referred to as *-one* (as in ket*one*). The term *deoxy-* indicates the absence of a hydroxyl group. The double bonds in the rings are denoted as Δ, with an appended number that refers to the lower numeral of the two carbons involved. *Dehydro-* indicates removal of two hydrogen atoms yielding a double bond. *Dihydro-* has a meaning opposite of dehydro-, i.e., indicates saturation of a double bond with two hydrogen atoms. The fully saturated C-27 steroid molecule is termed *cholestane.* A double bond in the ring structure is referred to by changing the ending to *-ene* (cholestene). Thus, the chemical name of cholesterol is Δ^5-*cholestene-3β-ol.* The names of certain precursors and metabolites are derived from the *trivial names* of the steroid hormones (e.g., 11-deoxycortisol).

The biosynthesis of steroid hormones follows a *general scheme* (Fig. 12-8), which is *modified in a cell type-specific manner* due to differential expression of the enzymes, and the organ-specific use of isoenzymes and/or different promoters. Tumors of steroidogenic tissues may express an altered set of enzymes and secrete hormones uncharacteristic for the normal tissue. Steroids associate with proteins and penetrate lipid bilayers with ease. Thus, steroid hormones leave the cell immediately upon their synthesis, which implies a tight synthesis-secretion coupling. Figure 12-8 may give the impression that steroidogenic pathways generate several molecules, which serve only as inert intermediary metabolites that are finally processed within the same cell into biologically active end products. This impression is mistaken for several reasons:

A

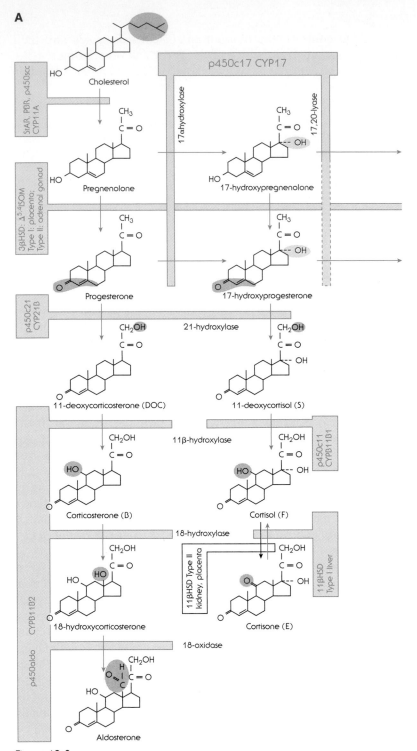

Figure 12-8.

B

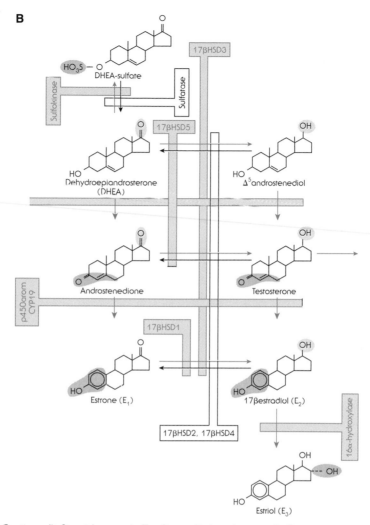

Figure 12-8. (*Continued*) Steroidogenesis. The figure displays the metabolites, enzymes, and reactions irrespective of the cell types in which they occur. The moieties of the structures highlighted in *gray* represent the change(s) from top to bottom, those highlighted in *color* represent the changes from left to right. HSD is hydroxysteroid dehydrogenase. The zona glomerulosa performs all reactions from cholesterol to aldosterone (first column on the left), but no other reactions. The zona fasciculata and reticularis perform the reactions leading to corticosterone, cortisol (in the first two columns), and to DHEA/DHEA-sulfate and androstene-dione (in the first two rows). In the first two columns, all reactions starting with 21-hydroxylase are specific for the adrenal cortex. The dashed line indicates that 17OH-progesterone is normally not converted into androstenedione in the adrenal cortex because it is rapidly used up by 21-hydroxylase. The cortisol-cortisone conversions are performed in peripheral tissues. The gonads process the "adrenal androgens" further into testosterone and estradiol by a preferential Δ4 pathway which follows the steps in the second row. DHT is produced by 5α-reductase in peripheral tissues and is reversibly inactivated by 3αHSD. Estriol is the main sexual steroid product of the placenta.

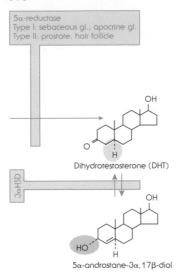

Figure 12-8. (*Continued*)

• Intermediary metabolites of the steroidogenic pathways may be secreted ("escape" from the cells) and enter the circulation. The escape route is based on the same principle as the secretion of the end products. The escape of intermediary metabolites, however, is normally minimized by the presence of enzymes, which process them very rapidly. A compound, which is the end product in one cell type, may be an intermediary metabolite in another cell type.

• Either the intermediary metabolites or certain end products of a cell population may be taken up and processed by other steroid hormone-producing cells. Thus, the complete synthetic process may involve cooperation between distinct cell populations and/or organs.

• Some of these intermediary metabolites display significant biologic activities without further processing.

Measurement of intermediary metabolites is useful in the diagnosis of enzyme deficiencies in the steroidogenic pathways. The rule of thumb is that the amount and/or plasma concentration of the metabolites *preceding* the site of the enzyme defect in the pathway *accumulate,* whereas the metabolites, which would normally be generated by the involved enzyme, either decrease or (in case of partial defects) may remain normal.

The Rate-Limiting Step of Steroid Hormone Synthesis Is the Regulated Transfer of Cholesterol from the Cytoplasm to the Matrix Side of the Inner Mitochondrial Membrane   Most steroidogenic enzymes belong to the *cytochrome P450 family* encoded by various *CYP* genes (Table 12-6). Steroid hormone synthesis is performed by the sER and the inner mitochondrial membrane. The first step of steroidogenesis is the conversion of cholesterol

Table 12-6 The Main Components of the Steroidogenic Pathway

Enzyme	Gene	Chromosomal location	Enzyme activity (or activities)	Subcellular localization	Characteristic features of normal tissue-specific expression
StAR	StAR	8p11.2	Activation of PBR	Outer mitochondrial membrane	All steroid hormone-producing cells except the placenta, Schwann cells, and the brain
PBR	PBR	22q13.31	Regulated cholesterol channel	Forms channel at the contact sites between the outer and inner mitochondrial membranes	All steroid hormone-producing cells
P450scc	CYP11A	15q23–24	Cholesterol-20,22-desmolase	Matrix side of inner mitochondrial membrane	All steroid hormone-producing cells
3βHSD/ISOM	3βHSD type I	1p13, the HSD3B1 and HSD3B2 loci are located 1–2 cM of the centromeric marker D1Z5	3β-hydroxysteroid dehydrogenase, $\Delta^{5,4}$-oxosteroid isomerase	sER	Expressed in syncytiotrophoblast cells, sebaceous glands
	3βHSD type II				Expressed in the definitive adrenal cortex and the gonads. Absent from the fetal zone of the adrenal cortex.
P450c21	CYP21B	6p21.3 (close to HLA locus)	21-hydroxylase	sER	Only in adrenal cortex (all zones); low levels in fetal zone
	CYP21A	6p21.3 (close to HLA locus)	Pseudogene	N/A	N/A
P450c11	CYP11B1	8q21–22	11 β-hydroxylase	Matrix side of inner mitochondrial membrane	Only expressed in zona fasciculata and zona reticularis of the adrenal cortex; low levels in fetal zone
P450aldo	CYP11B2	8q24.3	Aldosterone synthase: 11 β-hydroxylase, 18-hydroxylase, 18-oxidase	Matrix side of inner mitochondrial membrane	Only expressed in the zona glomerulosa of the adrenal cortex; low levels in fetal zone
P450c17	CYP17	10q24–25	17 α-hydroxylase 17,20-lyase	sER	Absent from the zona glomerulosa in adults, the placenta, and the definitive zone of fetal adrenal cortex until the third trimester
P450arom	CYP19	15q	Aromatase	sER	See Table 13-2

ABBREVIATIONS: StAR, steroidogenic acute regulatory protein; PBR, peripheral-type benzodiazepine receptor; HSD, hydroxysteroid dehydrogenase; sER, smooth endoplasmic reticulum; HLA, human leukocyte antigen or histocompatibility locus antigen; cM, centimorgan; scc, side chain cleavage; ISOM, isomerase; arom, aromatase.

into *pregnenolone (pregnene-3β-ol-20-one)* by the sidechain-cleaving enzyme *P450scc*. This enzyme is an integral protein of the inner mitochondrial membrane with its active site *facing the mitochondrial matrix*. The function of P450scc is supported by a mini electron transport chain located in the mitochondrial matrix involving *adrenodoxin*, which receives electrons from the cyclic AMP-regulated flavoprotein *adrenodoxin reductase* and transfers them to P450scc.

Cholesterol exists in cells as a *membrane pool* and a *steroidogenic cytoplasmic pool*. The first step in the steroidogenic process is the liberation of *free cholesterol* from *cholesteryl esters* stored in lipid droplets. For sidechain cleavage, cholesterol must be delivered from the cytoplasmic compartment to the matrix side of the inner mitochondrial membrane. Cholesterol is highly hydrophobic; thus the hydrophilic compartment between the inner and outer mitochondrial membranes presents a barrier against cholesterol transport. *The delivery of cholesterol to P450scc is the rate-limiting step of steroid hormone biosynthesis*. The process of cholesterol delivery involves at least two regulatory proteins:

- *Steroidogenic acute regulatory protein* (StAR) is transiently incorporated into the outer mitochondrial membrane upon exposure of steroidogenic cells to their adequate tropic hormone. StAR appears to activate PBR.
- *Peripheral-type benzodiazepine receptor* (PBR) is a multifunctional transmembrane protein, which probably serves as a regulated *cholesterol channel*. It is associated with a *voltage-dependent anion channel* (VDAC) also known as *mitochondrial porin* at the contact sites between the outer and inner mitochondrial membranes. The StAR-activated PBR allows the passage of cholesterol to the mitochondrial matrix, where it is exposed to the active site of P450scc. StAR-mediated steroidogenesis is inhibited either by the benzodiazepine compound *flunitrazepam* or by targeted disruption of the PBR gene.

PBR is ubiquitous and is constitutively expressed in all steroidogenic tissues. StAR therefore confers the *inducibility* of steroidogenesis by tropic hormones. ACTH (in the zonae fasciculata and reticularis), LH/hCG (in the Leydig cells of the testis, theca interna, and lutein cells of the ovary) acting via cyclic AMP, and angiotensin II (in the zona glomerulosa) acting via increasing intracellular Ca^{2+}, induce the rapid de novo synthesis of StAR thereby stimulating steroidogenesis. These tissues require the mandatory presence of StAR for steroid hormone synthesis. Upon termination of the stimulus by the tropic hormone, further synthesis of StAR stops and StAR is rapidly eliminated. All known cases of *congenital lipoid adrenal hyperplasia* (also known as *type VI congenital adrenal hyperplasia;* Box 12-6), which were formerly thought to be due to P450scc-deficiency, are *inactivating mutations of StAR*.

The brain, the Schwann cells of peripheral nerves (the sites of neurosteroid production), and the placenta are active steroidogenic tissues with-

BOX 12-6   Congenital Adrenal Hyperplasia

ACTH, the main regulator of zona fasciculata/reticularis, is under a negative feedback suppression by a *single* product of the adrenal cortex, namely cortisol. Any biochemical defect leading either to complete or partial impairment of cortisol production results in an increased pituitary secretion of ACTH. ACTH not only stimulates StAR (and thus steroidogenesis), but it is also a growth factor for its target cells. The prolonged stimulation by increased plasma ACTH results in hyperplasia of the adrenal cortex. The inborn biochemical defects leading to decreased cortisol and increased ACTH secretion are known as *congenital adrenal hyperplasia* (CAH, also known as *adrenogenital syndrome*). In cases of partial enzyme deficiencies, the increased cortical mass may be able to produce normal amounts of cortisol *at the expense of overproducing other biologically active steroid hormones.* Depending on the site of the block in the steroidogenic pathway, six main types of CAH are distinguished, some of which present as life-threatening emergencies in the newborn. The specific outcomes of the enzyme defects will be discussed later. In general, the defects cause well-defined constellations of contrasting clinical and laboratory symptoms such as

- overproduction of androgens leading to *virilization,* or lack of sex steroid production leading to *sexual infantility* (primary hypogonadism); both alterations in sex steroids may result in intersex development.
- mineralocorticoid deficits leading to *salt wasting,* or overproduction of mineralocorticoids leading to *hypertension* and *hypokalemic alkalosis.*
- *adrenal insufficiency* involving glucocorticoid and/or mineralocorticoid deficiency.

out expressing StAR. These tissues do not respond to hormonal stimuli by increased steroid hormone synthesis. It is assumed that in these tissues PBR is activated by a different mechanism, possibly involving endogenous benzodiazepines (*endozepines*).

Pregnenolone May Be Processed Either by the Δ^5 or the Δ^4 Pathway
Pregnenolone is the substrate of two different enzymes. These enzymes perform the initial steps of the Δ^5 and the Δ^4 pathways, respectively. The Δ^5 pathway is the preferred route in the zonae fasciculata and reticularis of the definitive adrenal cortex, and the only pathway in the fetal zone of the adrenal cortex. The synthesis of testosterone requires the joint action of both pathways. Although the synthesis may start with either route, it appears that the preferred initial route in the human gonads is the Δ^4 pathway. This explains why (in contrast with the adrenal cortex) the gonads

secrete more *andostenedione* than *dehydroepiandrosterone* (DHEA; Fig. 12-8).

- *P450c17* is the first enzyme of the Δ^5 pathway. The *CYP17* gene is expressed in the gonads, the fetal adrenal cortex, the zonae fasciculata and reticularis of the definitive adrenal cortex. P450c17 is a single enzyme with two catalytic activities:

    - *17α-hydroxylase* generates 17α-hydroxypregnenolone. This activity is required for the biosynthesis of both glucocorticoids and androgens (all sex steroids are derived from androgens). Note that the 17α-hydroxylase activity also converts progesterone (the initial product of the Δ^4 pathway) into 17α-hydroxyprogesterone.

    - *17,20-lyase*, which converts 17α-hydroxypregnenolone into DHEA and (mainly in the gonads where the Δ^4 pathway predominates) 17α-hydroxyprogesterone into androstenedione. *This is the first step in the biosynthesis of sex steroids* (the conversion of C-21 steroids into C-19 compounds). The 17,20-lyase activity is regulated separately from the 17α-hydroxylase. The 17,20-lyase activity significantly increases in the adrenal cortex at a developmental milestone known as *adrenarche* at the age of 6 to 8 years. The adrenarchal increase in 17,20-lyase activity is not associated with an increase in 17α-hydroxylase activity. Certain mutations of the *CYP17* gene abolish the 17,20-lyase activity, while retaining the 17α-hydroxylase activity.

The zona glomerulosa and the placenta are unable to synthesize either glucocorticoids or androgens because of the physiologic absence of *CYP17* expression (the absence of P450c17). Thus, these organs do not utilize the Δ^5 pathway, and by definition must rely on the Δ^4 pathway.

Loss-of-function mutations of the *CYP17* gene are known as *type V congenital adrenal hyperplasia.* In this condition, neither glucocorticoids nor sex steroids are produced. However, the zona fasciculata will produce the potent mineralocorticoids *11-deoxycorticosterone* (DOC) and corticosterone, which explains the hypertensive presentation of the disease.

- *3β-hydroxysteroid dehydrogenase:$\Delta^{5,4}$-oxosteroid isomerase* (3βHSD), which converts pregenenolone into progesterone, is by definition the first enzyme of the Δ^4 pathway. This enzyme has two isoenzymes: *type II 3βHSD* is expressed in the gonads and in all layers of the definitive zone of the adrenal cortex. The placenta (and the sebaceous glands) express *type I 3βHSD.*

In *type IV congenital adrenal hyperplasia only the type II 3βHSD activity is absent.* Thus, although the production of adrenal corticosteroids and the gonadal and adrenal synthesis of post-DHEA sex steroids is blocked, the placental production of progesterone (a hormone essential in maintaining pregnancy) remains normal.

- In addition to pregnenolone, 3βHSD acts on three additional substrates:

    - 3βHSD converts 17α-hydroxypregnenolone into 17α-hydroxyprogesterone and DHEA into androstenedione. These steps utilize substrates generated in the Δ^5 pathway by the successive prior actions of P450c17. Thus, these steps occur in the zonae fasciculata and reticularis of the adrenal cortex and, due to the preferential use of the Δ^4 pathway, to a lesser extent in the gonads.

- 3βHSD converts androstenediol into testosterone. Androstenediol is a minor substrate generated by the testis-specific type 3 17βHSD (17β-hydroxysteroid dehydrogenase; see Chap. 13).

The main adrenal androgens are DHEA and androstenedione. Their physiologic functions and further processing will be discussed in Chap. 13.

Progesterone and 17α-Hydroxyprogesterone Are Further Processed by the Adrenal-Specific Enzyme P450c21 Expression of *P450c21* (21-hydroxylase) is specific for the adrenal cortex: 21-hydroxylation is the step that commits steroid hormone precursors to the synthesis of mineralocorticoids as well as glucocorticoids.

- In the zona glomerulosa, the only substrate available to P450c21 is progesterone, which is converted into DOC.
- In the zona fasciculata/reticularis, due to the preferential Δ^5 pathway, little progesterone is produced, and the main substrate of P450c21 is 17α-hydroxyprogesterone. Thus, the main product of P450c21 is *11-deoxycortisol*.

The progesterone generated by the type I 3βHSD in the placenta cannot be further processed because the placenta expresses neither P450c17, nor P450c21. This explains why progesterone is the only de novo synthesized steroid hormone of the placenta. Note, however, that the placenta produces estrogens by converting fetally produced androgens taken up from the circulation (see fetoplacental unit, Chap. 13).

Mutations of P450c21 Are the Most Frequent Causes of Congenital Adrenal Hyperplasia The congenital deficiency of P450c21 results in *types I and II congenital adrenal hyperplasia* (CAH), which account for about 90% of all CAH cases. (The original clinical designation as type I and II has been replaced by novel classification based on molecular analysis; see below.) In 21-hydroxylase deficiency, the immediate precursor of 11-deoxycortisol 17α-hydroxyprogesterone accumulates both intracellularly and also in plasma. The elevated plasma *17α-hydroxyprogesterone* is utilized in the laboratory diagnosis of 21-hydroxylase deficiency. The intracellularly accumulating 17α-hydroxyprogesterone is shunted to the androgen biosynthetic pathway and converted into *androstenedione* by the 17,20-lyase activity of P450c17. Thus, a major consequence of 21-hydroxylase deficiency is the ACTH-driven hypersecretion of adrenal androgens. 21-hydroxylase deficiency is classified as follows:

- *Classical forms* are very rare, and present with clinical symptoms at birth. The virilization is sometimes severe and may result in ambiguous external genitalia in females.
    - In the *salt-wasting type,* virilization is associated with subnormal plasma levels of aldosterone. The mutations in this form completely inactivate P450c21.
    - In the *simple virilizing type,* plasma levels of aldosterone are normal. In these patients, the point mutations yield enzymes with 1 to 2% of the normal activity.
- The *nonclassical form* is characterized by late-onset virilization in females, which presents in childhood or adolescence (Fig. 12-9). In males, the condition imitates precocious puberty (see Chap. 13). This form has a

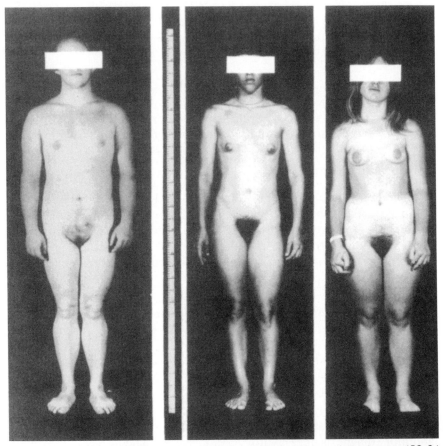

Figure 12-9. Habitus of pubertal girls with congenital adrenal hyperplasia due to p450c21 deficiency. The treatment of the condition is the suppression of ACTH-driven adrenal androgen production by exogenously administered glucocorticoids. From left to right, the glucocorticoid therapy was started at the ages of 16, 9, and 4 years. Note the progressively more feminine habitus with earlier treatment. (*Source:* Fig. 104-16 in New MI, Levine LS: Congenital adrenal hyperplasia, in Harris H, Hirschhorn K (eds): *Advances in Human Genetics,* vol. 4. New York, Plenum, 1973, pp 251–326.)

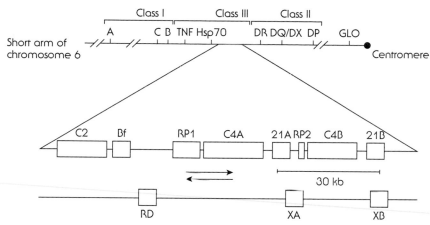

Figure 12-10. Map of the short arm of chromosome 6. The top line shows the organization of the class I, III, and II regions of the human leukocyte antigen (HLA) locus. The enlarged segment shows two strands of DNA with opposite transcriptional orientation of the genes. *CYP21A* (21A) is a pseudogene, therefore it is not transcribed. *CYP21B* encodes for p450c21 (21-hydroxylase). The horizontal bar indicates the 30-kb region that is deleted in approximately 20% of the chromosomes carrying 21-hydroxylase deficiency. Certain HLA haplotypes are associated with an increased risk for specific autoimmune diseases, including Addison's disease in which an adrenal-specific target of the immune reaction is the p450c21 enzyme. The HLA association of p450c21 deficiency, however, is explained by the chromosomal location of the *CYP21B* gene. C2, complement factor 2; C4A, C4B, nonallelic genes for complement factor 4; Bf, properdin factor Bf; RP1, nuclear protein of unknown function; RP2, a pseudogene corresponding with RP1; XB, the TNXB gene encoding for tenascin-X and extracellular matrix protein; XA, TNXA, a pseudogene; A, C, B, DR, DQ/DX, and DP, histocompatibility loci; TNF, tumor necrosis factor; Hsp70, heat shock protein 70. (*Source:* Modified from Fig. 5, p 738 in Miller WL: Congenital adrenal hyperplasia. Endocrinol Metab Clin North Am 20:721, 1991; and Fig. 2 in Speiser PW, White PC: Congenital adrenal hyperplasia due to steroid 21-hydroxylase deficiency. Clin Endocrinol 49:411–417, 1998.)

very high frequency among Ashkenazi Jews. The point mutations involved in this form yield P450c21 proteins with 20 to 60% of normal enzyme activity.

P450c21 is encoded by the gene *CYP21B*, which is found on the short arm of chromosome 6 in tandem with the closely related pseudogene *CYP21A*. *CYP21B* and *CYP21A* are 98% identical, but the pseudogene has accumulated a number of point mutations that would inactivate the putative gene product. The chromosomal localization of these genes has several consequences:

• *CYP21B* and *CYP21A* are found between the human leukocyte antigen (HLA)-B and the HLA-D locus, closely associated with two complement-coding genes (*C4A* and *C4B*, Fig. 12-10). This explains the association of P450c21 deficiency with certain HLA haplotypes. It is noteworthy that P450c21 is a major target of the autoimmune reaction destroying the adrenal cortex in Addison's disease. The association of Addison's disease with certain HLA haplotypes is related to the immunological dysfunction and not to mutations of P450c21.

- Almost all 21-hydroxylase deficiencies are caused by two types of mutations:
    - *Gene conversion* is responsible for about 75 to 80% of 21-hydroxylase deficiencies, and involves microgene conversions. This process changes a portion of *CYP21B* to the corresponding but mutated portion of *CYP21A*. The imported mutations are heterogenous point mutations, some of which partially, whereas others completely, inactivate the putative gene product.
    - *Deletions* of a 30-kb DNA segment, which includes the 3' end of *CYP21A*, the entire *C4B*, and the first 5 to 7 exons of *CYP21B*. This deletion yields a nonfunctional *chimeric pseudogene* by fusing portions of *CYP21A* and *CYP21B*.

P450c21 deficiency is an autosomal recessive disorder. Quite often the maternal and the paternal *CYP21B* genes carry different mutations of P450c21. This condition is known as *compound heterozygosity*. The phenotype of these patients is usually determined by the allele carrying the less severe defect.

The overproduction of androgens can be suppressed by exogenously administered glucocorticoids via the suppression of ACTH. Thus, the condition could be viewed as *glucocorticoid-remediable hyperandrogenism*. The salt-wasting forms require treatment with mineralocorticoids.

The Biosynthesis of Aldosterone and Cortisol Are Performed by Distinct Mitochondrial Enzymes Encoded by Two Genes Closely Associated on Chromosome 8q   The conversion of DOC to aldosterone involves three chemical reactions (11β-hydroxylase, 18-hydroxylase, 18-oxidase) all catalyzed by the multifunctional enzyme *P450aldo*, encoded by *CYP11B2*. P450aldo expression is specific for the zona glomerulosa and induced by angiotensin II and/or elevated plasma potassium. P450aldo is also known as P450c11AS (for aldosterone synthase) and P450cmo. The first catalytic activity (11β-hydroxylase) is identical with that of P450c11. The 18-hydroxylase and 18-oxidase activities are also called corticosterone *methyl-oxidase* I and II (CMO-I and II, respectively). These two activities jointly introduce a unique aldehyde group to C18, hence the name aldosterone (aldehydesterone).

Deoxycortisol is converted to *cortisol* (also known as *hydrocortisone*) by the 11β-hydroxylase activity of *P450c11*, encoded by *CYP11B1*. P450c11 expression is specific for the zonae fasciculata and reticularis, and induced by ACTH. P450c11 may also convert DOC into corticosterone, albeit this function does not occur to a significant degree under physiologic circumstances.

CYP11B2 and *CYP11B1* are 95% identical genes closely linked on chromosome 8. Both P450aldo and P450c11 are localized in the *inner membrane* of mitochondria. Mutations of the genes may produce a wide variety of clinical presentations:

- The classic form of type III CAH is due to a variety of inactivating mutations of *CYP11B1*. The classical presentation of type III CAH includes:
  - *hypertension with hypokalemic alkalosis* due to the accumulation and secretion of DOC (a potent mineralocorticoid); and
  - *virilization* due to shunting of the accumulating 17α-hydroxyprogesterone toward androgen synthesis.

  In suspected 11-hydroxylase deficiency, three precursor metabolites are used routinely in the laboratory diagnosis of the condition:
  - 17α-hydroxyprogesterone is elevated both in 21-hydroxylase and 11-hydroxylase deficiencies,
  - DOC and 11-deoxycortisol are elevated only in 11-hydroxylase deficiency.

- Defects of P450aldo due to mutations of *CYP11B2* cause *salt-wasting without virilization*. Two forms have been described as *CMO-I* and *CMO-II deficiencies,* which led to the mistaken conclusion that the three enzymatic reactions involved in the conversion of DOC to aldosterone were carried out by three different gene products. In actuality, the various mutations of *CYP11B2* have a differential impact on the catalytic activities of P450aldo. Both conditions are associated with increased production of corticosterone. The two subtypes can be distinguished by the plasma levels of *18-hydroxycorticosterone:*
  - In CMO-I deficiency, plasma levels of 18-hydroxycorticosterone are subnormal.
  - In CMO-II deficiency, 18-hydroxycorticosterone is overproduced.

- *Glucocorticoid-remediable* (hyper)*aldosteronism* (GRA) is an autosomal *dominant* disease, which is due to a fusion between the regulatory portion of *CYP11B1* and the protein-coding portion of *CYP11B2*. The resulting chimeric gene is ACTH-regulated, expressed in the zonae fasciculata and reticularis, but the expressed enzyme processes 11-deoxycortisol (and DOC) along the pathway of aldosterone synthesis. This results in the appearance of high levels of the abnormal adrenal steroids 18-oxocortisol and 18-hydroxycortisol. Aldosterone is also generated by this chimeric enzyme. Because these metabolic processes cause an initial decrease in circulating cortisol, ACTH becomes elevated. However, normalization of plasma cortisol levels is achieved at the expense of overproducing mineralocorticoids. Administration of exogenous glucocorticoids suppresses ACTH and resolves the hypertension.

Mineralocorticoids

The Transport, Action, and Biologic Effects of Mineralocorticoids

About One Third of Circulating Aldosterone Is Free Hormone Leading to a Plasma Half-Life of 15 to 20 Minutes The *total* plasma levels of aldosterone and DOC (11-deoxycorticosterone) are comparable, but their carrier protein-binding and cellular sources are different.

• Aldosterone is secreted by the zona glomerulosa, and its plasma levels are influenced by postural changes (supine, 80 to 440 pM [30 to 160 pg/mL]; upright, 190 to 830 pM [70 to 300 pg/mL]).
• The main source of DOC is the zona fasciculata/reticularis. Its normal secretion is ACTH-dependent and, therefore, follows a circadian rhythm with peak levels in the morning (61 to 576 pM [20 to 190 pg/mL]).

In vitro, DOC is almost as potent a mineralocorticoid as aldosterone. In vivo, however, aldosterone functions as the predominant physiologic mineralocorticoid. Compared to cortisol, DOC or progesterone, aldosterone has low affinity for binding with *cortisol-binding globulin* (CBG). About 20% of plasma aldosterone is bound to CBG, 40% is bound loosely to albumin and the remainder is in a free, biologically active form. In contrast, less than 3% of DOC circulates as a free hormone (see Table 4-2).

Aldosterone is cleared rapidly from the circulation in part by its main target organ, the kidney, by filtration of the free hormone. Because plasma DOC is mostly protein bound, only trace amounts of free DOC appear in urine. Most of the aldosterone and practically all of DOC are eliminated by the liver. Inactivation of mineralocorticoids as well as glucocorticoids in the liver primarily involve reduction of the A-ring and the 3-oxo group. The resulting 3-hydroxy group is then conjugated either with glucuronic acid or sulphate. Thus, the liver converts aldosterone and DOC to tetrahydroaldosterone 3-glucuronide and tetrahydro-DOC-3-glucuronide, respectively. The conjugated compounds are highly hydrophilic and do not bind with plasma carrier proteins. Thus, they are readily eliminated by renal filtration.

Aldosterone Stimulates Sodium Reabsorption and Potassium Secretion in the Renal Cortical Collecting Duct, Promotes Alkalosis Indirectly by Systemic K⁺/H⁺ Exchange, and Directly by Enhancing Renal Proton Secretion   Aldosterone is a sodium-conserving hormone, which serves a major regulator of the volume and the electrolyte composition of ECF. Although aldosterone has other sites of action (see below), its main target is the cortical collecting duct of the kidney.

Sodium is freely filtered by the renal glomerulus. Thus, plasma concentration of sodium and the glomerular filtration rate (GFR) determine the amount of sodium delivered into the tubular lumen. Changes in the GFR provoke parallel changes in sodium reabsorption by the proximal tubule, a phenomenon known as the *glomerulotubular balance*. This adjustment of sodium reabsorption assures that the proximal tubules reabsorb approximately 65% of the filtered sodium.

The thick ascending limb of the loop of Henle and the distal convoluted tubules are lined by water-tight epithelial cells (i.e., devoid of aquaporins). These segments of the nephron are responsible for the reabsorption of about 20 to 25% of the filtered sodium. This sodium reabsorption is important in the generation of the *corticomedullary osmotic gradient,* which is essential for the concentrating function of the kidney. The sodium-reabsorption in these water-tight epithelia is regulated by antidiuretic hormone (ADH) acting on V_2 receptors (see Fig. 10-6).

About 10% of the filtered sodium reaches the *cortical collecting duct.* On a normal sodium diet, less than 1% of the filtered sodium appears in urine. Thus, the cortical and the medullary collecting ducts reabsorb about 9% of the filtered sodium. *The cortical collecting duct (CCD) is a shared site of action of ADH and aldosterone.*

- *Aldosterone maintains the ADH responsiveness of the cortical collecting duct* by inducing the expression of the ADH-regulated adenylyl cyclase. ADH regulates the water permeability of the cortical as well as the medullary collecting ducts by mobilizing aquaporin-2 (AQP2; see Chap. 10).
- *Aldosterone stimulates sodium reabsorption in the cortical collecting duct. The reabsorption of about 2% of the filtered sodium is aldosterone-regulated.* Calculating with a 180 L/d GFR and an average plasma sodium concentration of 145 mM, the maximal aldosterone-regulated reabsorption equals about 30 g NaCl per day. Thus, the *discretionary sodium loss or retention* significantly exceeds the typical dietary sodium intake (6 to 8 g/d).

By these mechanisms, aldosterone increases sodium reabsorption and, by acting in concert with ADH, increases water reabsorption. The net effect is *expansion of the volume of isosmotic ECF and increased blood pressure.* Similar to the situation with ADH, the volume of ECF is involved in a negative feedback regulatory loop of aldosterone secretion.

The aldosterone-regulated reabsorption of sodium is functionally coupled with K^+ secretion into the tubular lumen. The urinary potassium losses lower the potassium concentration in the ECF. As discussed later, K^+ is a physiologic regulator of aldosterone secretion; thus, the hypokalemic action of aldosterone is also regulated in a negative feedback loop. Potassium in the ECF is replenished from the large potassium reserve of the intracellular fluid (ICF) by exchanging intracellular K^+ with extracellular H^+. This *systemic K^+/H^+ exchange* is the main mechanism behind the alkalosis-promoting action of aldosterone. Thus, *aldosterone promotes hypokalemic metabolic alkalosis.*

The cellular action of aldosterone is mediated by the mineralocorticoid receptor, a ligand-regulated transcription factor. The expression and activity of several proteins involved in electrolyte transport are regulated by aldosterone (see Fig. 10-6 inset showing CCD):

- Aldosterone stimulates the de novo synthesis and activity of *amiloride-sensitive Na^+-channels* in the *apical* membrane. These channels allow the influx of Na^+ into the cell driven by the electrochemical gradient. The resulting depolarization of the luminal (but not the basolateral) membrane (i.e., the lumen becomes negatively charged) is the driving force of K^+

secretion into the lumen via *ATP-sensitive potassium channels* in the apical membrane. These channels are closed in the presence of high intracellular concentrations of ATP. Aldosterone stimulates the activity of the $3Na^+/2K^+$-ATPase in these cells (see below), thereby lowering intracellular concentrations of ATP and opening the potassium channels (see also insulin secretion, Chap. 9).

• Aldosterone stimulates the de novo synthesis and activity of the electrogenic *$3Na^+/2K^+$-ATPase* in the *basolateral* membrane. The exchange mechanism delivers Na^+ from the cytosol to the interstitial fluid, and replenishes the intracellular pool of K^+. The effects of aldosterone on Na^+ and K^+ transport are exerted on the *principal cells,* which comprise about 75% of the epithelial lining of the cortical collecting ducts.

• In the *intercalated cells* of the cortical collecting ducts, aldosterone induces the expression of the *N*-ethylmaleimide (NEM) sensitive *proton-pump* (H^+-ATPase) in the apical membrane and the *Cl^-/HCO_3^--exchanger* in the basolateral membrane. These cells express carbonic anhydrase, and contribute to the acidification of urine and concomitant alkalinization of plasma.

The sodium-retaining action of aldosterone is limited by the *escape phenomenon,* which is observed either during prolonged administration of supraphysiologic doses of mineralocorticoids or in patients suffering from *hyperaldosteronism*. The escape phenomenon refers to the observation that *in spite of the sustained presence of mineralocorticoids, the initial sodium retention is followed by a new equilibrium that is maintained by increased sodium excretion*. Thus, the volume expansion related to sodium retention becomes limited, which explains the *absence of overt edema* formation in hyperaldosteronism (see also at atrial natriuretic peptide). The escape phenomenon does not apply to potassium and protons: their increased excretion persists during prolonged mineralocorticoid exposure. Thus, hyperaldosteronism is characterized by *hypertension* and *hypokalemic alkalosis*.

The actions of aldosterone are antagonized by the potassium-sparing diuretic drug *spironolactone,* and to a lesser degree by endogenously produced *progesterone*. The latter becomes physiologically relevant mainly during pregnancy.

The Actions of Aldosterone on the Ducts of Salivary and Eccrine Sweat Glands and on the Intestinal and Respiratory Mucosa Are Similar to Those on the Distal Nephron   In each of these target organs, aldosterone exerts an effect on the epithelium that promotes sodium conservation and potassium secretion. In these tissues, the sodium-retaining effect of aldosterone does not display the escape phenomenon.

The sodium secreted by the acini and reabsorbed by the ducts of salivary glands is an arrangement comparable with that of the glomerulus and the cortical collecting duct. The reabsorption of sodium and the associated secretion of potassium in salivary ducts are regulated by aldosterone.

The concentration of these ions, however, are also influenced by the production rate of the saliva: increased production rate is associated with a definite increase in sodium and slight decrease in potassium. *A salivary sodium : potassium ratio of less than 0.25 indicates excessive mineralocorticoid effects.*

Aldosterone affects sodium and potassium in eccrine (but not in apocrine) sweat glands in a manner similar to its action on salivary glands. Sweat is normally hypotonic. Sodium and potassium concentrations in sweat are rarely used for the assessment of mineralocorticoid status. Increased concentrations of sodium chloride in sweat may indicate cystic fibrosis, which is due to the mutation of a chloride channel termed cystic fibrosis transmembrane regulator (CFTR).

The quantitatively most important potassium-excreting extrarenal target organ of aldosterone is the colon. Hypokalemia in hyperaldosteronism and hyperkalemia in Addison's disease (hypadrenia) are in part related to alterations of colonic potassium handling.

Aldosterone also exerts direct effects on heart function. In addition to a positive inotropic effect, it has been implicated in the development of *myocardial fibrosis* during ventricular hypertrophy.

The Ligand-Specificity of the Mineralocorticoid Receptor Is Assured by Type II 11β-Hydroxysteroid Dehydrogenase

The mineralocorticoid receptor is closely related to the glucocorticoid, progesterone and androgen receptors (see Chap. 5). This is reflected by a similar ligand specificity of the hormone-binding domain (HBD) and sequence-specificity of the DNA-binding domain (DBD) of the mineralocorticoid and glucocorticoid receptors. Specificity of hormone action is achieved mainly by two mechanisms:

- *distinct cellular expression patterns* of mineralocorticoid and glucocorticoid receptors, and
- *protection* of the mineralocorticoid receptor by *11β-hydroxysteroid dehydrogenase* (11β-HSD) from being activated by the glucocorticoids cortisol and corticosterone.

Two isoforms of 11β-HSD have been cloned and characterized (Table 12-7, Fig. 12-8). In the target tissues of aldosterone, *the mineralocorticoid receptor is coexpressed with type II 11β-HSD,* which converts cortisol into *cortisone* and corticosterone into 11-dehydrocorticosterone. These compounds are devoid of mineralocorticoid activity. Although 11β-HSD is a microsomal enzyme, it is also present within the cell nucleus.

Mutations of the type II 11β-HSD are responsible for the syndrome of *apparent mineralocorticoid excess* (AME). In this autosomal recessive condition, physiologic levels of cortisol act on the unprotected mineralocorticoid receptor and mimic hyperaldosteronism. The acquired form of AME is due to the ingestion of large quantities of *licorice,* which contains *glycyrrhizin,* an inhibitor of type II 11β-HSD.

Glucocorticoid excess is a potent inhibitor of growth in children (see

Table 12-7   11β-Hydroxysteroid Dehydrogenase Isoenzymes

Type	Chromosomal localization	Coenzyme	Tissue distribution	Remarks
11β-HSD type I	1q32.2-41 (HSD11B1)	NADP$^+$	Glucocorticoid target tissues: liver, adrenal, pituitary, gonad, lung, decidua	Low-affinity enzyme; catalyzes dehydrogenase and mainly reductase reactions; produces cortisol from cortisone, enhances glucocorticoid receptor activation
11β-HSD type II	16q22 (HSD11B2)	NAD$^+$	Mineralocorticoid target tissues: adult and fetal kidney (cortical collecting duct); placenta; excretory ducts of salivary and eccrine sweat glands; mammary gland during pregnancy; absorptive epithelial cells of the small intestine and colon; ciliated epithelial cells of the respiratory tract; heart	High-affinity enzyme; catalyzes the dehydrogenase reaction only; protects the mineralocorticoid receptor from exposure to cortisol in the kidney and other tissues; protects the fetus from maternal cortisol; mutated in AME patients; glycyrrhizin-(licorice-) sensitive

ABBREVIATION: AME, apparent mineralocorticoid excess.

Chap. 10). Fetal tissues are also sensitive to this action of cortisol. The fetal adrenal cortex produces very low quantities of cortisol, starting after midgestation. Total as well as free cortisol increases in the maternal circulation during pregnancy. Because cortisol as a lipophilic hormone could penetrate the placental barrier, the fetus is protected against its transfer by *type II 11β-HSD,* which is expressed in the placenta. This mechanism is comparable with the expression of type III deiodinase in the placenta, which limits the placental transfer of thyroid hormones (see Chap. 11). The history of AME patients usually includes low birth weight.

The capacity of type II 11β-HSD can be saturated by extremely high levels of cortisol, such as seen in certain cases of *Cushing's disease,* especially those caused by ectopic production of ACTH. Under these circumstances, the hypertensive action of cortisol includes apparent mineralocorticoid excess, which is typically associated with a significant increase in urinary free cortisol excretion. In Cushing's disease, the excess ACTH stimulation of the adrenal cortex also increases the production and free plasma levels of DOC; thus, Cushing's disease usually involves true mineralocorticoid excess.

Regulation of the Zona Glomerulosa

The Zona Glomerulosa Is Directly Regulated by the Renin-Angiotensin Axis and Potassium   The main regulatory mechanisms of aldosterone secretion from the zona glomerulosa are summarized in Fig. 12-11. The

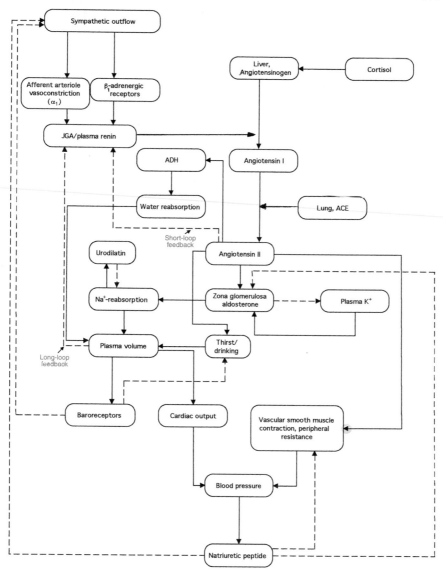

Figure 12-11. Regulation of the renin-angiotensin-aldosterone axis. Solid arrows indicate stimulation/increase; dashed arrows indicate inhibition/decrease. Compare with Figs. 10-7 and 12-6. Note that the osmotic regulation of antidiuretic hormone (ADH) is not displayed; nevertheless, the aldosterone-induced sodium reabsorption is *initially* not accompanied by water, and the resulting hypernatremia and increased osmolality promptly stimulate ADH secretion, which leads to isosmotic volume expansion. Note that aldosterone directly enhances ADH responsiveness in both the cortical and medullary collecting ducts. The cardiac output is also stimulated by sympathoadrenal activity via β_1-adrenergic receptors and heart rate (not shown). The circled area is a reminder of target cell responsiveness, which is maintained by glucocorticoids. JGA, juxtaglomerular apparatus.

Table 12-8   Normal Plasma Values of the Renin-Angotensin-Aldosterone Axis
in Adults on a Normal Sodium Diet

Compound	Normal range
PRA (generation of A-I acting from either endogenous or exogenous angiotensinogen)	Supine (30 min): 0.2–1.6 ng A-I/mL/h Standing (4 h): 0.7–3.3 ng A-I/mL/h
Angiotensin-II	Supine (30 min): 10–60 pg/mL
Aldosterone	Supine: 80–440 pM [30–160 pg/mL] Standing: 190–830 pM [70–300 pg/mL]
Urinary aldosterone 18-glucuronide (sodium replete patients)	5–20 μg/24 h (14–56 nmol/24 h)
Potassium	3.5–5.1 mM

ABBREVIATIONS: PRA, plasma renin activity; A-I, angiotensin-I.

normal values of the diagnostically relevant substances are shown in Table 12-8. There are two physiologically important *direct* regulators of zona glomerulosa cells:

- *Angiotensin II*, an octapeptide generated by successive cleavage of *angiotensinogen* by the proteolytic enzymes *renin* and *angiotensin I converting enzyme* (ACE).
- Similar to angiotensin II, *hyperkalemia* stimulates aldosterone synthesis and secretion by increasing intracellular levels of Ca^{2+} in zona glomerulosa cells.

The cellular effects involve the induction of StAR and P450aldo.

The involvement of ACTH in the regulation of aldosterone secretion is controversial. In spite of an acute, transient stimulation of aldosterone secretion, ACTH does not appear to be involved in the physiologic regulation of aldosterone. Nevertheless, prolonged excess of ACTH may stimulate cell proliferation in the entire adrenal cortex, including the zona glomerulosa.

The Renin-Angiotensin System Is an Extracellular Prohormone Processing Machinery   Protein hormones are usually produced as preprohormones (see Chap. 3). After cleavage of the signal peptide, the prohormone is further processed by *intracellular* enzymes called proprotein convertases. The renin-angiotensin system may be viewed as a modification of this general scheme, whereby the prohormone (angiotensinogen) is secreted by the liver, and the two "proprotein convertases" (renin and angiotensin converting enzyme) process it in the circulation. Dispersal of an intracellular machinery to different organs aids coordinated regulation within the framework of whole-body processes.

Renin is a 46-kDa glycosylated aspartyl proteinase encoded by chromosome 1q32-42. Renin is highly specific for a single substrate, angiotensinogen. The plasma half-life of renin has a rapid initial component ($\approx$12 min) and a slow delayed component ($\approx$60 to 120 min). It is degraded mainly in the liver and the kidney. Because *renin is the rate-limiting step in the generation of angiotensin II,* its short half-life is essential in the minute-to-minute regulation of aldosterone secretion. The source of renin is the JGA, which consists of the *macula densa,* the *extraglomerular mesangium,* and the *juxtaglomerular afferent arterioles.* The macula densa is a modified portion of the distal convoluted tubule, which is anatomically associated with the vascular pole of the very glomerulus from which the tubule originates (see Fig. 10-6).

Angiotensinogen is a member of the *serpin* (serine-protease inhibitor) *family* of proteins: depending on its carbohydrate content, it is a 59- to 64-kDa glycoprotein related to cortisol-binding globulin (CBG), thyroxine-binding globulin (TBG), and α_1-antitrypsin. The single gene encoding human angiotensinogen is closely associated with that of renin on chromosome 1q42.3. The liver maintains an ample supply of angiotensinogen in the plasma. The half-life of plasma angiotensinogen has two components: the rapid initial component ($\approx$10 min) is due to cleavage by renin, the slow delayed component (4 to 8 h) is due to its clearance primarily by the kidney. Angiotensinogen is processed only by renin. The N-terminal decapeptide of angiotensinogen is cleaved by renin to yield *angiotensin I.*

ACE is a membrane-anchored zinc metalloproteinase that functions as a promiscuous *dipeptidyl carboxypeptidase* ectoenzyme. It converts angiotensin I into the biologically active angiotensin II. In addition, ACE is responsible for the rapid inactivation of bradykinin and kallidin (see Chap. 4), enkephalins, gonadotropin-releasing hormone (GnRH), substance P, and other peptides. *Using different promoters,* two isoenzymes are expressed from the ACE gene (found on chromosome 17q23):

* *Somatic ACE* has two internally homologous zinc-binding catalytic domains (N- and C-domains) that arose from the duplication of an ancestral gene. The domains display somewhat different substrate preferences. Somatic ACE is expressed in the *endothelium* (especially in the lungs), the epithelium of renal proximal tubules, activated macrophages and several areas in the brain.
* *Spermatocyte* (germinal) *ACE* essentially lacks the N-terminal domain and, therefore, is about half the size of somatic ACE. Testicular ACE has a short N-terminal domain expressed from a testis-specific first exon (located within an intron of somatic ACE) and the C-domain, which is anchored in the membrane of *postmeiotic spermatocytes.* Experiments with transgenic mice suggest that absence of testicular ACE (but not the absence of angiotensinogen) results in decreased fertility secondary to a yet undefined impairment of spermatozoon function.

ACE inhibitor drugs such as *captopril* are used in the treatment of hyperreninemic forms of hypertension. Note that these drugs do not penetrate the blood-testis barrier and have no significant impact on fertility.

Due to their action on kallikrein degradation, ACE inhibitors may cause angioedema and persistent coughing.

Angiotensin II is the main biologically active angiotensin. Its plasma half-life is extremely short, less than 1 min. Thus, both the rate limiting enzyme of angiotensin II production (renin) and angiotensin II per se have short half-lives. The biologically less potent heptapeptide angiotensin III is generated from angiotensin II by *aminopeptidase A*. Angiotensin III can be further processed by *aminopeptidase B* to yield the hexapeptide angiotensin IV.

Two types of *angiotensin receptors* have been identified. Both belong to the G-protein-coupled heptahelical family, but use different postreceptor mechanisms. The clinically recognized effects of angiotensin II are mediated by the type 1 angiotensin receptors (AT_1). The *AT_1* gene is located on chromosome 3; its expression in vascular smooth muscle is induced by glucocorticoids. Angiotensin II stimulates PLC and increases intracellular levels of Ca^{2+}, thereby stimulating aldosterone synthesis and secretion in zona glomerulosa cells. By the same mechanism, angiotensin II functions as a *potent vasoconstrictor* acting on vascular smooth muscle. In part by activating PKC and the MAP-kinase pathways, and perhaps by activating tyrosine kinases, stimulation of AT_1 receptors causes *proliferation of zona glomerulosa and vascular smooth muscle cells*. AT_1-receptor specific angiotensin II antagonist drugs, such as *losartan,* are effective alternatives to ACE inhibitors. The *AT_2 receptors* appear to oppose the proliferative action mediated by tyrosine kinases: these receptors activate intracellular tyrosine phosphatases via a pertussis toxin-sensitive mechanism. Targeted disruption of the mouse *AT_2* gene results in a significant increase in blood pressure and increased sensitivity to the pressor action of angiotensin II. Thus, AT_2 mediates a depressor effect and antagonizes the AT_1-mediated pressor action of angiotensin II. Angiotensin IV appears to act on its cognate (as yet unidentified) receptor and cause vasodilatation.

Renin Secretion Is Regulated by the Tension in the Afferent Glomerular Arteriole, the Sympathoadrenal System, and Feedback Mechanisms Involving the Macula Densa and Angiotensin II The classic experiments of Goldblatt revealed that narrowing of the renal artery results in an increased secretion of renin. The clinical equivalent of these experiments is seen in *renovascular hypertension*. Indeed, any condition that leads to a decreased renal blood flow, and a *decreased tension of the glomerular afferent arteriolar wall,* will also increase renin secretion from the JGA.

The *macula densa* functions as a sodium sensor. The luminal concentration of NaCl at the macula densa modulates two interrelated functions: the glomerular arteriolar resistance through tubuloglomerular feedback and renin secretion.

• *Tubuloglomerular feedback* is the negative feedback relationship between macula densa NaCl concentration and the GFR, which stabilizes the minute-to-minute salt delivery to the distal nephron. *In response to an increase in the luminal NaCl concentration, the macula densa secretes adenosine,* which causes constriction of the afferent arteriole of the glomerulus and a consequent decrease of GFR. This myogenic response is the main mechanism of rapid, short-term adaptation to alterations of sodium balance.

- The adenosine released by the macula densa *decreases renin secretion by the JGA*. Modulation of renin secretion is the dominant mechanism of long-term adaptation to sustained alterations of sodium balance.

Both macula densa effects can be blocked by theophylline and *adenosine$_1$- (A$_1$-) receptor-specific antagonists.*

Neuronal nitric oxide synthase (nNOS) is highly expressed in the macula densa cells. *NO produced by the macula densa blunts the tubuloglomerular feedback response.* The blunted feedback equals a relatively enhanced production of renin. The activity of nNOS is stimulated by salt restriction and angiotensin II.

As discussed, the amount of sodium entering the renal tubules depends on the plasma concentration of sodium and the GFR. In case of volume depletion, less sodium is filtered, which leads to a decrease of NaCl concentration in the luminal fluid *at the macula densa*. This results in an increased secretion of renin from the JGA. In addition, volume depletion and/or standing up from a reclining position activates the sympathoadrenal system via the baroreceptor reflex. The sympathoadrenal system stimulates renin secretion by two mechanisms:

- Stimulation of α_1-adrenergic receptors causes vasoconstriction mainly in the afferent arterioles and decreases GRF.
- Stimulation of β_1-adrenergic receptors directly stimulates renin secretion from the JGA.

The increased plasma renin activity results in a significant increase in the circulating concentration of angiotensin II. Thus, the pressor response achieved by the sympathoadrenal system is augmented by the vascular effect of angiotensin II. Within the kidney, the vasoconstrictor action of angiotensin II is preferentially exerted on the *efferent* arterioles, thereby antagonizing the effect of α_1-adrenergic receptor stimulation on the glomerular filtration pressure and GFR.

Angiotensin II inhibits renin secretion from the JGA. This is referred to as the *short-loop feedback of renin secretion*. The *long-loop feedback* is provided by the angiotensin II-stimulated aldosterone via sodium retention. Note that the sodium retention is accompanied by ADH-regulated water retention, and thus plasma sodium levels remain normal.

Plasma renin activity displays a *sleep-associated pattern*. There is a minor decrease in plasma renin activity during REM sleep. During the non-REM (NREM) phases of sleep, plasma renin activity markedly increases. During NREM, the vasoconstrictor sympathetic tone is decreased, which results in a fall of blood pressure. The decrease in blood pressure stimulates renin secretion. During NREM sleep plasma renin activity increases over that observed during wakefulness, suggesting that renin is more important in maintaining blood pressure during NREM sleep. The variations in plasma levels of aldosterone follow those of plasma renin activity with a lag time of about 20 min.

The Sodium-Retaining and Hypertensive Actions of the Renin-Angiotensin-Aldosterone Axis Are Functionally Antagonized by Natriuretic Peptides   Atrial natriuretic peptide (ANP) defends against mineralocorticoid-induced and diet-related salt retention, and the consequent hypertension. ANP is produced by atrial cardiomyocytes, especially those in the right atrium. Increased central venous pressure, which indicates fluid retention, results in stretching of atrial cardiomyocytes thereby releasing ANP. ANP exerts most of these effects by acting on the type A natriuretic peptide receptor (NPR-A), which is a single membrane-spanning receptor guanylyl cyclase (see Chap. 5). ANP has multiple targets:

- In the kidney, ANP exerts effects on hemodynamic, tubular, and JGA functions.
    - By a differential action on afferent and efferent arterioles, *ANP increases* hydrostatic pressure in the glomerular capillaries thereby increasing *GFR*.
    - *ANP inhibits sodium reabsorption in the inner medullary collecting duct.* This action, however, is mainly related to *urodilatin*. ANP and urodilatin are the products of the same gene. Due to a different renal processing, urodilatin is missing the four N-terminal amino acid residues of mature ANP. Urodilatin does not appear in plasma, and is secreted by distal tubular cells directly into the tubular lumen. Urodilatin binds to luminal NPR-A receptors in the collecting duct and causes a cyclic GMP-mediated inhibition of the *amiloride-sensitive sodium channel* thereby *inducing diuresis and natriuresis*.
    - ANP *inhibits renin secretion* from the JGA.
- ANP *inhibits aldosterone secretion* by a direct effect on the zona glomerulosa.
- By acting on the circumventricular organs (subfornical organ [SFO], area postrema), ANP *decreases salt appetite, ADH secretion, and sympathetic outflow*.
- By acting on the vasculature, ANP causes
    - dilatation of arteries and decreasing total peripheral resistance;
    - dilatation of veins, thereby increasing venous capacitance;
    - increasing capillary permeability to fluids, thereby shifting intravascular fluid into the interstitial compartment and increasing hematocrit.
- ANP is antimitogenic and/or antihypertrophic in most target tissues including the heart and vascular smooth muscle.

The physiologic role of ANP is supported by experiments with transgenic and knockout mice. Overexpression of ANP decreases blood pressure. Homozygous ANP-knockout mice kept on a low-salt diet have only slightly elevated blood pressure, which is markedly elevated upon increasing dietary salt intake. Even the heterozygous ANP-knockout mice are more susceptible to salt-induced hypertension than wild-type mice. ANP-knockout mice display an accentuated cardiac hypertrophy.

The normal defensive mechanism by ANP is insufficient to normalize blood pressure and ECF volume, but limits the increase of these parameters under several pathophysiologic conditions, such as congestive heart failure or hyperaldosteronism. Indeed, the increased ANP secretion is in part responsible for the *aldosterone escape phenomenon*. The rise in the concentration of plasma ANP coincides with the onset of escape.

Major Pathologic Conditions Involving the Renin-Angiotensin-Aldosterone Axis

Whereas Secondary Hyperaldosteronism Is Caused by Hyperreninemia, Primary Hyperaldosteronism Suppresses Plasma Renin Activity by Feedback Mechanisms Both primary and secondary hyperaldosteronism present as hypertension (systolic and diastolic pressures may exceed 200 and 110 mmHg, respectively), which is associated with hypokalemic alkalosis. Hyperaldosteronism is usually confirmed from urine samples by measuring aldosterone liberated from the acid-labile metabolite *aldosterone-18-glucuronide* (see Table 12-8), which reflects about 5 to 15% of aldosterone secretion. (Urinary excretion of tetrahydroaldosterone is about 4 times higher than that of aldosterone-18-glucuronide.)

Assessment of aldosterone is usually prompted by hypokalemia or low-normal potassium levels observed on routine serum chemistry profile. The degree of hypokalemia (and alkalosis) depends on the dietary sodium intake: the higher the sodium intake the more severe the hypokalemia. Thus, for proper laboratory evaluation, patients may need to be instructed to consume extra salt (1 g of NaCl with each meal for 4 days).

The alkalosis may manifest as muscle cramps due to a shift from free to albumin-bound fraction of plasma calcium (see Chap. 8). Plasma potassium alterations impact excitable tissues, which may manifest in the electrocardiogram (EKG) (Box 12-7). For the same reason, hypokalemia may blunt insulin secretory responses and cause *insulinopenic* impaired glucose tolerance.

The differential diagnosis of primary and secondary types of hyperaldosteronism follow the same logic used for hyperthyroidism. *Primary hyperaldosteronism* (also known as *Conn's syndrome*) is the autonomous production of aldosterone, which is most often due to adrenocortical adenoma or bilateral nodular hyperplasia of the zona glomerulosa. This condition results in *feedback suppression of plasma renin activity*. The autonomous nature

BOX 12-7   EKG Symptoms of Altered Plasma Potassium Levels

Dale Dubin in his classic book *Rapid Interpretation of EKG's* compared the T-wave to a tent housing potassium ions. Thus, *hypokalemia* is associated with a *flat or* in extreme cases *inverted T-wave,* which is followed by a U-wave. In contrast, in *hyperkalemia* the P-wave flattens, the QRS-complex widens and the *T-wave becomes peaked.*

of aldosterone secretion is shown by the inability of ACE inhibitor drugs to suppress aldosterone secretion, a feature used in the *captopril test. Glucocorticoid-remediable aldosteronism* (see Biosynthesis of Adrenocorticoids) is classified as primary aldosteronism because it is independent of renin production.

In contrast, *secondary hyperaldosteronism* is renin-dependent. The condition is most often due to *renovascular disease* and rarely to *renin-producing tumors.* Secondary hyperaldosteronism may be the consequence of catecholamine overproduction, such as seen in pheochromocytoma (see also The Actions and Regulation of Catecholamines). *Plasma renin activity is high* and aldosterone secretion is significantly decreased either by ACE inhibitors or by angiotensin II antagonists acting on AT_1 receptors.

Pseudohyperaldosteronism (also known as AME) may be due to congenital defect of type II 11β-hydroxysteroid dehydrogenase, or its inhibition by licorice (see above). This condition has all the features of primary hyperaldosteronism, but aldosterone excretion is not elevated.

Bartter Syndrome Is Characterized by Salt Wasting-Induced Tertiary Hyperaldosteronism Associated with Low or Normal Blood Pressure *Bartter syndrome* comprises a set of autosomal recessive *NaCl-wasting renal disorders* affecting the thick ascending limb of the loop of Henle and/or the distal convoluted tubules. Because this part of the nephron is essential in generating the corticomedullary osmotic gradient, Bartter syndrome typically includes ADH-resistant impairment of renal concentrating ability.

The consequence of salt and volume loss is the activation of a compensatory mechanism: the chronic stimulation of the renin-angiotensin-aldosterone axis, which results in *hyperreninism* with hypertrophy and hyperplasia of the JGA and *hyperaldosteronism* with adrenal cortical hyperplasia. Hyperaldosteronism stimulates sodium reabsorption in the cortical collecting ducts and causes renal potassium wasting, which leads to hypokalemic, hypochloremic metabolic alkalosis.

Bartter syndrome is a reactive hyperreninism that could be classified as a *tertiary hyperaldosteronism* intended to normalize an initially low blood pressure. Thus, unlike secondary and primary hyperaldosteronism, which

BOX 12-8 Mutations Leading to Bartter Syndrome and Its Variants

- *Classic Bartter syndrome* results from defective chloride transport across the basolateral membrane in the distal nephron due to mutations in the chloride channel gene *CLCNKB* (see Fig. 10-6). The condition presents during infancy and childhood with polyuria and growth retardation, which are not accompanied by nephrocalcinosis.
- The *antenatal hypercalciuric variant* (also termed *hyperprostaglandin E syndrome*) results from
    - mutations in the *SLC12A1* gene encoding the *bumetanide-sensitive sodium-potassium-2 chloride cotransporter* (NKCC2) resulting in defective reabsorption of NaCl in the thick ascending limb of the loop of Henle.
    - mutations in the *KCNJ1* gene encoding the luminal *ATP-sensitive inwardly rectifying K channel* (ROMK) disrupt potassium recycling back to the tubule lumen thereby inhibiting the activity of NKCC2 and causing loss of NaCl.

    Antenatal Bartter syndrome is a life-threatening condition beginning in utero, with marked fetal polyuria that leads to *polyhydramnios* and premature delivery. Life-threatening episodes of dehydration and fever occur during the early weeks of life. Antenatal Bartter syndrome is characterized by growth retardation, marked hypercalciuria and, as secondary consequences, nephrocalcinosis and osteopenia.
- The *hypocalciuric-hypomagnesemic variant*, also known as *Gitelman syndrome,* is due to mutations in the *SLC12A3* gene encoding the *thiazide-sensitive sodium-chloride cotransporter*, leading to impaired reabsorption of NaCl in the distal convoluted tubule. Gitelman syndrome is observed in older children and adults presenting with intermittent episodes of muscle weakness and tetany, hypokalemia, and hypomagnesemia.

are hypertensive diseases, hyperaldosteronism in Bartter syndrome is associated with persistently low or normal blood pressure. In contrast with *pseudohypoaldosteronism,* aldosterone is effective in increasing sodium reabsorption. Bartter syndrome can be treated with increased dietary salt intake combined with the ACE inhibitor captopril, the angiotensin II antagonist losartan, or the aldosterone antagonist spironolactone. Three clinical phenotypes of Bartter syndrome, which are due to different mutations, have been distinguished (Box 12-8).

Hypermineralocorticoid States May Arise from Excessive Secretion of DOC   As seen, normal plasma levels of DOC are unable to stimulate the mineralocorticoid receptor because of extensive binding of DOC to plasma CBG. Excessive production of DOC may occur in several conditions:

- Cushing's disease;
- Certain types of CAH:
    - 11β-hydroxylase deficiency (in association with virilization);
    - 17α-hydroxylase deficiency (in association with sexual infantilism).
- Glucocorticoid resistance. In this case, due to mutations of the glucocorticoid receptor, the feedback to ACTH is impaired, which has consequences similar to that of 11β-hydroxylase deficiency (i.e., DOC-mediated hypertension and virilization by adrenal androgens). However, in glucocorticoid resistance these symptoms are milder and usually manifest later in life than in 11β-hydroxylase deficiency.

Hypoaldosteronism Is Associated with Hyperkalemic Acidosis and Hypotension   Primary hypoaldosteronism is most commonly due to *Addison's disease,* which usually involves the autoimmune destruction of the entire adrenal cortex (see Major Pathologic Conditions Involving the CRH-ACTH-Adrenocortical Axis). The hypotension in Addison's disease has multiple causes:

- Volume depletion due to salt loss.
- Decreased epinephrine synthesis due to glucocorticoid deficiency.
- Decreased vascular reactivity due to glucocorticoid deficiency, which involves lower receptor levels of α_1-adrenergic receptors and AT_1 receptors. Thus, although plasma angiotensin II levels are high and contribute to the maintenance of peripheral resistance, the effectiveness of angiotensin II is blunted.
- In the absence of glucocorticoids, the production of the vasodilator bradykinin is increased.

Inborn errors of steroid hormone synthesis may also cause hypoaldosteronism, including type VI congenital adrenal hyperplasia (StAR deficiency), inactivating mutations of P450c21 (21-hydroxylase deficiency), and P450aldo (CMO-I and CMO-II deficiencies).

Pseudohypoaldosteronism Is a Heterogenous Disorder that Mainly Involves the Effectors of the Activated Mineralocorticoid Receptor Rather Than the Receptor Per Se   The term *pseudohypoaldosteronism* implies resistance to mineralocorticoids. In contrast with most hormone resistance syndromes, this condition is usually unrelated to mutations of the hormone receptor: the mineralocorticoid receptor gene (found on chromosome 4q31.1-31.2) is intact in most patients. Most mutations involve the *amiloride-sensitive sodium channel,* which is normally induced and activated by aldosterone in the cortical collecting duct. The primary salt loss is associated with a feedback-related elevation of plasma renin activity, angiotensin II, and aldosterone concentrations, but a key effector (i.e., the sodium channel) is unresponsive, which explains why the sodium loss is accompanied by hyperkalemic acidosis. Therefore, this condition is different from Bartter's syndrome, in which the primary salt loss activates aldosterone-mediated sodium reabsorption, which leads to hypokalemic alkalosis.

Glucocorticoids: The CRH-ACTH-Adrenocortical Axis

The Transport and Metabolism of Glucocorticoids

The Cortisol-Binding Capacity of Plasma CBG Is Approximately 25 μg/dL   The main glucocorticoid hormone, cortisol, circulates in plasma mainly in association with CBG and has a half-life of about 70 to 90 min (see Table 4-2). CBG does not bind certain synthetic glucocorticoids such as dexamethasone; dexamethasone is transported mainly in an albumin-bound form. Plasma CBG levels are increased by thyroid hormones and estrogens, and decreased by glucocorticoids and androgens (see Table 4-3). The concentration of free cortisol is usually in the range of 4 to 10% of its total plasma concentration. Due to the absence of binding proteins in the saliva, the concentration of salivary cortisol is an excellent estimate of *free* cortisol in the plasma and the general ECF. The cortisol-binding capacity of plasma CBG becomes saturated at the concentration of about 25 μg/dL, which coincides with the normal circadian peak plasma levels of cortisol. Any further increase in plasma cortisol concentration dramatically increases the free fraction, which carries the biologic activity and is also cleared faster from the circulation. Normally less than 1% of the secreted cortisol appears in the urine in a chemically unchanged form (*urinary free cortisol*). This fraction sharply increases upon saturation of CBG. For this reason, urinary free cortisol is considered to be one of the most reliable tests in the diagnosis of Cushing's disease (excessive cortisol production).

Cortisol Is Primarily Metabolized by the Liver and the Conjugated Products Are Excreted in the Urine   Similar to the degradation of mineralocorticoids, the quantitatively dominant pathway of cortisol metabolism involves reduction of the A-ring. This irreversible inactivation of cortisol by Δ^4-reductases yields dihydrocortisol, which is converted to *tetrahydrocortisol*. As discussed earlier (see apparent mineralocorticoid excess), cortisol is converted to the inactive *cortisone* by the type II 11β-hydroxysteroid dehydrogenase usually *in the target tissues of mineralocorticoids*. After being transported to the liver, cortisone may be processed by two pathways:

- it may be processed as described for cortisol to yield *tetrahydrocortisone;* or

- it may be converted to cortisol by type I 11β-hydroxysteroid dehydrogenase, and act as a glucocorticoid. This mechanism is taken advantage of in clinical practice when cortisone (an inactive steroid) is used as an orally active glucocorticoid drug.

Tetrahydrocortisol and tetrahydrocorticosterone are conjugated with glucuronic acid. As is the case with DOC, the conjugated compounds are hydrophilic, do not bind with carrier proteins, and are rapidly excreted by renal filtration. *Urinary 17-hydroxycorticosteroids* are 17α,21-dihydroxy-20-one compounds, which include cortisol, cortisone, 11-deoxycortisol, 6β-hydrocortisol and their tetrahydro/conjugated derivatives, which are measured in a single colorimetric assay *(Porter-Silber reaction)*. This classic method (and some related assays such as 17-ketogenic steroids, 17-ketosteroids, see later) have been replaced by more specific hormone measurements. However, these methods are inexpensive, suitable for gross assessment of steroid hormone metabolism and are still used in some countries.

About 10% of cortisol is converted in the liver to 17-ketosteroid derivatives, which are sulfated and excreted with urine. *Urinary 17-ketosteroids,* however, are mainly derived from the degradation of androgens (see Chap. 13).

The Action and Biologic Effects of Glucocorticoids

Most Actions of Cortisol Are Mediated by the Intracellular Glucocorticoid Receptor Via Altering Gene Expression   The main function of glucocorticoids is to aid the adaptation of the body to adverse situations, which requires a coordinated response involving several organs (the stress response of Selye). Accordingly, the glucocorticoid receptor is widely expressed. Because glucocorticoids are relatively lipophilic hormones, they have access to transcellular fluid compartments and penetrate the BBB with ease. As noted earlier, endogenous maternal glucocorticoids have limited access to the fetal compartment because of the placental expression of type II 11β-hydroxysteroid dehydrogenase. Certain synthetic analogs of glucocorticoids such as *dexamethasone* may escape inactivation and gain access to the fetus.

The glucocorticoid receptor is encoded by chromosome 5q31. In addition to its classical mode of action which involves binding as a homodimer to glucocorticoid response elements (GREs) in target gene promoters and subsequent activation or suppression of transcription (see Chap. 5.2), a second mode of action is based on *transcriptional cross-talk* (see also Chap. 5). This transcriptional cross-talk may involve various mechanisms:

- Protein-protein interactions between the activated glucocorticoid receptor and another transcription factor, thereby *regulating the expression of a gene which has a cis-acting element binding only one of them*. Such interaction has been observed between the glucocorticoid receptor and the

AP-1 (c-Fos/c-Jun) transcription factor, which results in a mutual inhibitory effect. Another example of such a cross-talk with the glucocorticoid receptor is *nuclear factor-κB* (NF-κB), an important regulator of several cytokine genes such as *tumor necrosis factor-α* (TNF-α). The ability of NF-κB to bind DNA is inhibited by the activated glucocorticoid receptor. The DNA-binding zinc finger domain of glucocorticoid receptor is necessary for the inhibition of both NF-κB and AP-1. *This mechanism is important in the immunosuppressive and antiinflammatory actions of glucocorticoids.*

• Protein-protein interactions between the activated glucocorticoid receptor and another *activated* transcription factor, thereby *regulating the expression of a gene which has cis-acting elements binding both of them.* In this case, *the glucocorticoid receptor-binding sites are distinct from the classical half-palindromic GRE sequences,* and do not function without the other activated transcription factor. Such a transcriptional cross-talk has been described between glucocorticoid receptors and STAT-5, a prolactin-activated transcription factor. *This mode of interaction restricts gene expression to sites and conditions where both STAT-5 and the glucocorticoid receptor are activated, like the mammary epithelium during lactation.* The Jak–STAT pathway is used by several cytokine receptors including those of the GH/prolactin family, and thus serves as a potential target for cross-talk with glucocorticoid receptors.

The glucocorticoid receptor may be activated in a *ligand-independent* manner. This has been demonstrated in human lung fibroblast and smooth muscle cells upon stimulation by β_2-adrenergic receptor agonists. This mechanism may contribute to the antiasthmatic actions of β_2-adrenergic receptor agonists such as *salbutamol.*

The effects of glucocorticoids can be classified as *direct actions* (e.g., inducing enzymes involved in gluconeogenesis) and *permissive* (indirect) *actions* such as maintaining vascular reactivity to catecholamines and permitting the actions of lipolytic hormones (catecholamines, growth hormone) in adipose tissue.

The best characterized *nongenomic actions* of glucocorticoids are the fast (but transient) feedback inhibition of ACTH secretion which occurs within 10 min of exposure, and the induction of PNMT *activity* in the adrenal medulla.

In spite of the detailed understanding of the molecular mechanisms of glucocorticoid action and the wide array of well-established biologic effects of glucocorticoids, the coupling mechanism between receptor activation and the biologic response is often unknown. The main targets and actions of glucocorticoids are listed in Table 12-9. The table compares and contrasts two disease entities that serve as prototypes of the excess and absence of glucocorticoids:

• *Cushing's syndrome* is a condition of overt glucocorticoid exposure irrespective of the etiology. Cushing's syndrome may be a manifestation of *Cushing's disease,* which is caused by an ACTH-secreting pituitary adenoma

Table 12-9 The Main Targets and Actions of Glucocorticoids, and the Consequences of Cushing's and Addison's Diseases

Target system	Specific target	Physiologic function	Cushing's disease	Addison's disease
Intermediary metabolism	Liver	Increased expression of gluconeogenic enzymes PEPCK, glucose-6-phosphatase and fructose-2,6-bisphosphatase	Increased hepatic glucose output; together with insulin, increased hepatic glycogen stores	Diminished hepatic glucose output and glycogen stores
	Adipose tissue	Permissive for lipolytic signals (catecholamines, GH) leading to elevated plasma FFA to *fuel* gluconeogenesis.	Overall effect (together with insulin): central obesity (truncal obesity, moon facies, and buffalo hump)	Decreased adiposity and decreased lipolysis
	Skeletal muscle	Degradation of fibrillar muscle proteins by activating the ubiquitin pathway thereby providing *substrate* for gluconeogenesis	Muscle weakness and wasting mainly in proximal muscles; increased urinary nitrogen excretion (urea from amino acids)	Muscle weakness, decreased muscle glycogen stores; decreased urinary nitrogen excretion
	Plasma glucose	Maintains plasma glucose during fasting (antihypoglycemic action), increases plasma glucose during stress (hyperglycemic action)	Impaired glucose tolerance, insulin-resistant diabetes mellitus; increased plasma glucose is mainly due to decreased peripheral glucose utilization	Hypoglycemia, increased insulin sensitivity
Calcium homeostasis	Kidney	Decreased reabsorption of calcium	Hypercalciuria without hypercalcemia leading to secondary hyperparathyroidism; retardation of bone growth and bone age by direct action and by decreasing GH; osteoporosis in adults	Retardation of bone growth mainly through decreased GH; hypercalcemia possible
	Bone/cartilage	Inhibition of collagen synthesis and bone deposition		
	GI tract	Inhibition of calcium, magnesium and phosphate absorption by antagonizing calcitriol		
Other endocrine systems	Hypothalamus/pituitary	Decreases endogenous opioid production; decreases gonadotroph responsiveness to GnRH; stimulates GH gene expression by pituitary action; inhibits GH secretion via the hypothalamus	Scanty menses by suppressed gonadotroph sensitivity to GnRH; suppressed GH secretion by hypothalamic action; minimal suppression of the TRH-TSH axis	Scanty menses by upregulated CRH-endogenous opioid pathway-mediated suppression of GnRH; suppressed GH secretion; hypothyroidism (if present) is due to direct autoimmune action
	Pancreas	Inhibits insulin secretion by decreasing the efficacy of cytoplasmic Ca^{2+} on the exocytotic process	*Absolute* hyperinsulinemia with *relative* hypoinsulinemia (lower plasma insulin than expected for the degree of hyperglycemia)	*Absolute* hypoinsulinemia with *relative* hyperinsulinemia
	Adrenal medulla	Increases PNMT expression and activity (adrenaline synthesis)	Increased responses to sympathoadrenal activation	Decreased responses to sympathoadrenal activation
	Carrier proteins (CBG, SHBG, TBG)	Decreases all major hormone-binding proteins	Decrease in total T_4, free T_4 remains normal	
Immune system	Thymus, lymphocytes	Causes age-related involution of the thymus. Induces apoptosis of T lymphocytes; suppresses lymphocyte proliferation, IL-2 production	Immunocompromised state; lymphocytopenia in peripheral blood	Relative lymphocytosis in peripheral blood

Table 12-9 The Main Targets and Actions of Glucocorticoids, and the Consequences of Cushing's and Addison's Diseases

Target system	Specific target	Physiologic function	Cushing's disease	Addison's disease
	Monocytes	Inhibits monocyte proliferation and antigen presentation; decreased production of IL-1, IL-6, and TNF-α	Monocytopenia in peripheral blood	Monocytosis in peripheral blood
	Granulocytes	Demargination of neutrophils by suppressing the expression of adhesion molecules	Peripheral blood: granulocytosis, eosinopenia	Peripheral blood: granulocytopenia, eosinophilia
	Inflammatory response	Inhibition of inflammation by inhibiting PLA$_2$, thereby inhibiting production of leukotrienes and prostaglandin synthesis; suppresses COX-2 expression		
	Erythrocytes (RBCs)	No significant effect	Increased hemoglobin and hematocrit are due to ACTH-mediated overproduction of androgens	Anemia is more pronounced in women, and is due to loss of adrenal androgens; anemia may be related to direct autoimmune targeting of gastric parietal cells
Skin and connective tissue		Antiproliferative for fibroblasts and keratinocytes	Easy bruisability due to dermal atrophy; striae at sites of increased tension, especially sites of adipose tissue accumulation; poor wound healing; hirsutism and acne are due to ACTH-mediated increase of adrenal androgens; hyperpigmentation is a direct effect of ACTH on MC1 receptors	The darkening of the skin is due to ACTH-mediated stimulation of epidermal MC1 receptors; vitiligo may occur due to direct autoimmune destruction of melanocytes in circumscribed areas
Breast	Mammary epithelium	Mandatory requirement for lactation	Cushing's disease may be associated with galactorrhea	Addison's disease is not associated with galactorrhea
Lung	Type II alveolar cell	Stimulation of surfactant production	—	—
Cardiovascular system	Heart Vasculature	Increased contractility Increased vascular reactivity to vasoconstrictors (catecholamines, angiotensin-II)	Hypertension	Low peripheral resistance; hypotension with further postural decrease in blood pressure (orthostatic hypotension); low voltage EKG
Na$^+$, K$^+$, and ECF volume	Kidney	Increased GFR and nonphysiologic actions on mineralocorticoid receptors	Hypokalemic alkalosis, increased ECF volume due to mineralocorticoid activity (increased DOC, saturation of type II 11β-HSD by extreme cortisol)	Hyponatremia, hyperkalemic acidosis, and decreased ECF volume are mainly due to loss of mineralocorticoid activity
	Posterior pituitary	—	—	SIADH mainly via hypovolemia-related baroreceptor mechanism

Table 12-9   (*Continued*)

Target system	Specific target	Physiologic function	Cushing's disease	Addison's disease
Psychiatric parameters of CNS function	Mood	Eucortisolemia maintains emotional balance	Initial, euphoria; long-term, depression	Depression
	Appetite	Increases appetite	Hyperphagia	Decreased appetite in spite of improved taste and smell
	Sleep	Suppression of REM sleep	Sleep disturbances	—
	Memory	Sensitizes hippocampal glutamate receptors, induces atrophy of dendrites	Impaired memory, bilateral hippocampal atrophy	—
Eye		Increasing intraocular pressure	Cataract formation; increased intraocular pressure	Decreased intraocular pressure

ABBREVIATIONS: PEPCK, phosphoenolpyruvate carboxykinase; GH, growth hormone; FFA, free fatty acids; GI, gastrointestinal; GnRH, gonadotropin releasing hormone; TRH, thyrotropin-releasing hormone; TSH, thyroid-stimulating hormone; CRH, corticotropin-releasing hormone; CBG, cortisol-binding globulin; PNMT, phenylethanolamine-N-methyltransferase; SHBG, sex hormone-binding globulin; TBG, thyroxine-binding globulin; IL, interleukin; PLA, phospholipase A; RBC, red blood cell; ACTH, adrenocorticotroph hormone; EKG, electrocardiogram; ECF, extracellular fluid; DOC, deoxycorticosterone; HSD, hydroxysteroid dehydrogenase; SIADH, syndrome of inappropriate antidiuretic hormone secretion; MC, melanocortin; TNF, tumor necrosis factor; T_4, thyroxine; COX, cyclooxygenase; GFR, glomerular filtration rate; REM, rapid eye movement.

(Fig. 12-12). Thus, Chushing's disease includes certain symptoms which are unrelated to glucocorticoid excess, but are due to either the direct effects of ACTH or the ACTH-induced adrenal androgens and mineralocorticoid activities, such as DOC.

• *Addison's disease* is also known as *primary adrenocortical insufficiency*. Most often it is caused by the autoimmune destruction of the cortex. Tuberculosis may destroy both the cortex and the medulla. Adrenocortical insufficiency involves the absence of glucocorticoids, mineralocorticoids, and adrenal androgens, and the effects of the excessive plasma levels of ACTH, which are due to the loss of feedback suppression by cortisol.

The manifestations of Cushing's and Addison's diseases related to endocrine mechanisms other than glucocorticoids are specified in Table 12-9. Most actions of glucocorticoids have already been discussed in earlier chapters.

Cortisol Supports the Increased Energy Requirements During Stress

During stress, adrenaline initially mobilizes glucose by increasing glycogenolysis. However, the hepatic glycogen stores (which may contribute to circulating glucose) are limited and become rapidly depleted. The largest energy store in the body is found in adipose tissue in the form of triglycerides. Catecholamines, glucagon and growth hormone mobilize this energy by activating the hormone-sensitive lipase thereby increasing circulating levels of FFA and glycerol. *A major action of glucocorticoids is to facilitate the action of these lipolytic agents by a permissive action on adipose tissue.*

Peripheral tissues utilize FFA by generating acetyl-coenzyme A in the process of β-oxidation. Acetyl-coenzyme A then enters the Krebs cycle

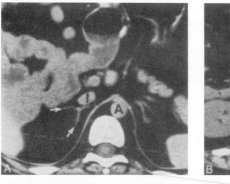
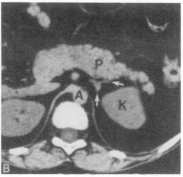
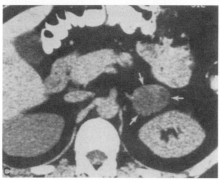
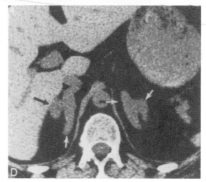

Figure 12-12. Computed tomographic (CT) scan images of the adrenal gland. By convention, the transverse section images are viewed *from below*. Normal conditions are shown in A and B; note that although the right kidney is positioned lower than the left kidney, the adrenal glands are opposite to this arrangement. This is mainly due to the medial (rather than superior) position of the left adrenal relative to the kidney. The adrenals appear as Y-shaped structures. A. The medial limb of the right adrenal gland curves posteriorly; the lateral limb extends horizontally (arrows). Note the position of the aorta (A) and the inferior vena cava (I). B. The left adrenal (arrows) is found medial to the kidney (K), anterolateral to the aorta (A) and posterior to the pancreas (P). C. Adenoma of the left adrenal gland (arrows), which resulted in Cushing's syndrome due to ACTH-independent hypercortisolemia. D. Bilateral adrenal hyperplasia (arrows) in a patient with ectopic Cushing's syndrome having extremely high plasma ACTH. In Cushing's disease due to pituitary adenoma, ACTH is less elevated, and as many as 50% of the patients may present with normal size adrenal glands as assessed by CT scan. (*Sources:* Figs. 98-1, 98-6B, and 98-7B, pp 1711–1730 in Doppman JL: Adrenal imaging, in DeGroot LJ (ed): *Endocrinology,* vol 2. Philadelphia, Saunders, 1995.)

and ultimately yields ATP, which in turn slows down the glycolytic pathway. Thus, *the increased FFA supply inhibits peripheral glucose utilization.* This interplay between FFA and glucose is part of the *glucose-fatty acid cycle,* also known as the *Randle mechanism.* FFA-induced insulin-resistance and the Randle mechanism are the main reasons of hyperglycemia during *chronic* hypercortisolemia in Cushing's disease.

The main *acute* hyperglycemic action of glucocorticoids is due to stimulation of gluconeogenesis. Glucocorticoids support hepatic gluconeogenesis by several mechanisms:

• Cortisol induces the expression of key gluconeogenetic enzymes, especially phosphoenolpyruvate carboxykinase (PEPCK), which is the rate-limiting step of gluconeogenesis.

• Cortisol provides FFA for the liver. It is important to emphasize that acetyl-coenzyme A cannot be converted to pyruvate, and thus will not be available for gluconeogenesis as a substrate. However, utilization of FFA promotes gluconeogenesis by

      • providing ATP as an energy source and as an allosteric regulator of enzyme activities;

      • supplying NADPH and GTP (see Chap. 9).

• Cortisol provides the *substrate* for gluconeogenesis by mobilizing amino acids primarily from the contractile proteins of skeletal muscle. Amino acid mobilization involves the *ubiquitin* mechanism (Box 12-9). Alanine is the main gluconeogenic amino acid. The first step of amino acid utilization for gluconeogenesis is their deamination (usually by a transaminase enzyme). The liberated nitrogen is processed in the hepatic urea cycle and appears in urine. Thus, glucocorticoids increase excretion of urea and

BOX 12-9   Ubiquitin

Ubiquitin is a 76-amino-acid highly conserved polypeptide. Tagging cytoplasmic proteins with a chain of polymerized ubiquitin is utilized as a *degradation signal*. The tagged proteins are recognized by the *26S proteasome*, which consists of a 19S cap complex and a 20S proteasome. The 20S proteasome is a cylindrical particle composed of four stacked rings. The rings form a tunnel in which ubiquitinylated proteins are hydrolyzed. Ubiquitin is recycled in the proteolytic pathway. Proteolysis mediated by the ubiquitin-proteasome pathway has been shown to be involved in a wide variety of biologically important processes, such as metabolism, development, immune response, endocytosis, cell cycle progression, apoptosis, signal transduction, receptor downregulation, transcriptional regulation, and protein quality control. Abnormalities in ubiquitin-mediated processes have been shown to cause pathologic conditions, including malignant transformation.

In contrast with either the lysosomal (e.g., cathepsin D) or the Ca^{2+}-dependent (e.g., m-calpain) processes, the ubiquitin-dependent protein breakdown is ATP-dependent and influenced by nutritional manipulation (fasting and dietary protein deficiency), muscle activity and disuse (denervation atrophy and simulated weightlessness), as well as pathologic conditions (sepsis, cancer, trauma, and acidosis). Glucocorticoids activate the ATP-ubiquitin-dependent proteolytic system in skeletal muscle during fasting. Increased mRNA levels for ubiquitin, the 14-kDa ubiquitin-conjugating enzyme E2 (involved in the ubiquitinylation of protein substrates) and subunits of the 20 S proteasome are present in skeletal muscle upon glucocorticoid exposure. Hyperinsulinemia and hyperaminoacidemia decrease ubiquitin mRNA levels in skeletal muscle.

promote a negative nitrogen balance (protein catabolic state). *In Cushing's disease patients the activation of the ubiquitin mechanism is severely attenuated* in comparison with an acute cortisol challenge. The attenuation is most probably mediated *by the increased plasma levels of insulin,* which result in a decreased rate of muscle wasting. This mechanism explains the decreased contribution of gluconeogenesis to hyperglycemia in Cushing's disease patients.

Cortisol maintains and acutely increases circulating levels of amino acids by mobilizing them from contractile skeletal muscle proteins via the proteasome pathway, and in the case of glutamine, by active synthesis. The catabolism of branched chain amino acids provides the carbon and the nitrogen for glutamine synthesis, a pathway enhanced by the cortisol-induced expression of *glutamine synthetase.* Plasma glutamine is the main fuel of immune cells, the intestinal and renal epithelia. Glutamine is also important as a major precursor of purine nucleotide synthesis, especially in rapidly proliferating cells, such as those involved in immunological responses. Glutamine supports the function of neutrophil granulocytes by serving as a source of NADPH.

Glucocorticoids Support Lipolysis and Cause Obesity: A Paradox Resolved by the Nutritional Status and Interaction with Insulin During fasting or starvation, cortisol becomes a preeminent antihypoglycemic hormone, which *restores* euglycemia. In these hypoglycemic conditions insulin secretion is inhibited and glucocorticoids stimulate lipolysis by a permissive action. This mechanism depletes fat stores.

When cortisol is liberated by stimuli other than hypoglycemia (such as stress or alcohol consumption) or administered exogenously, it causes hyperglycemia which in turn results in elevated insulin secretion. Moreover, cortisol increases appetite, and the resulting food intake contributes to the *combination of hypercortisolemia, hyperglycemia and hyperinsulinemia.* Insulin promotes glucose uptake by adipocytes and inhibits the hormone-sensitive lipase. Thus, in conjunction with hyperphagia, hyperglycemia, and hyperinsulinemia, cortisol achieves shifting glucose to adipocytes and storing the energy as triglycerides. This mechanism promotes obesity. The obesity of Cushing's syndrome displays a characteristic *central distribution of fat,* which includes *moon facies, buffalo hump,* and *truncal obesity* (Fig. 12-13).

These processes and the mutual reliance between glucocorticoids and insulin are dramatically exemplified by the following conditions:

• In the absence of insulin (in type I diabetic patients), the classical image is a severe weight loss, which is in part due to the marked decrease in adiposity (see Fig. 9-2). Cortisol released in type I diabetic patients upon stress (such as infections) will not promote adiposity but causes diabetic ketoacidosis.

• Intensive insulin therapy, which is intended to keep HbA_{1c} levels in the normal range, causes weight gain. In the absence of endogenous

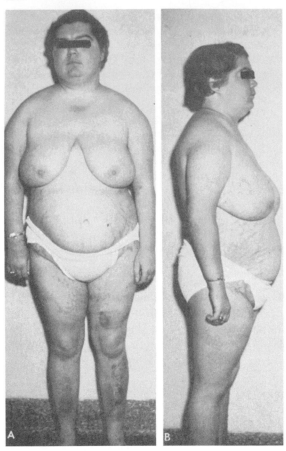

Figure 12-13. Physical appearance of a patient with Cushing's syndrome due to a cortisol-producing adrenocortical adenoma without an androgenic component. Truncal obesity, buffalo hump, moon facies, purple striae, and bruises are evident. Note the absence of hirsutism. (*Source:* Fig. 22-32 in Wilson JD, Foster DW (eds): *Williams' Textbook of Endocrinology,* 7th ed., Philadelphia, Saunders, 1985; originally appeared in Bondy PK, Rosenberg LE: *Metabolic Control and Disease,* 8th ed., Philadelphia, Saunders, 1980.)

cortisol (such as in Addison's disease), insulin will not promote adiposity but causes severe hypoglycemia.

Although hyperglycemia in Cushing's disease results in hyperinsulinemia, the degree of hyperinsulinemia is less than expected from the plasma glucose levels. This phenomenon is referred to as *relative hypoinsulinemia,* which is due to a direct inhibitory action of cortisol on the pancreatic β-cell.

Cortisol Is a Major Physiologic Regulator of Immune Responses and Inflammatory Reactions Glucocorticoids are potent antiinflammatory and immunosuppressive agents. Cortisol achieves these effects by acting on multiple target cell populations and by modulating several cellular functions.

The transcriptional cross-talk that provides the basis of antagonism between glucocorticoids and proinflammatory cytokines was discussed previously. In addition, cortisol suppresses the production of proinflammatory cytokines.

Cortisol *directly* inhibits prostaglandin synthesis by suppressing the transcription of the inducible prostaglandin synthase (cyclooxygenase-2 [COX-2]). A major action of cortisol is the induction of *lipocortins*. Lipocortins belong to the family of *annexins,* which are calcium-dependent phospholipid-binding proteins. *Annexin I* (lipocortin-1), is a 346-amino acid 37-kDa protein, which mediates local antiinflammatory effects of cortisol (Fig. 12-14). Lipocortin-1 exerts its effects in an *unphosphorylated* state; its phosphorylation by PKC (e.g., on activation of IL-1 β receptors) decreases the antiinflammatory effect of cortisol. The mechanism of action of lipocortin-1 includes the following:

- Lipocortin-1 inhibits phospholipase A_2 activity *in the cytoplasmic compartment,* thereby inhibiting the production of all types of arachidonate derivatives (prostaglandins, leukotrienes, lipoxins).
- Lipocortin-1 acts as an *autocrine* inhibitor of neutrophil, eosinophil, and monocyte extravasation process including the adhesion, chemotaxis, and diapedesis in response to stimuli such as IL-8. These effects of glucocorticoids are mimicked by exogenously administered recombinant lipocortin-1 This implies that lipocortin (an essentially cytoplasmic protein which has no signal peptide sequence as a secretory signal) may become secreted (externalized).

Glucocorticoids cause apoptosis in T lymphocytes, suppress IL-2 production, and suppress proliferation of lymphocytes. Glucocorticoids are involved in the physiologic involution of the thymus. Persistent thymus is usually an indication of hypadrenia.

Cushing's and Addison's diseases are characteristically associated with altered immune status and *complete blood count* (CBC). In Addison's disease, lymphocytosis, monocytosis, and eosinophilia are accompanied by granulocytopenia. The opposite is seen in Cushing's disease, stress, and upon exogenous administration of glucocorticoids.

Cortisol is transported in plasma by CBG, a member of the serpine family of proteins. CBG is a substrate of neutrophil elastase: it is cleaved at a single site close to its carboxy terminus, and this reduces its affinity for cortisol resulting in an over 80% release of CBG-bound cortisol. The capillary permeability is increased at sites of inflammation; thus, CBG-bound cortisol is effectively delivered to tissue neutrophils. This mechanism is important in limiting the inflammatory response.

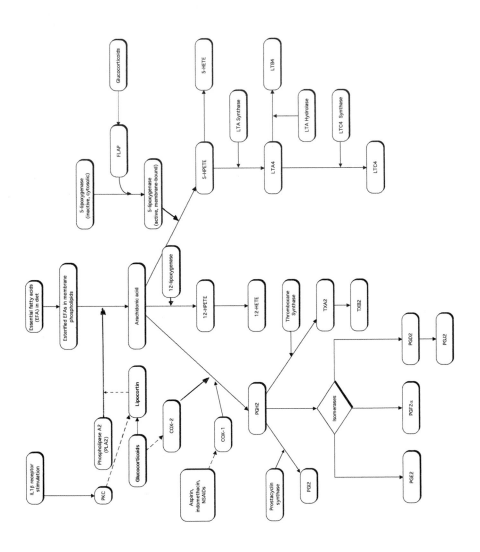

The Lipocortin Mechanism Is Also Involved in Noninflammatory Responses Such as the Rapid Feedback of Cortisol on Corticotropin-Releasing Hormone-Induced Release of ACTH Lipocortin-1 is present in pituitary tissue. A small proportion of lipocortin-1 is attached to the outer surface of the cell membranes by a Ca^{2+}-dependent mechanism. Exposure to glucocorticoids increases the proportion of lipocortin-1 attached to the outer surface of the cells without a change in the total amount of pituitary lipocortin-1. This response develops in parallel with the inhibitory effect of the glucocorticoids on corticotropin-releasing hormone- (CRH-) induced release of ACTH. The acute inhibition of CRH-stimulated release of ACTH by glucocorticoids can be reversed by a monoclonal antilipocortin antibody. The glucocorticoid-induced externalization of lipocortin-1 in the pituitary gland and the resultant inhibition of ACTH release are sensitive to cyclo-heximide but not to actinomycin D, indicating that this glucocorticoid effect does not involve transcriptional regulation. This mechanism is involved in the rapid feedback inhibition of ACTH secretion by cortisol (see details of feedback regulation below).

Cortisol Inhibits the Function of Fibroblasts and Fibroblast-Related Cells Cortisol inhibits the proliferation and collagen synthesis of fibro-blasts, chondroblasts, and osteoblasts. This results in easy bruisability of the skin, poor wound healing, development of *purple striae* at sites of stretching (sites of adipose tissue deposition), decreased rate of bone growth, and deposition in the process of bone remodeling. Because cortisol inhibits renal calcium reabsorption and intestinal absorption of calcium, excess cortisol induces secondary hyperparathyroidism, which results in increased bone resorption. The combination of decreased bone deposition and increased bone resorption explains the often severe degree of osteopo-rosis seen in Cushing's disease patients. The inhibitory effect on bone growth is in part related to suppression of pituitary GH secretion. Even a relatively minor excess in glucocorticoids may cause significant growth retardation and delayed bone age in children.

Cortisol Exerts Direct Effect on CNS Function Cortisol as a lipo-philic hormone penetrates the BBB with ease, and is also filtered by the

---

Figure 12-14. The biosynthesis of eicosanoids and the inhibitory action of glucocorticoids. Cortisol induces the expression of lipocortin-1 (annexin-1). Lipocortin is mobilized (in part externalized) by a nongeomic action of glucocorticoids, thereby inhibiting PLA_2 and decreas-ing the entire arachidonic acid metabolism. Lipocortin is active only when unphosphorylated; phosphorylation of lipocortin by protein kinase C (PKC) antagonizes the nongenomic action of cortisol. Cortisol directly suppresses the COX-2 gene (cyclooxygenase-2); thus, the synthesis of prostaglandin H_2 (PGH_2) derived products becomes significantly inhibited. The effect of glucocorticoids on leukotriene (LT) synthesis is influenced by two factors: inhibition of PLA_2 which decreases the activity of both 12- and 5-lipoxygenase pathways, and induction of FLAP (5-lipoxygenase activating protein) which may counterbalance the decrease in arachidonic acid by increasing the activity of 5-lipoxygenase.

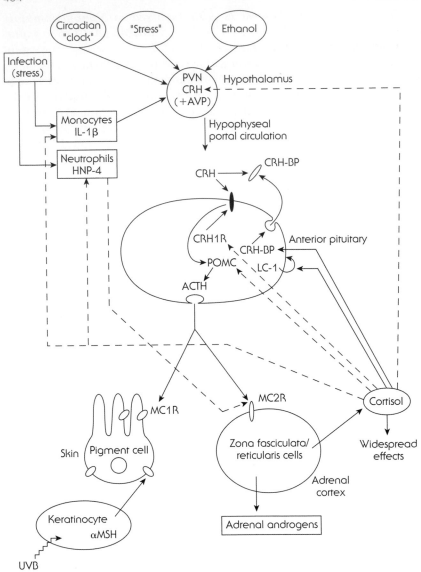

Figure 12-15. Regulation of the CRH-ACTH-adrenocortical axis. Corticotrophin-releasing hormone (CRH) is cosecreted with arginine vasopressin (AVP) from neurons residing in the parvocellular paraventricular nucleus (PVN). CRH activates the CRH1 receptors (CRH1R) of the corticotroph cells in the anterior pituitary gland. Its binding to the receptor can be prevented by CRH-binding protein (CRH-BP). Stimulation of CRH1R induces the expression of POMC (proopiomelanocortin), i.e., the precursor of ACTH (adrenocorticotroph hormone). ACTH normally activates only MC2R (melanocortin 2 receptors) in the adrenal cortex, which results in increased cortisol and androgen secretion. When plasma ACTH is excessive, it may cross react with the MC1Rs of epidermal melanocytes, which are normally stimulated by locally produced α-MSH (melanocyte stimulating hormone). Adrenal androgens do not participate in the feedback regulation of ACTH. The negative feedback by cortisol has a rapid, nongenomic component that acutely regulates the *rate* of ACTH secretion mainly by

choroid plexus. Cortisol levels in the cerebrospinal fluid reflect the concentration of free cortisol in plasma.

Therapeutic doses of exogenous glucocorticoids and overproduction of endogenous cortisol cause memory impairment. Cushing's syndrome is associated with an initially reversible bilateral hippocampal atrophy, which is in part due to a decreased resistance of hippocampal neurons to ischemia, an increased sensitivity to stimulation by glutamate, and an involution of neuronal dendrites. Hippocampal atrophy has been documented in *posttraumatic stress disorders,* such as in combat veterans and victims of child abuse.

Cortisol acts on limbic structures and has a major impact on mood. Normal levels of plasma cortisol are required for normal mood. Both Addison's and Cushing's disease patients are depressed. Cushing's disease patients may have sudden emotional outbursts. Therapeutic doses of glucocorticoids may induce initial euphoria, which is typically followed by depression. A confounding factor of mood disorder is the sleep disturbance, which is related to suppression of REM sleep by excessive glucocorticoids.

Glucocorticoids stimulate appetite. Hyperphagia is characteristic in Cushing's syndrome and is a major contributor to the development of obesity (see Chap. 15).

The Regulation of the Zonae Fasciculata and Reticularis

Glucocorticoid Secretion Is Stimulated by Exogenous and Endogenous Stress Signals and the Plasma Levels of Cortisol Are Stabilized by a Negative Feedback Regulatory System The secretion of cortisol is regulated by the *corticotropin-releasing hormone* (CRH)–ACTH axis (Fig. 12-15). This axis has to fulfill a dual role:

- It must be activated by different stimuli, which all represent potential harm to the organism and a need for an adaptational response (stress). Cortisol is vitally important in the mobilization of energy resources required for the adaptational response.
- Because most actions of cortisol involve transcriptional regulation (i.e., the biologic responses are slow), *long-term normocortisolemia is required* for maintaining an acute responsiveness to other stress hormones, such as adrenaline (permissive action). The stress-induced release of corti-

---

Figure 12-15. (*Continued*) mobilizing lipocortin (LC-1). Via a slower, genomic action, cortisol inhibits expression of CRH1R and POMC, and induces the expression of CRH-BP, which all contribute to the direct pituitary negative feedback by cortisol. Cortisol also inhibits CRH expression in the hypothalamic PVN. These genomic actions are the main regulators of the *long-term absolute concentrations* of the hormones in the axis. Note that infections (a special type of stress) active the CRH-ACTH axis mainly via IL-1β. Because cortisol inhibits the synthesis of several cytokines (including IL-1β), this operates as a separate feedback loop. Neutrophils secrete corticostatin (HNP-4), which functions as a competitive antagonist of ACTH on MC2R.

sol functions within the framework of a negative feedback regulatory system.

The spontaneous activity as well as the stress sensitivity of the CRH–ACTH–cortisol axis follows a circadian rhythm with highest cortisol levels and responsiveness in the early morning (6:00 to 8:00 A.M.) and lowest levels in late afternoon/evening (6:00 to 10:00 P.M.). This circadian rhythm is organized by the suprachiasmatic nucleus via its action on the CRH neurons in the paraventricular nucleus, and is entrained by environmental cues such as light and the timing of meals (see Chap. 14). An early manifestation of Cushing's disease is the loss of the circadian rhythm in plasma cortisol (i.e., plasma cortisol does not decrease by the afternoon).

Stressful stimuli typically activate the CRH-ACTH-cortisol axis by increasing the secretion of CRH. Stressful stimuli include:

- Emotional stress: situations associated with the subjective sensation of *anxiety*.
- Hypoxia, hypercapnia.
- Hypoglycemia.
- Decreased blood pressure and depletion of ECF volume.
- Infections leading to increased production of IL-1β.
- Changes in environmental temperature (either cold or hot); fever.
- Consumption of ethanol.

We shall now turn our attention to the components of the regulatory system: CRH, ACTH, and related peptides.

CRH Generates an Integrated Stress Response, Which Includes Stress-Induced ACTH Release as Well as Complimentary Stress-Related Endocrine, Autonomic, and Behavioral Responses CRH is a 41-amino acid polypeptide hormone structurally related to frogskin *sauvagine*, fish *urotensin I*, and the CRH-like mammalian neuropeptide *urocortin*. CRH is widely expressed in the CNS, especially in the cortex, limbic system, hypothalamus, and central arousal-sympathetic system in the brainstem and spinal cord. Urocortin is primarily expressed in the Edinger-Westphal nucleus in the midbrain and in the superior olive; its involvement in stress responses is unlikely.

The CRH neurons involved in the regulation of pituitary ACTH secretion are located in the parvocellular portion of the hypothalamic paraventricular nucleus, and project to the median eminence. These are the neurons, whose CRH production is suppressed by glucocorticoids as a part of the negative feedback regulation of cortisol secretion. These hypophysiotrophic CRH neurons coexpress ADH, which also stimulates ACTH secretion and potentiates the action of CRH (see also Chap. 10). ACTH is derived from by proteolytic processing of the prohormone proopiomelanocortin (POMC). The relationship between CRH and POMC-positive cells extends beyond the regulation of pituitary ACTH secretion: CRH neurons regulate POMC positive neurons within the hypothalamus, and CRH stimulates ACTH-production by lymphocytes.

Two CRH-receptors have been discovered: *CRH1R* and *CRH2R*, both of which are G-protein-coupled heptahelical receptors. It appears that CRH is not a physiologic ligand of CRH2R. Urocortin has equally high affinity to both CRH1R and CRH2R. CRH stimulates the CRH1R of adenohypophyseal corticotroph cells (a periodic acid Schiff [PAS]-positive subset of pituitary basophils), thereby increasing the activity of adenylyl cyclase and the synthesis and the release of ACTH. This effect of CRH can be antagonized with the CRH analog *astressin*. CRH1R is a target of negative feedback by cortisol: the expression of CRH1R mRNA is suppressed by glucocorticoids in corticoptroph cells. In mice lacking CRH1R, the stress-induced release of adrenocorticotropic hormone (ACTH) is attenuated and the *medulla* of the adrenal gland is atrophied. The latter finding reflects the involvement of *CRH in the regulation of preganglionic sympathetic outflow* in response to stress. This mechanism involves CRH-stimulated activity of oxytocin neurons that form a descending tract from the hypothalamus to the intermediolateral column of the spinal cord.

CRH is released upon stress also at sites not involved in the regulation of ACTH secretion. CRH1R is highly expressed in the neocortex, hippocampus, amygdala and cerebellum. Some of the extrahypophysiotropic CRH sites are responsible for mediating the stress-related psychological sensation of anxiety. Overproduction of CRH and increased levels of CRH in the CSF have been demonstrated in *major depression* and other affective disorders such as *anorexia nervosa*. Experiments with CRH1R-knockout mice indicate the essential role of CRH in anxiety: these knockout mice display increased level of exploratory behavior in a strange (i.e., potentially dangerous) environment. The increased CRH neuronal activity is believed to mediate certain behavioral symptoms of depression such as *sleep and appetite disturbances* (see also in Chaps 14 and 15) and decreased libido. The activity of CRH neuronal systems can be used as a state marker for depression because the CRH–ACTH–cortisol axis hyperactivity normalizes upon successful antidepressant treatment.

Additional endocrine effects of CRH include the stress-related inhibition of GnRH-secretion via POMC-positive interneurons in the medial basal hypothalamus. These POMC neurons secrete the endogenous opioid β-endorphin. This mechanism explains the well-established antigonadotroph actions of stress and morphine, and is apparently involved in the amenorrhea or the male hypogonadism of highly trained runners and ballet dancers.

CRH is also produced outside the CNS. At certain sites CRH acts as a proinflammatory signal and stimulates the synthesis of prostaglandins. This action via CRH1 receptors is involved in *the initiation of parturition by placentally produced CRH* (see Chap. 13). Stimulation of CRH2R mainly by urocortin results in vasodilatation and decreased edema formation in injured tissues.

CRH and urocortin are among the few peptide hormones, which have a binding protein (*CRH-BP*). Plasma CRH-BP is secreted mainly by the liver and the placenta. Membrane-associated CRH-BP is expressed near certain target cells of CRH such as neurons and astrocytes in the cerebral cortex and pituitary corticotrophs. *CRH-BP* is structurally unrelated to the CRH receptors. Its function is to prevent the biologic action of CRH and facilitate its elimination ("CRH sink").

ACTH, α-Melanocyte-Stimulating Hormone (α-MSH), Endogenous Opioid Peptides, and β-Lipotropin Are Derived by the Cell Type-Specific Proteolytic Cleavage of POMC   POMC is a large (26-kDa) glycoprotein that serves as a precursor for several biologically active peptides (Fig. 12-16). In the corticotroph cells of the anterior pituitary gland, *proprotein convertase 3* (PC3) processes POMC into ACTH and the weak lipolytic hormone β-lipotropin (β-LPH). The production of α-MSH and β-endorphin requires the processing of POMC by both PC2 and PC3. The intermediate lobe of adult humans is rudimentary and, unlike in rodents, does not produce appreciable amounts of α-MSH. However, α-MSH is produced by:

- the human intermediate lobe during fetal life, and might recruit PRL-producing cells from the somatotrophs;
- keratinocytes of the skin in response to ultraviolet B (UVB) irradiation, and stimulates the synthesis of *eumelanin* by melanocytes (Box 12-10);
- monocytes, for which α-MSH is an autocrine/paracrine anti-inflammatory agent;
- certain POMC-expressing neurons, such as those involved in leptin-mediated appetite suppression or those involved in decreasing body temperature.

According to chromatographic analysis, authentic α-MSH of extrahypophyseal origin is present in human plasma. The N-terminal 13 amino acids of ACTH are identical to α-MSH. As a consequence, ACTH cross-reacts with the receptors of α-MSH (see below), and states of ACTH hypersecretion such as Addison's disease are associated hyperpigmentation of the skin and sometimes mucosal surfaces such as the buccal mucosa and the gingiva.

ACTH, a 39-amino-acid peptide, is the most important secretory product of the pituitary corticotrophs. The full biologic activity of ACTH is carried by its N-terminal 24 amino acids. ACTH circulates in plasma in an unbound form with a half-life of about 7 to 12 min. ACTH is unstable in blood and avidly binds to glass surfaces; for measurement of circulating ACTH, blood must be collected in chilled plastic tubes containing the calcium chelator ethylenediaminetetraacetic acid (EDTA) and the protease inhibitor aprotinin.

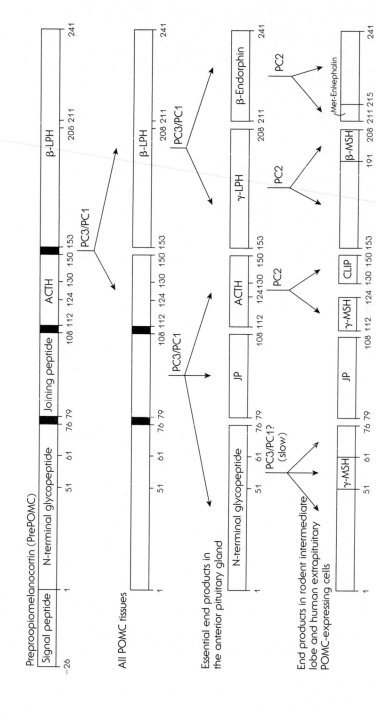

Figure 12-16. Schematic representation of preproopiomelanocortin (prePOMC), and its processing in various tissues. PC, Proprotein convertase; JP, joining peptide; ACTH, adrenocorticotroph hormone; LPH, lipotrop hormone (lipotropin); MSH, melanocyte-stimulating hormone; CLIP, corticotropin-like intermediate lobe peptide.

439

BOX 12-10   Skin Pigmentation

Two types of melanin pigment are present in human skin: the brown-to-black *eumelanins* and the yellow-to-reddish-brown *pheomelanins*, both of which are heterogenous polymer molecules. Individuals with red hair have a predominance of pheomelanin in their hair and skin, and a reduced ability to produce eumelanin, which explains why they fail to tan and are at risk for ultraviolet radiation-induced cutaneous malignancies. Eumelanin protects the skin from the damaging effects of ultraviolet radiation. Eumelanin and its precursor, *5,6-dihydroxyindole,* possess a potent photoprotective property. Pheomelanin and its precursor, *5-S-cysteinyldopa,* are complexed with Fe^{3+} and produce free radicals upon exposure to ultraviolet radiation, thereby promoting *cutaneous photoaging*, which includes lipid peroxidation, DNA damage, and the liberation of matrix metalloproteinases with consequent connective tissue damage. The switch from one type of melanin to the other is regulated by the levels of the copper enzyme *tyrosinase* (which produces L-DOPA from tyrosine) and thiols such as cysteine and glutathione. The relative proportions of pheomelanin and eumelanin are regulated by α-MSH, which is secreted mainly by keratinocytes upon exposure to ultraviolet radiation. It acts via the MC1R on melanocytes to increase the expression of tyrosinase and the synthesis of eumelanin. *The MC1R is an allelic protein: the sequence variant in individuals with red hair and/or fair skin has a limited ability to promote eumelanin synthesis.* In mice, the agouti protein antagonizes the receptor binding of α-MSH, thereby promoting the production of pheomelanin leading to a yellow coat color. Antagonism of MSH on MC4R in the brain by *agouti* or the protein encoded by *agouti-related transcript* (ART) increases food intake (see Chap. 15). In disease states associated with high levels of circulating ACTH, ACTH may promote the production of eumelanin by cross-reacting with the MC1R. This mechanism is also influenced by the allelic type of the MC1R.

ACTH secretion displays a pulsatile pattern, which is mainly driven by the pulses of CRH released from the median eminence. ACTH gene expression, synthesis, and secretion are stimulated by CRH, ADH and, under certain circumstances, cholecystokinin (CCK). ACTH secretion is suppressed by glucocorticoids (mainly cortisol) and by increased expression of CRH-BP by corticotroph cells. The feedback by glucocorticoids therefore includes both hypothalamic and direct pituitary actions. The feedback follows a particular timecourse: the prompt inhibition of ACTH secretion is probably a nongenomic, membrane receptor-mediated effect on hypothalamic CRH neurons followed by another nongenomic action: cortisol-induced lipocortin-externalization in pituitary corticotrophs. The slowest

Table 12-10 Melanocortin Receptors

Receptor	Ligands	Distribution	Function	Natural receptor antagonist
MC1-R (α-MSH-R) encoded by the "extension" locus	α-MSH = ACTH > β-MSH > γ-MSH (γ-MSH is not a physiological ligand)	Melanocytes, monocytes, neutrophil granulocytes	Stimulation of melanocyte proliferation and synthesis of eumelanin. Affinity for MC1-R and biological activity of ligands correlate; antiinflammatory	Agouti (expressed in skin, hair follicle)
MC2-R (ACTH-R)	ACTH only	Adrenal cortex: fetal zone; Z. fasciculata and reticularis of the definitive zone; zona glomerulosa: transient effect; adipocytes	Stimulation of glucocorticoid and adrenal androgen secretion; lipolytic	Agouti inactive Corticostatin (defensin)
MC3-R	γ-MSH > α-MSH	CNS, heart	Promotion of hypotension, bradycardia, hypothermia	?
MC4-R	β-MSH > α-MSH > ACTH (1–39) > γ1-MSH > γ2-MSH	CNS	Tonic inhibition of feeding behavior	Agouti, ART (agouti-related transcript)
MC5-R	α-MSH > γ-MSH	Adipocytes, adrenal gland, leukocytes, gonads, CNS, pituitary	Lipolysis	Agouti inactive

feedback response is the suppression of gene expression of both CRH and POMC, and the increased expression of CRH-BP.

The ACTH receptor belongs to the family of melanocortin receptors (Table 12-10), all of which are G-protein-coupled heptahelical membrane receptors. As discussed, ACTH stimulates adrenocortical steroidogenesis and is important in maintaining normal tissue mass of the adrenal cortex (growth factor function). Upon treatment with exogenous glucocorticoids (as short a duration as a few days), the zonae fasciculata and reticularis of the adrenal cortex atrophy because of the suppressed plasma levels of ACTH. *It is imperative to gradually taper the dose of exogenous glucocorticoids.* Abrupt discontinuation of glucocorticoids would lead to a sudden rise of ACTH; however, ACTH would not have the appropriate tissue mass to act on, and the patient could face a life-threatening Addisonian crisis. We have already seen the consequence of *chronically* elevated plasma ACTH on adrenocortical mass in CAH.

The Activity of CRH-ACTH-Cortisol Axis Is Integrated with Immunoregulation by Multiple Mechanisms of Action   As discussed, cortisol is a major antiinflammatory hormone, which inhibits the synthesis as well as the action of several cytokines, including IL-1β, an endogenous pyrogen. IL-1β (which is produced in response to endotoxin) is a potent stimulator of CRH secretion. Thus, infections may provoke an inflammatory reaction as well as activate the CRH-ACTH-cortisol axis. The latter supports the fight against infection by mobilizing energy resources including glutamine (an important fuel for immune cells), and limits the inflammatory response, which in part serves as a negative feedback loop of glucocorticoid secretion.

The effect of ACTH is functionally antagonized by a group of conserved 29-35 amino acid cationic peptides known as *corticostatins* (a subgroup of the family of *defensins*). These peptides are produced either by epithelia or by neutrophils in response to infections, and they exert direct antimicrobial and antiviral actions. Especially one of the corticostatins, *human neutrophil peptide-4* (HNP-4) inhibits cortisol secretion antagonizing ACTH mainly by directly competing with the ACTH[14-18] sequence for binding to the MC2 receptor.

Developmental Aspects of Adrenocortical Function

The Fetal Zone of the Adrenal Cortex Produces DHEA   The adrenal gland is a source of weak androgens in both sexes during fetal life and after adrenarche. In contrast, between the ages of 6 months and about 6 to 8 years, the adrenal cortex produces only minute quantities of androgens.

As discussed earlier, the fetal zone does not express 3β-hydroxysteroid dehydrogenase/isomerase (3βHSD/ISOM); thus the Δ^5 pathway is the only steroidogenic pathway in this tissue. The CYP17 gene encoding P450c17 is expressed in the cells of the fetal zone. Both catalytic activities of p450c17 (17α-hydroxylase and 17,20-lyase) are high in this tissue, leading to the production of dehydroepiandrosterone (DHEA) and its sulfated form (DHEAS). Most of the sulfation of DHEA occurs in the fetal liver. The fetal production of DHEAS is essential for providing precursors for estrogen synthesis by the placenta (see Chap. 13, Fig. 13-24). The placenta expresses neither 3βHSD/ISOM nor P450c17. Thus, it can synthesize progesterone from LDL-derived cholesterol, but can synthesize estriol *only* by processing fetally produced DHEAS.

Adrenarche Is Due to the Increased 17,20-Lyase Activity of P450c17
With the involution of the fetal zone of the adrenal cortex, circulating levels of DHEA and DHEAS decrease. Although the zona fasciculata (and the zona reticularis when it develops) of the definitive zone expresses P450c17, the enzyme displays very little 17,20-lyase activity. Thus, only minimal adrenal androgen production occurs. *Adrenarche* is a developmental event characterized by an increased adrenal production of DHEA and androstenedione without a concomitant increase either in cortisol or in ACTH secretion. Adrenarche occurs at the age of 6 to 7 years in girls and 7 to 8 years in boys. Peak levels of DHEA and DHEAS are attained in late

puberty/young adulthood; thereafter plasma concentrations of these hormones continuously decrease with age (see Fig. 13-52). The decrease in DHEA has been implicated as a causative factor in aging. Exogenous DHEA has been demonstrated to exert some beneficial antiaging effects unrelated to sex steroid actions and unusual for a steroid hormone, such as improved glucose tolerance and enhanced resistance against infections.

Adrenarche involves an upregulation of the 17,20-lyase activity of P450c17. To catalyze 17α-hydroxylase and 17,20-lyase reactions, P450c17 must receive reducing equivalents from electron donors (redox partners). Increasing the molar ratio of the redox partner *P450 oxidoreductase* to P450c17 *increases the ratio of 17,20-lyase to 17α-hydroxylase activity*. Phosphorylation of serine and threonine residues of P450c17 selectively increases its 17,20-lyase activity because of an increase in the affinity of P450c17 for redox partners. The signal leading to the developmental activation of the 17,20-lyase activity is currently unknown. In addition to the mandatory presence of ACTH, a distinct (yet uncharacterized) pituitary hormone termed cortical androgen-stimulating hormone (CASH) and stimulation of type I IGF-1 receptors have been implicated in the process.

Major Pathologic Conditions Involving the CRH-ACTH-Adrenocortical Axis

The main pathologic conditions of the zona fasciculata/reticularis function can be classified as syndromes of hypofunction, hyperfunction, and dysfunction. As described, the prototypes of deranged adrenocortical function are Addison's and Cushing's diseases and the various forms of congenital adrenal hyperplasia. Adrenocortical dysfunctions due to the overproduction or the absence of ACTH are referred to as secondary; those related to innate derangements of adrenal function are referred to as primary.

- Adrenal insufficiency is categorized as follows:
  - *Primary* adrenal insufficiency is characterized by low levels of plasma cortisol and supranormal plasma ACTH. Addison's disease, which is usually due to the autoimmune destruction of the entire adrenal cortex is a *chronic* primary adrenal insufficiency. A major target of the autoimmune reaction is the P450c21 enzyme, an adrenal-specific antigen expressed by all layers of the cortex. Thus, primary adrenal insufficiency includes decreased levels of plasma aldosterone, supranormal plasma renin activity, and increased concentrations of angiotensin II. Autoimmune Addison's disease may be the manifestation of *Schmidt's syndrome* (see Chap. 11). Adrenal insufficiency secondary to adrenal metastases of various tumors (such as bronchial, mammary, renal and gastrointestinal cancers) also develops slowly and gradually, and manifests clinically only when about 90% of the adrenal cortex is destroyed. In contrast, acute destruction of the adrenal glands, such as seen in *Waterhouse-*

Friderichsen syndrome (usually due to meningococcal sepsis) presents with a life-threatening Addisonian crisis.

• *Secondary* adrenal insufficiency is due to a diminished secretion of ACTH. This condition is seen in craniopharyngioma, pituitary infarction, or pituitary apoplexy. Unlike primary adrenal insufficiency, this condition spares the mineralocorticoid function of the adrenal cortex.

• A common feature of adrenal hyperfunction (Cushing's *syndrome*) is an increased urinary excretion of free cortisol. Adrenal hyperfunction is categorized as follows:

• *Primary* adrenal hyperfunction is an ACTH-independent hypersecretion of glucocorticoid(s) leading to *suppressed* plasma levels of ACTH. This condition may be due to tumors and nodular hyperplasia of the adrenal cortex. Nodular hyperplasia of the cortex may be a manifestation of McCune-Albright syndrome (see Chap. 8). Iatrogenic Cushing's syndrome (which is due to high dose glucocorticoid therapy) may be viewed as a subset of primary "adrenal" hyperfunction.

• *Secondary* adrenal hyperfunction is an ACTH-driven hypersecretion of glucocorticoid(s), which may cause bilateral symmetrical adrenal hyperplasia (Fig. 12-12). If the cause of ACTH hypersecretion is a pituitary tumor, the condition is termed Cushing's *disease*. In *ectopic Cushing's syndrome* the source of ACTH is extrahypophyseal, usually a small cell bronchial cancer or a carcinoid tumor. Note that in ectopic Cushing's syndrome several classical manifestations of Cushing's disease (see Table 12-9) may be missing: these are often highly malignant tumors, which are rapidly fatal and do not allow time for the gradual development of the classical symptoms. In addition, increased production of TNF-α effectively antagonizes the hyperphagic action of cortisol in these patients, thereby preventing the development of central obesity.

Similar to the differential diagnosis of primary versus secondary hypothyroidism, the initial evaluation relies on the association of laboratory parameters connected by feedback regulation. The most relevant laboratory normal values are shown in Table 12-11.

A major diagnostic problem is related to the pulsatile nature of ACTH secretion: ACTH concentration in a randomly collected blood sample may not be informative. This may necessitate the use of *provocation* and *suppression tests* in the evaluation of the ACTH-adrenocortical axis. These tests include:

• Acute stimulation of pituitary ACTH secretion with synthetic CRH may distinguish hypothalamic versus pituitary causes of decreased ACTH reserve. The CRH test is also used in the differential diagnosis of Cushing's syndrome.

• A normal cortisol response to acute stimulation by ACTH validates the presence of appropriate adrenocortical tissue mass and ACTH sensitivity.

Table 12-11   Normal Laboratory Values Used In the Evaluation of the ACTH-Adrenocortical Axis

Compound	Normal range
Plasma ACTH	08:00 h (a.m.): 10–120 pg/mL
	16:00–20:00 h (p.m.): <10 pg/mL
Plasma cortisol (total)	08:00 h (a.m.): 5–23 μg/dL
(Compound F)	16:00 h (p.m.): 3–16 μg/dL
	20:00 h (p.m.): ≤50% of the a.m. value
Urinary-free cortisol	20–90 μg/24 h
Serum DHEA	After 6 months of age, before adrenarche: 18–130 ng/dL (mean: ≈30 ng/dL)
	After adrenarche, before puberty: 20–345 ng/dL (mean: ≈100–150 ng/dL)
	Young adult: Male: 180–1250 ng/dL, Female: 130–980 ng/dL
Serum	Prepubertal: 8–50 ng/dL
androstenedione	Adult male: 75–205 ng/dL; female: 85–275 ng/dL
11-deoxycortisol	08:00 h: 12–158 ng/dL
(Compound S)	
17-hydroxy-	Prepubertal: 3–90 ng/dL
progesterone	Adult male: 27–199 ng/dL
	Adult female, follicular phase: 15–70 ng/dL; luteal phase: 35–290 ng/dL; pregnancy: 200–1200 ng/dL

- Tests of ACTH reserve:
    - The *overnight metyrapone test* relies on the drug-induced inhibition P450c11, which simulates 11-hydroxylase deficiency in an acute setting. The inhibition of cortisol synthesis increases ACTH secretion, which in turn results in an increased adrenal secretion of 17-OH-progesterone and (mainly) 11-deoxycortisol. In a patient who responds to exogenous ACTH with normal cortisol secretion, a subnormal response to metyrapone indicates diminished ACTH reserve, i.e., secondary adrenocortical insufficiency.
    - Insulin-induced hypoglycemia is an alternative to the metyrapone test in the assessment of pituitary ACTH reserve. This test is suitable for the simultaneous evaluation of GH in cases of suspected panhypopituitarism.
- *Dexamethasone suppression tests* are usually used in the differential diagnosis of Cushing's syndrome of various etiologies. The various versions of this test rely on the different sensitivity of pituitary tumors and ectopic ACTH-production to the feedback action of glucocorticoids. As a rule of thumb, ACTH and thus cortisol secretion are not suppressed even by the high-dose dexamethasone test if ectopic ACTH-producing tumor is the source of ACTH. In Cushing's disease, the high-dose dexamethasone test is expected to suppress ACTH and cortisol secretion. However, it has been discovered that ACTH-producing pituitary adenomas sometimes harbor somatic mutations of the glucocorticoid receptor, which makes their ACTH secretion less suppressible by dexamethasone than that of normal corticotroph cells. In such conditions, sampling of the inferior petrosal sinus (by catheterization via the internal jugular vein) for assessment of pituitary ACTH secretion may be necessary.

It is important to remember that laboratory results must be interpreted within the framework of the clinical presentation of the disease. Diagnostic procedures are also aided by radiologic imaging studies, such as computed tomography and MRI of the adrenal glands and the pituitary, and ^{111}In-labeled octreotide scintigraphy for the localization of ectopic sources of ACTH.

The clinical presentation is not simply related to an excessive or diminished glucocorticoid activity, but may also be due to direct action of ACTH (pigmentation), and alterations in mineralocorticoid and androgenic activities. Stimulation of mineralocorticoid receptors may modify plasma renin activity, and increased androgen production may interfere with the regulation of gonadotroph function.

Nelson's syndrome is an important disease entity related to Cushing's disease. Cushing's disease is treated by the removal of the pituitary adenoma. The removal of the tumor may be incomplete, which leads to regrowth of the tumor, and may ultimately necessitate adrenalectomy. The adrenalectomized patient receives hormone replacement therapy to achieve a eucorticoid state which, however, is inappropriate for suppressing the function of the adenoma cells. Due to the somatic mutation of glucocorticoid receptor in the monoclonal adenoma cell population, supranormal doses of glucocorticoids would be required to suppress the ACTH secretion and the proliferation of these cells. Thus, the adenoma usually grows rapidly and causes excessive hyperpigmentation of the skin and the oral mucosa. More importantly, the growing adenoma may cause defects due to its local expansion, such as visual field defects, invasion of the cavernous sinus leading to extraocular muscle palsies, and severe headaches. The enlargement of tumor may result in a life-threatening apoplexy.

Adrenocortical tumors may secrete either "normal" or abnormal steroid hormones. Unilateral cortisol-secreting adenomas cause suppressed plasma ACTH and atrophy of *normal* zona fasciculata and reticularis cells in both glands. Abnormal hormones may include various androgens and estrogens leading to virilization and feminization, respectively. Selective hypersecretion of these sex steroids does not directly influence pituitary ACTH production.

There are certain adrenocortical diseases that cannot be simply classified as hypo- or hyperfunctional syndromes. These include certain compensated states of congenital adrenal hyperplasia and generalized glucocorticoid resistance.

- In the *nonclassic form of P450c21 deficiency,* normal levels of plasma cortisol are achieved at the expense of hypersecretion of ACTH, bilateral adrenal hyperplasia, and excessive adrenal androgen production.
- *Partial defects of P450c11* are compensated: normal cortisol is attained at the expense of ACTH-driven hypersecretion of DOC (leading to excess mineralocorticoid action) and androgens (leading to virilization).

- Decreased affinity of the glucocorticoid receptor results in a *compensated generalized glucocorticoid resistance*. In this case, the mutant receptor is less able to exert any biologic action, including the negative feedback regulation of ACTH. Thus, ACTH increases and bilateral adrenal hyperplasia develops, which results in excessive cortisol production. However, in spite of a Cushing's disease-like arrangement, no biologic manifestations of glucocorticoid excess are present. In contrast, the high levels of cortisol overwhelm the type II 11β-HSD and produce apparent mineralocorticoid excess. In addition, the overstimulated cortex produces supranormal quantities of androgens (just like in Cushing's disease), which may result in varying degrees of virilization and/or gonadal dysfunction.

13

REPRODUCTIVE ENDOCRINOLOGY

INTRODUCTION

Phylogeny is the evolutionary process of speciation, i.e., the development of new species. A *species* is defined as the population of individuals capable of producing fertile offspring. These definitions mean that new species arise and become established when the reproductive function of a population diverges from its ancestors. Because this precludes exchange of genetic material between the two populations, additional (nonreproductive) genetic and biologic differences may arise. However, due to the very nature of speciation, the least conserved of all biologic functions is reproduction.

This book is primarily focused on *human* endocrine physiology. This chapter is no exception. However, like most life sciences, endocrine research heavily relies on experimental animal models. Quite understandably, the clinical applicability of animal research in the field of reproductive endocrinology is far more restricted than in any other area of endocrinology. For this reason, we must frequently rely on human disease entities for explaining the normal regulatory processes. In spite of major advances in our understanding of human reproductive endocrinology, the explanation of several physiologic processes remains circumstantial at best.

Reproductive endocrinology involves the most intricate and complex regulatory system. We first discuss the biosynthetic pathways of sexual steroids in both sexes. This topic will be followed by the reproductive endocrinology of the adult male. The next subject, the adult female, has various reproductive states: menstrual cycle, pregnancy, and lactation. Finally, we discuss and compare the ontogeny of reproductive endocrine function in males and females: sexual differentiation, puberty, and menopause. Because of the complexity and amount of information related to reproductive function, the learning objectives are listed separately for each major area.

THE BIOSYNTHESIS, MECHANISM OF ACTION, AND METABOLISM OF SEXUAL STEROIDS

OBJECTIVES

1. Review the biosynthesis of adrenocortical steroids (see Chap. 12) and steroid hormone receptors (see Chap. 5).
2. Identify the cells involved in the gonadal biosynthesis of sexual steroids. Discuss the interplay between *granulosa* and *theca interna* cells in steroidogenesis before and after luteinization.
3. Describe the roles and cellular targets of *gonadotropins* as the main regulators of gonadal steroidogenesis. Compare and contrast the roles of *luteinizing hormone* (LH) and *follicle-stimulating hormone* (FSH) in males versus females in steroidogenesis and gametogenesis.
4. Discuss the contribution of peripheral (extragonadal) conversion in the biosynthesis of sexual steroids: identify the enzymes, their isoforms, sites of expression, tissue-specific regulation, and their roles in local versus systemic action.
5. Discuss the actions of *testosterone* in males without peripheral conversion and its actions after being converted either into *dihydrotestosterone* or into *estradiol* (E_2). Identify the laboratory parameter most closely related to the activity of *5α-reductase* and *hirsutism* in females.
6. Discuss the molecular relationship between *sex hormone-binding globulin* (SHBG) and *androgen-binding protein* (ABP). Describe the mechanism of prostatic androgen receptor activation via the SHBG receptor.
7. Discuss the mechanism of degradation and elimination of sexual steroids, and its consequences on the oral administration of these lipophilic hormones.

Sexual Steroids Are Synthesized by the Leydig Cells in Males and by the Cooperative Function of Granulosa and Theca Cells in Females

The two main functions fulfilled by the gonads are *gametogenesis* (production of germ cells) and *hormonogenesis*. The hormones produced by the gonads play an essential role in supporting all aspects of reproduction. These hormones influence other physiologic functions, such as mineral and electrolyte homeostasis, fuel and protein metabolism, adiposity, and muscle mass. In addition to the gonads, the adrenal cortex contributes to the pool of circulating androgens. *The relative importance of adrenal androgens is greater in females than in males*, whose predominant androgen source is the testis.

In the testis, the physiologic source of all steroid hormones is the *Leydig cell*, which is found in the connective tissue stroma near the seminiferous tubules and the fenestrated capillaries (Fig. 13-1). The Leydig cells primarily secrete *testosterone* and small amounts of *17β-estradiol* (E_2). *Leydig cells* show the characteristic structural features of steroid hormone-

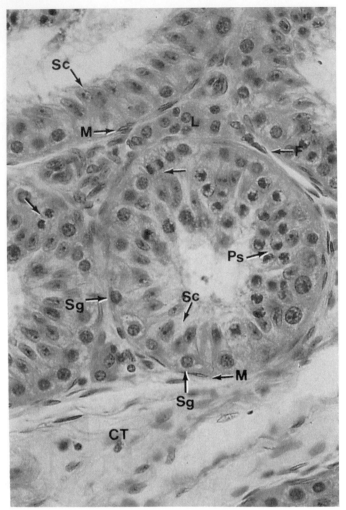

Figure 13-1. The Leydig cells of the testis (L) are located near fenestrated capillaries in the interstitium of the seminiferous tubules. The seminiferous tubules are lined by Sertoli cells (Sc) resting on a basal lamina. The tubules are encircled by the myoid cells (M). Within the tubular epithelium, various developmental forms of sperm are seen in this section, including spermatogonia (Sg) and primary spermatocytes (Ps). The arrows indicate spermatogia in mitosis. CT, connective tissue; F, fibroblast. (*Source:* Fig. 18-5, p 275 in Berman I: *Color Atlas of Histology,* Stamford, CT, Appleton & Lange, 1993.)

producing cells: they have extensive smooth endoplasmic reticulum (sER), tubulovesicular mitochondria, and several cytoplasmic lipid droplets. *Reinke's crystalloids* are cytoplasmic and sometimes intranuclear inclusions specific for Leydig cells and their female equivalents, the *hilar cells* (see the section on The Ovary (Adnexum)). The function of the crystalloids is obscure; their numbers increase with age and their appearance depends on functional androgen receptors expressed by the Leydig cells. Thus, they are absent from the Leydig cells of patients with *androgen insensitivity syndrome* (androgen receptor defect).

In the ovary, the *maturing ovarian follicles* and (after ovulation) the *corpus luteum* are the major steroidogenic tissues. The maturing ovarian follicle consists of two adjacent steroidogenic cell populations: the epithelial *granulosa cells*, and the mesenchyme-derived *theca interna* cells (Fig. 13-2; see details in the section on the female reproductive system). The corpus luteum develops from the ovarian follicle upon ovulation. Its steroidogenic cells are derived from their preovulatory counterparts and are termed *granulosa lutein* and *theca lutein cells*, respectively (Fig. 13-3). The main secreted sexual steroid hormone before ovulation is E_2. The main steroid hormones produced by the corpus luteum are *progesterone* and E_2. During pregnancy, progesterone and *estriol* (E_3) are the main steroid products of the fetoplacental unit. Thus, even though the masculine and feminine secondary sexual characteristics are related to androgens and estrogens, respectively, *the most distinctive hormone between males and females is progesterone*, which is secreted in significant quantities only by the corpus luteum and the placenta.

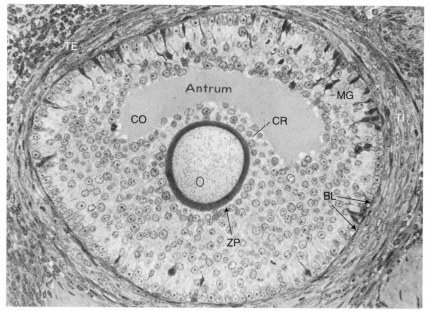

Figure 13-2. Tertiary (antral) follicle. The primary oocyte (O) surrounded by the zona pellucida (ZP) and corona radiata (CR) is found in the developing cumulus oophorus (CO). The follicular antrum is bordered by multiple layers of granulosa cells as membrana granulosa (MG). The vascular theca interna (TI) is separated from the avascular MG by a basal lamina (BL). These two cell populations contribute to sex steroid synthesis. The theca externa (TE) is not involved in hormone production. Compare with Fig. 13-15 (developing follicles). (*Source:* Modified from Fig. 32-13, p 860 in Fawcett DW: *Bloom and Fawcett's Textbook of Histology;* 11th ed., Philadelphia, Saunders, 1986.)

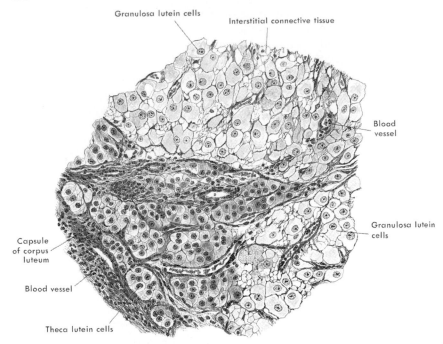

Figure 13-3. Corpus luteum. The image shows a small area of the convoluted surface of the corpus luteum at high magnification. After ovulation, the granulosa cell layer became vascularized, and connective tissue stroma developed. Both the granulosa and the theca interna cells are "luteinized" and function as granulosa lutein cells and theca lutein cells, respectively. The two cell populations essentially retain the proportions and relative positions found in the preovulatory follicle. (*Source:* Modified from Fig. 32-21, p 868 in Fawcett DW: *Bloom and Fawcett's Textbook of Histology,* 11th ed., Philadelphia, Saunders, 1986.)

In females, normal sex hormone production is achieved by the *coordinated* function of the granulosa and theca cells both before and after ovulation (Fig. 13-4):

• Theca interna and theca lutein cells express P450scc and produce pregnenolone, which is converted into progesterone by the preferentially Δ^4 steroidogenic pathway. Progesterone produced by the theca interna and the theca lutein cells is mainly used as a precursor of androgen synthesis involving P450c17.

• Theca interna cells express *aromatase* (P450arom, see below), the enzyme that converts androgens into estrogens. Upon ovulation/luteinization, aromatase expression ceases and theca lutein cells cannot secrete estrogens.

• The granulosa and granulosa lutein cells are unable to produce androgens because they lack the P450c17 enzyme. Thus, they must rely on androgens produced by the theca interna and theca lutein cells, respectively, and convert the androgens into estrogens by their aromatase activity. These cells are the most important *immediate* sources of E_2.

- In contrast with theca interna cells, the granulosa cells lack the P450scc enzyme and are unable to synthesize pregnenolone from cholesterol. After ovulation, granulosa *lutein* cells express P450scc and synthesize pregnenolone. Due to the continued absence of P450c17:
  - pregnenolone may only proceed to the production of progesterone. Thus, the main source of progesterone secreted by the corpus luteum is the granulosa lutein cell.
  - the granulosa lutein cells still rely on theca cell-derived androgenic precursors for their estrogen synthesis.

An intricate cooperation among various fetal, placental and maternal cells is involved in the generation of estrogens present in pregnant females, which is reminiscent of the cooperation between granulosa lutein and theca lutein cells. Similar to the granulosa lutein cells, the syncytiotrophoblast cells of the placenta may synthesize progesterone (but not androgens) de novo (see The Fetoplacental Unit). Most actions of androgens, estrogens and progesterone are mediated by their respective intracellular receptors involving a genomic action (see Chap. 5).

After Puberty, Steroidogenesis Is Regulated by LH in Males, and by Both FSH and LH in Females

Before puberty, the gonads secrete very low quantities of sexual steroids. This is in part related to the *basal, gonadotropin-independent steroid synthesis and secretion* of Leydig cells and of the maturing follicles (see the Female Reproductive System, below). The low levels of gonadal sexual steroids play an essential role in inhibiting gonadotropin secretion in prepubertal children, whose hypothalamus is exquisitely sensitive to negative feedback regulation by sexual steroids. This explains why, in *Turner's syndrome* (45,X gonadal dysgenesis) patients, who have *streak gonads* without follicles, plasma concentrations of gonadotropins are elevated in comparison with healthy children (see Fig. 13-43).

After puberty, the main determinants of gonadal steroid hormone secretion are the pituitary gonadotropins. The rate-limiting step of steroidogenesis in the gonads is the *LH-* or *human chorionic gonadotropin (hCG)*-stimulated and protein kinase A (PKA)-mediated induction of *steroidogenic acute regulatory protein* (StAR). LH receptors mediate this action in all gonadal cells that express P450scc: Leydig cells, theca interna, theca lutein, and granulosa lutein cells.

In males, the only target of LH is the Leydig cell, the source of all testicular steroid hormones. The only target of FSH is the nonsteroidogenic *Sertoli cell*, which provides the epithelial lining of the seminiferous tubules. The Sertoli cells secrete the protein hormone *inhibin B* (see Regulation of the Gonadotropin–Gonad Axis in Postpubertal Males) in response to FSH. As we shall see, the Sertoli cell is developmentally homologous with the granulosa cells, which explains the similarities in their endocrine function.

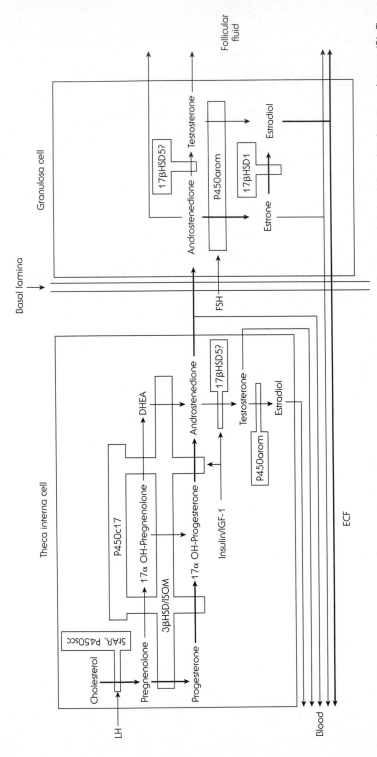

Figure 13-4. Cooperation between theca interna and granulosa cells in steroidogenesis in *preovulatory* follicles (A) and in the corpus luteum (B). The ovary produces small but physiologically relevant amounts of testosterone; however, the isoenzyme of 17β-hydroxysteroid dehydrogenase (17βHSD) converting androstenedione to testosterone is uncertain. As indicated by the thickness of the arrows, estradiol is preferentially produced by the androstenedione—estrone pathway involving aromatase (P450arom) and 17βHSD1. In nondominant follicles, FSH receptors are downregulated, androgens accumulate in the follicular fluid, and atresia ensues. Note that after ovulation of the dominant follicle, two parallel steroidogenic pathways operate leading to the secretion of estradiol and progesterone. LH not only leads to luteinization of the granulosa cells but becomes the regulator of their steroidogenic activity.

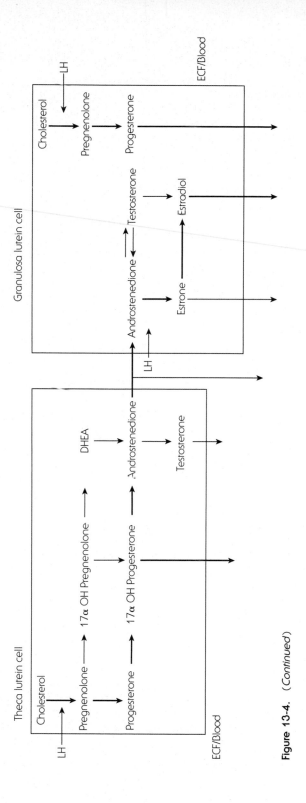

Figure 13-4. (*Continued*)

Although FSH is an important stimulator of *spermatogenesis* (see Spermato-genesis), it has no direct stimulatory action on either the de novo synthesis or the conversion of steroid hormones.

In contrast, in females FSH is the physiologic stimulus of estrogen secretion before ovulation. The only target of FSH in females is the granu-losa cell. FSH stimulates the proliferation of granulosa cells, the secretion of *inhibin B,* and the expression of *aromatase. At advanced stages of follicular maturation, granulosa cells also express small numbers of LH receptors, which are important in luteinization.* The *preovulatory surge of LH* initiates luteinization in the theca interna and granulosa cells and causes ovulation, the development of the corpus luteum, and the completion of the luteiniza-tion process. Starting with the appearance of the *luteinized* granulosa and theca cells (i.e., shortly before ovulation), LH stimulates streoidogenesis in both cell populations. In granulosa lutein cells, LH stimulates aromatase activity, progesterone and *inhibin A* secretion. Because LH increases the secretion of androgens by the adjacent theca lutein cells, the increased aromatase activity in granulosa lutein cells results in increased estrogen se-cretion.

Dehydroepiandrosterone and Androstenedione Are Processed by Isoenzymes of 17β-Hydroxysteroid Dehydrogenase and a Single Aromatase Enzyme (P450arom)

We followed the biosynthesis of androgens to dehydroepiandrosterone (DHEA) and androstenedione in the adrenal cortex (see Fig. 12-8). In contrast with the adrenal cortex, which preferentially secretes DHEA over androstenedione (i.e., preferential Δ^5 pathway), the biosynthesis of andro-gens in the gonads follows the Δ^4 pathway. Thus, the gonads secrete rela-tively small quantities of DHEA, especially in females (see Fig. 13-4). The two key enzymes involved in the further processing DHEA and androstene-dione in the gonads and peripheral (extragonadal) locations are

- the isoenzymes of *17β-hydroxysteroid dehydrogenase* (17βHSD), which convert androgens and/or estrogens either into their less or into more potent forms (Table 13-1); and
- a single *aromatase* enzyme (P450arom), which converts C19 steroids (androgens) into C18 steroids having an aromatic A-ring (estrogens).

The 17βHSD1, 17βHSD3, and 17βHSD5 isoenzymes constitute an *activator subfamily* that produces more potent sex steroids from substrates having lower biologic activities.

- *17βHSD1* is an *estrogen-specific* enzyme that produces 17β-estradiol from estrone. This isoenzyme is present in the main sources of circulating

Table 13-1   17β-Hydroxysteroid Dehydrogenase Isoenzymes

Type	Gene	Chromosomal localization	Preference for substrate(s) and product(s)	Tissue distribution
1	17βHSD1	17q11-21	Estrone to estradiol (18OH-steroid-specific); produces more active estrogens by a reductive reaction	Primarily in the ovary (granulosa cells, granulosa lutein cells), placenta, mammary gland
2	17βHSD2	17q11-21	Estradiol to estrone ≈testosterone to androstenedione; possesses 20α-HSD activity: converts 20α-dihydroprogesterone to progesterone; normally unidirectional oxidative function; limits estrogen effects on endometrium by oxidizing estradiol into estrone	Liver, secretory endometrium, placenta, small intestine, prostate
3	17βHSD3	9q22	Androstenedione to testosterone > DHEA to 5-androstenediol > estrone to estradiol; mainly produces more active androgens by a reductive reaction	Testis
4	17βHSD4	5q21	Estradiol to estrone, androst-5-ene-3β,17β-diol to DHEA; unidirectional oxidative function	Liver, heart, prostate, testis
5	17βHSD5	10p14-15	Androstenedione to testosterone; low activity	Liver, adrenal gland, prostate, ovary (?)

estrogens: the granulosa and granulosa lutein cells of the ovary and the trophoblast cells of the placenta.

• The expression of *17βHSD3* is *required for normal testicular androgen secretion* both in utero and after puberty. The main substrate of 17βHSD3 is androstenedione, which is converted into testosterone. The congenital absence of 17βHSD3 results in *male pseudohermaphroditism* (Box 13-1 and Sexual Development).

• The physiologic importance of *17βHSD5* is uncertain. Hepatic 17βHSD5 might be an important determinant of circulating testosterone levels in women by conversion of androstenedione produced by the adre-

BOX 13-1   Hermaphroditism and Pseudohermaphroditism

In Greek mythology, Hermaphroditos was a son of Hermes and Aphrodite who possessed both male and female external genitalia. Today, the medical term *true hermaphroditism* refers to the condition when both ovarian and testicular tissues are present in the same individual. This rare condition is associated with a highly variable presentation of the external genitalia. In *pseudohermaphroditism* the gonad is either male or female (*not* both); the external genitalia and the gonad are mismatched (the external genitalia are either ambiguous or appropriate for the *opposite* gonadal sex). The gender in these cases is designated by the gonadal sex. Thus, male pseudohermaphrodites have testes (and female-like external genitalia), and female pseudohermaphrodites have ovaries (and male-like external genitalia).

nals. 17βHSD5 is a minor enzyme in the adrenal cortex, which explains the usually negligible adrenal testosterone production. The theca and granulosa cells may convert androstenedione to testosterone, but the type of 17βHSD involved has not yet been elucidated; 17βHSD5 is a candidate for this function.

The 17βHSD2 and 17βHSD4 isoenzymes mainly function as unidirectional *inactivators* of potent sex steroids.

*   *17βHSD2 is equally potent in decreasing the activity of E_2 and testosterone. Its function is to limit the action of these hormones on their major target cells such as the endometrium, liver, and prostate.* In combination with aromatase, 17βHSD2 in the placenta protects the fetus from maternally derived testosterone.
*   The functions of *17βHSD4* in the liver and the prostate are similar to those of 17βHSD2. However, 17βHSD4 is less active converting its androgenic than its estrogenic substrate. Thus, 17βHSD4 *mainly protects against estrogen receptor stimulation.*

Aromatase is a membrane-anchored heme glycoprotein found in the sER. Aromatase is associated with the ubiquitous *NADPH-cytochrome P450 reductase*, which transfers reducing equivalents from NADPH to *any* microsomal cytochrome P450. The aromatase reaction uses 3 moles of oxygen and 3 moles of NADPH for every mole of C19 steroid metabolized. The first two oxygens oxidize the C19 methyl group by standard hydroxylation mechanisms. The third oxidative reaction is a *peroxidative attack* on the C19 methyl group, which (by cleaving the methyl group as formic acid from the steroid frame) leads to the aromatization of the A-ring. This is the only known reaction in vertebrates that introduces an aromatic ring into a molecule.

Aromatase is encoded by the *CYP19* gene localized on chromosome

15q. It is 27.4 cM telomeric to the closely linked *CYP11A* and *CYP1A1* genes. *CYP11A* encodes the mitochondrial P450scc enzyme (see Chap. 12). *CYP1A1* encodes an *aryl hydrocarbon receptor*-regulated microsomal monooxygenase, which is involved in hepatic detoxification processes.

The *CYP19* gene consists of 10 exons and uses multiple promoters in a tissue-specific manner (Table 13-2); various first exons are regulated by these promoters. Because the AUG start codon is located on exon II, this arrangement results in a heterogeneity of the transcripts only in their 5′ untranslated regions, and the protein encoded by the various transcripts is identical. The usage of different promoters allows a tissue-specific regulation of the aromatase activity.

Depending on gender and reproductive stage, significant contribution to circulating estrogens by aromatase activity is provided by the gonads and/or certain peripheral (extragonadal) tissues. In males, under most physi-

Table 13-2 Tissue-Dependent Regulation of Aromatase Expression via Multiple Promoters

Tissue	Main promoter(s)	Main regulator(s)
Placenta	I.1	Retinoids acting via RXR/RAR; SF-1 is absent
Ovary	II	FSH, granulosa cells; LH, theca interna and granulosa lutein cells (cyclic AMP/CREB; action is SF-1-dependent)
Leydig cells of the testis	II (LH-induced) ? (SRY-induced)	LH (cyclic AMP/CREB; action is SF-1-dependent), SRY
Adipose tissue (preadipocytes, mesenchymal stromal cells in adipose tissue)	I.4 >> I.3, II	Glucocorticoids + class I cytokines (e.g., oncostatin-M, LIF, IL–6, IL–11) via the JAK1 STAT3 pathway and the GAS element; TNF-α, involving sphingomyelinase and an AP1 site; PGE$_2$ via cyclic AMP, PKC and CREB
Preadipocytes in breast tissue near breast cancer cells	II, I.3	PGE$_2$ via cyclic AMP/CREB and PKC
Bone, epiphyseal cartilage	I.4 >> I.3 > I.6	Glucocorticoids and class I cytokines, IL-1β, TNF-α
Brain (appears to be region-specific usage of promoters)	1f > II, I.4	Androgens; PKC and PKG pathways, α_1-adrenergic agonists, substance P, cholecystokinin, natriuretic peptide
Pituitary gland	Similar to brain (?)	Androgens (?)

ABBREVIATIONS: SF-1, Steroidogenic factor-1, a transcription factor that is an orphan member of the steroid hormone receptor superfamily; JAK, Janus kinase (a receptor-associated tyrosine kinase); STAT, signal transducer and activator of transcription (a phosphorylation-dependent transcription factor); GAS, γ-interferon-activated sequence (a cis-acting element); RXR, retinoid X receptor; RAR, retinoic acid receptor; FSH, follicle-stimulating hormone; LH, luteinizing hormone; SRY, a transcription factor encoded by the sex-determining region of the Y chromosome; LIF, leukemia inhibiting factor; IL, interleukin; TNF-α, tumor necrosis factor α; CREB, cyclic AMP response element-binding protein.

ologic circumstances, 80% of 17β-estradiol and 98% of estrone in plasma is derived from peripheral conversion of androgens primarily in adipose tissue. In contrast, in females during the menstrual cycle direct ovarian secretion is the main source of circulating estrogens. The specific C18 steroid produced in each tissue depends on the presentation of the C19 steroid.

- Although *Leydig cells* primarily produce testosterone, they also secrete small quantities of estrogens (mainly 17β-estradiol) because of the presence of aromatase. *Supranormal production of estrogens by Leydig cells occurs when their LH receptors are hyperstimulated*. This is the cause of LH-induced *gynecomastia* (female-breastedness), which affects 60 to 70% of *adolescent males*, and the cause of hCG-induced gynecomastia in *testicular choriocarcinoma* patients. Unlike in most animal species, the Sertoli cells of adult men do not express significant aromatase activity in vivo. However, Sertoli cell *tumors* may express aromatase, which may lead to feminization (including gynecomastia).
- Similar to the testis, the ovary may produce 17β-estradiol from testosterone. However, the preferred route of ovarian production of 17β-estradiol involves the aromatization of androsetenedione followed by the conversion of the resulting estrone into 17β-estradiol by 17βHSD1. The aromatase activity is very high in the granulosa cells, and normally the follicular secretion of androgens (mainly as androstenedione) is minimal. Overt stimulation of insulin and/or IGF-1 receptors of theca cells, however, increases the secretion of androgens, including testosterone, as seen in *polycystic ovary disease* (see Regulation of the Ovarian Cycle: The Hypothalamic–Pituitary–Ovarian Axis).

The *peripheral tissues* that significantly contribute to *circulating* estrogens by their aromatase activities include adipose tissue and the placenta.

- *Preadipocytes*, rather than mature adipocytes filled with a triglyceride droplet, *are the sites of aromatase expression*. However, *the amount of preadipocyes in the body is proportionate to the degree of adiposity*. Aromatase activity in preadipocytes displays a regional distribution: higher aromatase activity is present in the adipose tissue of the *buttocks* and *thighs* than in the abdominal subcutaneous fat or in the (nontumorous) breast. The cytokine-dependent expression of aromatase in adipose tissue requires the mandatory presence of glucocorticoids. The age-dependent increase of these cytokines explains the age-dependent increase of adipose tissue aromatase activity in both sexes even in the absence of obesity.
  - In females, adipose tissue mainly produces estrone from androstenedione primarily secreted by the adrenal cortex. The physiologically higher adipose tissue mass in females and its feminine distribution explain the higher peripheral aromatase activity in females compared to males. Obese postmenopausal women have an *increased risk for endometrial cancer* and a *decreased risk for osteoporosis*.

- In males, adipose tissue converts both testicular androgens (testosterone) and adrenal androgens (androstenedione). Obesity increases the estrogen:androgen ratio in both sexes. Body mass index (BMI; see Box 10-4) is positively correlated with gynecomastia in males.
- The *trophoblasts* of the placenta mainly produce estriol from 16α-OH-DHEA, a product of the combined activities of the fetal adrenal cortex, the fetal liver and placental steroid sulfatase (see The Endocrine Physiology of the Pregnant Woman and the Fetoplacental Unit). Placental aromatase prevents the masculinization of the female fetus by androgens generated by the fetal adrenal cortex and an unidentified placental 17βHSD isoenzyme. Placental aromatase deficiency is one of the causes of *female pseudohermaphroditism* (see The Endocrine Physiology of the Pregnant Woman and the Fetoplacental Unit).

In certain peripheral tissues, the conversion of androgens into estrogens by aromatase has no significant impact on circulating levels of estrogens, but plays essential roles in several *local actions*. These *estrogen receptor-mediated actions of circulating androgens* include:

- The prevention of *osteoporosis* and mediation of *epiphyseal closure* in males (osteoblast and chondroblast aromatase).
- Participation in the *feedback* of androgens on gonadotropin secretion via the hypothalamus (conversion by brain aromatase) and the gonadotroph (conversion most probably by pituitary aromatase). Aromatase expression in the human pituitary gland has not yet been confirmed. At least in rodents, pituitary aromatase expression is significantly higher males than in females. The difference is presumed to be related to expression from androgen-induced promoter site.
- Stimulation of *breast cancer* growth. This mechanism involves a local positive feedback, whereby breast cancer cells stimulate aromatase in preadipocytes via a paracrine mechanism involving prostaglandin E_2 (PGE_2), and the locally generated estrogens stimulate the proliferation of the cancer cells. Inhibitors of aromatase such as *letrozole* are used in the treatment of breast cancer.

Testosterone May Be Converted to the More Potent Dihydrotestosterone by Two Isoenzymes of 5α-Reductase Expressed in Target Tissues

In addition to its conversion by aromatase, testosterone is subject to conversion into *dihydrotestosterone* (DHT) by two isoenzymes of *5α-reductase* (see Fig. 12-8; Table 13-3). Almost all circulating DHT is generated in peripheral tissues. Pharmacologic evidence obtained in men suggests that the *type II* (*finasteride-sensitive*) *5α-reductase* generates three times as much DHT as the type I (MK-386-sensitive) isoenzyme. The skin (dermal fibroblasts, keratinocytes, hair follicles, sebaceous and apocrine sweat glands)

Table 13-3   5α-Reductase Isoenzymes

Type	Chromosomal localization	Tissue distribution	Inhibitor(s)
5α-reductase type I	5p	*Sebaceous glands, apocrine sweat glands,* epidermal keratinocytes, dermal papilla cells, fibroblasts, dermal papilla cells, fibroblasts from genital and nongenital skin, brain, rat Leydig cell	MK-386, LY191704
5α-reductase type II	2p	*Prostate,* epididymis, seminal vesicles, fetal genital skin, *inner root sheath of hair follicles,* fibroblasts from normal adult genital skin, gonadotropin feedback (brain?)	Finasteride

NOTE: italicized are the clinically most important features.

is the main source of circulating DHT; the cutaneous production is complemented by the prostate in men. The distribution and activity of 5α-reductase associated with hair follicles displays racial differences: in general, the activity is highest in Caucasians especially of Mediterranean origin, and the lowest in Orientals. Unlike testosterone, *DHT is not a substrate for aromatase,* and therefore, the biologic actions of DHT are not mediated by estrogen receptors.

DHT is the most potent activator of the androgen receptor; it is about 2.5 times more potent than testosterone. Certain actions of androgens, such as the masculinization of external genitalia and the development of benign prostatic hypertrophy, have an absolute requirement for 5α-reductase activity. Although not mandatory, 5α-reductase activity significantly contributes to the proper embryonic development of the prostate, descent of the testes, phallic growth, male-pattern balding (in individuals with genes predisposing for baldness), the development of terminal body hair, pubic and underarm hair, *hirsutism* (excessive terminal hair growth usually with a male pattern observed in females), and the activity of sebaceous and *apocrine* sweat glands. Other androgenic actions are mediated by testosterone per se irrespective of peripheral conversion, such as the embryonic development of Wolffian duct-derived structures and their postpubertal secretory activity; the pubertal growth of the larynx (deepening of the voice); the anabolic effect on eythropoiesis and muscle (increased muscle protein and lean body mass, positive nitrogen balance); inhibition of breast development; the stimulation of spermatogenesis; libido; and possibly the sexual orientation toward females. The various mechanisms of actions of androgens in males are summarized in Table 13-4.

DHT acts mainly in an *intracrine* manner, i.e., it activates the androgen receptor within the 5α-reductase-expressing cell. These cells also express

Table 13-4   Physiologic Actions of Androgens in Males Without and With Peripheral Conversion of Testosterone

Testosterone-mediated actions without peripheral conversion	Absolute requirement for 5α-reductase activity	Significant but nonmandatory involvement of 5α-reductase activity	Aromatase-dependent actions
Mostly androgen-receptor mediated genomic actions			Mostly estrogen receptor-mediated genomic actions
Embryonic development and postpubertal secretory activity of Wolffian duct-derived structures: epididymis, vas deferens, seminal vesicle	Masculinization of external genitalia: labioscrotal fusion, *normal* phallic development	Proper embryonic development of prostate	Epiphyseal closure
Laryngeal growth (Adam's apple)	Development of benign prostatic hypertrophy	Phallic growth	Prevention of osteoporosis
Stimulation of erythropoiesis (mainly via erythropoietin)	—	Descent of the testes	
Anabolic effect on muscle	Male-pattern distribution of hair (mustache, beard, chest, escutcheon)[a]	Male-pattern balding (with predisposing genetic background)	Prevention of Alzheimer's disease (direct trophic action in the CNS)
Decreased HDL		Ambisexual hair growth (pubic, underarm)	Fluid retention
Stimulation of spermatogenesis	—	Activity of sebaceous glands	—
Inhibition of breast development	—	Activity of apocrine sweat glands	—
Behavioral responses: libido, aggresion, sexual orientation toward females	—	Erection	—
—	—	Feedback regulation of gonadotropin secretion	Feedback regulation of gonadotropin secretion

[a] The assignment of male-type hair distribution into this column is based on the typical clinical picture of type II 5α-reductase deficiency in postpubertal male pseudohermaphrodites, who develop ambisexual hair, but no male escutcheon, beard or mustache. Male-type hair distribution, however, could also qualify as only partially dependent on 5α-reductase activity.

ABBREVIATIONS: CNS, central nervous system; HDL, high density lipoprotein.

Table 13-5   Assessment of 5α-Reductase Activity

5α-androstane-3α,17β-diol glucronide (normal concentration range in serum)	Potential causes of supranormal concentration	Potential causes of subnormal concentration
Prepubertal children: 10–60 ng/dL (0.21–1.28 nM) Adult male: 260–1500 ng/dL (5.54–31.95 nM) Adult female: 60–300 ng/dL (1.28–6.39 nM)	Hirsutism, acne, conditions associated with virilization such as certain types of congenital adrenal hyperplasia and polycystic ovary syndrome	5α-reductase deficiency, non-Caucasian race (adult males)

3α-hydroxysteroid dehydrogenase (3αHSD; see Fig. 12-8). 3αHSD catalyzes the *reversible* reduction of DHT to *5α-androstane-3α,17β-diol* (a weak androgen). The equilibrium between the reductive and oxidative activities of 3αHSD is an important factor in the regulation of intracellular levels of DHT and androgen receptor stimulation. There are at least three isoenzymes of 3αHSD (designated as types 1 through 3).

Although DHT is primarily an intracrine/paracrine hormone, DHT also enters the circulation and is present in plasma in significant quantities (about 10% of testosterone levels); thus, DHT may exert androgenic action on 5α-reductase negative tissues. The liver expresses type 2 3αHSD, which is important in the inactivation of *circulating* DHT. The 5α-androstane-3α,17β-diol generated in the liver and by peripheral tissues is glucuronidated by the liver and excreted by the kidneys. *Plasma levels and urinary excretion of 5α-androstane-3α,17β-diol glucuronide (3α-diol-G) are the best markers for assessing peripheral formation of DHT* (Table 13-5).

In Addition to Being the Carrier Protein of Androgens and Estrogens in Plasma, SHBG Acts on a Membrane Receptor in a Steroid Hormone-Dependent Manner

As lipophilic compounds, androgens, estrogens, and progesterone circulate in plasma mainly in association with carrier proteins (see Chap. 4 and Table 4-2).

Plasma SHBG (mainly produced by the liver) and testicular *androgen-binding protein* (ABP, secreted by Sertoli cells into the lumen of the seminiferous tubules) are homodimeric glycoproteins with a single steroid-binding site. SHBG and ABP are products of a single gene (chromosome 17p12-13), which is expressed in several tissues including liver, testis, brain, endometrium, and placenta. The transcripts and amino acid sequences of *plasma* SHBG and *testicular* ABP are identical and differ only in their oligosaccharides. The SHGB gene is widely expressed in the brain, where several transcripts result from differential exon utilization; their biologic functions are unknown.

The glycosylation of SHBG and other hormone-binding globulins in the liver is increased by estrogens, which leads to their prolonged half-life and accumulation in plasma (Fig. 13-5). Due to the higher affinity of androgens than estrogens to SHBG, the increased plasma concentration of SHBG shifts the estrogen:androgen ratio of the free (biologically active) hormones toward estrogens. This mechanism contributes to the protection of the developing female fetus from the masculinizing action of maternal androgens. Cirrhosis of the liver is associated with an increased glycosylation of SHBG, which (by the above mechanism) results in estrogen excess and gynecomastia in males.

Plasma SHBG and testicular ABP are modular proteins comprised of an N-terminal steroid-binding and dimerization domain, and a C-terminal domain containing a highly conserved consensus sequence for glycosylation. The C-terminal domain may be required for recognition of cell surface receptors. The *SHBG receptor* has been partially characterized. Because its action on cell function is mediated by activation of adenylyl cyclase and PKA, it is presumed to be a heptahelical transmembrane receptor.

Only the unliganded SHBG/ABP may bind with its cognate receptor: *prior* binding of steroid ligands prevents interaction of SHBG with its receptor. Binding of unliganded SHBG results in a mild increase of cytosolic cyclic AMP. Whereas prior steroid ligand binding of SHBG prevents the activation of the SHBG receptor, the cyclic AMP-increasing effect of the receptor-bound SHBG is markedly enhanced by the *subsequent* binding of certain steroid ligands (Fig. 13-6). The increased cyclic AMP results in a PKA-mediated phosphorylation and the modulation of several signal transduction mechanisms, including *androgen-independent activation of the androgen receptor*. The steroid ligands that may bring about this alternate route of androgen receptor activation in the prostate include 5α-androstane-3α,17β-diol (a degradation product of DHT) and 17β-estradiol. This explains how estrogens cause *benign prostatic hypertophy* by an androgen receptor *dependent* mechanism.

Progesterone, as a C21 steroid, does not bind to SHBG but circulates in association with *cortisol-binding globulin* (CBG, a member of the serpin family; see Chap. 12) and albumin.

The Degradation Products of Sexual Steroids and Progesterone Are Conjugated with Glucuronic Acid or Sulfate in the Liver and Mainly Excreted in the Urine

The degradation of sexual steroids and progesterone is similar to that of corticosteroids. Thus, more hydrophilic derivatives are formed that are not bound by plasma proteins and are therefore readily filtered by the kidney. The degradation is primarily performed by the liver. The rapid and extensive breakdown during a single passage through the hepatic circulation explains

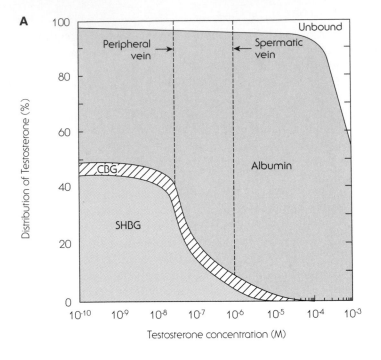

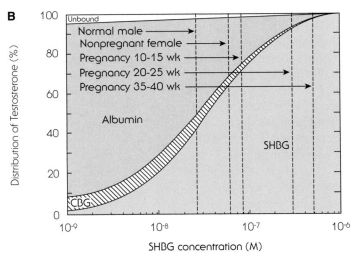

Figure 13-5. Computer-simulated effects of increasing concentration of testosterone (A) and sex hormone-binding globulin (SHBG; B) on the distribution of testosterone in plasma. Note the logarithmic scale of the concentrations. A. The high concentration of testosterone in spermatic vein nearly saturates the binding capacity of plasma SHBG, but leaves most binding sites of plasma SHBG unoccupied in the systemic circulation. With increasing concentrations of testosterone, the proportion of albumin-bound and free testosterone increases, provided the concentrations of carrier proteins remain unchanged. B. The increasing concentration of SHBG decreases free testosterone levels in plasma. Because the affinity of SHBG for estrogens is lower than for androgens, increasing plasma SHBG has less impact on free estrogens. Thus, the estrogen : androgen ratio shifts toward estrogens with increasing plasma

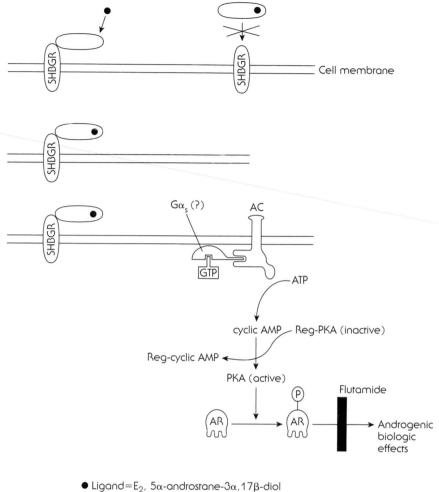

Cell membrane

Gα$_s$ (?)

AC

GTP

ATP

cyclic AMP — Reg-PKA (inactive)

Reg-cyclic AMP ←

PKA (active)

Flutamide

AR → AR → Androgenic biologic effects

 Ligand = E$_2$, 5α-androstane-3α,17β-diol

SHBG

Figure 13-6. Model of signaling via the sex hormone-binding globulin receptor (SHBGR). The SHBGR is not activated by preformed SHBG-ligand complexes. Binding of unliganded SHBG to its receptor results in a weak activation of protein kinase A (PKA), which is significantly augmented by subsequent binding of the ligand, such as estradiol (E$_2$) or 5α-androstane-3α,17β-diol (the degradation product of dihydrotestosterone). The activation of PKA is presumed to involve a trimeric G-protein mechanism (see details in Fig. 5-4). PKA activates the androgen receptor (AR) by phosphorylation. Thus, E$_2$-provoked benign prostatic hypertrophy can be antagonized by antiandrogens, such as flutamide. Reg, regulatory subunit of PKA; AC, adenylyl cyclase.

Figure 13-5. (*Continued*) SHBG. Compared to men, women especially during pregnancy have significantly elevated plasma SHBG. CBG, cortisol binding globulin. (*Source:* Figs. 4 and 5 (with slight modification) from Dunn JF et al: Transport of steroid hormones: Binding of 21 endogenous steroids to both testosterone-binding globulin and corticosteroid-binding globulin in human plasma. J Clin Endocrinol Metab 53:58–68, 1981.)

that natural sexual steroids and progesterone (unlike their synthetic analogues) are not suitable as oral drugs. The degradation of androgens may
follow several routes:

- aromatization followed by degradation of the resulting estrogens;
- degradation of DHT by 3αHSD;
- degradation of testosterone through androstenedione. This mechanism may include the action of 17βHSD2 (and 17βHSD4) in the liver (see
above). Androstenedione is then reduced into any of three closely related
compounds: *etiocholanolone*, *epiandrosterone*, or *androsterone*, which are
conjugated with glucuronic acid via their 3-hydroxyl groups and end up in
urine as the main *17-ketosteroids* (Fig. 13-7).

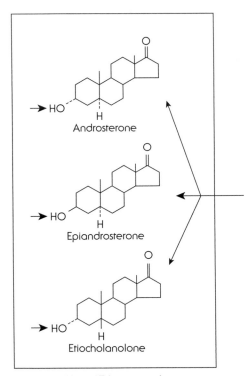

Main 17-ketosteroids

Figure 13-7. The metabolism of sexual steroids and progesterone. The reactions shown
are mainly performed by the liver. The end products are hydrophilic, do not bind with SHBG,
and are excreted with urine. Note that the degradation of dihydrotestosterone is neglected
(see Fig. 12-8). The color arrows indicate targets of glucuronidation, the black arrowheads
show targets of sulfation. The central precursor in the degradative pathway of androgens is
androstenedione, which is either broken down into 17-ketosteroids, or becomes aromatized.
Estrone plays a similar central role in the degradative pathway of estrogens as androstenedione does for androgens. It may be metabolized into 3-sulfated 16-hydroxyestone, double-
conjugated estriol, or catecholestrogens which are inactivated by catechol-O-methyltransferase (COMT, compare with Fig. 12-5). A simplified flowchart of the rapid degradation of
progesterone is shown on the right.

Figure 13-7. (Continued)

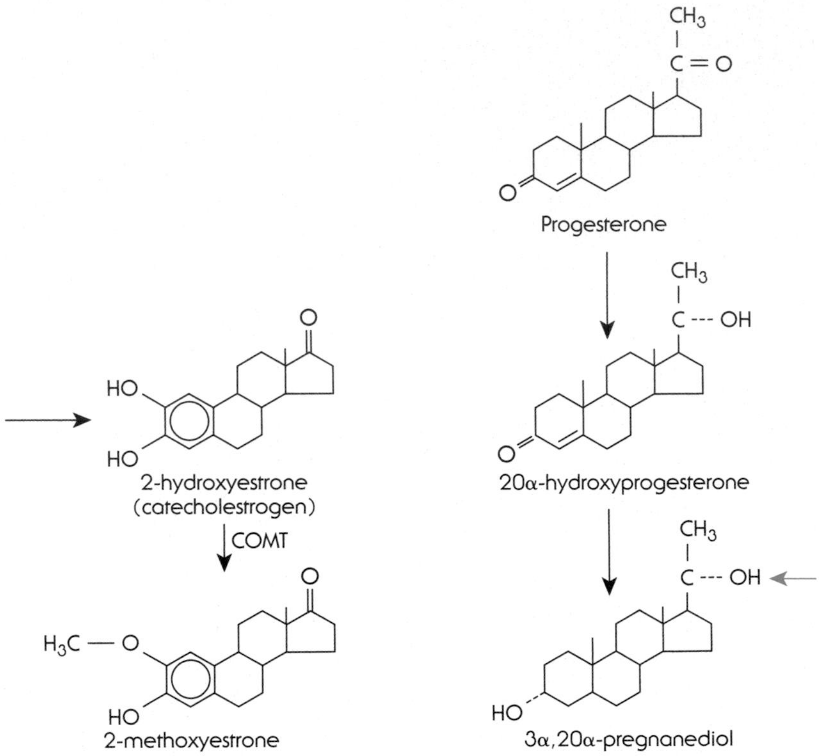

Figure 13-7. (*Continued*)

In adult men, about one-third of urinary 17-ketosteroids are derived from testosterone, and two-thirds from the less potent adrenal androgens, DHEA and androstenedione. In adult women, the ovarian contribution to *total urinary 17-ketosteroids* is minimal, compared to the amount derived from adrenal androgens. This explains why the normal urinary ketosteroid production in women is about two-thirds of that in men. It is important to note, however, that ovarian contribution to *the total androgenic activity in the circulation* is significant. The explanation for the difference lies in the fact that testosterone as well as androstenedione are metabolized into 17-ketosteroids, but testosterone has more androgenic activity. The ovaries significantly contribute to the circulating pool of testosterone by direct secretion from theca cells.

The inactivation of 17β-estradiol (the most potent estrogen) starts in the liver with conversion to estrone by 17βHSD2 and 17βHSD4. Some 17β-estradiol and estrone is directly conjugated and excreted. Estrone is mainly converted either into biologically active *catecholestrogens* (2- or 4-hydroxyestrone) or 16α-hydroxyestrone (see Fig. 13-7). The catecholestrogens are processed by the catechol-O-methyltranferase (COMT) enzyme, which is involved in the degradation of catecholamines. The 16α-estrone is converted to estriol, which is excreted as estriol 3-sulfate,16-glucuronide. Plasma and urinary *estriol is the main estrogen during pregnancy* (see The Endocrine Physiology of the Pregnant Woman and the Fetoplacental Unit).

The breakdown of progesterone is extremely rapid. The main route of degradation involves two successive reduction reactions to 20α-hydroxy-progesterone and pregnanediol. The latter is excreted as *pregananediol-20-glucuronide* (see Fig. 13-7).

THE MALE REPRODUCTIVE SYSTEM

OBJECTIVES

1. Discuss the anatomy of the testis, the excurrent duct system, and the male accessory glands. Describe the main functions of each organ. Identify the sources of semen and preseminal fluid. Discuss the coagulation system of semen and its relationship with the *prostate-specific antigen* (PSA).

2. Discuss the stages and the timeframe of *spermatogenesis*. Identify the relationship between developing sperm and the blood-testis barrier, and the functions Sertoli cells in spermatogenesis. Discuss the hormonal regulation of spermatogenesis; identify hormonal targets, sources, and the importance of high local concentrations of testosterone.

3. Discuss the composition of semen, sperm count, the parameters of sperm quality, *azoospermia,* and the mechanism of the regulation of spermatogenesis by temperature.

4. Describe the structure of the penis and the endocrine regulation of its growth. Explain the mechanism of erection, the role of parasympathetic nerves, nitric oxide, and its relationship with androgens.

5. Discuss ejaculation, its phases, its regulation by sympathetic nerves, and its relationship with erection and orgasm.

6. Discuss the regulation of the hypothalamic–pituitary–testicular axis in adult (postpubertal) males. Discuss in detail: *gonadotropin-releasing hormone* (GnRH), pituitary *gonadotropins,* testicular hormones (including steroids and the members of the *transforming growth factor β* [TGF-β] family), their secretory patterns, receptors, cellular targets, and the mechanisms of feedback action. Distinguish *pulse frequency* and *pulse amplitude* of the pulsatile release of GnRH, and identify hypothalamic mechanisms regulating these parameters. Identify mechanisms whereby the pulse amplitude of LH may dissociate from changes in the pulse amplitude of GnRH. Discuss differential regulation of LH and FSH secretion, the role of pulse frequency, and the downregulation/desensitization of GnRH receptors. Describe the impact of *hyperprolactinemia* and *leptin* on the hypothalamic–gonadal axis.

7. Discuss selected pathologic conditions, such as *Kallmann's syndrome, McCune–Albright syndrome,* and *testotoxicosis.*

Anatomic Overview of the Male Reproductive System

Testis   The *testis* (*orchis*) is an egg-shaped organ (see Fig. 13-8). At the time of birth, the testicles are normally found in the scrotum; their absence from the scrotum is termed *cryptorchidism* (cryptic orchidism = hidden testicles), a condition *associated with increased risk for testicular malignancies*. The scrotal temperature is about 2 to 4°C lower than the normal core body temperature, which is essential for normal spermatogenesis and fertility.

Inside the scrotum, the outermost sheath enveloping each testicle is the *cremasteric fascia*, which also serves as a sheath and attachment site of the cremaster muscle. The *cremaster muscle* lifts the testis; in certain seasonal breader species, the testis is pulled back into the abdominal cavity during periods of sexual inactivity, thereby inhibiting spermatogenesis. The sheath immediately enveloping the testis is the *tunica vaginalis*, a double layer of serosal membrane derived from the peritoneum during development. *Hydrocele* is the condition when clear fluid accumulates in the tunica vaginalis. The visceral layer of the tunica vaginalis covers the dense connective tissue capsule of the testis (*tunica albuginea*), which sends septa toward the hilar region of the testis known as the *mediastinum testis*. Coils of *seminiferous* (semen-carrying) *tubules* and their connective tissue stroma occupy the space between the septa. Occasionally, ectopic vestigial adrenocortical tissue cortical tissue may be present (*"adrenal rest tissue"*) as a consequence of the close relationship between the development of the gonads and the adrenals.

The coiled seminiferous tubules, which provide approximately 80 to 90% of the testicular volume, are the site of *spermatogenesis* (see the section titled Spermatogenesis). The Leydig cells are found in the connective tissue stroma between the seminiferous tubules. Before puberty, the testes are small and have a rubbery consistency. During puberty, the testes increase in size, mainly under the influence of FSH, and their consistency becomes comparable to muscle. The consistency is due to an arrangement that could be compared to a moderately inflated tire: the material of the tire is the dense connective tissue of the tunica albuginea and the septa, which is "inflated" by the seminiferous tubules and their luminally secreted fluid. *The size and the consistency of the testes reflect testicular function and fertility* (Box 13-2).

The continuation of each seminiferous tubule near the mediastinum is devoid of germ cells. This short portion is known as the straight tubule (*tubulus rectus*). The tubuli recti coalesce within the mediastinal connective tissue to form a reticular network termed *rete testis*, whose content is drained by the *efferent ductules* of the testis to the head of the *epididymis* (see Excurrent Duct System).

The testes and the ovaries develop from the same primordial tissues

BOX 13-2 The Relationship between Testicular Size and Function

- The testicular volume (in milliliters) is calculated as $V = 0.52 \times L \times W^2$, where L = length and W = width of the testis in centimeters. The normal length ranges between 3.6 and 5.5 cm; a length of <2.5 cm usually indicates infertility and/or hypogonadism in adults. The normal testicular volume is >15 mL (18.6 ± 4.8 mL). Testicular volume in clinical practice is often estimated with the *Prader orchidometer,* which consists of a series of plastic "reference testicles" with volumes ranging between 1 and 25 mL.
- Patients with *Klinefelter's syndrome* (47,XXY; see Ontogeny of the Reproductive System) present with bilaterally small testes, which have a firm consistency. In this condition, the seminiferous tubules are hyalinized and replaced by fibrotic tissue. Postpubertal mumps may lead to a similar condition, which may be unilateral.
- In *postpubertal testicular atrophy* (e.g., due to pituitary dysfunction), the testes become smaller and soft to the touch. This condition resembles a deflated tire.
- A sudden unilateral increase in testicular size usually indicates tumor. Most testicular tumors are malignant. Similar sudden enlargement of the testicle may be due to orchitis (inflammation) accompanying mumps. The outcome of postpubertal mumps may include postinflammatory testicular atrophy (firm testicular consistency with diminished size) and decreased fertility.

(see Intrauterine Sexual Development). During their descent into the scrotum, the testes bring along their blood and lymphatic vessels through the *inguinal canal.* The *testicular* and *ovarian arteries* are direct branches of the aorta (see Fig. 12-1). The lymphatic vessels follow the course of arteries. This explains that the lymph of both the male and female gonads is filtered by *para-aortic lymph nodes.* Thus, the metastases of malignant gonadal tumors are inconspicuous. The veins of the gonads initially follow the course of the arteries and surround them as the *pampiniform plexus,* which coalesce to form a *testicular* (or *ovarian*) *vein* on each side. The venous drainage of the gonads is similar to that of the adrenal glands: the right testicular vein joins the inferior vena cava, the left testicular vein empties into the left renal vein. Due to the higher pressure in the renal vein than in the inferior vena cava, the hydrostatic pressure is higher in the left than in the right testicular vein. This has two consequences:

- the left testicle is normally positioned somewhat lower than the right testis (physiologic asymmetry);
- venous varicosities of the testicular vein (*varicocele testis*) are more frequently encountered on the left than the right side. Varicocele results

in decreased venous return, thereby contributing to elevated scrotal temperature, which may decrease fertility.

During development, both the ovaries and the testes descend from their original position. The *further* descent of the testes from this common site is an androgen-dependent process, which relies on the testosterone secretion of the fetal testes. The descent is influenced by both testosterone and DHT; in type II 5α-reductase deficient *male pseudohermaphroditism*, the testes are found variably in the inguinal canal or in the nonfused labia majora. The descent is probably mediated by the androgen-induced involution of the *gubernaculum*, a fibrous ligament that ties the inferior pole of the testis to the inner surface of the *labioscrotal swelling* (the primordium of the scrotum). During the 28th week of gestation, the testis reaches the deep inguinal ring and descends through the inguinal canal in a matter of 2 to 3 days. The descent from the superficial inguinal ring to the scrotum is completed by the 32nd week of gestation. Testicular descent may be provoked in cryptorchid boys by stimulating endogenous testosterone secretion with injections of hCG.

Due to the descent of the testes and/or the failure of the peritoneal *processus vaginalis* to close, the inguinal canal has a larger diameter in males than in females. This explains why *inguinal hernias* are far more common in males, and why females (especially children before menarche) presenting with inguinal hernias need to be evaluated for *androgen insensitivity syndrome* (testicular feminization, see Intrauterine Sexual Development).

Excurrent Duct System and Accessory Glands   The excurrent duct system includes the efferent ductules, the epididymis, the vas (ductus) deferens, the ejaculatory duct, and the urethra. The efferent ductules and the epididymis are not simple drainage tubes but have important functions in the maturation of spermatozoa. The accessory glands are the seminal vesicle, the prostate, and the bulbourethral glands of Cowper, all of which open into the excurrent duct system. The seminal vesicle and the prostate provide the bulk of the ejaculate. *The development and function of these organs are androgen-dependent.* The Cowper's glands produce mucus, which lubricates the glans penis thereby aiding its intromission into the vagina (see details that follow).

Because spermatozoa do not move actively until ejaculation, their delivery must be assured by the undulating movement of the ducts. This movement is performed by the *myoid cells* of the seminiferous tubules (see Fig. 13-1) and the *smooth muscle layers* of the excurrent duct system. The excurrect duct system starts with approximately 20 *efferent ductules* (Fig. 13-8), which drain the content produced by the seminiferous tubules to the initial portion of the *ductus epididymis* found in the *caput epididymis*. The efferent ductules are lined by a pseudostratified columnar epithelium, which

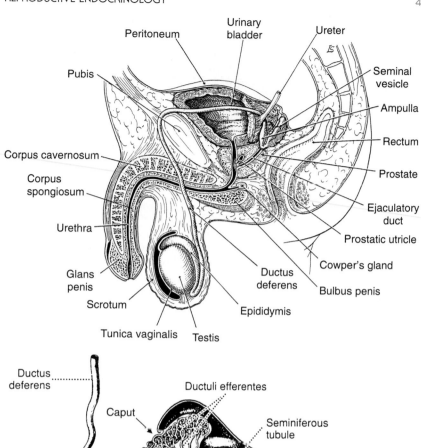

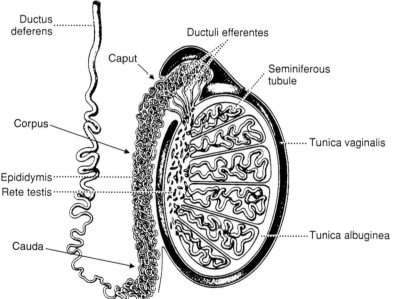

Figure 13-8. The anatomy of the male reproductive system. A. Sagittal pseudosectional diagram of the male urogenital system. B. Schematic presentation of the longitudinal section of the testis and its excurrent ducts. (*Source:* A: *modified* from Fig. 31-1, p 797 in Fawcett DW: *Bloom and Fawcett's Textbook of Histology,* 11th ed., Philadelphia, Saunders, 1986. B: *modified* from Fig. 30-3, p 932 in Dym M: The male reproductive system, in Weiss L (ed): *Cell and Tissue Biology,* 6th ed, Urban & Schwarzenberg, 1988.)

reabsorbs most of the fluid secreted by the seminiferous tubules, thereby increasing the concentration of spermatozoa.

The *epididymis* consists of three anatomic parts: *caput* (head), *corpus* (body) and *cauda* (tail). The *ductus epididymis* is a highly coiled tube with a length of 4 to 6 meters. It is lined by a *pseudostratified stereociliated columnar epithelium*. The epithelium modifies the composition of the luminal fluid both by absorption and active secretion. The secretion includes the action of the *proton pump* (H⁺-ATPase) which acidifies the luminal fluid. The acidic environment is essential for both the maturation and the storage of spermatozoa. The stereocilia are large nonmotile microvilli that provide the surface area for interaction between the membrane of spermatozoa and the epithelium. As a result of this interaction, the spermatozoa

- acquire the *ability* of active directional movement;
- become "incapacitated," i.e., a receptor-masking glycoconjugate is added to their surface, which is later removed during capacitation. *Capacitation* is the process that enables the spermatozoon to fertilize the ovum (see Fertilization).

The cauda of the epididymis serves as a reservoir of mature spermatozoa. The average time between spermiation (the release of spermatozoa from the seminiferous epithelium) and ejaculation is about 12 days (range: 1 to 21 days). Unejaculated, aging spermatozoa (i.e., older than 17 to 21 days) are phagocytosed by "foam cells," presumably derived from the epithelial lining. During ejaculation, the stored spermatozoa are propelled by the wave of smooth muscle contraction starting in the ductus epididymis and continuing in the vas deferens.

The well-developed smooth muscle layers surrounding the ductus epididymis become a thick muscular wall in the vas deferens. The vas deferens is palpable under the skin before it passes through the superficial inguinal ring: it is a pencil-thick tube with a consistency similar to that of cartilage (due to the thick layer of muscle). A widely used method of irreversible male contraception is *vasectomy*, which involves the excision of a segment of the vas deferens and interposition of a fascial barrier between the occluded cut ends to prevent recanalization.

The *seminal vesicles* are located behind the urinary bladder. Their highly convoluted secretory epithelium is embedded in thick smooth muscle layers. The lumen of the gland is drained by the short *excretory duct*, which joins the vas deferens. After these two tubes merge, their continuation is termed *ejaculatory duct*. The secretory product of the seminal vesicle is rich in fructose (the primary fuel of spermatozoa in their active movement), prostaglandins, ascorbic acid, fibrinogen-like, and thrombin-like proteins (Box 13-3). The lumen of the seminal vesicle stores the secretory product, which is propelled by smooth muscle contraction at the time of ejaculation

BOX 13-3 The Coagulation System of Semen and Prostate Specific Antigen

At ejaculation, the epididymal spermatozoa become mixed with the secretions produced by the seminal vesicles and the prostate. The ejaculate immediately turns into a gel-like structure that entraps the spermatozoa. The spermatozoa become progressively motile as the gel dissolves. *Semenogelin I* and *II* are products of two separate genes on chromosome 20 with 80% identity in their primary structures. They are mainly responsible for the immediate gel formation of freshly ejaculated semen. The proteolytic degradation of coagulated semenogelins is performed by *prostate-specific antigen* (PSA, a kallikrein-like serine protease), which results in the liquefaction of semen and the progressive release of motile spermatozoa within 5 to 15 min after ejaculation. PSA is a glycoprotein composed of 93% amino acids and 7% carbohydrates, with a molecular weight of about 30 kDa. The *PSA* and the *human kidney glandular kallikrein-1 (hKGK1)* genes are tandemly located on chromosome 19q13. These two genes display a high degree of homology reflecting a common phylogenetic origin. PSA appears in the circulation especially in patients with prostate cancer, benign prostatic hyperplasia, and after palpation of the prostate. PSA is also elevated in the extremely rare cancer cases of the *Skene's periurethral glands* in women, which indicates the developmental homology between Skene's glands and the prostate. PSA is secreted by the lactating mammary gland into milk.

and flushes the spermatozoa from the downstream portion of the excurrent duct system.

The ejaculatory ducts penetrate the *prostate* and join the prostatic portion of the *urethra*. The opening of each ejaculatory duct is found on either side of the *prostatic utricule* (the remnant of the Müllerian duct) at a posterior fold of the urethral mucosa known as the *colliculus seminalis*. The prostatic glands open into the urethra mainly at the grooves on either side of the colliculus. The prostate consists of 20 to 30 tubuloalveolar glands embedded in a thick fibromuscular tissue. The urethra penetrates the anterior portion of the prostate; prostatic enlargement may cause obstruction of urine flow. Due to the close relationship between the prostate and the rectum (Fig. 13-8A), prostatic enlargement can easily be diagnosed by rectal digital examination. The prostate secretes a fluid rich in proteins such as *acid phosphatase* and *prostate-specific antigen* (PSA), a kallikrein-like protease (see Box 13-3). Similar to the seminal vesicles, the prostate stores its secretory product in the lumen and suddenly propels it into the urethra at the time of ejaculation. The high-protein secretory product may precipitate as prostatic *concretions* (*corpora amylacea*) in the glandular lumen, especially in elderly individuals.

The male urethra has three segments: the *prostatic, membranous,* and *penile urethra.* The membranous urethra penetrates the *urogenital diaphragm,* which contains the *external (voluntary) sphincter of the urethra,* a skeletal muscle. The *internal sphincter of the urethra* (also known as *sphincter vesicae*) is an involuntary smooth muscle surrounding the initial portion of the urethra at the bladder. At the time of ejaculation, the external sphincter opens, whereas the internal sphincter contracts. When the internal sphincter fails to contract, semen is ejected into the lumen of the urinary bladder. The condition, known as *retrograde ejaculation,* is often due to diabetic neuropathy.

The *Cowper's glands* open into the initial portion of the penile urethra. These compound tubuloalveolar mucous glands are similar to salivary glands. Under the influence of parasympathetic nerves, they secrete mucus into the urethra upon erotic arousal. Their function is to lubricate the urethra and the glans penis with *preseminal fluid* before ejaculation takes place. The female equivalents of the Cowper's glands are the Bartholin's glands (great vestibular glands).

The structure of the penis is discussed together with the mechanism of erection.

Spermatogenesis

Spermatogenesis Is a Sertoli Cell-Supported Process of Mitotic Proliferation, Meiosis, and Maturation of Spermatogonia to Produce and Release Spermatozoa The gametogenesis normally occurring in *postpubertal* males is termed *spermatogenesis.* Spermatogenesis takes place in the convoluted seminiferous tubules. The tubular wall consists of *germ cells* associated with a simple columnar epithelium of *Sertoli cells* and surrounded by a basal lamina and a few layers of contractile *myoid cells,* whose function is to propel the tubular fluid by undulating peristaltic movement (see Fig. 13-1).

The Sertoli cells form the *blood-testis barrier,* which involves tight junctions and the expression of the P-glycoprotein (see also Chap. 4). Tight junctions are typically found near the apical surface of epithelial cells. Although in a geometric sense the Sertoli cell tight junctions are closer to the basal surface, in a functional sense they still demarcate the apical and basolateral plasma membrane surfaces. The space between adjacent Sertoli cells is divided by the tight junctions into an *abluminal* (away from the lumen) and a *luminal* (or adluminal [toward the lumen]) *compartment,* which are occupied by the various developmental stages of spermatogenesis. The premeiotic *spermatogonia* are found in the abluminal compartment bordered by the basal lamina of the seminiferous tubules. As the spermatogonia divide and detach from the basal lamina, tight junctions are organized at their basal aspect and dissolved at their apical aspect. Each *cohort* of cells derived from a single spermatogonium and entering meiosis remains interconnected by *cytoplasmic bridges* until the latest stage of spermiogenesis, when their excess cytoplasm becomes *collectively* shed. The cytoplasmic bridges assure synchronous development of spermatozoa in any patchlike area of the seminiferous tubules. Postmeiotic cells (*spermatocytes, spermatids* and *spermatozoa*), which express "foreign" antigenic epitopes, are located only in the luminal compartment, where they are inaccessible for immunologic surveillance.

Spermatogenesis involves four key elements:

- *Spermatocytogenesis* is the proliferation of spermatogonia by mitosis. The proliferation of the stem cells, known as *type A dark (Ad) spermatogonia*, yields type Ad, Ap (pale) and *type B spermatogonia*. *Preleptotene primary spermatocytes* arise by division of type B spermatogonia, which heralds the second phase of spermatogenesis.
- *Meiosis* is the process whereby the four chromatids (two for each chromosome) present in the diploid primary spermatocytes segregate into four daughter cells (*spermatids*) by two successive divisions. The first division (i.e., that of the primary spermatocytes) reduces the chromosome number to a haploid set ($n = 23$), the second division (i.e., that of the *secondary spermatocytes*) results in the separation of the *sister chromatids*.
- *Spermiogenesis* is the maturation of spermatids into *spermatozoa* that takes place in the apical folds of the plasma membrane of Sertoli cells (see details below).
- *Spermiation* is the release of spermatozoa from their attachment to Sertoli cells.

The process of spermatogenesis from spermatogonia to spermiation takes place over a period of 64 to 74 days. Based on the cross-sectional appearance of the seminiferous epithelium, six stages of its spermatogenic cycle can be distinguished (Fig. 13-9).

The Process of Spermiogenesis Is Characterized by a Progressive Condensation of the Nuclear Chromatin Structure, the Elongation of the Nucleus, and the Development of the Acrosome, Flagellum, and Mitochondrial Sheath   Throughout the process of spermiogenesis, the maturing spermatids are attached to the Sertoli cell membrane by specialized junctions. The process of spermiogenesis consists of four phases:

- The *Golgi phase* involves two major maturational events that determine the anterior and posterior poles of the developing spermatozoon:
    - The Golgi complex generates the *acrosomal vesicle*, which is a glycoprotein-rich membrane-cased organelle positioned near the nuclear envelope. Its position signals the future *anterior pole*.
    - The two centrioles (diplosome) of the spermatid migrate to the opposite side of the nucleus (*posterior pole*), and the distal

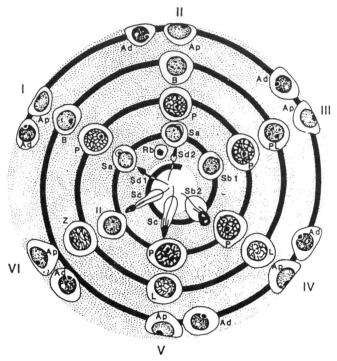

Figure 13-9. Schematic diagram of the constellations of developing germ cells based on which six stages of the spermatogenic cycle in the seminiferous tubule can be identified. The spiral indicates the time required from division of stem cells (dark type A spermatogonia [Ad]) to spermiation. The spiral portrays a total time of about 74 days, and each complete turn of the spiral indicates 16 days. The six constellations (labeled with Roman numerals) are due to the kinetics of the process. Note for example that type B spermatogonia (B) enter meiosis as preleptotene primary spermatocytes (PL) at stage III, but complete the first meiotic division 1-⅓ turns (~21–22 days) later as pachytene (P) primary spermatocytes at stage V. By this time, the next wave of primary spermatocytes arrived to the leptotene stage of meiosis (L). Secondary spermatocytes (II) complete the second meiotic division within 8 hours; their short-lived nature is indicated by their single spot on the spiral time-line at stage VI. Ap, pale type A spermatogonia; Z, zygotene primary spermatocytes; S, spermatogonia at various stages of spermiogenesis. (*Source:* From Kerr JB: Functional cytology of the human testis. Bailliere's Clin Endocrinol Metab 6:235–250, 1992.)

centriole initiates the development of the tail as the *axonemal complex*.

• During the *cap phase*, the acrosomal vesicle flattens and spreads over the anterior half of the condensing nucleus as the *acrosomal cap*. The axonemal complex continues to grow.

• The *acrosome phase* starts with the repositioning of the spermatids. Up until this phase, the anterior pole of the spermatid was oriented toward the lumen of the seminiferous tubule, and now becomes deeply embedded into the membrane folds of the Sertoli cell with its anterior pole oriented toward the basal lamina. This provides space for the elongation of the *flagellum* (a modified cilium) developing from the axonemal complex.

- The proximal centriole attaches to the nucleus and grows nine coarse fibers that connect the nucleus with the flagellum. This structure developing from the proximal centriole is known as the *connecting piece* or *neck region*.
- The *acrosome* develops: the space between the juxtanuclear acrosomal cap and the anterior plasma membrane diminishes; the cytoplasm is displaced posteriorly.
- With the posteriorly placed cytoplasm, mitochondria migrate to form a *mitochondrial sheath* around the coarse fibers in the *middle piece* of the flagellum.
- The distal portion of the flagellum consists of the *principal piece* and the *end piece*.

- During the *maturation phase*, the excess cytoplasm of the interconnected spermatids is collectively shed and becomes phagocytosed by the Sertoli cells.

The spermatozoa thus acquire key elements for their function (Fig. 13-10):

- *Haploid, supercoiled chromatin.* Half of the cells carry the X, the other half carry the Y sex chromosome. Unlike most somatic cells, gametes have a heterogenous genome due to meiotic crossing over and the random assignment of maternal and paternal chromosomes to each gamete.
- *Acrosome*, which contains enzymes necessary for the penetration of cervical mucus, the mucoid component of the corona radiata, and the zona pellucida of the oocyte.
- *Flagellum*, which provides active, fast, and independent movement.
- *Mitochondria*, which form a sheath in the neck region and provide adenosine triphosphate (ATP) for the flagellar movement. The GLUT5 transporter in the cell membrane of spermatozoa enables fructose uptake from semen upon ejaculation (see also Chap. 9).

Spermatogenesis Is Regulated by FSH, Testosterone, and Locally Acting Humoral Factors Spermatogenesis is a gonadotropin-dependent process. FSH stimulates spermatogenesis only indirectly: the sole target of FSH is the Sertoli cell which (among other responses) secretes ABP into the lumen of the seminiferous tubules. LH stimulates testosterone secretion by the Leydig cells. The concentration of testosterone in the testis is about 200-fold higher than in plasma; this is due to the local production and the testosterone-sequestering action of ABP. Testosterone stimulates spermatogenesis in part via an androgen receptor-mediated action on the Sertoli cells. *The locally high concentration of testosterone is a mandatory requirement of normal spermatogenesis.* An unusual and important feature is that the high local testosterone concentration does not suppress androgen receptor expression in the Sertoli cells, the peritubular myoid cells, or the Leydig cells. One of the functions of ABP is to mediate the membrane-receptor

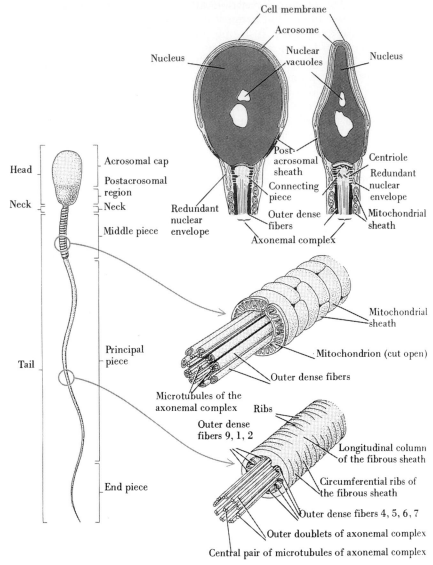

Figure 13-10. Structural features of the human spermatozoon. The regions of the spermatozoon are indicated on the left. Key features of the head (viewed in its major and minor dimensions), the middle piece and the principal piece are illustrated on the right. Note that the cell membrane covering the middle and principal pieces is not shown. (*Source:* Fig. 2-11, p 646 in Ross MH et al: *Histology. A Text and Atlas*, 3rd ed. Baltimore, Williams & Wilkins, 1995.)

(nongenomic) actions of testosterone, which include an increased protein secretory activity by spermatocytes but no effect on spermatids. Because the germ cells do not express androgen receptors, this effect is distinct from that involved in benign prostatic hypertrophy (see Fig. 13-6).

FSH stimulates the *proliferation* as well as the *secretory activity* of the Sertoli cells. The Sertoli cells secrete *inhibin B*, an inhibitor of pituitary FSH-β synthesis. Inhibin and the structurally related activin (see Regulation of the Gonadotropin–Gonad Axis in Postpubertal Males) have important local actions. *Inhibin antagonizes the proliferative action of FSH on the Sertoli cells*, thereby limiting the FSH-induced growth of the seminiferous tubules.

Additional locally acting factors mainly produced by the Sertoli and Leydig cells have been implicated in the regulation of spermatogenesis. One of the few identified factors that has a crucial role in supporting spermatogenesis is *transferrin*, which is secreted into the lumen of the seminiferous tubules by the Sertoli cells. Testicular transferrin acts as an iron shuttle system to transport ferric ions around the tight junctions to the germ cells inside the blood-testis barrier. The ferric ions are essential for the production of mitochondrial cytochromes. Spermatogenesis is defective in transferrin-deficient mutant mice. The concentration of seminal fluid transferrin is proportional to sperm production in humans.

The Normal Ejaculate Contains 80 to 120 Million Spermatozoa Per Milliliter and Has a Volume of 2 to 5 mL After 1 to 3 Days of Sexual Abstinence
Human semen is a white opalescent fluid with a pH close to that of plasma (pH 7.35 to 7.50). Most of its volume is the product of the seminal vesicle (60%) and the prostate (20 to 30%). These secretions counterbalance the acidic pH of the epididymal fluid.

Sperm count and *quality* are essential for fertility. After a sexual abstinence of at least 1 to 3 days, the normal sperm count is 80 to 120 $\times$ 10^6 per milliliter of semen, with up to 20% morphologically abnormal and/or immotile spermatozoa. Some reports suggest that in Western countries sperm quality (including sperm count, the proportion of normal spermatozoa, and motility indices) has declined during the past decades. Men with sperm counts below 20 $\times$ 10^6 per milliliter are infertile, and about 50% of men are infertile with sperm counts between 20 to 40 $\times$ 10^6 per milliliter.

Whereas the seminal vesicles and the prostate may relatively rapidly (within hours) replenish their secretory products and produce ejaculates with normal volume (2 to 5 mL), spermatogenesis is unable to replenish sperm counts as rapidly. Thus, with repeated ejaculations, sperm counts decline. In the clinical evaluation of sperm, a single sample with high sperm count and quality is sufficient for excluding gonadal dysfunction. In contrast, at least three samples collected at 2- to 3-month intervals are necessary to establish the diagnosis of gonadal dysfunction because spermatogenesis and passage through the epididymis require approximately 70 to 80 days.

This time allows recovery from conditions leading to temporary decrease in spermatogenesis such as nutritional factors and fever.

The absence of spermatozoa in semen is known as *azoospermia*. This condition has multiple etiologies, such as Klinefelter's syndrome, vanishing testes syndrome, ductal obstruction, or *Sertoli cell-only syndrome*. In Sertoli cell-only syndrome, mutations of genes encoding RNA-binding proteins have been implicated. An *azoospermia factor* (AZF) is present in the euchromatic region of the long arm of the Y-chromosome (Yq11), where clusters of two gene families, *RBM* and *DAZ*, have been identified.

- The *RNA-binding motif* (RBM) *genes RBM1, RBM2, RBM3* and the closely related *cold-inducible RNA-binding protein* (CIRP) are members of the *glycine-rich RNA-binding protein* (GRP) *family*. In contrast with RBMs, CIRP is autosomal (19p13.3). CIRP is an 18-kDa *cold-shock protein* that plays an essential role in cold-induced suppression of cell proliferation by prolonging the G1 phase of the cell cycle. In cultured somatic cells, the levels of CIRP mRNA and protein increase after a temperature downshift from 37°C to 32°C. Experimental overexpression of CIRP in cells cultured at 37°C decreases cell proliferation. In cultured human cells, RBM3 is also induced by cold stress. CIRP is expressed in all cell types of the seminiferous epithelium, except in elongated spermatids. *CIRP expression is downregulated in varicocele patients, and may be a major component of temperature-related infertility*. It has been proposed that CIRP is involved in diverting male germ cells from mitotic toward meiotic division.

- A cluster of *deleted in azoospermia* (DAZ) *genes* encode proteins that are found only in late spermatids and in sperm tails. A *DAZ-like autosomal* (DAZLA) also known as DAZ-homologue (DAZH) *gene* maps to 3p24. DAZLA/DAZH is also expressed in male germ cells. It has been proposed that the DAZ cluster on the Y chromosome arose from the autosomal DAZLA/DAZH during evolution. The autosomal localization of DAZLA/DAZH and CIRP may explain why the Y chromosome is involved in the pathogenesis of only a fraction of idiopathic male infertility.

Regulation and Function of the Penis

Erection   The size of the penis varies with the age, endocrine status, and erectile state. Penile length is measured on the dorsal aspect of the penis from the symphysis to the tip of the glans. In postpubertal men, the average *flaccid* length is 8.8 cm, the *stretched* length is 12.4 cm (10th percentile, 11 cm; 90th percentile, 16 cm) and the *erect* length is 12.9 cm. In contrast with the flaccid length, the stretched length is closely correlated with the erect length and is the better clinical indicator of genital development. Men with a stretched or erect length of <7.5 cm are candidates for penile lengthening.

At birth, the stretched dorsal penile length is normally >2.0 cm. Phallic growth is promoted by the GH–IGF-1 axis and testosterone both in utero and during pubertal growth. Accordingly, male patients with GH deficiency, GH resistance (Laron dwarfism), or hypogonadism present with *microphallus*. The microphallus of hypogonadal infants can be treated with hCG, which usually induces a rapid growth (up to 0.75 cm in 5 days) by increasing testosterone production. It is unknown what causes the cessation of penile growth after puberty; conflicting reports have been published regarding a decreased phallic expression of androgen receptors in postpubertal men.

On a cross section, the penis consists of three areas: two dorsal *corpora cavernosa* surrounded by a dense connective tissue layer (*tunica albuginea*), and a ventral *corpus spongiosum* that is devoid of a tunica albuginea.

- The *corpus spongiosum* houses the penile portion of the urethra, starts at *bulbus penis* at the inferior (superficial) surface of the urogenital diaphragm, and ends as the *glans*. The urethra normally opens at the tip of the glans. The ventrally positioned external orifice of the urethra is known as *hypospadias*, which is due to incomplete fusion of the urogenital folds (see Intrauterine Sexual Development).
- Each *corpus cavernosum* takes its origin from the pubic bone as the *crus penis*; its distal end is covered by the glans.

The corpora cavernosa and the corpus spongiosum consist of sinusoid systems lined by endothelial cells. Blood enters the sinusoids from the centrally positioned *helicine arteries* (branches of the *profunda penis* artery). Erection depends on the increased arterial blood flow into the corpora cavernosa of the penis. The necessary flow to provoke erection ranges between 80 and 120 mL/min. During erection, the corpora cavernosa become enlarged rigid columns, whereas the corpus spongiosum (including the glans) enlarges but remains pliable. This difference prevents compression of the urethra and permits the passage of semen during ejaculation. The rigidity of the erect corpora cavernosa is related to the increased influx of blood, the presence of the tunica albuginea, and veno-occlusion. Venous blood is primarily drained from the *subtunical venous plexus* (positioned on the *inner* surface of the tunica albuginea) by the *emissary veins* that traverse the tunica albuginea *at an angle*. The sudden influx of blood into the sinusoids has an effect comparable to inflating a tire with air. The *subtunical venous plexus* becomes pressed against the tunica albuginea and the emissary veins become compressed within the tinuca albuginea, which result in decreased venous efflux. The congestion of blood maintains erection.

Erection is induced by a *nitric oxide* (NO) mechanism (see also in Chap. 5). *Neuronal type NO synthase* (NOS) is expressed by the *parasympathetic nervi erigentes* under the stimulatory influence of testosterone. The nerves reach the penis escorting the profunda penis artery within the internal pudendal neurovascular bundle. When action potentials reach the axon terminals, NOS is activated by the influx of Ca^{2+}, and NO diffuses from inside the axon to the cytoplasm of neighboring vascular smooth muscle cells. This mechanism is similar to the endothelium-dependent vasorelaxation induced by acetylcholine (see Fig. 5-7) except that a distinct NOS isoenzyme is involved, which resides within the axon rather than the endothelium. NO activates the soluble guanylyl cyclase, and the increased cytoplasmic cyclic GMP concentration provokes smooth muscle relaxation, i.e., vasodilatation. Cyclic GMP causes vasorelaxation by several mechanisms that involve decreasing cytoplasmic concentration of Ca^{2+}, dephosphorylation of light chain myosin (the target of the contractile action of Ca^{2+}), and opening K^+-channels. *Sildenafil citrate* (Viagra) enhances (rather than causes) erection by inhibiting the degradation of cyclic GMP by type 5 cyclic phosphodiesterase (see Chap. 6). The parasympathetic nervi erigentes also synthesize vasoactive intestinal peptide (VIP), a potent vasodilatator agent, as a neurotransmitter. The physiologic role of VIP in erection is uncertain.

The preganglionic fibers of the erectile parasympathetic nerves originate from the sacral plexus (S_{2-4}). The preganglionic nerves receive input from penile mechanoreceptors as a spinal reflex arch and from corticospinal fibers that mediate *psychosexual* activation of the erectile mechanism, including *sleep-associated* (also known as nocturnal) *penile tumescence*, which occurs 4 to 8 times each night. The penile mechanoreceptors also send signals through the spinal cord to cortical sensory areas.

Alpha adrenergic sympathetic activation, such as stress, is an inhibitor of erection due to its vasoconstrictor effect on the helicine arteries. *Because ejaculation involves activation of sympathetic nerves, ejaculation usually results in the physiologic termination of erection*. For this reason, premature ejaculation is often perceived as an erectile dysfunction.

The regulation of bulbourethral gland secretions involves parasympathetic mechanisms. Preseminal fluid appears in the urethra during erection, usually when it is associated with erotic arousal.

Androgens enhance libido, the frequency of sexual acts, and sleep-associated erections. Its involvement in erections produced by erotic images or situations shows significant variations among subjects. Although postpubertal castration decreases libido and spontaneous erectile function, erotic images may continue to produce erections sufficient for intercourse. It is noteworthy that erotic images provoke physiologic sexual arousal irrespective of the subject's moral/ethical attitude toward viewing such images.

Erectile dysfunction (impotence) may have psychogenic and organic causes. *In contrast with organic erectile dysfunction, in psychogenic impotence the sleep-associated tumescence is preserved*. The organic causes of impotence include:

• Any endocrine disease that leads to decreased androgen production, such as Kallman syndrome, Klinefelter's syndrome, hyperprolactin-

emia, acromegaly, and hyper- and hypofunction of the thyroid or the adrenal glands.
- Cirrhosis of the liver via SHGB-mediated decrease in free testosterone and relative estrogen excess.
- Diabetic neuropathy by hyperglycemia-related activation of the polyol pathway. Other neuropathies may also be involved, such as multiple sclerosis.
- Drugs, mainly psychotropic agents and drugs used in the treatment of prostate cancer: estrogens, anti-androgens, 5α-reductase inhibitors, the GnRH agonist leuprolide, or progesterone. Several antihypertensive drugs may interfere with sexual function, including erection.
- Systemic illnesses such as cancer, chronic renal failure or chronic obstructive pulmonary disease.

The Ejaculation of Semen   The ejaculation of semen is a spinal reflex involving two distinct components:

- *Emission* is the process of moving all components of semen into the urethra by a coordinated smooth muscle contraction of the vas deferens, seminal vesicle, and prostate under the influence of *sympathetic* noradrenergic nerves acting on α_1-adrenergic receptors. The preganglionic fibers originate from the upper lumbar segments of the spinal cord. The postganglionic fibers are located in the genital branch of the genitofemoral nerve, which escorts the vas deferens. The nerves of the seminal vesicle and the prostate are derived from the inferior hypogastric plexus.
- *Ejaculation proper* is the ejection of semen out of the urethra. This process involves the coordinated action of several skeletal muscles and the smooth muscle internal sphincter of the urethra. The urogenital diaphragm, the external sphincter of the urethra, and the *bulbospongiosus muscle* (a superficial perineal muscle surrounding the bulbus of the corpus spongiosum) perform involuntary reflexogenic rhythmic contractions. These contractions, together with the peristaltic waves of the vas deferens, result in fractionated ejections of semen. The simultaneous contraction of the internal urethral sphincter prevents retrograde ejaculation into the bladder.

The first fraction of ejaculated semen contains the highest sperm count, indicating that the contraction of the vas deferens slightly precedes that of the accessory glands, and that the secretions of the accessory glands tend to flush out the spermatozoa from the urethra.

Similar to erection, ejaculation is provoked by the stimulation of the penile mechanoreceptors. Partial inhibition of sensory nerve function may delay ejaculation. Thus, topical application of lidocain or similar local anesthetics may be used for the treatment of premature ejaculation. The stimulation of mechanoreceptors on the dorsal aspect of the penis tends to prolong erection before provoking ejaculation. In contrast, the stimulation of mechanoreceptors on the ventral aspect of the penis and the glans hastens the onset of ejaculation.

Ejaculation is normally accompanied by *orgasm*, a sensation of pleasure that is prolonged for about 1 minute by continued mechanical stimulation of the glans. Orgasm is followed by a *refractory period*, when males are incapable of orgasm. The mechanism of the refractory period is unknown. Orgasm is in part due to the release of endogenous opioids in the hypothalamus and the limbic system. Certain drugs may result in the dissociation of orgasm from ejaculation. Orgasm is associated with the release of several hormones such as oxytocin (OT) and prolactin (PRL) in both sexes.

Regulation of the Gonadotropin-Gonad Axis in Postpubertal Males

The regulation of testicular function includes the following main components:

- Hypothalamic GnRH also known as *luteinizing hormone-releasing hormone* (LHRH) acting on its cognate receptor expressed by pituitary gonadotroph cells.
- Pituitary gonadotropins: LH and FSH acting on their specific receptors expressed by Leydig and Sertoli cells, respectively.
- Testicular hormones:
  - steroid hormones: *testosterone* and its derivatives,
  - polypeptide hormones: *inhibin, activin, follistatin*. Note that activin and follistatin are important autocrine/paracrine regulators *also in the pituitary gland*.
- SHBG, a determinant of the free (biologically active) concentration of androgens and estrogens.

Various models describe the regulation of the hypothalamic–pituitary–gonad axis in both males and females. Due to conflicting findings, the existing models often differ in the details. In general terms, the regulation of testicular function can be summarized as follows (Fig. 13-11):

- Pulsatile hypothalamic GnRH stimulates the secretion of both FSH and LH from the anterior pituitary gland. The pulsatile secretion of GnRH and LH display high concordance. FSH pulsatility is less pronounced and may appear dissociated from the LH pulses.
- LH stimulates testosterone secretion from the Leydig cells. Free (non-SHBG-bound) testosterone exerts biologic actions (see Table 13-4), including a negative feedback on the secretion of gonadotropins both at the hypothalamic and the pituitary level. *Most of the negative feedback action is mediated by estrogen receptors after the local aromatization of testosterone into 17β-estradiol, but full negative feedback also requires androgen receptor-mediated action.*
  - *Progesterone* is not secreted in significant quantities in males, and thus (unlike in females) does not participate in the physiologic regulation of gonadotropin secretion. However, admin-

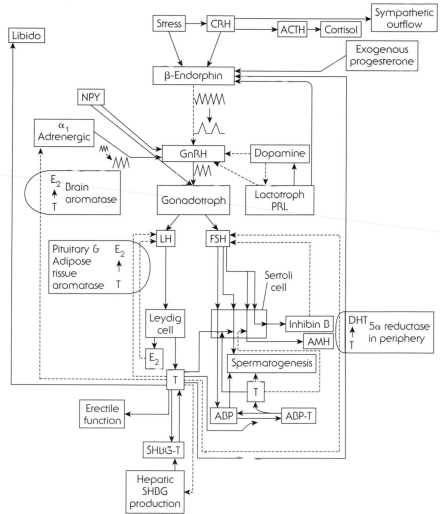

Figure 13-11. Postpubertal regulation of the GnRH-gonadotropin-testicular axis. Solid arrows indicate stimulation/increase; dashed arrows indicate inhibition/decrease. The bidirectional arrows show exchange between free and protein-bound testosterone. SHBG, sex-hormone-binding globulin; ABP, androgen-binding protein. Only free steroid hormones mediate genomic effects. The gonadotroph-Leydig cell axis involves luteinizing hormone (LH)-induced secretion of testosterone (T) and its feedback is mainly mediated by estradiol (E_2) generated by aromatase in the hypothalamus. The gonadotroph-Sertoli cell axis is based on follicle stimulating hormone (FSH)-induced secretion of inhibin B, which provides a feedback only at the pituitary gland. The gonadotroph-Sertoli cell axis receives input from Leydig cells: T acting on pituitary androgen receptors inhibits secretion of FSH. Note that gonadotropin-releasing hormone (GnRH) does not receive direct negative feedback. Instead, neurons regulating either GnRH pulse amplitude or pulse frequency (as shown near the arrows) receive the direct negative feedback input. Spermatogenesis is stimulated by FSH only indirectly via its actions on the Sertoli cell. T promotes spermatogenesis mainly by a similar Sertoli cell-mediated indirect action, and in part by a nongenomic action on spermatocytes. ABP maintains local levels of T about 200-fold higher than in the circulation. This is important for both spermatogenesis and the suppression of anti-Müllerian hormone (AMH). The mechanisms of suppressed GnRH-gonadotropin-gonad axis by excessive secretion of prolactin (PRL) is displayed. This mechanism is shared by excessive growth hormone (GH) secretion.

Table 13-6   Normal Values of the
Hormones of the Pituitary–Testicular Axis
in Adults[a]

Compound	Normal value
FSH	1.42–15.4 mIU/mL
LH	1.24–7.8 mIU/mL
Inhibin B	≈120 pg/mL
Testosterone	280–1100 ng/dL
Dihydrotestosterone	30–85 ng/dL
17β-estradiol	1.0–5.0 ng/dL
SHBG	59–472 μg/dL
Progesterone[b]	13–97 ng/dL
Urinary 17-ketosteroids	10–25 mg/d

[a] Except for 17-ketosteroids, all values refer to plasma/serum.
[b] Not involved in the physiologic regulation of the pituitary–testicular axis.
ABBREVIATIONS: FSH, follicle-stimulating hormone; LH, luteinizing hormone; SHBG, sex hormone-binding globulin.

istration of exogenous progesterone has a potent GnRH-inhibiting action just as in females (see Regulation of the Ovarian Cycle: The Hypothalamic–Pituitary–Ovarian Axis) and may be used for the suppression of the pituitary-testicular axis.

• FSH stimulates the Sertoli cells, which provide feedback action mainly by secreting inhibin B. Inhibin acts on the pituitary gonadotroph cell to selectively suppress FSH synthesis.

• Activin of mainly pituitary origin is a functional antagonist of inhibin and may selectively stimulate FSH. The biologic activity of activin is limited by follistatin of pituitary origin, which binds activin with a high affinity and prevents its binding to the activin receptor.

The normal values involved in the pituitary–testicular axis are shown in Table 13-6. We now discuss the components of this regulatory system in more detail.

GnRH Neurons Develop in the Olfactory Placode and Migrate to the Medial Basal Hypothalamus Under the Influence of Anosmin, a Cell Adhesion Protein Missing in Kallmann's Syndrome Patients   Two different forms of GnRH have been identified in humans (Box 13-4). The classic form of GnRH (now also called GnRH-I) is a decapeptide encoded by a gene on chromosome 8p21-8p11.2. The anatomic distribution of GnRH neurons displays significant species specificity. In humans, the GnRH neurons that project to the *median eminence* are mainly found in the *arcuate nucleus* of the hypothalamus. Fewer GnRH neurons are located in the *medial preoptic area* (the main location of GnRH neurons in rodents). During ontogeny, GnRH neurons develop in the *olfactory placode*, and

BOX 13-4   GnRH Genes in Humans

The GnRH (also referred to as GnRH-I) expressed from chromosome 8p21-p11.2 has the primary structure of *mammalian type* GnRH, and is a well-established regulator of reproductive function. A distinct gene on chromosome 20p13 encodes GnRH-II, a decapeptide of unknown physiologic function. The genomic and mRNA structures of GnRH-II parallel those of GnRH-I. Outside the brain, GnRH-II is expressed at up to thirtyfold higher levels than GnRH-I, particularly in the kidney, bone marrow, and prostate. In the brain of rhesus monkeys, GnRH-II mRNA is expressed mainly in the midbrain, hippocampus and discrete nuclei of the hypothalamus, including the suprachiasmatic, supraoptic, paraventricular and arcuate nuclei.

migrate via the olfactory bulb to their final destination under the influence of anosmin, the protein product of the *KAL* gene (chromosome Xp22.3). *Anosmin* is a 680-amino-acid cell surface-attached glycoprotein homologous with the family of *neural cell adhesion molecules* (N-CAMs). Anosmin regulates the migration of GnRH cells as well as the axons of the olfactory epithelium, including those originating from the *vomeronasal organ* (i.e., the pheromone-sensing olfactory area, see Regulation of the Ovarian Cycle: The Hypothalamic–Pituitary–Ovarian Axis). Deletions of the *KAL* gene result in *Kallmann syndrome*, an X-linked GnRH-deficient *hypogonadotrophic hypogonadism* associated with anosmia (absence of the sense of smell). The condition mainly affects males but cases of Kallman syndrome in females have also been reported. In a significant portion of reported cases, Kallmann syndrome is associated with *unilateral renal agenesis* and cerebellar dysfunction (nystagmus, ataxia, and/or mirror movements) probably reflecting the lost local actions of anosmin at these sites. A cluster of genes is found on Xp22.3 (next to the pseudoautosomal region), including the *chondrodystrophia punctata*, *steroid sulfatase* and *KAL* genes. The close apposition explains the association between Kallman syndrome, *X-linked ichthyosis* (absence of steroid sulfatase; see The Endocrine Physiology of the Pregnant Woman and the Fetoplacental Unit) and chondrodystrophia punctata.

The GnRH Pulse Generator Is Modulated by Hypothalamic Neurons and Peripheral Hormones   The GnRH neurons have an *intrinsic* rhythmic activity referred to as the *GnRH pulse generator*, which assures pulsatile secretion of GnRH into the pituitary portal circulation. In postpubertal men, the GnRH and GnRH-driven LH pulses occur with a period time of 90 to 140 min. Hormones modulating the *frequency* of pulsatile LH secretion by definition act at the hypothalamic level. Hormones modulating the *amplitude* of LH pulses may act either at the hypothalamic and/or the pituitary level; their site of action is problematic to ascertain in human studies.

Altered pituitary LH release in response to a fixed GnRH challenge indicates a pituitary site of action.

GnRH activity is modulated by stimulatory and inhibitory neurons (see Fig. 13-11):

- *Stimulatory input* to the pulsatile GnRH release are provided by *neuropeptide Y* (NPY, a neurotransmitter related to pancreatic polypeptide) and *noradrenergic neurons* acting on α_1-*adrenergic* receptors. The release of NPY and norepinephrine (NE) is intrinsically pulsatile; their pulses either precede or occur simultaneously with GnRH pulses. Centrally administered antagonists of NPY and NE suppress GnRH pulses in primates indicating that these transmitters may either entrain or override the intrinsic rhythm of GnRH neurons.
  - *Inhibitory input* to the GnRH neurons is provided by
    - *GABAergic neurons* acting on $GABA_A$ receptors. The *tonic* inhibitory action of these GABAergic neurons is involved in suppressing gonadotropin secretion before puberty.
    - A subset of NPY neurons apparently inhibits GnRH release. The activity of these NPY neurons is inhibited by circulating leptin (see following).
    - POMC-positive neurons producing the opioid peptide β-endorphin. These neurons have been implicated in stress/CRH-mediated inhibition of gonadotropin secretion and the negative feedback action of androgens (DHT) and progesterone, which *decrease the frequency of GnRH pulses*. The negative feedback of estrogens does not involve the opioid pathway. Consistent with this, *estrogens decrease pulse frequency only if sufficient amounts of androgens (or progesterone) are present*.
    - *Dopaminergic* neurons.

Certain *circulating hormones* may influence the activity of GnRH neurons in the arcuate nucleus.

- The negative feedback action of *sex steroids* is in part mediated by a hypothalamic action. Because the GnRH neurons lack the receptors for sexual steroids and progesterone, the negative feedback involves indirect mechanisms. As pointed out, the negative feedback of androgens is mainly mediated via estrogen receptors after local aromatization.
  - Stimulation of *estrogen* receptors decreases the *pulse amplitude* of GnRH. The reports on the effect of estrogens on the pulse frequency are conflicting. It appears that *in the presence of androgens (or progesterone)*, estrogens decrease GnRH pulse frequency (see above). *Clomiphene citrate* (an estrogen antagonist used for *ovulation induction*) increases both the frequency and amplitude of LH pulses in both sexes, albeit its effect on pulse frequency in females is inconsistent. The pulse amplitude is primarily suppressed via inhibiting the *noradrenergic* input to GnRH.

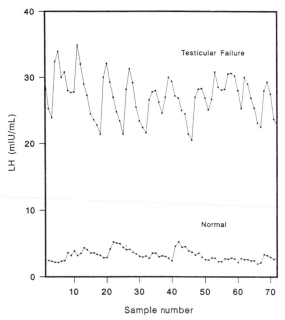

Figure 13-12.   LH levels in serum samples drawn every 10 minutes for 12 hours beginning at 8:00 A.M. in a normal 21-year-old man and in a 35-year-old man with bilateral cryptorchidism. The cryptorchidism led to testicular failure, and loss of negative feedback: note the increased pulse amplitude as well as pulse frequency. The high-amplitude pulses start from an elevated baseline. (*Source:* Fig. 131-11, p 2387 in Winters SJ: Clinical disorders of the testis, in De Groot LJ (ed): *Endocrinology,* 3rd ed., Philadelphia, Saunders, 1995.)

- *Progesterone* (which is *physiologically* relevant only in females), and DHT (which is *physiologically* relevant only in males), mainly exert their hypothalamic negative feedback action via endogenous opioids by decreasing the *frequency* (but not the amplitude) of GnRH pulses.

Removal of sex steroid feedback by castration increases the frequency and the amplitude of LH pulses (Fig. 13-12). The increased amplitude of LH pulses in castrated individuals also involves enhanced pituitary responses to fixed quanta of GnRH.

- High levels of PRL and GH (cross-reacting on PRL receptors) inhibit GnRH secretion. Thus, *hyperprolactinemia and acromegaly may cause amenorrhea in women and hypogonadism/impotence in men.* Three mechanisms have been identified: direct action of PRL on GnRH neurons and indirect inhibition of GnRH via the release of either dopamine or opioids. In women, these mechanisms are involved in the suppression of GnRH and the menstrual cycle during pregnancy (in part by PRL, in part by placental lactogens) and by PRL during lactation.

- *Leptin* is an adipose tissue-derived hormone that signals the state of nutrition and energy (lipid) reserves to the hypothalamus. Leptin is a required, albeit in itself an insufficient, positive signal of GnRH secretion, which serves as a metabolic gate to the reproductive system. The leptin

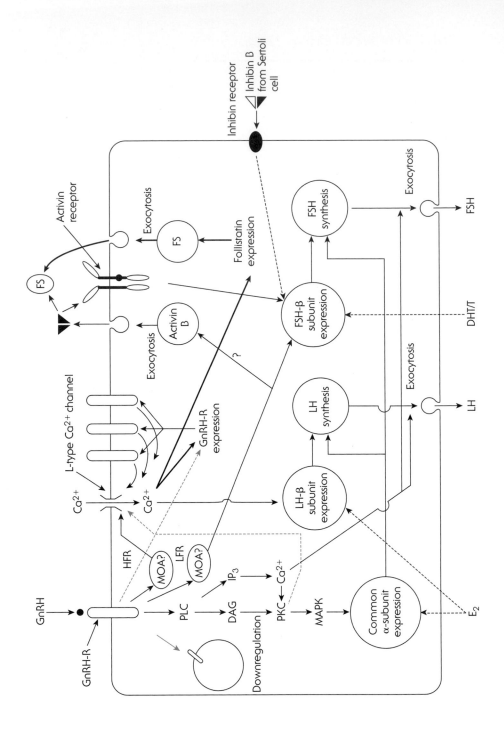

mechanism involves the GnRH-inhibiting subset of NPY neurons. *Leptin assures that the energy-demanding reproductive function proceeds only if adequate energy stores are available.* Commencement of puberty requires a minimal level of adiposity and the associated increase in plasma leptin levels. After puberty, when lipid stores are severely depleted (e.g., in certain athletes), the decrease in leptin shuts down reproductive function via GnRH.

The GnRH Receptors of Pituitary Gonadotrophs Are Rapidly and Extensively Dowregulated/Desensitized by Continuous Exposure to GnRH

Both the N- and C-termini of GnRH decapeptide are involved in receptor binding. This is due to a β-turn in the secondary structure of GnRH, which creates a hairpin loop bringing the two termini in close proximity. In response to GnRH pulses, the GnRH receptors are activated, leading to cosecretion of *LH* and *FSH* by pituitary gonadotroph cells. GnRH pulses stimulate both the *release* and the *biosynthesis* of gonadotropins.

GnRH acts on the *GnRH-receptors* encoded by chromosome 4q13.2-13.3. Several *cis acting elements* have been identified in the GnRH receptor gene that regulate its expression, including AP-1 sites and response element sequences for glucocorticoid, progesterone, thyroid hormones, and CREB (cyclic AMP response element binding protein). The GnRH receptor is a member of the G-protein-linked heptahelical transmembrane receptor family. The GnRH receptor is coupled with $G\alpha_{q/11}$, and activates the *PLC-β pathway*, which involves IP_3-Ca^{2+} and DAG-PKC-MAP kinase (Fig. 13-13). The activation of GnRH receptors results in the opening of *L-type (voltage-gated) Ca^{2+}-channels* and an influx of *extracellular* Ca^{2+}. The increased intracellular Ca^{2+} is essential for the exocytosis of secretory granules, that is, the *release* of gonadotropins. The ratio of LH and FSH within the secretory granules is determined by the differential regulation of their biosynthesis (see under next heading on p. 496).

GnRH or its long-acting *agonist* peptide analogues (such as *leuprolide*) *inhibit* the secretion of gonadotropins when administered in a *continuous* (as opposed to pulsatile) manner. The inhibitory action is due to *receptor*

Figure 13-13. Differential regulation of luteinizing hormone (LH) and follicle stimulating hormone (FSH) in the gonadotroph cell. Solid arrows indicate stimulation/increase; dashed arrows indicate inhibition/decrease. The effects of continuous exposure to gonadotropin-releasing hormone (GnRH) are shown in color. The precise mechanism of action (MOA) of high frequency (HFR; 1/hour) and low frequency (LFR; 1 per 3–4 hours) GnRH pulses are uncertain. HFR GnRH pulses activate L-type Ca^{2+}-channels, induce preferential expression of the LH-β subunit, increase GnRH receptor (GnRH-R) expression/numbers, and stimulate follistatin (FS). The increased GnRH-R numbers lead to favored production of LH over FSH, increased GnRH-sensitivity and responsiveness, and amplify the LH pulse amplitude. Activin B is an autocrine positive regulator of the FSH-β subunit; its action can be prevented by autocrine FS (a competitive binder of activin) and antagonized by Sertoli cell-derived inhibin B. The expression of the gonadotropin subunits is inhibited by sexual steroids. Note that in reality LH and FSH molecules are packaged together in the secretory vesicles. PLC, phospholipase C; PKC, protein kinase C; DAG, diacylglycerol; MAPK, mitogen activated protein kinase; T, testosterone; DHT, dihydroT; E_2, estradiol.

downregulation (internalization) and *desensitization.* GnRH receptor desensitization involves

- the inhibition of the L-type Ca^{2+}-channels probably due to their PKC-mediated phosphorylation. This mechanism explains in part why the biosynthesis of the LH β-subunit is preferentially inhibited upon prolonged GnRH receptor stimulation (see below).
- the inhibition of GnRH receptor gene expression.

The *GnRH test* is used in the evaluation of hypothalamic–pituitary–gonad axis. An acute challenge with an intravenous GnRH bolus injection (100 μg over 15 seconds) results in an age- and sex-dependent gonadotropin response. The normal response in adult men includes a more rapid and larger increase of LH and a delayed FSH increase with lower amplitude.

The Biosynthesis of LH and FSH Is Regulated Differentially by the Frequency of GnRH Pulses, Activin, Follistatin, Inhibin, and Sex Steroids

The pituitary gonadotropins are glycoprotein hormones structurally similar to thyroid-stimulating hormone (TSH) and hCG. As such, they share a *common α subunit* (localized on chromosome 6), and have *hormone-specific β-subunits* (see Chap. 10). Although the α-subunit is required for receptor binding, the β-subunit provides the receptor-specificity. The β-subunit of FSH is localized on chromosome 11. A single LH β-subunit and several highly homologous hCG β-subunit genes and pseudogenes are localized on chromosome 19. The β-subunits of LH and hCG recognize the same LH-receptor. Nevertheless antibodies distinguish the epitopes of the hCG and LH β-subunits (Box 13-5). The expression of the α-subunit gene is under multihormonal control, which varies in a cell type-specific manner in pituitary gonadotropes, thyrotropes, and the placenta, and is coordinated with the expression of different β-subunit genes. The expression of the α-subunit gene in the pituitary gonadotroph is stimulated by GnRH, inhibited by estrogens, and remains unaffected by a direct thyroid hormone action. The GnRH postreceptor signaling mechanisms exert a differential impact on the expression of the α- and β-subunit genes (see Fig. 13-13). The activation of the

- DAG-PKC-MAP kinase pathway selectively induces the expression of the *common α-subunit* gene in gonadotrophs.
- L-type (voltage-gated) Ca^{2+}-channels results in a selective expression of the *LH-β* subunit.

The molar ratio of LH and FSH in the secretory granules of the gonadotrophs is variable. This is achieved by the differential regulation of the biosynthesis of the β-subunits of LH and FSH. The frequency of the GnRH pulses has a differential effect on LH and FSH:

BOX 13-5   β-Subunit-Specific Immunoassay for the Detection of hCG

Absence of menses in women with previously established menstrual cycle is known as *secondary amenorrhea*. (*Primary amenorrhea* is diagnosed in a 16-year-old or older female, who never had a menstrual bleeding [see Table 13-9]. Note that the terms "primary" and "secondary" in this developmental setting are used in a context different from the one referring to the site in a regulatory system, such as the term "primary hypothyroidism.") The most prevalent causes of secondary amenorrhea are pregnancy and (typically after the age of 45 to 52 years) menopause. Both conditions are accompanied by increased concentration of LH-like biologic activity in urine. An outdated pregnancy test relied on the demonstration of this activity: male frogs released sperm upon injection with urine obtained from a pregnant woman. However, the test was relatively insensitive, and did not help the differential diagnosis between pregnancy and menopause. The immunologic demonstration of β-hCG in urine or plasma circumvents both problems. Measurements of β-hCG in postpartum women are essential in the diagnosis of *choriocarcinoma*.

In men, measurement of β-hCG is useful in the diagnosis and monitoring of certain testicular malignancies: all cases of *choriocarcinoma*, about 50% of *teratocarcinoma* and 5 to 10% of *seminoma* cases test positive for hCG. In *infantile embryonic carcinoma* (a yolk sac tumor of the testis usually seen in children under 3 years of age) another pregnancy-associated protein, *alpha fetoprotein* (AFP), appears in the plasma of most patients.

- FSH β gene expression is highest when gonadotrophs are stimulated by *low-frequency* pulses of GnRH, becomes relatively suppressed when GnRH is applied at higher frequencies, and absolutely suppressed upon continuous exposure to GnRH. *Activin*, a member of the TGF-β family, is a dimeric protein closely related to inhibin (see page 500). *Activin B* by an autocrine mechanism increases the concentration of FSH-β (but not LH-β) mRNA in the gonadotroph cells. Rodent experiments suggest that the higher GnRH pulse frequencies induce the production of pituitary *follistatin,* which binds activin and prevents its FSH-stimulating action.

- The LH-β gene is stimulated when GnRH is applied at higher frequencies and amplitudes. Because sexual steroids (mainly androgens and, in females, progesterone) inhibit the frequency of GnRH pulses, their *hypothalamic* feedback is a more effective suppressor of LH than FSH secretion. In addition, the LH-β gene is suppressed by a direct pituitary action of estrogens. Testosterone provides an *estradiol-mediated* physiologic feedback suppression of LH secretion in men. The main site of conversion by aromatase is presumed to be the pituitary gland, although systemic levels of estradiol (mainly determined by adipose tissue) appear to be sufficient to inhibit LH secretion by a pituitary action.

The mechanisms involved in the differential stimulation of FSH and LH by GnRH pulse frequency are only partially understood. GnRH receptor expression is upregulated at higher GnRH pulse frequencies. When GnRH receptor concentration in the plasma membrane is increased, LH is preferentially synthesized over FSH in response to GnRH. In addition to the GnRH pulse frequency, additional mechanisms are involved in modulating the FSH/LH ratio in the secretory granules:

- The inhibin/activin system is the main regulator of FSH-β expression. The action of pituitary activin B and follistatin as autocrine/paracrine regulators has been discussed. *Inhibin B*, a product of the testicular Sertoli cells delivered to the pituitary gonadotrophs by blood plasma, selectively inhibits the expression of FSH-β by a direct action. Because secretion of inhibin B is stimulated by FSH, this mechanism represents a separate, FSH-specific feedback loop (Fig. 13-11). In castrated men and in Klinefelter's syndrome patients whose Sertoli cell population is progressively destroyed, circulating levels of FSH are elevated. Because the Leydig cell population is less affected than the Sertoli cells in Klinefelter's syndrome, FSH becomes disproportionately more elevated than LH. The disproportionate increase is in part due to the different half-lives of LH and FSH (see following).
- *Testosterone* and/or DHT, by acting on androgen receptors of the pituitary gland, may suppress the expression of FSH-β.

Due to Its Shorter Half-Life, Plasma LH Displays a More Pulsatile Secretory Pattern than FSH   Under the influence of GnRH pulses, the pituitary gonadotropins are secreted in a pulsatile manner. LH and FSH circulate in plasma as free (unbound) hormones with initial half-lives of 30 min and 1 to 3 h, respectively. Within this range, the more heavily sialylated FSH has longer half-life but a decreased biologic activity. Due to its short half-life, plasma LH displays high-amplitude fluctuations ranging from very low to high concentrations. In contrast, plasma FSH levels are more stable and display lower amplitude fluctuations. Due to the difference in plasma half-lives and the variable FSH/LH ratio in the secretory vesicles, the secretory profiles of LH and FSH may appear dissociated in serially collected blood plasma samples.

Gonadotropins are used both in diagnostic tests and as therapeutic agents. Human recombinant FSH and LH have recently become available. The classic natural gonadotropins used in clinical practice are hCG (prepared from the urine of pregnant women) which is used as LH, and *human menopausal gonadotropin* (HMG, *menotropin*) which is used for its predominant FSH activity. The combination of HMG and hCG is used for the treatment of infertility in *hypogonadotropic hypogonadism* (Box 13-6). Cryptorchidism may be resolved by hCG treatment.

The Receptors of Gonadotropins Are Closely Related to Each Other and to the Receptor of TSH   The FSH and two LH receptor genes are

BOX 13-6   Exogenously Administered Androgens and Fertility

Testosterone is a required stimulatory factor of spermatogenesis. As discussed earlier, its biologic action mandates very high concentrations *in the seminiferous tubules,* which are provided by the local production of testosterone by Leydig cells and the presence of Sertoli cell-derived ABP. When testosterone is administered exogenously (e.g., as an intramuscular depot injection) as a treatment of hypogonadism, the dosage is aimed at achieving normal *systemic* levels of testosterone. This will normalize secondary sexual characteristics (hair, libido, erectile function, volume of the ejaculate) and exert a negative feedback on pituitary LH and FSH secretion. Under these circumstances, Leydig cells will not provide the necessary high local concentration of testosterone and Sertoli cells do not receive the appropriate stimulation by FSH. Thus, whereas sexual performance is normalized by testosterone, fertility is not achieved. Exogenous testosterone may therefore be used as a male contraceptive. Its usage is not widespread because of its negative impact on lipoprotein metabolism. Administration of decreased doses of testosterone combined with progesterone has been advocated as an alternative. Due to the negative feedback on the hypothalamic–pituitary–gonad axis, body builders who abuse *anabolic steroids* (chemically modified androgens) may have decreased fertility and, due to decreased androgenic activity, may experience erectile dysfunction.

   In the treatment of infertility, doses of testosterone that would increase systemic levels to the required testicular concentration are not feasible because of toxic side effects, such as *cholestatic hepatitis.*

all localized on chromosome 2p21, whereas the TSH-R gene is found on chromosome 14q31. These receptors are members of the heptahelical G-protein coupled receptor family and stimulate adenylyl cyclase activity via $G\alpha_s$.

   Postzygotic activating mutations of this G-protein subunit during embryonic development result in *McCune–Albright syndrome* (Chaps. 8 and Puberty in this chapter, see Fig. 13-51), which more often affects females and usually includes precocious puberty due to ligand-independent activation of both FSH and LH receptors. In females, activation of both receptors results in follicular maturation and increased hormone production.

   The activating mutation of the LH receptor, which is inherited in an autosomal dominant manner and affects segments of the receptor interacting with $G\alpha_s$, results in *male-limited familial precocious puberty* (*testotoxicosis*). The moderate ligand-independent activation of the postreceptor signaling cascade is sufficient to stimulate testosterone secretion by Leydig cells and cause precocious puberty. However, in the absence of FSH receptor stimulation and the resultant follicular growth, the ligand-independent

LH receptor stimulation is apparently insufficient to stimulate the secretion of ovarian steroids.

Loss-of-function mutations of either the FSH receptor or the FSH β-subunit result in infertility in both males and females; the presentation in females includes *primary amenorrhea* (see Table 13-9 in the section The Endometrial Cycle) indicating the mandatory involvement of FSH in follicular maturation. Males, however, do not present with hypogonadism because the LH–testosterone axis remains functional.

Members of the TGF-β Family Such as Inhibin, Activin, and Anti-Müllerian Hormone, and the Activin-Binding Protein Follistatin Play Essential Roles in Reproductive Function, the General Regulation of Mitogenesis and Morphogenesis   The Sertoli cells perform several hormonal functions:

- Sertoli cells produce hormones of the TGF-β family, which include
  - *Anti-Müllerian hormone* (AMH, also known as *Müllerian inhibitory hormone* [MIH]). AMH is secreted in utero and until about 8 to 10 years of age. The age-dependent termination of AMH secretion is related to the high local concentrations of testosterone in the seminiferous tubules; circulating levels of androgens are insufficient to suppress AMH. During puberty, intratubular levels of androgens increase to high levels before a major increase in systemic circulation occurs. The AMH-suppressing effect of androgens is so potent that it completely counteracts the AMH-stimulating effect of pubertally high levels of FSH. In patients with androgen insensitivity syndrome (androgen receptor mutation), plasma AMH levels do not decrease in early puberty but significantly increase due to the unopposed action of FSH. Sertoli cells during early development do not express androgen receptors; thus, testosterone produced by the fetal testis may masculinize the external genitalia without suppressing AMH production (see details in Intrauterine Sexual Development).
  - *inhibin*, an inhibitor of FSH secretion by a direct pituitary action.
  - *activin*, a locally acting hormone structurally related to inhibin and usually opposing inhibin's actions.

Except for inhibin, which acts both locally and also as a classic endocrine hormone, *the other hormones in this group act almost exclusively as local paracrine/autocrine regulators*.
- Sertoli cells secrete ABP into the lumen of the seminiferous tubules.

Inhibin is a disulfide-linked dimeric glycoprotein hormone that exists in two forms: a shared common α *subunit* is linked to one of two distinct β *subunits* (βA or βB). *Inhibin A* and *inhibin B* consist of α-βA and α-βB heterodimers, respectively. In addition to its function as a selective inhibitor of FSH-β expression, inhibin acts as a *tumor suppressor*. Inhibin α-knockout mice develop gonadal sex-cord stromal tumors (granulosa/Sertoli cell tumors) and adrenocortical tumors. An unusual feature of these adrenocortical tumors is that they often secrete estradiol.

Activins are either homodimers (βA-βA, βB-βB) or heterodimers (βA-βB) of the β subunits. The β subunits display extensive sequence homology with TGF-β. The α subunit, which is unique to inhibins, is encoded by chromosome 2q33-qter. The β subunits, which are shared by inhibins and activins, are localized on chromosomes 2cen-q13 (βB) and 7p15-p14 (βA).

Activins function as locally acting stimulators of β-FSH expression in the pituitary gland, as *mitogens* and, similar to the related bone morphogenetic proteins, as *morphogens*. As members of the TGF-β family, the action of acitivins involves two types of single membrane-spanning receptor serine/threonine kinases (see Chap. 5). The high-affinity ligand-specific binding to a type II receptor is followed by the recruitment of type I receptors. The recruitment relies on low-affinity and less ligand-specific binding via the exposed subunit of the ligand; the ligand thus functions as a bridge leading to the formation of a receptor heterodimer. The phosphorylated type I receptor serves as a docking site and acts as the only transducer of the intracellular signaling cascade (see Fig. 5-6). The immunophilin *FKBP-12* (see insulin action in Chap. 9) interacts with the serine/threonine kinase domain of the type I receptor, and plays a key role in the downstream signal transduction events of activin and also other members of the TGF-β family. This might explain a shared biologic action of activins, insulin, and IGF-1R agonists: they all promote androgen production in various target cells, including the adrenal cortex, theca and Leydig cells.

- The type I receptors include *ActRI* (activin receptor I, also called *ALK-2*), *ActRIB* (ALK-4), and *ALK-1* (shared by activins and TGF-β), which are related to Alk 6, a bone morphogenetic protein receptor (see Chap. 8).
- Two subtypes of the type II receptors have been described: ActRII, which recognizes the βA subunit, and ActRIIB, which preferentially binds the βB subunit. ActRII, the main mediator of activin's reproductive effects, is expressed in the pituitary gland, testis (including germ cells), the epididymis/vas deferens, male accessory glands, ovary, and uterus.

Ligand-specific *inhibin receptors* have been identified in the pituitary gland and other tissues, and the cDNA of an inhibin receptor has recently been cloned from bovine pituitary glands. The inhibin receptor binds inhibin with high affinity (20–40 pM). Inhibin antagonizes the actions of activin in several target cells. Upon binding its ligand, the inhibin receptor associates with type I activin receptors (such as Alk2 and Alk4), thereby preventing the recruitment of type I receptors by ligand-activated type II or type IIB activin receptors. Inhibin receptors do not associate with type II or type IIB activin receptors. At least in vitro, inhibin may also antagonize activin by acting on activin receptors. Inhibin A binds with the ActRII with low affinity and, in case of inhibin excess, may compete with activin. Because ActRII-bound inhibin does not recruit type I receptors, the binding of inhibin A with ActRII may antagonize the biologic action of activin.

The biologic action of activin is modulated by *follistatin*. Mature follistatin is a single-chain protein that contains four contiguous domains; three of the domains are highly similar to each other, as well as to human epidermal growth factor and human pancreatic secretory trypsin inhibitor. Follistatin is a local regulator, whose plasma concentration is relatively steady in both sexes and does not change during the menstrual cycle.

- Follistatin was originally discovered as a substance that specifically inhibits FSH. Follistatin inhibits FSH secretion by binding activin and preventing activin from binding to its (type II) receptor (see Fig. 13-13).
- Follistatin interacts with the β-subunits of activins. Because inhibin also contains a β-subunit, follistatin also binds inhibin. However, inhibin binds to follistatin with a lower affinity. In addition, the α-subunit of inhibin remains exposed. These factors may explain why follistatin does not eliminate the biologic activity of inhibin.
- Under certain circumstances, *follistatin is required for the biologic activity of activins*. Follistatin may bind to cell surface heparan sulfate proteoglycan. This *cell-surface-associated follistatin* may *present* activin to type II activin receptors by a mechanism similar to the action of the type III TGF-β receptor (betaglycan). The role of follistatin as an activin-supporting entity has been demonstrated in knockout mice. Mice deficient in the subunit βA (and thus deficient in activin A, activin AB, and inhibin A) display a phenotype shared by follistatin-deficient mice: although they survive to term, they die within 24 h of birth due to severe, multiple craniofacial abnormalities, including cleft palate, absent lower incisors and absent vibrissae. These actions exemplify the morphogenic nature of activins.

THE FEMALE REPRODUCTIVE SYSTEM

Functional Anatomic Overview of the Female Reproductive System

OBJECTIVES

1. Discuss the gross anatomy and histology of the ovary. Describe the morphologic process of follicular maturation: define primordial, primary, secondary, tertiary, and Graafian follicles. Describe the fate of the follicles after ovulation.
2. Describe the anatomic components of the female genital tract: the oviduct, the uterus, and the vagina. Compare the corpus/fundus and the cervix of the uterus. Describe the layered structure of the uterus. Identify the anatomic

relationship of the ovary and the female genital tract with the peritoneum and the peritoneal cavity.

3. Discuss the female external genitalia.

The Ovary (Adnexum)

Gross Anatomy   The ovaries are found close to the lateral wall of the lesser pelvis at the angle formed by the *external* and *internal iliac arteries*, and *in close association with the ureter* separated from these structures by the parietal peritoneum (Fig. 13-14). The right ovary is usually in the immediate vicinity of the *appendix*. During development, the ovary reaches its final position by a descent that is more limited than that of the testis. The location of the ovary becomes variable in parous women.

Each ovary is an approximately 1-cm thick almond-shaped organ, with a length of 3 cm and a width of 1.5 cm. The ovary is an essentially *intraperitoneal* organ as indicated by its peritoneal doubling known as the *mesovarium*, which is found on the posterior aspect of the *broad ligament* of the uterus. The portion of the broad ligament that is superior to the attachment site of the mesovarium is the *mesosalpinx*, the peritoneal doubling that reaches the *Fallopian tube* (*uterine tube, oviduct, salpinx*). At the *line of Farré*, a thin white line that encircles the ovarian attachment site of the mesovarium, the mesothelial cover of the ovary is replaced by a simple cuboidal epithelium termed *germinal epithelium*. This term is a misnomer because the germinal epithelium is not the source of germ cells; instead, the *follicular epithelium* (see Fine Structure below) is derived from it during intrauterine development.

During intrauterine development, the *inferior pole* of the ovary is tied to the dermis of the labioscrotal folds (the future labia majora) by the *gubernaculum*. The interposition of the uterus divides the fibrous gubernaculum into the caudal *round ligament* of the uterus and the more cranial *ovarian ligament*.

The *suspensory ligament* is attached to the *superior pole* of the ovary. Nerves, blood, and lymphatic vessels reach the ovary through the suspensory ligament and the mesovarium. The ovarian vessels are homologous with those of the testis and follow the same course in the retroperitoneum. The *ovarian artery* divides into a direct *ovarian* and a *salpingeal branch*, each of those forming an anastomosis with similar branches derived from the *uterine artery*; unless ligations are placed properly, this anastomosis may become the source of life-threatening bleeding during ovariectomy.

Fine Structure   In prepubertal females, the surface of the ovary is smooth. Underneath the germinal epithelium, a dense connective tissue layer (*tunica albuginea*) is found, which is thinner, less organized, and mechanically weaker than its male counterpart. The tunica albuginea envelops the thick outer layer of the ovary known as the *cortex*, which *contains the ovarian follicles and their derivatives* embedded in a cell-rich connective tissue. The tunica albuginea and the cortex form a shell that surrounds a small *medulla*, which contains highly vascular loose connective tissue. At the hilus, which is found at the mesovarium, the cortex is missing; through the hilus the nerves and vessels of the ovary directly enter (or leave) the medulla. The medulla contains variable numbers of *hilar cells*, which produce limited quantities of testosterone. The hilar cells are the female equivalents of the Leydig cells and usually contain *Reinke's crystalloids*.

The details of follicular maturation as related to the regulation of the pituitary-gonad axis are discussed in Regulation of the Ovarian Cycle: The Hypothalamic–Pituitary–Ovarian Axis. The discussion here follows the general maturational events of a single follicle destined for ovulation (Figs. 13-

A

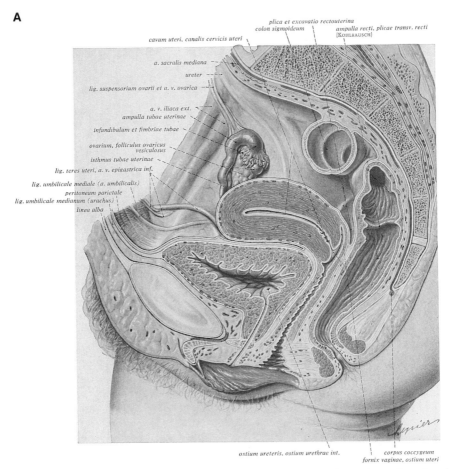

Figure 13-14. The anatomy of the female reproductive system. A. Sagittal pseudosectional diagram of the female urogenital system. B. Cutaway posterior view diagram of the internal female reproductive organs. (*Source:* A: modified from Fig. 303, p 229 and B from Fig. 300, p 226 in Ferner H, Straubesand J (eds): *Sobatta/Becher Atlas of Human Anatomy,* vol 2, 9th English ed., Urban & Schwarzenberg, 1975.)

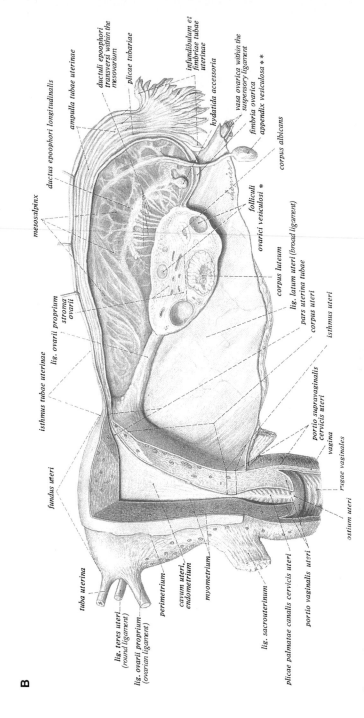

B

Figure 13-14. (Continued)

ductuli epoophori transversi within the mesovarium

ductus epoophori longitudinalis

ampulla tubae uterinae

plicae tubariae

infundibulum et fimbriae tubae uterinae

hydatida accessoria

vasa ovarica within the suspensory ligament

fimbria ovarica

appendix vesiculosa **

corpus albicans

mesosalpinx

folliculi ovarici vesiculosi *

corpus luteum

lig. latum uteri (broad ligament)

pars uterina tubae

corpus uteri

isthmus uteri

isthmus tubae uterinae

lig. ovarii proprium

stroma ovarii

fundus uteri

portio supravaginalis cervicis uteri

vagina

rugae vaginales

ostium uteri

tuba uterina

lig. teres uteri (round ligament)

lig. ovarii proprium (ovarian ligament)

perimetrium

cavum uteri, endometrium

myometrium

lig. sacrouterinum

plicae palmatae canalis cervicis uteri

portio vaginalis uteri

505

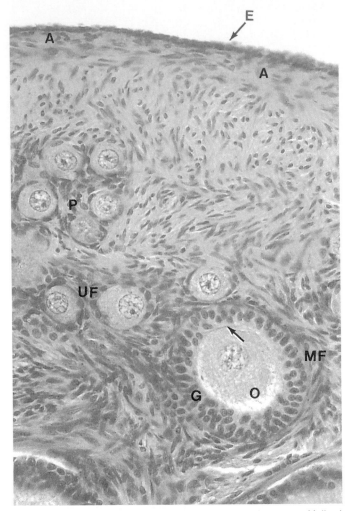

Figure 13-15. Ovarian histology displaying the early stages of follicular maturation. Primordial follicles (P) contain small primary oocytes covered by a single layer of squamous (flat) epithelium. Primary follicles (UF) have larger oocytes and the epithelium, which became cuboidal, is termed granulosa cell. Secondary follicles are also known as preantral follicles (MF). The oocyte is further enlarged, the granulosa cell layer is stratified, the basal lamina (BL) surrounding the granulosa layer is prominent, and the theca is already organized. E, the germinal epithelium covering the ovarian surface; A, Tunica albuginea; arrow, forming zona pellucida. Compare with Fig. 13-2 (antral follicle). [Fig. 19-3, p. 291 in Berman I: *Color Atlas of Histology,* Stamford, CT, Appleton & Lange, 1993.]

15 and 13-2). The diameters of the developing antral follicles can be determined by ultrasonography. This can be used in clinical practice for several purposes, such as evaluation for *polycystic ovary syndrome*, monitoring follicular development during *induced ovulation*, and in attempts to collect oocytes for *in vitro fertilization*. The terminology describing the morphologic stages

of follicular development and maturation is somewhat inconsistent in the literature. In this text the following definitions are used:

- The *primordial follicle* consists of a *primary oocyte* surrounded by a single layer of *squamous follicular epithelium*. The follicular epithelium (which later develops into *granulosa* cells) is separated from the ovarian stroma by a basement membrane, but the stroma does not yet form a recognizable *theca* around it. The growth of the follicle mandates the basal lamina/membrana limitans externa to be constantly remodeled. Primordial follicles are quiescent and are up to 40 μm in diameter. The diameter of the oocyte within the primordial follicle is 15 to 25 μm.
- The *primary follicle* is already engaged in follicular development. *The first sign of follicular development is the enlargement of the oocyte*, which grows from the original 15 to 25 μm to its maximum size of 80 to 100 μm in late secondary (preantral) follicles. The follicular epithelium assumes a *simple cuboidal* morphology and the cells are henceforth called *granulosa cells*. A *glycoprotein-rich* eosinophilic material known as the *zona pellucida* begins to be deposited between the oocyte and the granulosa cells. At this stage the ovarian stroma *begins* to organize as a fibroblast-like *theca*. These follicles are 40 to 100 μm in diameter.
- The *secondary* or *preantral follicles* develop when the granulosa cells further proliferate and become stratified. The granulosa cell layer (as a true epithelium) is *avascular*. Its basement membrane develops into a prominent *membrana limitans externa*. The granulosa cells are connected by well-developed *gap junctions*, which synchronize their function and allow the transfer of nutrients to the innermost layers. A definitive *theca* layer appears only when at least six layers of granulosa cells are present in the follicle; however, the *theca interna* and *externa* are not yet recognizable as separate layers. These follicles are 100 to 200 μm in diameter.
- The *tertiary follicles* are the antral follicles. The *antrum* (chamber) appears *within* the highly stratified granulosa cell layer and contains a hormone-rich *liquor folliculi* (follicular fluid). A number of granulosa cells are anchored in the zona pellucida and form the *corona radiata*. Outside the membrana limitans externa, the stroma is organized as concentric layers around the core of the follicle; this stromal component is termed *theca folliculi* (capsule, sheath). Unlike the epithelial granulosa layer, the mesenchymal theca is vascularized. Two cell types can be recognized in the theca:
    - the *theca interna* cells are characteristic steroid hormone-producing cells;
    - the *theca externa* cells are fibroblast-like cells, which display some contractility and are generally regarded as hormonally inactive.

The size of those tertiary follicles which are destined to regress without ovulation ranges between 200 μm and usually 5 mm (maximum 8 mm). The differential role of theca interna and granulosa cells in steroidogenesis is discussed in The Biosynthesis, Mechanism of Action and Metabolism of Sexual Steroids.

Some texts define the primary follicle as having the characteristics of both the primary and the secondary (preantral) follicles in the above description. In that terminology, the term *secondary follicle* means antral follicle, and the term *tertiary follicle* is not used. Thus, the terms primary and secondary follicles are ambiguous and their definitions must be sought when reading an unfamiliar text.

•   The single follicle in an ovarian cycle that can be recognized as the *dominant* follicle is called the *preovulatory* or *Graafian follicle*. This is typically the largest antral follicle at any given stage of the cycle. During the midfollicular phase, the dominant follicle can usually be identified by a diameter of 5 to 9 mm. By the time of ovulation, it usually reaches a diameter of 20 to 22 mm. In the Graafian follicle the oocyte with its corona radiata emerges into the antrum as the *cumulus oophorus* (ovum-carrying hill). As the time of ovulation approaches, hyaluronic acid accumulates in the interstitial space between the corona radiata cells and loosens the attachment of the cumulus oophorus with the surrounding granulosa cells. This process is known as *mucification*. At the time of ovulation, the base of the cumulus oophorus detaches from the underlying layer of granulosa cells and the oocyte is expelled with its corona radiata remaining attached to it. The preovulatory LH surge induces the completion of the first meiotic division of the oocyte, which yields the *secondary oocyte* and the first *polar body*, both of which are encased by the zona pellucida. The second meiotic division is prompted by fertilization (see Fertilization).

At the time of *ovulation*, which is induced by the preovulatory surge of LH, the entire wall of the follicle ruptures, including the (1) granulosa cell layers around the antrum, (2) membrana limitans externa, (3) theca interna, (4) theca externa, (5) general ovarian stroma, (6) tunica albuginea, and (7) germinal epithelium. This mechanism has several consequences:

•   The oocyte/corona radiata is expelled into the peritoneal cavity.
•   Due to its sensory innervation, the rupture of the tunica albuginea is painful.
•   After puberty, the originally smooth surface of the ovary becomes progressively scarred because ovulation repeatedly disrupts the tunica albuginea; the germinal epithelium regenerates and covers the sometimes deep fissures of the ovarian surface.
•   Between the membrana limitans externa and the germinal epithelium, all layers are vascularized. Thus, ovulation results in a small bleeding that fills the antral space previously occupied by the liquor folliculi. This modified follicle-containing clotted blood is known as the *corpus hemorrhagicum*.

The luteinization of the granulosa cells is *initiated* by the preovulatory LH surge. After ovulation, the granulosa lutein cells become vascularized, which leads to the *completion* of their luteinization process. The granulosa lutein cells, theca lutein cells, and the associated microvasculature form the corpus luteum. The function of these cells in steroidogenesis is discussed in The Biosynthesis, Mechanism of Action and Metabolism of Sexual Steroids. *The corpus luteum* has a defined life-span: unless rescued by stimulation of LH-receptors by hCG (i.e., in pregnancy), it *involutes and undergoes apoptosis in 14 ± 2 days after being formed.* When this happens, the cell debris is removed by macrophages, and the space occupied by the corpus luteum is filled with hormonally inactive fibrotic scar tissue: this is known as *corpus albicans* (white/glistening body). Eventually the corpus albicans is eliminated by degradation of the collagenous deposit.

The Female Genital Tract   The female genital tract consists of a pair of Fallopian tubes (oviducts), the uterus, and the vagina (see Fig. 13-14). Except for the lower two-thirds of the vagina, which is derived from the *urogenital sinus*, the female genital tract develops from the *Müllerian (para-mesonephric) ducts* (see details in Intrauterine Sexual Development). The Fallopian tube is intraperitoneal, the uterus is mainly intraperitoneal and in part *infra*peritoneal. The vagina is below the peritoneal sac.

The *Fallopian tubes* are 10- to 13-cm long visceral canals that develop from the *nonfused* (cranial) portion of the Müllerian duct. The Fallopian tube has four segments:

- The *infundibulum* is a funnel-shaped expansion of the abdominal end of the oviduct, which is surrounded by narrow irregular processes called *fimbriae*. The *ovarian fimbria* is attached to the ovary near the suspensory ligament. Due to their smooth muscle, the fimbriae are motile and may engulf the ovary at the time of ovulation, thereby aiding the attachment of the expelled ovum (covered with the corona radiata) to the inner surface of the Fallopian tube.
- The *ampulla* is the longest portion of oviduct. The highly folded mucosal surface of the ampulla is the usual site of fertilization.
- The *isthmus* is the narrowing of the Fallopian tube, which constitutes about one third of the length of the canal near the uterus. The folds of the oviduct diminish at the isthmus.
- The *intramural* (within the wall) *uterine part* is a short portion of the canal widening toward the uterine cavity, where it joins the uterus at the junction of the fundus and corpus.

The smooth muscle wall of the oviduct performs an active undulating movement. The mucosa of the oviduct is similar to that of the uterus. On occasion, implantation may take place in the oviduct (*ectopic pregnancy*). Neither the mucosa nor the space are sufficient for supporting normal development, and these tubal pregnancies abort amidst a rupture that may lead to life-threatening bleeding. The epithelial lining of the Fallopian tube contains *secretory* (peg) and *ciliated cells*. The active beating of cilia keeps a thin layer of mucous film flowing toward the vagina. This *mucous escalator* serves three major functions:

- keeps the mucosal lining germ-free by constant flushing;
- contributes to the orientation of the movement of spermatozoa, thereby aiding fertilization;
- carries the developing zygote (which is incapable of active movement) to its site of implantation.

The *uterus* is a modified oviduct, which (together with the upper one-third of the vagina) develops by the fusion of the caudal portion of the Müllerian ducts. Anatomically the uterus is an approximately pear-shaped organ, which has two main portions:

- The *corpus uteri* is the broader upper part of the uterus. The convex anterosuperior surface of the corpus between the joining oviducts is the *fundus*. The corpus surrounds the *uterine cavity*, a flat triangular space. The base of this triangle is the fundus, the downward-pointing tip of the triangle is the *internal orifice* of the cervical canal. The length of the corpus in nulliparous women is about 4.5 cm; in parous women, the corpus is longer (~5.5 cm).
- The *cervix uteri* is the lower, narrow cylindrical part of the uterus, which surrounds the *cervical canal*. The cervical canal is about 2.5 cm long both in nulliparous and parous women. Its *internal orifice* opens into the uterine cavity at the *isthmus uteri*. The cervix has two anatomic portions:
    - The *supravaginal portion* is cranial to the insertion of the vaginal fornix into the uterine cervix.
    - The *vaginal portion* (*portio vaginalis*) protrudes into the vagina. The *external orifice* of the cervical canal opens at the center of the vaginal portion; its shape varies with the parous state from round opening (nulliparous) to a transverse horizontal narrow slit (multiparous).

The *uterine cavity* is surrounded by three layers of the corpus and fundus of the uterus:

- *The endometrium* is the mucosal layer that consists of a simple columnar epithelium and an underlying connective tissue stroma (*lamina propria*). The simple tubular *uterine glands* span the entire thickness of the endometrium, and are lined by nonciliated as well as ciliated columnar epithelium identical with those of the surface. Unlike the cervical mucosa, the apical layers of the endometrium (*stratum functionale*) in the corpus/fundus region are shed during menstruation, leaving behind the *stratum basale,* a thin layer of lamina propria without surface epithelium and the blind ends of uterine glands. The stratum functionale is supplied by *spiral arteries* of the endometrium; the stratum basal receives a separate, parallel supply from the *basilar (straight) arteries*. The entire surface epithelium regenerates from the remnants of the glands, which explains the identical morphology of the glandular and surface epithelia. The endometrium is the site of implantation. Its involvement in the formation of the placenta is discussed in Implantation and the Placenta.
- The *myometrium* is the thickest layer of the uterine wall and consists of smooth muscle and vasculature. The enlargement of the uterus during pregnancy mainly involves *hypertrophy* of existing smooth muscle cells, but *hyperplasia* (proliferation of the smooth muscle cells) also contributes. This muscle is important in delivering the newborn. The permanent enlargement of the corpus in parous women is due to the incomplete postpartum involution of the myometrium. In older, especially multiparous women, the myometrium often contains benign smooth muscle tumors (*leiomyoma*). Be-

cause the blood vessels reach the endometrium via the myometrium, these tumors may cause irregular menstruation.

• The *perimetrium* is the connective tissue (within the broad ligament and the subserosal layer) and the associated mesothelium lining of the peritoneal cavity. The nerves, blood vessels, and lymphatics reach the uterus through the perimetrium mainly via the broad ligament. The arterial supply is provided by the *uterine artery*, a branch of the internal iliac artery.

The layers are modified in the *uterine cervix*.

• The *cervical mucosa* contains large, expanded branched glands. These glands produce the *cervical mucous plug* that is rich in hyaluronic acid and serves as a barrier against bacterial invasion. Because the acrosome of spermatozoa contains *hyaluronidase*, they can penetrate the mucous plug. Although the cervical mucosa is not shed at the time of menstruation, it shows important cycle-dependent functional changes that affect the amount and consistency of the cervical mucus, and influence fertility. The mucosal glands are sometimes obliterated leading to the development of *Nabothian cysts*, which are usually asymptomatic accidental findings in clinical practice. At the external orifice, the simple columnar epithelial lining of the cervical canal abruptly changes into the stratified squamous epithelium of the portio vaginalis uteri. The *Papanicolaou (Pap) smear* used in the screening for *cervical cancer* (a malignant tumor of the epithelium of the cervical canal probably caused by human papilloma virus) is taken from the external orifice, where shed cells of the cervical canal appear as a part of normal epithelial turnover.

• In lieu of the myometrial layer, the cervix has a thick dense connective tissue wall. This structure is important for parturition: contraction of smooth muscle would narrow the birth canal. Near parturition, the dense connective tissue is softened by the action of *relaxin* (see Box 13-11 in The Endocrine Physiology of the Pregnant Woman and the Fetoplacental Unit). This phenomenon is known as *cervical ripening*, which enables the cervix to dilate, "disappear," and allow the passage of the fetus.

• The peritoneal cover of the uterus leaves the uterine surface at the insertion of the anterior and posterior vaginal fornices.

The *vagina* is an approximately 9 cm long, flattened muscular canal that connects the uterine cervix with the opening of the urogenital diaphragm. The anterior wall of the vagina is closely associated with the urethra. Through the rectum and the posterior wall of the vagina the portio vaginalis can be palpated. In pregnant women this association can be used in the assessment of cervical dilation without increasing the risk of infection of the fetal membranes. The superior end of the vagina forms an anterior and a posterior fornix. These are in association with two recesses of the peritoneal sac: the vesicouterine and the rectouterine recesses. In cases of ruptured tubal pregnancy, blood accumulates in the *rectouterine recess [of Douglas]*, which can be detected by needle aspiration upon piercing through the posterior vaginal fornix.

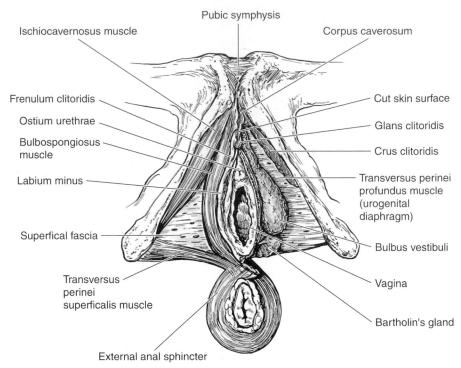

Pubic symphysis

Ischiocavernosus muscle

Corpus caverosum

Frenulum clitoridis

Ostium urethrae

Bulbospongiosus muscle

Labium minus

Superfical fascia

Transversus perinei superficalis muscle

External anal sphincter

Cut skin surface

Glans clitoridis

Crus clitoridis

Transversus perinei profundus muscle (urogenital diaphragm)

Bulbus vestibuli

Vagina

Bartholin's gland

Figure 13-16. Anatomy of the female external genitalia. The skin including the labia majora has been removed. The cut diagram shows the bulbus vestibuli underneath the bulbospongiosus muscle. The transversus perinei superficialis represents the posterior (in this figure, inferior) edge of the urogenital diaphragm. The voluntary sphincter of the urethra is embedded in the tissue layer of the urogenital diaphragm (not shown). (*Source:* Modified from Fig. 297, p 223, in Ferner H, Staubesand J (eds): *Sobotta/Becher Atlas of Human Anatomy,* vol 2, 9th English ed., Urban & Schwarzenberg, 1975.)

The mucosal lining of the vagina is devoid of glands. The moist environment is provided by the cervical glands, the vestibular glands, and (during sexual arousal) filtration of fluids due to vascular congestion in the vaginal wall (*transudate*). The vagina must resist harsh mechanical forces, such as childbirth and intercourse. The mechanical resistance is achieved by the adaptation of three constituents:

- Stratified squamous epithelium.
- A thin layer of lamina propria that decreases the shearing effect of tangential mechanical forces.
- Thick layers of smooth muscle.

The Female External Genitalia   Physical examination may reveal ambiguous external genitalia and provide evidence of endocrine dysfunction. The female external genitalia consist of three main components (Fig. 13-16):

- The *clitoris* is the homologous organ of the penis. Its *crura* and *corpora cavernosa* are erectile and correspond to those of the penis. The urethra opens at the base of the *glans clitoridis*.
- The *labia minora* (the inner longitudinal pair of skin folds) border the *vestibule*. They develop from the *urogenital folds* without fusion, and are homologous with the skin of the penis. The labia minora are covered by a thin, hairless, highly pigmented epidermis. In their deeper tissue layer is found the *bulbus vestibuli*. This erectile tissue is homologous with the bulbus penis (the root of the corpus spongiosum), but unlike its male counterpart, it is a paired organ on either side of the vestibule. The bulbus vestibuli continues anteriorly into the *frenulum clitoridis*, and fuses with the contralateral bulbus to form the glans. The *greater vestibular (Bartholin's) gland*, which is the female equivalent of the Cowper's gland is located posterior to the bulbus and opens into the vestibule.
- The *labia majora* (the outer longitudinal pair of skin folds) develop from the *labioscrotal swellings* without fusion and are homologous with the scrotum. They contain adipose tissue that spreads to the anterior surface of the symphysis pubis and forms the *mons pubis*. At puberty, pubic hair grows on the mons and the outer surface of the labia majora.

The vagina opens to the vestibule through the *urogenital diaphragm*. On the external surface of the diaphragm, on either side of the vestibule, a triangle is formed by a group of *superficial perineal muscles*. These include the *bulbospongiosus, ischiocavernosus*, and *trasversus perinei superficialis* muscles.

The Menstrual Cycle

OBJECTIVES

1. Discuss the regulation of the ovarian cycle: the hypothalamic–pituitary–ovarian axis. Identify the relationship between the *ovarian cycle* and the *endometrial cycle*. Identify the time-course of the plasma levels of gonadotropins and ovarian hormones during the menstrual cycle, and the feedback mechanisms operating during the *follicular phase, preovulatory surge* of gonadotropins (positive feedback), and *luteal phase*. Compare and contrast the feedback regulation of gonadotropin secretion in males and females.
2. Discuss *oogenesis,* the gonadotropin-independent, and the gonadotropin-dependent phases of follicular growth and maturation. Discuss the timeframe of these processes, and the fate of the follicular pool during the lifespan of women. Discuss the roles of *Wilms' tumor 1* (WT1) and *growth differentiation factor-9* (GDF-9) in follicular growth. Define the terms *cohort, recruitment, selection,* and *dominance*. Compare and contrast bi-ovarial and mono-ovarial phases of feedback regulation during the menstrual cycle. Discuss the mechanism of *dizygotic twinning*.
3. Identify the role of *kit* and *kit ligand* in the LH-regulated resumption of meiosis. Discuss the mechanism of ovulation, and the role and regulation of proteases

in the process. Describe postovulatory neovascularization and its role in the completion of luteinization.

4. Describe the ovarian contribution to circulating androgens in healthy women. Discuss *hyperthecoses* and the *polycystic ovary syndrome*. Discuss hormonal contraceptives and their mechanism of action. Discuss ovulation induction.
5. Discuss the *pheromonal* regulation of the menstrual cycle.
6. Discuss the biologic actions of androgens, estrogens, and progesterone in cycling women. Describe the regulation of the endometrial cycle and the mechanism of *menstrual bleeding,* including the involvement of prostaglandins and *matrix metalloproteinases*. Describe the main types of abnormal menstrual bleeding and the endocrine background of *breakthrough bleeding*.
7. Discuss cyclic changes in the vagina and the uterine cervix/cervical mucus. Describe the normal flora of the vagina and its relationship with vaginal pH. Discuss the *maturation index, Spinnbarkeit,* and *ferning*.
8. Discuss the mechanism of *premenstrual syndrome*.

Regulation of the Ovarian Cycle: The Hypothalamic–Pituitary–Ovarian Axis

The Phases of the Endometrial Cycle Are Dictated by the Phases of the Ovarian Cycle   The regulation of the hypothalamic–pituitary–ovarian axis in postpubertal females typically follows a 28-day cycle (normal range 25 to 35 days). *Menstruation* (menses; from the Latin *mensa*, month) is the shedding of the *stratum functionale* of the endometrium, which is accompanied by mainly arterial bleeding. *The onset of menstrual bleeding is designated as the first day of the cycle.* Two cycles are distinguished:

- The *ovarian cycle* is related to the gonadotropin-dependent maturation of the ovarian follicles, including the formation and demise of the corpus luteum. The ovarian cycle has two phases:
  - The *follicular phase* is characterized by the absence of a functional corpus luteum, and the gonadotropin-dependent follicular maturation leading up to ovulation. The maturing follicles mainly secrete *17β-estradiol* (E_2) and *inhibin B*, but plasma progesterone remains very low. The length of the follicular phase is variable, and this variability accounts for the overall variability of the length of the menstrual cycle.
  - The *luteal phase* starts with the development of the corpus luteum. The characteristic and determinant hormone of the luteal phase is *progesterone*. However, the corpus luteum also secretes *17β-estradiol* and *inhibin A*. The length of the luteal phase is relatively invariable (14 ± 2 days) and determined by the life-span of the corpus luteum.
- The *endometrial cycle* is the cyclic change of the endometrium, which is essentially dictated by the ovarian hormones and the ovarian cycle. Three phases are distinguished:

BOX 13-7   Diagnostic Use of Progesterone

Exogenously administered progesterone or its analogs such as *medroxy-progesterone* can be used diagnostically for evaluating endogenous estrogen secretion. The test is useful as an inexpensive initial evaluation that does not require direct hormone measurements. Unlike hormone measurements, this biologic test takes tissue responsiveness into consideration. In *nonpregnant* women who present with *secondary amenorrhea,* progesterone is administered for 5 to 7 days. If menstrual bleeding occurs upon withdrawal of progesterone, it indicates the prior stimulation of the endometrium by sufficient exposure to endogenous estrogens. Sufficient (i.e., biologically relevant) amounts of estrogens are produced only in a gonadotropin-dependent manner. If menstrual bleeding does not occur upon withdrawal of progesterone, the cause of decreased estrogen action is identified by further tests.

Most contraceptive pills contain a combination of synthetic estrogen and progestin. In each 28-day cycle, tablets are taken for 21 days, followed by a 7-day pause of hormone exposure. Thus, the "menstrual" bleeding that follows is essentially a progesterone-withdrawal bleeding. This can be used as a test of uterine function.

• *Menstruation.* With the demise of the corpus luteum of the previous cycle, plasma levels of progesterone decrease and the endometrium is shed. Menstruation usually lasts 4 days (normal range: 2 to 7 days). The menstrual blood loss is approximately 30 mL; blood loss above 80 mL is abnormal.

• The *proliferative phase* is the estrogen-dependent regeneration and growth of the endometrial lining. The stimulation of estrogen receptors leads to proliferation of both stromal and epithelial cells. The epithelium regenerates from the basal portion of the endometrial glands left behind in the stratum basale during menstruation. *Both menstruation and the proliferative phase occur during the follicular phase of the ovarian cycle.*

• The *secretory phase* is the *progesterone-dependent* maturation of the endometrium that makes it suitable for the implantation of the blastocyst. The secretory phase of the endometrial cycle *coincides with the luteal phase* of the ovarian cycle. The action of progesterone requires the preparation of the endometrium by estrogens. Although 17β-estradiol is secreted together with progesterone by the corpus luteum, its continued presence is not required (Box 13-7).

The Feedback Regulation of the Hypothalamic–Pituitary–Ovarian Axis Varies with the Stage of the Ovarian Cycle   The regulatory mechanisms functioning in adult males (Regulation of the Gonadotropin–Gonad Axis in Postpubertal Males) are significantly modified in adult females:

• In males, the negative feedback action of circulating androgens on gonadotropins is mainly (but not exclusively) exerted via estrogen receptors after *local* aromatization. In contrast, in females the *circulating* estrogens (primarily 17β-estradiol) secreted directly from the ovaries serve in lieu of locally converted androgens. The stimulation of androgen receptors is not involved in the physiologic regulation of gonadotropin secretion in females.

• If the plasma levels of estrogens are high for a prolonged period of time (17β-estradiol exceeds approximately 150 to 200 pg/mL for at least 36 h), they exert a *positive feedback* action on gonadotropin secretion. The positive feedback mechanism is abolished in male rats by perinatally secreted androgens, which alter hypothalamic structures via stimulating estrogen receptors. Conflicting data exist as to whether the positive feedback mechanism is operational in men. Under physiologic circumstances, it is definitely a unique female mechanism of gonadotropin regulation.

• In females, hormone secretion follows an approximately 28-day cycle dictated by the growth, differentiation, and apoptosis of ovarian steroidogenic tissues.

> • The cellular mass of the androgen-producing Leydig cell is relatively constant. In contrast, in females *the cellular mass of theca and granulosa cells,* which cooperatively secrete 17β-estradiol, significantly increases during the follicular phase of the ovarian cycle.
>
> • With the cyclic development of the corpus luteum, females acquire a short-lived steroidogenic organ that secretes *progesterone.* Progesterone has multiple actions in the regulation of gonadotropin secretion, contributing to both the positive and negative feedback actions. In males, its negative feedback action can be demonstrated on exposure to *exogenous* progesterone.

The normal values of the hormones involved in the pituitary-ovarian axis are listed in Table 13-7. The typical profile of the hormones of the hypothalamic–pituitary–ovarian axis during the menstrual cycle is displayed in Figs. 13-17 and 13-18. Feedback regulation during the follicular phase, the preovulatory surge of gonadotropins, and the luteal phase are shown in Fig. 13-19. The regulation during these three phases can be briefly summarized as follows.

During the early *follicular phase*, due to the decreased feedback by the degenerating corpus luteum of the previous cycle, plasma concentration of FSH is elevated. This increase is required to engage follicles in gonadotropin-dependent maturation (*recruitment*). The main regulatory mechanisms during the follicular phase are similar to those observed in males: 17β-estradiol by acting on both the pituitary and the hypothalamus, and inhibin B by acting only on the pituitary (suppression of FSH-β synthesis), exert a negative feedback on gonadotropin secretion (Fig. 13-19A). During the follicular phase, the *GnRH pulses occur at about 90-min intervals* in spite of increasing levels of estradiol. The absence of a decrease in pulse frequency is related to the lack of sufficient concentrations of progesterone and androgens. (Androgens normally do not participate in the feedback regulation

Table 13-7   Normal Values of the Hormones of the Pituitary–Ovarian Axis in Adults[a]

Compound	Follicular phase	Midcycle peak	Luteal phase
FSH (mIU/mL)	1.37–9.9	6.17–17.2	1.09–9.2
LH (mIU/mL)	1.68–15.0	21.9–56.6	0.61–16.3
Inhibin B (pg/mL)	139–403		60–220
Inhibin A (pg/mL)	10–35		30–70
17β-estradiol (ng/dL)	Early: 2.0–15.0	15.0–75.0	3.0–45.0
	Late: 4.0–35.0		
Progesterone (ng/dL)	15–70	—	200–2500

	Mostly Independent of Menstrual Cycle Phase
SHBG (μg/dL)	118–797
DHEAS[b] (μg/dL)	19–30 y: 29–781
	31–50 y: 12–379
Androstenedione[b] (ng/dL)	85–275 (shows midcycle peak)
Testosterone[b] (ng/dL)	15–70 (shows midcycle peak)
Dihydrotestosterone[b] (ng/dL)	4–22
Urinary 17-ketosteroids[c] (mg/d)	6–14

[a] Except for 17-ketosteroids, all values refer to plasma/serum.
[b] Circulating androgens are not involved in the physiologic regulation of the pituitary–ovarian axis.
[c] Mainly reflects urinary excretion of androgen metabolites.
ABBREVIATIONS: FSH, follicle-stimulating hormone; LH, luteinizing hormone; SHBG, sex hormone-binding globulin; DHEAS, dehydroepiandrosterone sulfate.

of gonadotropins in females.) The exponential increase of estradiol during the second half of the follicular phase occurs in spite of decreasing levels of FSH and very low levels of LH. The increasing plasma concentration of estradiol is explained by the proliferation of theca interna and (mainly) the granulosa cells of the *dominant follicle*. This follicle is dominant because of its increased responsiveness to FSH; thus, in spite of a decrease in FSH, its granulosa cells continue proliferating, and producing about the same amount of estradiol *per cell*. The very high levels of estradiol lead to the next stage of the cycle.

The *preovulatory surge* of gonadotropins is due to a *transient positive feedback* regulation by 17β-estradiol and progesterone (Fig. 13-19B). In spite of intensive research, the mechanism of the positive feedback is only partially understood. The preovulatory surge of gonadotropins (LH and FSH) is *initiated* by the prolonged and robust elevation of circulating 17β-estradiol (see Fig. 13-17). The rising LH induces luteinization and progesterone secretion by preovulatory granulosa cells. This progesterone secretion, which precedes the LH peak by 12 to 42 h (see Fig. 13-18), is mandatory for the development of the preovulatory LH surge with normal amplitude and duration. The normal LH surge is required for ovulation and the formation of the corpus luteum. The antiprogestin *mifepristone* (RU486) disrupts the generation of a normal preovulatory LH surge and prevents ovulation by inhibiting the positive feedback effect of progesterone.

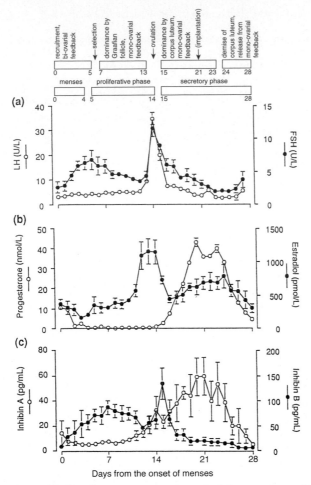

Figure 13-17. Plasma concentrations of pituitary and gonadal hormones during the menstrual cycle. Peak levels of biologically active inhibin coincide with the peak of inhibin A. (*Source:* Modified from Fig. 1, p 155 in Buffet NC et al: Regulation of the human menstrual cycle. Frontiers Neuroendocrinol 19:151–186, 1998.)

- The positive feedback by 17β-estradiol targets both the pituitary and the hypothalamus.
    - The pituitary responsiveness to GnRH is increased mainly because of estradiol-induced expression of GnRH receptors. Administration of GnRH *at constant pulse frequency* to GnRH-deficient women (such as in Kallmann's syndrome) elicits normal ovulation and may result in pregnancy. This finding suggests that the primary site of positive feedback is the pituitary gland. Note, however, that the exogenous dose of GnRH may achieve concentrations corresponding to peak levels of high-amplitude GnRH pulses.

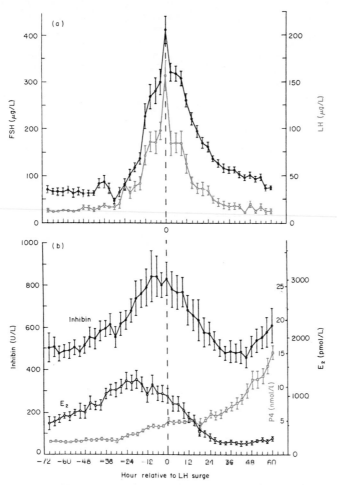

Figure 13-18. Midcycle dynamics of gonadotropin regulation. Data points were collected at 3-hour intervals; the timing of the LH/FSH peak is designated as zero. Note that the increase of LH starts about 27 hours prior to attaining peak levels (−27 h). The critical estradiol (E_2) threshold of 150 pg/mL (550 pmol/L) was reached at −69 h (i.e., 42 h before the initial rise of LH). Progesterone (P4) started to rise between −27 and −24 h in response to an initial LH stimulus. The rise in progesterone is critical in the development of the full-blown surge of gonadotropins. (*Source:* From MacLachlan RI et al: Serum inhibin levels during the periovulatory interval in normal women: Relationship with sex steroid and gonadotropin levels. Clin Endocrinol 32:44, 1990.)

- During the follicular phase, the GnRH pulse frequency does not display major changes. Each GnRH pulse is preceded by a burst of electrical activity of the GnRH neurons. During the estrogen-induced positive feedback, a *GnRH surge* is observed, which includes an *increased GnRH pulse frequency in spite of the electrical silence of the GnRH neurons*. The apparent discrepancy might be resolved by a NPY-mediated action. High levels of estrogens stimulate the secretion and pulse frequency of *NPY* via mechanisms

A

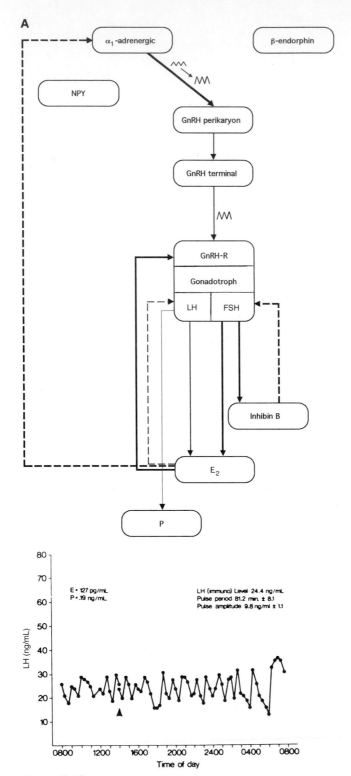

Figure 13-19.

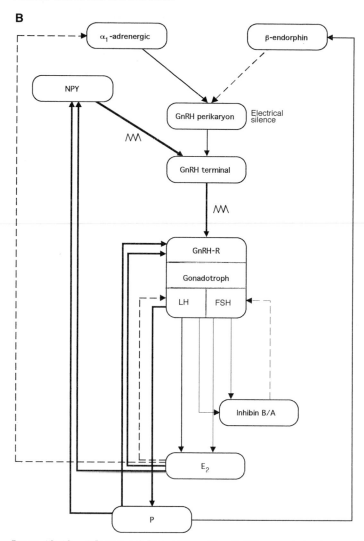

Figure 13-19. (*Continued*) Regulation of the GnRH–gonadotropin–ovarian axis during the menstrual cycle. Solid arrows indicate stimulation/increase; dashed arrows indicate inhibition/decrease. The thickness of the arrows indicates the relative importance of the mechanism. A. Midfollicular phase. B. Preovulatory surge of gonadotropins. C. Midluteal phase. Compare with the dynamic changes of plasma hormone levels shown in Fig. 13-17. Compare with the regulatory mechanisms in postpubertal men (Fig. 13-11). Secretion of estradiol involves the cooperation of theca interna and granulosa cells (see Fig. 13-4). For normal regulation, the concentration of sex hormone-binding globulin (SHBG) must not be elevated (not shown). The insets display secretory patterns of LH during the late follicular phase (panel A), and the same day of the follicular phase after administration of exogenous progesterone for 8 days (panel C). The latter condition induces an LH secretory pattern normally seen during the luteal phase. GnRH, gonadotropin-releasing hormone; GnRH-R, GnRH receptor; LH, luteinizing hormone; FSH, follicle stimulating hormone; E₂, estradiol; P, progesterone; NPY, neuropeptide Y. (*Source:* Insets from Soules et al: Progesterone modulation of pulsatile luteinizing hormone secretion in normal women. J Clin Endocrinol Metab 58:378–383, 1984.)

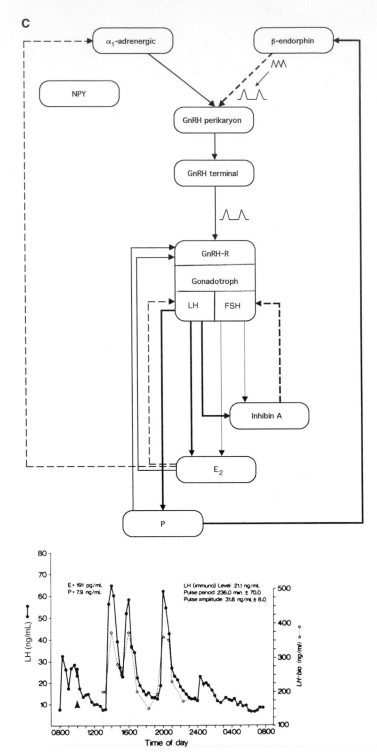

Figure 13-19. (*Continued*)

involving increased nitric oxide production and decreased opioid input. NPY acting on Y1 receptors *in the median eminence* provokes the release of GnRH from nerve terminals without evoking electrical activity of GnRH perikarya.

- The positive feedback by progesterone also involves dual targets.
    - After the priming action of estradiol, progesterone enhances pituitary sensitivity to the action of GnRH.
    - Progesterone increases the pulse frequency of NPY secretion after the priming action of estradiol. The coupling between the pulses of NPY and GnRH is maintained under the influence of progesterone.

- The termination of the preovulatory gonadotropin surge is poorly understood. The surge of pituitary gonadotropins is terminated well before the GnRH surge subsides. This may imply pituitary desensitization during the robust surge of GnRH. The declining LH and FSH, and the follicular events, result in decreased estradiol secretion, which eliminates an important signal of the positive feedback.

The regulation of gonadotropins during the *luteal phase* is similar to that of males, except that the role of androgenic action is replaced by progesterone, and that progesterone production is terminated by the demise of the corpus luteum (see Fig. 13-19C). Progesterone and 17β-estradiol acting on both the pituitary and the hypothalamus, and inhibin A acting only on the pituitary, exert a strong negative feedback on gonadotropin secretion. *GnRH/LH pulses occur at about 2- to 4-h intervals during the early luteal phase, then progressively slow down to 4- to 6-h intervals during the midluteal phase and 8- to 12-h intervals by the late luteal phase.* This pattern demonstrates the preeminence of progesterone's long-lasting inhibitory effect on the GnRH pulse generator. The potent negative feedback via decreased pulse frequency assures very low levels of LH, which leads to *luteolysis* (the demise of the corpus luteum), unless the LH receptors of the corpus luteum are stimulated by hCG, i.e., pregnancy occurs. Unlike pituitary gonadotropins, the secretion of hCG is not suppressed by ovarian steroids. In the absence of hCG, luteolysis terminates the negative feedback action on the hypothalamus and the pituitary, and a new cycle begins. This is heralded by menstrual bleeding, which is due to the decrease of progesterone secretion by the degenerating corpus luteum.

From the above description it is clear that the regulation involves events in the hypothalamo-hypophyseal system and in the ovaries. A crucial element is the dynamic coordination of these two poles of the axis. In the next section, we discuss ovarian regulatory mechanisms in more detail.

Oogenesis During Embryonic Life Generates a Nonreplenishable Pool of Primary Oocytes that Are Arrested in the Prophase of the First Meiotic Division up to 50 Years

Unlike spermatocytogenesis, *oogenesis* (the mitotic proliferation of oogonia) occurs only prenatally and is completed by the 7th gestational month (*ovum*, egg [Latin]). *Oogonia*, which are derived from the *yolk sac* about 24 days after conception, eventually generate *primary oocytes* that *enter meiosis during embryonic life* and *become arrested at the diplotene stage* of the first meiotic division for up to 12 to 50 years, i.e., the range between the average ages of *menarche* and *menopause*. The completion of meiosis and the maturation of the oocyte takes place as a component of *gonadotropin-dependent follicular maturation* (see below). Follicular maturation is classified into a *gonadotropin-independent phase* that occurs continuously from embryonic life until menopause and *gonadotropin-dependent phase* that commences with puberty.

The Gonadotropin-Independent Phase Involves All Maturation Stages up to Early Antral Follicles Having a Diameter of up to 8 mm (Usually 0.5 to 2 mm)   As mentioned earlier (The Biosynthesis, Mechanism of Action and Metabolism of Sexual Steroids), the prepubertal ovaries secrete very low quantities of sex steroids, which are insufficient to bring about the development of secondary sexual characteristics. Due to prepubertally enhanced hypothalamic responsiveness to sex steroids, the low concentrations are nevertheless sufficient to suppress pituitary gonadotropin secretion. This basal, gonadotropin-independent ovarian steroid synthesis and secretion requires the generation of steroidogenic theca interna and granulosa cells. Reaching the antral stage by a gonadotropin-independent follicular development assures that the cell types as well as the cell mass meet the requirements of gonadotropin-suppressing steroidogenesis.

The gonadotropin-independent maturation starts in utero as soon as the ovarian follicles are formed, and continues until the depletion of the ovarian follicular pool at menopause. After an initial rapid atresia, which decreases the number of primordial ovarian follicles from about 5–7 million to 2 million between the 7th gestational month and birth, the ovarian follicles are depleted with a predictable *half-life of about 5 to 6 years. The rate of depletion is irrespective of the reproductive stage and/or the endocrine milieu such as prepubertal life, pregnancy, or hormonal contraceptives.*

Follicular maturation is initiated by unknown local factors. The gonadotropin-independent maturation is *noncyclic*, i.e., the follicles are continuously engaged in maturation *in both ovaries*. The gonadotropin-independent growth and maturation of follicles is slow and takes approximately 250 days. At that stage, the follicles either undergo *atresia* (apoptosis), or (after puberty) some may be rescued by pituitary FSH and enter the gonadotropin-dependent phase (Fig. 13-20).

- Preantral follicles develop from primordial follicles over the course of about 180 days, and represent the last stage of maturation at which follicles do not undergo apoptosis.
- The first stage in the development of tertiary follicles is the last gonadotropin-independent process. This is known as the *phase of slow*

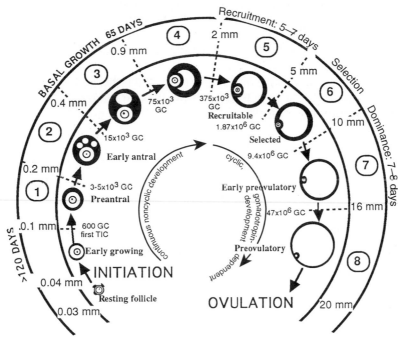

Figure 13-20. The scheme of gonadotropin-independent and gonadotropin-dependent follicular growth. The numbers in circles refer to "classes" of follicles not detailed in this text. Before puberty, follicular growth may proceed to recruitable follicles that, in the absence of an FSH stimulus, may reach sizes up to 8 mm in diameter as detected by ultrasonography. TIC, theca interna cell; GC, granulosa cell. (*Source:* Modified from Fig. 3 in Gougeon A: Regulation of ovarian follicular development in primates: Facts and hypotheses. Endocrine Rev 17:121–155, 1996.)

(*basal*) *growth:* the early antral follicles usually grow from about 200 μm to 2 mm (maximum, 8 mm) in diameter *over the course of about 65 to 70 days.* After puberty, about 35% of apoptosis (atresia) occurs at this stage of development. *Before puberty, this is the last stage of development and all follicles become atretic.*

The regulation of the gonadotropin-independent phase of follicular growth involves the *WT1* transcription factor and *GDF-9.*

• The *WT1* gene found on chromosome 11p13 (whose mutation is a cause of Wilms' tumor) encodes a zinc finger protein with transcriptional *repressor* activity on several growth factor and growth factor receptor genes, including the inhibin α subunit. Ovarian WT1 mRNA is expressed exclusively in the follicular epithelium of primordial follicles and the granulosa cells of primary and secondary follicles. WT1 mRNA levels decrease during follicle growth. *WT1 may inhibit the initiation of follicular growth.*

• GDFs are members of the TGF-β family (see Box 8-1). Follicular development is arrested at the stage of primary follicles in GDF-9 knockout mice, indicating a *mandatory role of GDF-9 in follicular development be-*

yond the primary stage. GDF-9 has been localized in the oocyte of primary, secondary, and preantral follicles. Growth of preantral follicles is enhanced by treatment with GDF-9 in vitro.

Several growth factors as well as their receptors are expressed by primary follicles, but not by the quiescent primordial follicles. These growth factors, such as IGF-1, IGF-2, EGF, and the closely related TGF-α may exert paracrine/autocrine effects and promote follicular growth.

Gonadotropin-Dependent Follicular Maturation Involves the FSH-Mediated Recruitment of a Cohort of Early Antral Follicles and the Selection of a Dominant Follicle, Which in Turn Causes Apoptosis of the Other Follicles in the Cohort by Feedback Suppression of FSH The *gonadotropin-dependent phase* starts with the second phase in the development of tertiary follicles, includes all subsequent maturation stages of follicular development, and ends with the involution of the corpus luteum. Thus, whereas the gonadotropin-independent phase required about 250 days, the gonadotropin-dependent growth and maturation is accomplished within a single ovarian cycle.

The gonadotropin-dependent phase occurs starting with puberty: it is *cyclic* and initially involves a *cohort* of FSH-dependent/FSH-recruited follicles from *both ovaries* during each menstrual cycle. A single follicle selected from either one of the two ovaries establishes *dominance* during the cycle and proceeds to ovulation. Between menarche and menopause, approximately 350 to 400 follicles mature to *Graafian follicles* and expel their oocytes in the process of ovulation. With *menopause*, the nonrenewable pool of primordial follicles becomes exhausted. Thus, nearly all of the 5 to 7 million follicles die in the apoptotic process of follicular atresia. The development of tertiary follicles has three distinct stages.

• As mentioned, the phase of slow growth is the last gonadotropin-independent phase. Although the granulosa cells at this stage express receptors for FSH, the follicles grow up to 8 mm in diameter even in the absence of FSH. However, their rescue from apoptosis is dependent on the presence of FSH.

• *Recruitment is the FSH-mediated rescue of a quasi-synchronous group of 1 to 15 follicles known as the cohort. Recruitment begins on the first day of the menstrual cycle (onset of menses) when FSH levels are elevated, and is completed by day 5 to 7 of the same cycle.* The follicles of the recruited (rescued) cohort are present in both ovaries, and there is no difference in the estradiol production by the two gonads. Recruitment means that the follicles have become sensitive to the action of gonadotropins, and their need to be rescued implies that they are *gonadotropin-dependent*. If FSH levels are low at the time when the follicle reaches this stage of development, it undergoes apoptosis. About 50% of atresia occurs at this stage of development in postpubertal women.

• *Selection* is the process whereby a single follicle of the recruited cohort *becomes dominant*, destined to ovulate and form the corpus luteum. Selection usually occurs at a follicular size of 2 to 5 mm. Typically the largest, fastest growing follicle is selected and dominates, probably because it has the highest level of FSH receptor expression. Experimental ablation of the largest follicle during the stage of recruitment has no impact on the cycle because another follicle can take over and reach dominance. However, once the selection has occurred and dominance is established, ablation of the largest (dominant) follicle prevents ovulation until the cycle is repeated.

• The dominant follicle is also known as *preovulatory* or *Graafian follicle*. *Dominance* is defined as the period of growth of a single follicle from its selection until its ovulation. This phase corresponds with days 7 to 14 of the menstrual cycle, during which the dominant follicle grows from about 5–8 to 20–22 mm in diameter. The granulosa cell population grows over 125-fold in an exponential manner, which (together with the growth of the theca interna) explains the rapid rise of 17β-estradiol in plasma (see Fig. 13-17). Once dominance is established, the estradiol secretion from the two ovaries becomes asymmetrical: *only the ovary containing the dominant follicle secretes significant amounts of estradiol and inhibin*. This also means that the negative feedback regulation of gonadotropin secretion that was accomplished jointly by the two ovaries during the first 7 days of the menstrual cycle is replaced by a *mono-ovarial (monofollicular) feedback*. The mono-ovarial feedback by estradiol includes both negative and positive feedback actions on pituitary gonadotropins. The negative feedback exerted by estradiol and inhibin from the dominant follicle leads to atresia of the other follicles in the cohort because the other follicles have lower expression levels of FSH receptors than the dominant follicle (see the concept of spare receptors in Chap. 5). This also means that the expression of aromatase in nondominant follicles declines, and the increasing concentrations of nonconverted local androgens induce atresia. The mechanism assures not only monofollicular feedback but also monofollicular ovulation (Box 13-8).

Gonadotropin-Dependent Follicular Maturation and Ovulation Results in the Cyclic Formation and Demise of the Corpus Luteum As discussed, about 36 to 48 hours after the onset of the preovulatory LH surge, the prolonged stimulation of LH receptors causes several events:

• The primary oocyte resumes and completes the first meiotic division. The function of LH is to suspend the mechanism responsible for meiotic arrest. *Kit* is a protooncogene receptor tyrosine kinase (RTK) expressed by oocytes. Two alternatively spliced *kit ligand* transcripts encoding 248- and 220-amino acid membrane-associated kit ligand proteins have been demonstrated in ovarian tissue and granulosa cells. The ligand-induced stimulation of kit (due to the interaction between the oocyte and the follicular epithelium) is responsible for meiotic arrest. LH suppresses the expression of *kit ligand* by granulosa cells.

• The LH surge halts the further proliferation of granulosa cells.

• The granulosa and theca interna cells become luteinized, which

BOX 13-8   Dizygotic Twinning

Heredity, older maternal age, and increased parity are associated with dizygotic twinning. In general, the cause of dizygotic twinning is that supranormal FSH prevents the apoptosis of more than one follicle. In hereditary dizygotic twinning, FSH levels are elevated because of the primary increase of stimulating mechanisms that regulate pituitary gonadotropin secretion. In most nonhereditary conditions, such as recovery from hypothalamic amenorrhea and older age, excessive FSH secretion occurs as a result of diminished ovarian feedback. Thus, dominance is shared by two (or sometimes more) follicles, and the two dominant follicles together provide sufficient suppression of FSH to cause apoptosis of the other rescued follicles in the cohort. This mechanism is operational in species normally giving birth to multiple sets of twins. In clinical practice, supraphysiologic doses of exogenous FSH are utilized for *induced ovulation* with the intent of collecting multiple ova for *in vitro fertilization.*

leads to increased secretion of progesterone mainly by the granulosa lutein cells (see Figs. 13-4 and 13-18). This involves an increase in cytoplasmic cyclic AMP concentration exceeding those achieved by the stimulation of FSH receptors.

- The Graafian follicle ruptures involving inflammatory mechanisms and leads to ovulation. The LH surge induces cyclooxygenase-2 (COX-2). In response to the preovulatory surge of gonadotropins, the granulosa cells secrete *tissue plasminogen activator* (tPA) into the follicular fluid, which activates plasminogen. The resulting plasmin may activate latent *matrix metalloproteinases* (MMPs). These enzymes degrade the perifollicular matrix and break down the collagen fibers, which provide the strength to the follicular wall. The increased synthesis of the protease inhibitors *plasminogen activator inhibitor-1* (PAI-1) and *tissue inhibitor of metalloproteinases-1* (TIMP-1) in the *theca* of growing follicles protects them from enzymes diffusing from neighboring ovulatory follicles.

The rupture of the follicle leads to the formation of the *corpus hemorrhagicum*. Marcophages and mesenchymal cells invade the corpus hemorrhagicum, which leads to rapid vascularization of the entire structure, including the formerly avascular granulosa cells. The *neovascularization* requires vascular endothelial growth factor (VEGF) mainly produced by luteinized granulosa and theca cells in an LH-dependent manner. The fenestrated endothelium makes the already luteinized granulosa cells accessible to low density lipoprotein (LDL) cholesterol as the precursor of pregnenolone synthesis. At this time, the luteinization of granulosa cells becomes complete: the *granulosa lutein* cells give the bulk of the *corpus luteum* (yellow body). Unlike granulosa cells, granulosa lutein cells express the P450scc (see The Biosynthesis, Mechanism of Action and Metabolism of Sexual Steroids), which is indicated by the change of mitochondrial morphology from shelflike to tubulovesicular cristae. The theca interna cells differentiate into lipid droplet-rich *theca lutein* cells that form a narrow layer on the lobulated surface of the corpus luteum (see Fig. 13-3).

As discussed, the steroid hormones of the corpus luteum suppress the secretion of LH and FSH by inhibiting the GnRH pulse generator and the mainly LH-driven inhibin A suppresses the synthesis of FSH-β in the pituitary gonadotrophs. The low levels of LH result in the demise of the corpus luteum in 14 days. This event removes suppression mainly from FSH secretion. The increased FSH leads to recruitment of a cohort from the pool of follicles that is continuously maturing in a gonadotropin-independent manner, and the cycle is repeated.

The Ovaries Contribute to Circulating Androgens
In women, androgens are not involved in the physiologic regulation of gonadotropin secretion. However, they are important in the development of sexual hair and body odor during puberty (underarm and pubic hair, apocrine sweat glands) and contribute to the maintenance of libido.

As discussed, the adrenal cortex is the main source of androgens and their degradation products (such as the 17-ketosteroids) in women. The significance of the ovarian contribution to the pool of circulating androgens is exemplified by the scanty development of sexual hair in Turner's syndrome patients, whose streak gonads are in essence hormonally inactive.

The source of ovarian androgens is primarily the *theca interna* cell population of developing *antral* follicles (Box 13-9). The contribution of hilar cells varies but is usually negligible. Because the theca interna cells produce these androgens as precursors of estrogen secretion, it is understandable that ovarian androgen secretion follows a pattern that parallels the profile of estradiol during the menstrual cycle. In contrast, adrenal androgen secretion shows no relationship with the menstrual cycle, but displays a circadian rhythm dictated by ACTH.

Due to the preferentially Δ^4 pathway, the ovaries contribute minimally to circulating DHEA and DHEAS. This is indicated by the lack of menstrual cycle-dependent changes in circulating DHEA and DHEAS. Androstenedione (a weak androgen) has the highest production rate among ovarian androgens. However, in terms of normal androgenic *action*, only testosterone and dihydrotestosterone are relevant. Under physiologic conditions, up to 300 μg testosterone is produced daily. On the average, 50 to 70% of the testosterone is generated by *peripheral conversion* of androstenedione by 17β-hydroxysteroid dehydrogenases. Because the adrenal gland has negligible ability to synthesize testosterone, the rest must be produced directly by the ovaries. The absolute concentration of androstenedione and testosterone, and the relative contribution of the ovary to both circulating androgens is increased during the preovulatory LH surge.

At the same *total* plasma concentration of testosterone, the concentration of *free* testosterone is lower in women than in men because of the

BOX 13-9   Polycystic Ovary Syndrome and Stromal Hyperthecosis

In *polycystic ovary syndrome* (PCOS also known as *Stein-Leventhal syndrome*), follicular development does not result in ovulation and formation of the corpus luteum. Instead, the hyperplastic theca interna cells of the aberrant cystic follicles (*follicular hyperthecosis*) produce overt quantities of androgens. The supranormal androgen secretion exerts a negative feedback on the hypothalamic–pituitary–gonad axis, and suspends the ovarian and menstrual cycle. In addition, male-type distribution of hair growth develops (hirsutism). Amenorrhea and hirsutism are therefore the leading features of this condition. As mentioned, PCOS patients are insulin-resistant and at least 40% present with obesity. The compensatory increase of insulin may normalize plasma glucose concentration. However, stimulation of insulin and IGF-1 receptors of theca interna cells increases androgen production mainly by inducing the expression of P450c17 and its 17,20-lyase activity.

In *stromal hyperthecosis,* the ovarian cortical stromal cells assume the morphology and function of theca interna cells. The condition, which results in the uniform enlargement of the ovaries and hypersecretion of androgens, is typically seen either in postmenopausal women or as a part of the presentation of PCOS.

higher plasma levels of SHBG (see Fig. 13-5). SHBG limits the availability of testosterone to target tissues, which may express 5α-reductase and produce DHT. A shift in the estrogen:androgen ratio toward androgens may cause a decrease of SHBG and increased biologic availability of testosterone. The increased androgenic activity may have mild clinical manifestations (hair growth, acne) before a clear elevation of total testosterone is observed.

Hormonal Contraception Prevents Ovulation by Suppressing Gonadotropin Secretion   Most orally active hormonal contraceptives contain a combination of synthetic estrogen and progestin. All preparations provide negative feedback suppression of gonadotropin secretion by an exogenous source. *The exogenous source of ovarian hormones fulfills the role of the dominant follicle, except that the preovulatory rise of estrogen is omitted.* The exogenous estrogens do not reach the levels necessary to provoke positive feedback, and prevent the rise of endogenous estrogen production by suppressing follicular growth via inhibiting FSH. Since the introduction of the first oral contraceptives, the dose of estrogen has been reduced to avoid severe side effects, such as thromboembolism and liver tumors (Table 13-8). The lower doses, however, occasionally prove insufficient to take over the role of the dominant follicle in providing the negative feedback to FSH. The efficacy of ovulation prevention is lower during first cycle of contraceptive pills because the recruitment may have occurred during the luteolysis of the previous (spontaneous cycle). To imitate the normal cycle, the pills are administered for 21 days followed by either a 7-day break or 7 days of hormonally inactive tablets. A fixed dose of both agents is used in *monophasic preparations*. *Sequential preparations* are designed to mimic the estrogen and progesterone pattern of the normal menstrual cycle. *Biphasic preparations* contain a fixed dose of estrogen, and after 10 days of a lower dose of progestin, the progestin dose is increased for the next 11 days to mimic the luteal phase. *Triphasic preparations* essentially follow the same concept with more graded doses of steroids. The progestin content of the pills also contributes to contraception by altering cervical mucus, making it less permeable for spermatozoa.

Progestins alone may also be used as oral contraceptives. However, in the absence of the negative feedback provided by estrogens, progestins are less effective in suppressing the GnRH pulse generator. Thus, progestin-only "minipills" are less effective in preventing pregnancy. However, unlike estrogen-containing pills, which suppress established milk production (*galactopoiesis*, see Functional Development of the Breast), these low-dose progestin pills are compatible with lactation and may be prescribed to breastfeeding women.

The observations with oral contraceptives indicate that steroid-mediated feedback is sufficient for suppressing pituitary gonadotropin secretion and preventing ovulation. Thus, the feedback provided by inhibin appears to be a redundant mechanism.

Hormonal contraception can be achieved with subcutaneous implants of superactive *agonists of GnRH*. This approach is similar to the treatment of prostate cancer and relies on the extensive downregulation and desensitization of the GnRH receptors.

Ovulation May Be Induced by Estrogen Antagonists, Pulsatile Administration of GnRH, or Sequential Administration of FSH and LH

Ovulation induction is used in the treatment of infertility. The common problem associated with ovulation induction is that the precise control of endogenous mechanisms is not matched by these exogenous hormonal interventions. This often leads to multiple ovulations and twin pregnancies.

Clomiphene citrate is an estrogen receptor antagonist that *prevents the negative feedback action* of endogenous estrogens, thereby inducing gonadotropin secretion. The action of clomiphene citrate requires an intact hypothalamic–pituitary unit. In conditions such as Kallmann's syndrome, idiopathic GnRH deficiency or posthypophysectomy states alternative means must be utilized.

The pulsatile administration of GnRH does not require an intact hypothalamic GnRH, only an intact pituitary gonadotroph cell population. This method, however, necessitates specialized equipment.

Table 13-8   The Physiologic Actions of Estrogens and Progesterone in
Postpubertal Cycling Women[a]

Target	Estrogens	Progesterone
Fallopian tube	Increases the numbers of ciliated cells in the oviduct	After an initial upregulation of ciliary beating activity, decreases the numbers of ciliated cells
Endometrium	Regeneration and proliferation of the endometrium	Inhibition of endometrial proliferation and induction of maturation to secretory endometrium
Uterine cervix	Increased production of low-viscosity cervical mucus with high content of hydrated hyaluronic acid	Decreased production of cervical mucus; viscosity of the mucus increases
Vagina	Increased proliferation, thickness, glycogen accumulation, and cornification of the epithelium; increased numbers of surface cells in vaginal smears	Increased contribution of polymorphonuclear leukocytes and parabasal epithelial cells in vaginal smears
Breast	Maintenance of connective/adipose tissue and turgor; minimal cyclic development of mammary ductal epithelium	Minimal cyclic development of alveolar epithelium
Bones	Prevention of osteoporosis (see Table 8-7)	?
Brain	Prevention of Alzheimer's disease	Increases body temperature by a hypothalamic action; increased ventilatory response to CO_2
Liver/metabolism	Increased production of vitamin K-dependent clotting factors (II, VII, IX, X) Increased glycosylation (and synthesis?) of SHGB, TBG, and CBG leading to increased plasma levels of carrier proteins Increases HDL, decreases LDL, with slight decrease of total cholesterol; slightly increases triglycerides	Mainly glucocorticoid-like effects: induces insulin resistance leading to increased insulin secretion
Electrolytes	Enhances movement of ECF from the intravascular to the interstitial compartment thereby activating the renin mechanism and leading to fluid retention	Decreased Na^+-retention by antagonizing aldosterone on the mineralocorticoid receptor (becomes prominent in pregnancy)

Table 13-8 (Continued)

Target	Estrogens	Progesterone
Smooth muscle	Sensitizes uterine smooth muscle to the action of oxytocin (relevant in pregnancy)	Decreases the contactility of smooth muscles in general: may cause constipation (GI smooth muscle), decreased uterine contractility, and contributes to the development of venous varicosities by vascular smooth muscle relaxation (mainly during pregnancy)
Pituitary/hypothalamus	Direct pituitary action: increased PRL gene expression; induces lactotroph hyperplasia	Upregulation of GnRH receptors in estrogen-primed pituitary
	Via the hypothalamus: increased synthesis and secretion of PRL in part by inhibiting the tuberoinfundibular dopaminergic activity	Coupling the pulsatile release of NPY with that of GnRH during the preovulatory surge of gonadotropins; luteal phase, inhibits the pulse frequency of the GnRH pulse generator via endogenous opioid mechanism
Skin, sebaceous gland	Looser consistency of sebum, decreased formation of acne	—

[a] The regulation of gonadotropins is not included in detail.

ABBREVIATIONS: SHBG, sex hormone-binding globulin; TBG, thyroxine-binding globulin; CBG, cortisol-binding globulin; HDL, high density lipoprotein; LDL, low density lipoprotein; ECF, extracellular fluid; GI, gastrointestinal; PRL, prolactin; NPY, neuropeptide Y; GnRH, gonadotropin releasing hormone.

The gonadotropins used for ovulation induction are HMG (menotropin) and hCG, which provide the FSH and the LH-like activities, respectively. These hormones need not be administered in a pulsatile manner to induce ovulation. Menotropin-induced follicular development may be monitored by ultrasonography. Ovulation is usually induced with hCG when the lead Graafian follicle reaches the diameter of at least 16 to 18 mm but less than 20 to 22 mm.

The Menstrual Cycle May Be Entrained by Pheromonal Signals
Pheromones are signaling molecules that communicate information *between individuals*. In mammals, most pheromones are odorous substances emitted by *apocrine sweat glands* of an individual (mainly the underarm, mammary, and perianal glands in humans), and provoke behavioral and/or physiologic changes in other individuals via a specialized olfactory epithelium known as the *vomeronasal organ*. As discussed related to the development of GnRH neurons, the olfactory epithelium (including the vomeronasal organ)

is directly connected to the anterior hypothalamus and the limbic system, an area of the brain involved with emotions and sexual function.

Human studies indicate the existence of a functioning vomeronasal organ–hypothalamic connection that regulates the gonadotropin–gonad axis in postpubertal women. Body odor collected on underarm cotton pads was wiped on the upper lip of recipient women for 6 h per day. When the donor was in her follicular phase, the follicular phase of the recipients became shorter and ovulated earlier. Axillary odors of women on the day of ovulation and the next 2 days delayed ovulation of recipients in their follicular phase. As mentioned, the function of the apocrine sweat glands, and presumably pheromone secretion, is androgen-dependent. The cyclic nature of ovarian androgen production may explain the phase-dependent pheromone composition of underarm sweat. Such phase-advancing and phase-delaying effects of pheromones may explain the *menstrual synchrony* experienced by women living in close relationship, such as roommates or members of a sports team.

The Effects of Ovarian Hormones During the Menstrual Cycle   The systemic effects of ovarian hormones produced during the menstrual cycle are listed in Table 13-8. Estrogen and progesterone are secreted in a sequential manner during the menstrual cycle. This is important for those actions of progesterone, which are exerted only in estrogen-primed tissues. The estrogen priming includes the induction of progesterone receptors. Conversely, progesterone decreases estrogen receptors in several target tissues.

In addition to the cyclic nature of their action, ovarian steroids exert chronic effects, which on the whole are irrespective of cyclicity. Examples of this type of action include the osteoporosis-preventing action of estrogens and the maintenance of normal sexual hair by ovarian androgens.

In addition to hirsutism, androgenic hyperactivity in women often presents as seborrhea and/or acne due to overactive sebaceous glands. Estrogens exert a direct anti-acne action on the sebaceous glands by decreasing the viscosity of sebum. Some women experience acne during their menstrual bleeding. This is related to the nadir of plasma estrogen during the cycle, which leads to a peak androgen : estrogen ratio.

The Endometrial Cycle   The phases of the endometrial cycle are discussed on page 514. Here we discuss selected mechanisms involved in the endometrial cycle. Abnormal menstruation often indicates endocrine dysfunction. The main types of abnormal menstrual bleedings are summarized in Table 13-9.

Menstrual bleeding is triggered by the decrease of progesterone exposure of an estrogen-primed endometrium. The bleeding is mainly caused by MMPs and prostaglandin-mediated ischemia, although additional factors such as the liberation of lysosomal proteases may play important roles.

Table 13-9   Abnormal Menstruation

Terminology	Manifestation/definition
Primary amenorrhea	Menarche (first menstrual bleeding) has never occurred and the patient is >16 years old.
Secondary amenorrhea	Absence of menstrual period after menstrual cycles have already occurred. Amenorrhea is usually diagnosed if menstruation is absent for at least 6 months.
Oligomenorrhea	Menstrual periods occur more than 35 days apart.
Polymenorrhea	Menstrual periods occur too frequently (<3 weeks apart).
Hypomenorrhea (cryptomenorrhea)	Unusually light menstrual flow.
Dysmenorrhea	Excessively painful menstruation.
Menorrhagia (hypermenorrhea)	Too heavy (>80 mL) or prolonged (>6 days) menstruation.
Metrorrhagia	Bleeding that occurs *between* menstrual phases within a cycle. Includes midcycle breakthrough bleeding. May be due to endometrial or cervical cancer.
Menometrorrhagia	Bleeding that occurs at irregular intervals.

- The degradation of the stromal extracellular matrix in the endometrium involves mechanisms similar to those causing follicular rupture during ovulation. Upon progesterone withdrawal, endometrial stromal cells express the mRNA of MMP-1, -2, -3, and -9, and secrete them as inactive proproteins that are subsequently activated by plasmin. Most of these MMPs are also induced by IL-1 and TNF-α, suggesting that progesterone suppresses MMP expression by suppressing locally acting cytokines. The endometrial expression of TIMP-1 and -2 (the inhibitors of MMPs) is unchanged during the menstrual cycle. Thus, decrease of progesterone induces matrix degradation by altering the balance between MMPs and their inhibitors.
- Similar to glucocorticoids, progesterone inhibits the synthesis of prostaglandins. With the luteolytic decrease of progesterone, the production of $PGF_{2\alpha}$ increases. The stratum functionale is supplied by the spiral arteries, which (unlike the straight arteries supplying the stratum basale) respond to these mechanisms with a sustained and strong vasoconstriction leading ischemia. The prostaglandins cause cramps related to smooth muscle contraction of the myometrium. These muscle contractions contribute to the expulsion of the sloughed off endometrium from the uterine cavity through the cervical canal.

The etiology of *breakthrough bleeding* is different from that of bona fide menstrual bleeding. Breakthrough bleeding occurs when the estrogen-stimulated endometrial growth yields such a thick mucosal lining that its innermost layers are not properly supplied by blood and undergo an ischemic necrosis. This mechanism implies that in the absence of progesterone (which normally stops endometrial proliferation), further growth is limited by the blood supply. During puberty, several of the initial "menstrual" cycles involve breakthrough bleeding. Pubertal development involves a gradual decrease in the hypothalamic sensitivity to the feedback action of gonadal steroids. This results in a gradual increase in gonadotropin secretion. Thus, FSH secretion may be sufficient to recruit/rescue early antral follicles, induce their growth, and increase estrogen production, but insufficient to reach the threshold of plasma estradiol necessary for provoking the preovulatory LH surge. The consequence is the absence of both ovulation and corpus luteum formation. In the absence of progesterone, the unopposed estrogen action leads to overproliferation of the endometrium and breakthrough bleeding. Thus, these breakthrough bleedings are associated with anovulatory cycles. Some women experience *"midcycle spotting."* This is essentially a breakthrough bleeding that occurs just before ovulation due to overt estrogenization of the endometrium.

The *unopposed action of estrogens* (i.e., absence of progesterone) is a risk factor for the development of endometrial cancer. Obesity is a hyperestrogenic state due to the conversion of adrenally derived androstenedione into estrone by adipose tissue aromatase. Obesity therefore predisposes postmenopausal women to endometrial cancer. This explains the clinical practice to supplement estrogen with progestin in the prevention of postmenopausal osteoporosis.

Unlike the menstrual cycle of primates, which is characterized by shedding the endometrium upon decreased progesterone exposure, most mammals follow an *estrous cycle*. Estrus coincides with ovulation, and is characterized by sexual receptivity ("heat"). The mechanism of midcycle breakthrough bleeding is involved in the bloody vaginal discharge seen in dogs during their estrus.

The Vagina and the Uterine Cervix   Under the influence of estrogens, the vaginal epithelium thickens and accumulates glycogen. This has several important consequences:

* The color of blood in the capillaries of the lamina propria shows through the thin vaginal epithelium of prepubertal girls. This red color turns pink after puberty due to the estrogen-induced epithelial thickening.
* The glycogen-rich surface cells are continuously shed, die, and release their content. This glycogen serves as the nutrient of *lactobacillus acidophilus* (also known as *Döderlein's bacilli*, which are used in active yogurt cultures), which is the normal flora of the postpubertal vagina. The activity of these bacteria turns the pH of the vagina acidic (pH 3.8 to 4.2), which protects against colonization by other bacteria.
* Vaginal cytology reveals three types of epithelial cells in postpubertal women: *parabasal cells* (small, round, thick noncornified cells with a large nucleus), *intermediate cells* (large, polyogonal cells with a relatively *large nonpyknotic nucleus*), and *superficial cells* (large, polygonal, flat, cornified cells with a *small pyknotic nucleus*). All cell types have a single nucleus.

The *maturation index* is the percentage of these cells in the vaginal smear preparation. Prepubertal and postmenopausal vaginal smears have a preponderance of parabasal cells. Normally superficial (>30 to 50%) and intermediate cells are dominant during the reproductive years. Whereas estrogens increase, progestins decrease the contribution of superficial cells. Due to other influencing factors (such as vaginal infections and personal hygiene), the maturation index is not a reliable measure of estrogen production and is now rarely used in clinical practice.

The quality and quantity of the cervical mucous plug is regulated by estradiol and progesterone and varies with the stage of the ovarian cycle.

- *Spinnbarkeit* is the elasticity of the mucus, which is examined by dropping a sample of cervical mucus on a glass slide, covering it with another slide, then stretching the mucus by lifting the upper slide until the thinning thread of mucus breaks.
- *Ferning* (arborization) refers to the microscopic pattern of mucus dried on a glass slide and is the consequence of the composition of cervical mucus (Fig. 13-21).

Estradiol promotes the secretion of copious amounts of watery mucus rich in hyaluronic acid. The production of this type of mucus peaks at peak levels of estradiol, i.e., at the time of the preovulatory surge of gonadotropins. The preovulatory midcycle mucus shows the most prominent ferning. During the follicular phase the Spinnbarkeit of mucus increases from about 2 cm (early follicular phase) to 14 cm (midcycle); the maximum Spinnbarkeit coincides with maximum ferning. This midcycle mucus is easily penetrated by spermatozoa.

Progesterone decreases the amount and increases the viscosity of the cervical mucus. The Spinnbarkeit decreases to its minimum (2 to 3 cm) within days after ovulation. The ferning pattern disappears and the mucus becomes highly cellular. This type of mucus represents a significant barrier against penetration by spematozoa. As noted, progestins present in oral contraceptives decrease fertility in part by altering the character of cervical mucus.

Premenstrual Syndrome   The recurrent mood and physical disturbances associated with the luteal phase of the menstrual cycle is known as the premenstrual syndrome (PMS).

- The mood symptoms include *negative affect* (depression, irritability, emotional lability), *food cravings,* and insomnia.
- The physical symptoms include *water retention* (bloating, ankle edema) and *pain* (headaches, breast tenderness).

The severity of these symptoms shows significant individual variability. About 5 to 10% of cycling women present with moderate to severe symp-

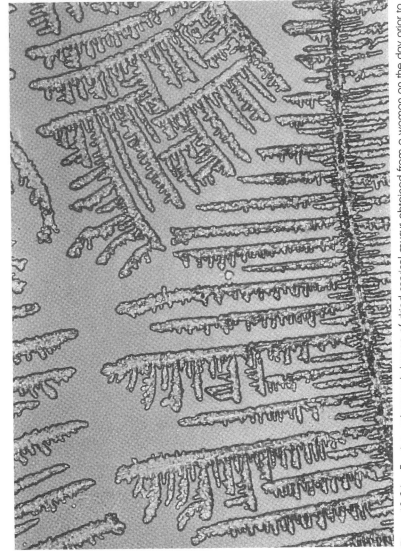

Figure 13-21. Ferning: microscopic image of dried cervical mucus obtained from a woman on the day prior to ovulation. The extensive ferning pattern is consistent with high Spinnbarkeit and high E_2 levels. (*Source:* Fig. 14-9, p 321 in Moore WT, Eastman RC (eds): *Diagnostic Endocrinology,* 2nd ed., St. Louis, Mosby, 1996.)

toms. The underlying cause of PMS is most probably a cyclic dysregulation of calcium homeostasis. PMS has a long-term association with the development of osteopenia/osteoporosis. Women presenting with PMS have lower plasma ionized calcium levels than women without PMS. The consequence is a cycle-dependent secondary hyperparathyroidism with an immunoreactive PTH peak during midcycle. PTH does not fluctuate during the menstrual cycle in women without PMS. Changes in plasma ionized calcium are reflected in the cerebrospinal fluid (CSF), and this may result in altered neuronal activity and mood. Ionized calcium acts upon the calcium-sensing receptors (CaR) in the thick ascending limb of the loop of Henle, where it antagonizes the action of antidiuretic hormone (ADH) on sodium reabsorption. By this action, increased ionized calcium decreases the corticomedullary osmotic gradient and may cause diabetes insipidus-like polyuria. Conversely, when ionized calcium is decreased (such as in women with PMS), fluid is retained. The etiology of the deranged calcium homeostasis is uncertain. However, the involvement of ionized calcium in the pathomechanism of PMS is supported by the finding that dietary calcium (1200 mg/d) or magnesium (200 mg/d) supplementation alleviates the symptoms of PMS in most patients.

Pregnancy

OBJECTIVES

1. Discuss the female aspects of intercourse, including arousal, orgasm, and its relationship with oxytocin secretion.
2. Describe fertilization. Discuss the timecourse of events from ejaculation to fertilization. Identify the mechanisms involved in *capacitation*, the interaction between spermal *fertilization antigen-1* and *zona pellucida receptors* (ZP3), *acrosomal reaction*, and *block to polyspermy*. Discuss the fusion of pronuclei, and its relationship with *trophoblastic disease*. Identify the mechanisms underlying the immunosuppressive action of semen.
3. Discuss implantation, the involvement of *leukemia inhibiting factor* (LIF), and *epidermal growth factor* (EGF). Describe the stage of embryonic development at the time of implantation, and the interaction between the trophoblast cells and the endometrial lining. Define the difference between embryonic/fetal age (postfertilization time) and gestational weeks counted from the last menstrual period (LMP).
4. Discuss human placentation, and the structure and development of the placenta. Describe the main functions of the placenta and the types of its endocrine function including the hormones synthesized, degraded, transported, or modified. Discuss the mechanisms leading to shallow placentation and *preeclampsia*. Describe the mechanisms preventing the rejection of the placenta/fetus as an *allograft*.

5. Discuss the regulation and role of the corpus luteum maintaining pregnancy. Identify the timing of placental development when the corpus luteum becomes expendable. Discuss the central role of hCG in placental endocrine function, including its impact on maternal and fetal targets. Identify markers of luteal function and discuss *relaxin*. Discuss steroidogenesis within the framework of the *fetoplacental unit*. Compare and contrast the fetoplacental unit with the function of granulosa lutein and theca lutein cells. Identify the role of the fetal adrenal in placental estrogen production, and the role of the placenta in corticosteroid production by the fetal zone of the adrenal cortex. Discuss *X-linked ichthyosis* and its relationship to placental estrogen production.

6. Discuss the causes and impact of altered endocrine function during pregnancy: the consequences of increased estrogens and progesterone, the nature of increased mineralocorticoid secretion, the Cushingoid features of pregnancy related to excess glucocorticoid production, the increased GH-like biologic activity and IGF-1 in plasma. Discuss calcium homeostasis during pregnancy. Describe the functions of the maternal pituitary gland during pregnancy: gonadotropins, PRL, GH, TSH, and ACTH. Discuss insulin during pregnancy, the concept of *accelerated starvation,* and the mechanisms potentially leading to *gestational diabetes mellitus.*

7. Discuss parturition, the *placental clock,* the role of placental corticotropin-releasing hormone (CRH) and its binding protein, prostaglandins, the *Ferguson reflex,* and oxytocin. Identify the role of estrogens and progesterone in uterine contractility. Discuss potential mechanisms of *tocolysis* to prevent premature delivery and pharmacologically induced uterine contraction to control postpartum bleeding.

8. Compare the timecourse of placental CRH secretion and uterine contractions. Define *Braxton-Hicks contractions.* Describe the changes in the uterine cervix during prelabor and labor.

Intercourse   Pregnancy starts with fertilization, which usually occurs subsequent to intercourse. Upon erotic arousal, the Bartholin's glands provide lubrication to aid the intromission of the penis. The bulbus vestibuli, the glans clitoridis and the corpora cavernosa are erectile tissues that swell with blood.

Orgasm is induced by a combination of stimuli:

- Tactile stimulation of the clitoris (especially the glans), the labia minora, and the *anterior* wall of the vagina. The existence of the *Grafenberg spot* (G spot, supposedly a small circumscribed hypersensitive orgastic area of the anterior wall) is uncertain.
- Activation of stretch receptors located in the *upper* portion of the vagina.
- Stimulation of the nipple and the areola of the breasts.
- Reinforcing olfactory, visual, and auditory stimuli.

Orgasm involves the activation of the sympathetic system, which results in rhythmic contractions of the vaginal wall. In addition, 3 to 15 involuntary rhythmic contractions of the bulbospongiosus and ischiocavernosus muscles are provoked by somatic motor fibers of the pudendal nerve. These contractions of smooth and skeletal muscles are similar to those observed in males. On the average, orgasm lasts approximately 30 seconds. Unlike in males, repeated orgasms may be achieved without a refractory period. Some females experience "ejaculation" during orgasm. The composition of the ejaculate is urine-like and does not support an origin from the Skene's paraurethral glands (the female prostate-equivalent).

It is notable that the mechanical stimuli leading to orgasm coincide with the stimuli of *oxytocin* secretion (see also Parturition and Lactation). During orgasm, oxytocin is released from the posterior pituitary gland. Oxytocin may cause contraction of the uterine smooth muscle. Upon relaxation, the uterine cavity expands and the expansion generates a slight vacuum that aspirates sperm and delivers spermatozoa faster to the site of fertilization. This mechanism, however, is not essential for successful fertilization.

Fertilization   At the time of ejaculation, semen is deposited in the vagina near the external orifice of the cervical canal. The rapid clotting of semen prevents its outflow. The spermatozoa migrate from the liquefying semen to the cervical mucus. This movement is directed by pH: spermatozoa avoid the acidic pH of the vagina and are attracted by the slightly alkaline (pH 8) mucus. With the aid of hyaluronidase, spermatozoa penetrate the abundant, low viscosity midphase cervical mucus. In part aided by uterine contraction-induced suction, in part by active flagellar movement, spermatozoa find their way to the ampullary portion of the Fallopian tube, where fertilization usually occurs. Spermatozoa reach the ampulla within 5 to 10 minutes after ejaculation. Of the approximately 200 to 300×10^6 ejaculated spermatozoa, about 200 to 300 reach the vicinity of the ovum.

Spermatozoa are capable of fertilizing the egg for up to 48 to 72 h after ejaculation. The ovum (at this stage, secondary oocyte) can be fertilized for about 24 to 48 h after ovulation. The time limits of fertilization serve as the basis of the traditional albeit unreliable "calendar method" of birth control. The efficacy of this method can be improved by regular monitoring of morning body temperature, which rises by approximately 0.5 to 0.7°C as an effect of progesterone, indicating the timing of ovulation.

A single spermatozoon out of the about 200 to 300 million present in the ejaculate fertilizes the ovum. The process of fertilization involves several steps:

- The spermatozoon must reach and attach to the zona pellucida. To achieve this goal, the hyaluronidase content of the spermatozoon is needed for penetrating the mucified intercellular space of the corona radiata.
- During the penetration of the corona radiata, the final steps of *capacitation* occur. This is in part supported by a nongenomic action of

progesterone produced by the corona radiata granulosa lutein cells. In the process of capacitation, epididymal glycoproteins that have masked binding sites of plasma membrane proteins are removed from the surface of the spermatozoon.

- Upon capacitation, the spermatozoon binds to the zona pellucida. The interaction involves several receptor proteins making the spermatozoon-zona pellucida interaction relatively species specific. A crucial factor supporting this process is a 51-kDa protein receptor tyrosine kinase in the spermatozoon membrane termed *fertilization antigen-1* (FA-1), which specifically reacts with the zona pellucida receptor *ZP3*. Affinity-purified antibodies targeting FA-1 completely block the sperm-zona pellucida interaction. Because FA-1 is a unique protein (its sequence is unrelated to other known protein families) and its expression is restricted to sperm, FA-1 is a potential target of male contraceptives.

- The binding of FA-1 with ZP3 results in the activation of the tyrosine kinase domain of FA-1 leading to autophosphorylation and tyrosine phosphorylation of other proteins. These events activate voltage-gated Ca^{2+}-channels and ultimately trigger the *acrosome reaction*, which includes the release and activation of *acrosin*, a trypsin-like enzyme needed for the penetration of the zona pellucida.

- Only the head of the spermatozoon fuses with the oocyte. The mitochondrial sheath of the middle piece, the centrioles, and the flagellum are left behind. Thus, mutations of mitochondrial DNA (such as mitochondrial diabetes) are passed on to the next generation only by the mother.

- The fusion triggers the *second meiotic division* of the oocyte, which leads to the formation of the mature oocyte and the *second polar body*. Note that the polar bodies contain minimal cytoplasm due to the inequal cytokinesis of these meiotic divisions.

- Fusion by a spermatozoon head triggers a cascade of events that block *polyspermy*, i.e., prevent the fusion with multiple spermatozoa. These events include

   - *Depolarization* of the oolemma (also known as *fast block to polyspermy*).
   - *Cortical reaction*. The oocyte contains cortical granules. The cortical reaction is their exocytosis, which is provoked by the increased cytoplasmic concentration of Ca^{2+}. The Ca^{2+} influx is due to the initial depolarization of the membrane.
   - The *zona reaction* is carried out by the exocytosed cortical granule proteins. This includes the proteolytic degradation of ZP3, and the crosslinking of proteins on the surface of the zona pellucida that yields the *perivitelline barrier*.

- The male and female *pronuclei* fuse, thereby reconstituting the diploid karyotype. This normally diploid cell is the *zygote* (Box 13-10).

- The mitotic proliferation of the zygote proceeds within the confines of the zona pellucida to yield a *morula* then a *blastocyst*. During this process, the developing embryo travels on the mucous escalator of the Fallopian tube toward the site of implantation in the endometrium near the opening of the oviduct.

BOX 13-10   Hydatidiform Mole

Hydatidiform mole is a proliferative *trophoblastic disease* characterized by the transformation of the conceptus into a mass of grape-like clusters. The "grapes" are aberrant, edematous chorionic villi. In the classic form, the entire conceptus is transformed (*complete mole*). In *partial mole,* the trophoblastic proliferation is focal and fetal parts develop. Ninety percent of complete moles develop from zygotes having a *uniparental, paternally derived diploid karyotype:* the oocyte loses the female pronucleus, and the 23 paternal chromosomes of a single fertilizing spermatozoon are duplicated. In contrast, partial moles are due to an imperfect block to polyspermy: two spermatozoa fertilize the egg yielding a triploid karyotype. Molar pregnancies typically present with a uterine growth exceeding the expected size for gestational age. Due to the abundance of trophoblasts, maternal plasma and urinary hCG levels are supranormal. The moles may have locally malignant character (invasive mole) or may give rise to distant metastases by hematogenous spread (*choriocarcinoma*). This condition may also arise in postpartum women after a normal pregnancy. Similar to the choriocarcinoma of the testis, the condition is characterized by the secretion of hCG. Monitoring plasma hCG is used for the assessment of tumor mass during chemotherapy.

In general, foreign cells (such as spermatozoa and viral infected cells) are eradicated by the killing activity of T cells and natural killer (NK) cells of the immune system. This cytotoxicity is stimulated by interleukin (IL)-12 and partially inhibited by IL-10. Human semen contains high concentrations of prostaglandins, especially PGE and 19-OH PGE. Either human seminal plasma or synthetic PGE/19-OHPGE increases the IL-10/IL-12 ratio. The seminal fluid prostaglandins thus can effect a cytokine-mediated switch away from a cell-mediated immune response. This effect, mediated via the antigen-presenting *Langerhans cells* of the genital mucosa, induces a state of non-responsiveness to sperm antigens in the female reproductive tract. It has been proposed that the induction of anergy to sperm antigen is needed for maintaining the fecundity of the female during repeated exposure to sperm. Although this immune system modulation benefits fertility, the response to infective agents present in semen, especially human immunodeficiency virus (HIV), will also be diminished and may play a critical role in the pathomechanism of sexually transmitted diseases.

Implantation and the Placenta

Implantation Requires Signaling to the Trophoblast by Uterine Leukemia Inhibiting Factor (LIF)   Ovulation occurs on about day 14 of the ovarian cycle followed by fertilization within 24 to 48 h. The rapidly proliferating zygote forms a *morula*, which transforms into the *blastocyst*. The *trophoblast* cells are the surface cells of the blastocyst, which eliminate the remnants of the zona pellucida and function as the active embryonic participants of implantation process.

Implantation requires signaling between the uterine epithelium and the trophoblast cells of the embryo.

- Mutant mouse embryos, which lack the EGF receptor, fail to attach to the endometrial epithelium, indicating that the EGF receptor is necessary for producing an implantation-competent embryo.
- LIF is a crucial factor in the uterine-trophoblast interaction. Knockout mice unable to express LIF in the endometrium fail to support implantation. Their blastocysts, however, are viable and, when transferred to wild-type pseudopregnant recipients, they can implant and develop to term. Recent evidence indicates that abnormal expression of LIF, or the related cytokine IL-6 in the endometrium may underlie some forms of human infertility.

Normally, human pregnancy lasts 280 days (40 weeks) *from the last menstrual period* (LMP). On the average, the actual pregnancy (i.e., *from fertilization*) is 2 weeks shorter. In clinical practice, the point of reference is the LMP. Embryology texts typically describe the early developmental events using fertilization as the point of reference ("fertilization days").

The implantation of the embryo begins 5 to 6 days after fertilization, i.e., on about the 21st day of the cycle. This event may be accompanied by a bleeding due to the trophoblastic invasion of the endometrium, and may be mistaken for an early-onset (albeit unusually light) menstrual bleeding, especially in women with irregular cycles.

Implantation coincides with peak production of progesterone by the corpus luteum, which has prepared the appropriately decidualized secretory endometrium for implantation. Even before implantation is complete, the anatomic arrangement is established to secrete hCG (the LH-like glycoprotein hormone product of the *syncytiotrophoblast*) directly into the maternal circulation, which is the key step in maintaining the corpus luteum, progesterone secretion, the endometrial lining, and thus pregnancy. The implantation process is complete by the 11th day after fertilization. The implantation of the blastocyst eventually leads to the development of the chorion and the placenta.

The Placenta Is a Transient Multifunctional Organ Consisting of Maternal and Fetal Components   The placenta is often described as the interface between maternal and fetal tissues, which functions as an *exchange organ*: it provides nutrients and oxygen to the fetus, and eliminates the byproducts of metabolism from the fetus. The placenta also functions as a *barrier*, which prevents passage of certain molecules (such as hydrophilic hormones) and blood cells between the fetal and maternal compartments (see also Chap. 4). Indeed, a crucial role of placental structure is *keeping the maternal and fetal intravascular fluid compartments separated*. The interface or barrier is primarily provided by the *trophoblast* cells that belong to the *fetal components* of the placenta (see below). The *maternal component* of the placenta is the *decidua* (decidualized endometrial stroma), which has no barrier function.

In many ways, the placenta functions as if it were an incomplete twin serving the fetus as an accessory gastrointestinal tract, lung, and kidney. The placenta has to fulfill two main additional roles:

- The placenta is a major *immunologic organ*. It is an interface between genetically distinct individuals, and as such it must prevent immunologic rejection of the fetus by the mother (see page 550). The trophoblastic barrier also prevents the transfer of most immunoglobulins, except IgG. Whereas the transfer of maternal IgGs is important in obtaining *passive immunity* against infectious agents as a preparation for adaptation to extrauterine life, it may also be harmful. Examples of the deleterious effects of IgG transfer include
    - Rh blood group-specific antibodies of an Rh-negative mother entering the circulation of the Rh-positive fetus may cause potentially fatal *erythroblastosis fetalis*.
    - TSH receptor-specific antibodies of Graves' disease mothers may cause *congenital hyperthyroidism*. The transfer of TSH receptor-blocking antibodies may cause *congenital hypothyroidism*.
- The placenta is a complex *endocrine organ* (Table 13-10) that coordinates the metabolism of the fetus and the mother, prepares the mother's body for lactation, regulates growth and several developmental processes of the conceptus, and is the main determinant of the onset of parturition. As an endocrine organ, the placenta
    - synthesizes hormones and hormone-binding proteins de novo and delivers them to the fetal and/or maternal intravascular fluid compartment;
    - produces hormones by processing precursors derived either from maternal or from fetal sources;
    - transports hormones between the maternal and fetal compartments;
    - degrades hormones, thereby altering maternal endocrine function and/or protecting the fetus from undue exposure to maternal and fetal hormones;
    - serves as a target of hormones mediating regulated transport mechanisms.

To understand these placental functions, we first briefly review the most important aspects of the development and structure of the placenta (Fig. 13-22).

Due to the invasive character of the trophoblast cells, the entire blastocyst penetrates the uterine epithelial lining and becomes encapsulated by the endometrial *stroma*. The blastocyst has an *inner cell mass* that develops into the *embryo proper*, and an outer cell mass that is the trophoblast. By

Table 13-10 The Main Endocrine Functions of the Placenta

Hormone group	Hormones synthesized de novo	Hormones produced by processing	Hormones transported through the placenta	Hormones degraded by the placenta
Steroids	Progesterone	Estriol	Progesterone, estriol, non-aromatizable androgens	Androgens by aromatase; cortisol by type II β-HSD
Thyroid hormones	—	—	T_4, T_3 (minimal but relevant transfer from mother to fetus)	T_4, T_3 by type III deiodinase
Monoamines	—	—	—	By MAO-A, MAO-B, and COMT (requires *uptake–1* mechanism)
Calcium homeostasis	PTHrP	Calcitriol, $24R,25$-$(OH)_2D_3$	Vitamin D and its derivatives	Calcitriol by 24-hydroxylase
Insulin and related hormones	IGF–1, IGF–2, relaxin (by decidual cells)	—	—	Insulin by insulinase
Growth factors	EGF, TGF–α, FGF, PDGF, TGF–β, activin, inhibin, follistatin	—	—	—
Anterior pituitary related hormones	hCG, hCS (hPL), hGH–V, PRL (by decidual cells); ACTH	—	—	—
Posterior pituitary related hormones	OT	—	—	—
Hypothalamic neurohormones	CRH, CRH–BP, GnRH, TRH, GHRH, SRIF, NPY, β–endorphin	—	TRH	—
Cytokines	TNF–α, IL–1, IL–2, IL–6, IL–8, IFN–γ	—	—	—

ABBREVIATIONS: MAO, monoamine oxidase; COMT, catecho-O-methyltransferase; IGF, insulin-like growth factor; EGF, epidermal growth factor; TGF, transforming growth factor; FGF, fibroblast growth factor; PDGF, platelet-derived growth factor; hCG, human chorionic gonadotropin; hPL, human placental lactogen; hCS, chorionic somatommotropin; hGH-V, human growth hormone variant; PRL, prolactin; ACTH, adrenocorticotropic hormone; OT, oxytocin; CRH, corticotropin-releasing hormone; CRH-BP, CRH binding protein; GnRH, gonadotropin-releasing hormone; TRH, thyrotropin-releasing hormone; GHRH, growth hormone-releasing hormone; SRIF, somatostatin; TNF, tumor necrosis factor; IL, interleukin; IFN, interferon.

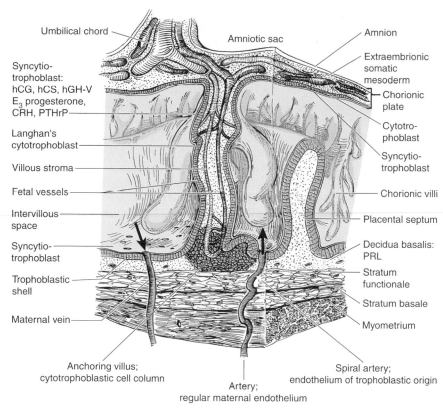

Labels (clockwise from top left):

Umbilical chord

Amniotic sac

Amnion

Syncytio-trophoblast:
hCG, hCS, hGH-V
E₃ progesterone,
CRH, PTHrP

Langhan's cytotrophoblast

Villous stroma

Fetal vessels

Intervillous space

Syncytio-trophoblast

Trophoblastic shell

Maternal vein

Anchoring villus; cytotrophoblastic cell column

Artery; regular maternal endothelium

Spiral artery; endothelium of trophoblastic origin

Extraembrionic somatic mesoderm

Chorionic plate

Cytotro-phoblast

Syncytio-trophoblast

Chorionic villi

Placental septum

Decidua basalis: PRL

Stratum functionale

Stratum basale

Myometrium

Figure 13-22. Placenta. The fetus is developing in the *amniotic sac*. Its blood vessels communicate through the *umbilical cord* to the *chorionic plate* and the *chorionic villi*. In early pregnancy, the chorionic villi are covered by two layers of trophoblast cells. The *Langhans cytotrophoblast*, which serves as a stem cell for developing the *syncytiotrophoblastic* surface layer, becomes depleted later in pregnancy. At the tip of the *anchoring villi*, the syncytiotrophoblast is absent, and the extravillous (peripheral) cytotrophoblast cells form a compact *cell column* that spreads to form the *trophoblastic shell*. These extravillous trophoblasts are in contact with the maternal decidua cells in the *decidua basalis*. The decidua basalis and the trophoblastic shell form *placental septa*, which demarcate the cotyledons (lobules) of the placenta but do not reach the chorionic plate. Modified extravillous cytotrophoblasts invade the maternal blood vessels as endothelium and intermingle with maternal endothelial cells. Maternal blood enters the intervillous spaces from *spiral arteries*, exchanges materials with fetal blood through a barrier of the villi, and leaves via *maternal veins*. The villous barrier includes two layers of trophoblast cells, the trophoblast basal lamina, the villous connective tissue stroma, endothelial basal lamina and the fetal endothelium. Maternal blood and decidua cells are in contact with the foreign trophoblastic tissue antigens. The trophoblast and the decidua are hormone-producing cells. (*Source:* Modified from Fig. 23-20, p 456 in Junquieira LC et al: *Basic Histology*, 6th ed., Norwalk, CT, Appleton & Lange, 1989; originally appeared in Duplessis GDT, Haegel P. *Embriologie*. Masson, 1971; English Edition Springer Verlag/Chapman & Hall/Masson, 1972.)

the 13th day of development, *extraembryonic somatic mesoderm* appears at the inner surface of the *trophoblasts,* which together form the *chorionic sac.* The trophoblasts of the chorion are in contact with the decidualized stromal cells of the endometrium. The decidua interpositioned between the implanted conceptus and the myometrium is known as the *decidua basalis,* which serves as the route of placental blood supply. The endometrium apical to the conceptus is referred to as *decidua capsularis*; the endometrium peripheral to the site of implantation is the *decidua parietalis.*

The chorionic trophoblast already has two cell populations:

- the *cytotrophoblast* is composed of mitotic individual cells. The cytotrophoblast cells are further classified as the *Langhans* (or *villous*) *cytotrophoblast* cells which form the inner trophoblastic layer of chorionic villi during early pregnancy, and *peripheral cytotrophoblast* cells that form the *trophoblastic cell columns* and the *trophoblastic shell.*
- the *syncytiotrophoblast* is a *postmitotic* surface layer derived by the fusion of the plasma membranes of cytotrophoblast cells. This multinuclear syncitium is highly differentiated with ultrastructural hallmarks of steroidogenesis, and may only grow by fusion of additional cytotrophoblast cells until the pool of cytotrophoblasts becomes depleted. The differentiation of cytotrophoblast into syncytiotrophoblast is probably induced by exposure to relatively high oxygen tension.

The syncytiotrophoblast forms an initial chorionic shell that erodes thin-walled endometrial capillaries and veins. The *lacunae* within the chorionic shell (which are the forerunners of the *intervillous spaces*) are filled with blood from the eroded veins. By the erosion of few small arterioles, the lacunae are sluggishly perfused by maternal blood (*lacunar phase*; fertilization days 9 to 13).

At the end of the second fertilization week, chorionic villi develop as proliferating solid epithelial cords of cytotrophoblasts (*primary villi*). *Secondary villi,* defined by the presence of embryonic mesenchyme, develop a few days later and start a branching pattern of growth. By the end of the third fertilization week, blood vessels appear in the core of the villi. The development of these *tertiary chorionic villi* coincides with the development of the primitive cardiovascular system, although blood cell formation in the islands of the yolk sac does not begin until the 5th week.

During the 6th fertilization week, chorionic villi start growing in an asymmetric manner: elaborate villi are grown toward the decidua basalis and form the *chorion frondosum* (leafy chorion), whereas the chorion facing toward the decidua capsularis remains smooth (*chorion laeve*). (The correct Latin spelling is *leve,* but the misspelled version used in anatomic texts is retained here as a time-honored tradition). The largest villi of the chorion frondosum attach to the endometrium as *anchoring villi* via solid columns of cytotrophoblast cells, which spread as the trophoblastic shell and secure the attachment of the placenta to the decidua basalis (see Fig. 13-22). The trophoblastic invasion of about 40 to 60 spiral endometrial arteries occurs at this time. The inner cell mass (by then the embryo within the amnion) is adjacent to the chorion frondosum. The allantois-associated blood vessels communicate with the vessels within the chorionic plate and the chorion frondosum; this communication elongates and develops into the *umbilical cord*.

The *cotyledons* (lobules of the placenta emerging from the chorionic plate) are clusters of branching chorionic villi separated from each other by placental septa. The *placental septa* are wedgelike protrusions of the decidua covered by trophoblastic shell. Formation of primordial cotyledons occurs during the 6th to 7th fertilization weeks. At this time, maternal circulation in the intervillous space is still sluggish with low pressure (5 to 8 mmHg). By the 11th to 12th fertilization week (about 13th week LMP), 10 to 12 large cotyledons develop that are flushed by high-pressure maternal blood (40 to 60 mmHg in the central intervillous space). This stage heralds the development of the *definitive placenta. The maturational increase in placental perfusion coincides with the peak plasma hCG concentrations.*

The name decidua (decidual membrane) refers to the fate of the endometrial lining: it falls off at the time of parturition. At parturition, the apical layer of the decidua is shed, which corresponds with the stratum functionale of the cycling endometrial lining. This is the layer supplied by the spiral arteries. The stratum basale supplied by the straight arteries is retained and the endometrium regenerates from it during the *puerperium* (early postpartum period).

Shallow Placentation Is Due to the Failure of Cytotrophoblast Cells to Express Adhesion Molecules of the Endothelial Phenotype, and Its Consequence Is Preeclampsia During the development of the placenta, cytotrophoblast cells of anchoring chorionic villi aggregate into cell columns and invade both the uterine interstitium and vasculature, thereby generating the basal plate, which anchors the fetus to the uterus and establishes maternal blood flow to the intervillous space. The *invasive character* of trophoblast cells is a result of several factors, including the expression of integrin $\alpha V\beta 3$, VE-cadherin, and MMP-9, which make trophoblasts functionally similar to osteoclast cells (see Chap. 8). Cytotrophoblasts colonizing the spiral arterioles replace the maternal endothelium as far as the luminal one third of the myometrium. The differentiating *cytotrophoblasts switch their adhesion receptor repertoire so as to resemble the endothelial cell phenotype they replace.*

- The cytotrophoblasts in cell columns display decreased expression of E-cadherin and express VE-cadherin, platelet-endothelial adhesion molecule-1, vascular endothelial adhesion molecule-1, and α_4-integrins.
- The cytotrophoblasts in the uterine interstitium and maternal vasculature express these receptors and integrin $\alpha V\beta 3$.

The phenotype switch is critical for endovascular invasion. The musculoelastic wall of the invaded spiral arterioles is replaced by a mixture of fibrinoid and fibrous tissue. These vessels become relatively large, low-resistance channels functionally similar to arteriovenous shunts. The decreased vascular resistance related to trophoblastic invasion can be demonstrated by *pulsed Doppler* ultrasound examination of the uterine *arcuate arteries* from which the spiral (and the straight) arteries originate.

In *preeclampsia*, a potentially life-threatening hypertensive disease (also known as *toxemia of pregnancy*) in which endovascular invasion is abrogated, cytotrophoblasts fail to adopt a vascular adhesion phenotype, including integrin, cadherin, and Ig superfamily members. The consequence is shallow placentation leading to placental ischemia, the release of vasoconstrictor substances, and a decrease of placental PGE_2 and prostacyclin production. Doppler examination may verify the abnormally high vascular resistance.

Preeclampsia occurs in approximately 6% of pregnant women, and mainly affects primigravida women during the last trimester. It is characterized by hypertension, edema, proteinuria, and fetal growth retardation. The endothelial dysfunction may proceed to *disseminated intravascular coagulation* (DIC) resulting in widespread organ damage (*eclampsia*).

Preeclampsia has a strong genetic component. It has been proposed that the condition is due to the mutation of a paternally imprinted, maternally active gene which must be expressed by the fetus in order to establish a normal placenta.

The Implanted Conceptus Avoids Immunologic Rejection by Trophoblastic Expression of Indoleamine 2,3-Dioxygenase (IDO), Which Rapidly Degrades Tryptophan, Thereby Suppressing T-Cell Activity

All tissues of the developing fetus are immunologically foreign to the mother due to the presence of paternally determined histocompatibility antigens. The human placenta is *hemochorial*, meaning that the syncytiotrophoblast cells are in direct contact with maternal blood. The syncytiotrophoblast cells form a barrier between maternal and fetal tissues on the surfaces of *chorionic villi*, the *chorionic plate*, and the *trophoblastic shell* (Fig. 13-22). Several mechanisms have been suggested for the explanation for the maternal immunologic tolerance for the "fetal allograft." Experimental evidence obtained in mice suggests the expression of *indoleamine 2,3-dioxygenase (IDO)* by the trophoblast is essential in the prevention of immunologic rejection. T cells have a mandatory requirement for tryptophan for their proliferation. Marcophages may express IDO upon stimulation with interferon-γ (IFN-γ), and inhibit T-cell responses by depriving them of tryptophan. Murine as well as human trophoblast cells express IDO, and the systemic concentration of tryptophan in maternal plasma decreases during normal pregnancy. Inhibition of IDO activity by 1-methyl-tryptophan has no impact on the survival of syngeneic concepti, but allogeneic concepti are rejected in a rapid T-cell mediated reaction.

Tryptophan is an essential amino acid that is required for fetal protein synthesis. Tryptophan is transported across the trophoblast barrier into the fetal circulation. Thus, the expression of IDO in the trophoblast had been puzzling until the discovery of its involvement in preventing fetal rejection.

It is currently uncertain how the IDO-mediated protection fits with the *trophoblast-lymphocyte cross-reactive* (TLX) *alloantigen system*, another regulatory mechanism involved in preventing rejection. TLX (also known as *membrane cofactor protein* [MCP] or CD46 antigen) is a complement regulatory protein that protects tissues from autologous complement damage. TLX is involved in maternal allogeneic recognition during pregnancy. Antibodies to paternal TLX allotypes are produced in women suffering from secondary recurrent abortions. Because of the allotypic nature of TLX antigens, a pregnant female must be able to regulate TLX immune responses to avoid rejection of the conceptus. The proposed mechanism of specific and systemic regulation of TLX immunity is the idiotype–anti-idiotype network. Seminal plasma contains high levels of allotypic TLX antigen produced by the seminal vesicle that could prime mothers prior to fertilization. Such priming effects for pregnancy acceptance are supported by improved implantation rates upon using timed vaginal exposure to semen during in vitro fertilization.

The Endocrine Physiology of the Pregnant Woman and the Fetoplacental Unit

Implantation Rescues the Corpus Luteum from Apoptosis Resulting in the Continued Maintenance of the Endometrium   Implantation coincides with peak plasma progesterone levels of the midluteal phase, i.e., the time when the function of the corpus luteum would start its spontaneous decline. However, the syncytiotrophoblast cells secrete hCG directly into the maternal circulation, which is detectable in maternal plasma within 24 h after the beginning of implantation (on about the 21st day of the cycle). The resulting maintenance of the endometrium is usually the first sign of pregnancy: women are alerted to pregnancy by missing their menstrual bleeding at the expected time. In fact, the most prevalent cause of *secondary amenorrhea* in women during the reproductive age is pregnancy. Usually the urine test for β-hCG (see Box 13-5) turns positive by the first day after the missed bleeding, (i.e. day 14 after fertilization and day 7 after implantation).

The syncytiotrophoblast cell mass at this time is very small. Plasma hCG may reach sufficient concentrations only because the half-life of hCG is unusually long among the glycoprotein hormones: about 9 to 24 h. The long half-life is due to the high sialic acid content of hCG (see also the half-life of FSH, Regulation of the Gonadotropin–Gonad Axis in Postpubertal Males). With the increasing mass of trophoblast, plasma concentration of hCG doubles approximately every 2 days, and peaks at the end of the first trimester (13th week LMP; Fig. 13-23). The time-course of plasma hCG explains several functions of hCG:

SYSTEM	HORMONE	PATTERN	AVERAGE PEAK CONCENTRATION (TIME)
Placenta and corpus luteum	Progesterone	Rises to term.	190 ng/mL (552 nmol/L) (term)
	17-Hydroxy-progester-one	Peaks at 5 weeks, then declines.	6 ng/mL (19 nmol/L) (5 weeks)
Adrenal	Cortisol	Increases to 3 times prepreg-nancy values at term.	300 ng/mL (0.83 μmol/L) (term)
	Aldosterone	Plateaus at 34 weeks with small rise near term.	100 ng/mL (277 nmol/L) (term)
	DOC	Increases to 10 times prepreg-nancy value at term.	1200 pg/mL (3.48 nmol/L) (term)
Thyroid	Total T_4	Increases during first trimester, then plateaus.	150 ng/mL (193 pmol/L)
	Free T_4	Unchanged.	30 pg/mL (38.6 pmol/L)
	Total T_3	Increases during first trimester, then plateaus.	2 ng/mL (3.1 nmol/L)
	Free T_3	Unchanged.	4 pg/mL (5.1 pmol/L)

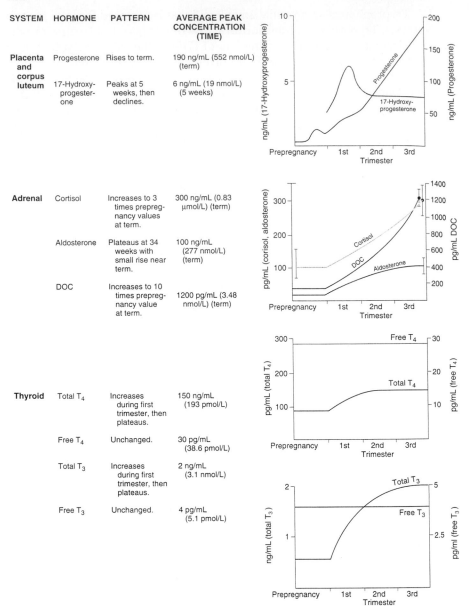

Figure 13-23. Maternal serum hormone changes during pregnancy. (*Source:* Modified from Fig. 16-1 in Taylor RN, Martin MC: The endocrinology of pregnancy, in Greenspan FS, Strewler GJ: *Basic & Clinical Endocrinology*, 5th ed., Stamford, CT, Appleton & Lange, 1997.)

SYSTEM	HORMONE	PATTERN	AVERAGE PEAK CONCENTRATION (TIME)
Anterior pituitary	LH, FSH	Low, basal levels.	
	ACTH	Unchanged.	
	PRL	Rise to term.	≈200 ng/mL (200 µg/L) (term)
Placental proteins	hCG	Peaks at 10 weeks, then decreases to a lower plateau.	5 µg/mL (5µg/L) (end of first trimester)
	hPL	Rises with placental weight.	5–25 µg/mL (5–25 µgl/L) (term)
Fetopla- central estrogens	Estriol	Increases to term.	15–17 ng/mL (55– 62 nmol/L) (term)
	Estradiol	Increases to term.	12–15 ng/mL (42– 52 nmol/L) (term)
	Estrone	Increases to term.	5–7 ng/mL (18.5– 26 nmol/L) (term)
Fetopla- central androgens	Testos- terone	Rises to 10 times pre- pregnancy values.	≈2000 pg/mL (6.9 nmol/L) (term)
	DHEA	Falls during pregnancy.	5 ng/mL (17.3 nmol/L) (pre- pregnancy)
	Andro- stenedione	Small increase.	2.6 ng/mL (9.0 nmol/L) (term)

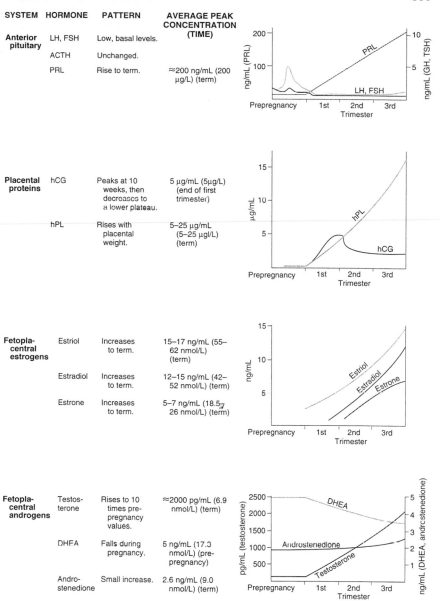

Figure 13-23. (*Continued*)

- stimulation of luteal function (see below).
- inducing "morning sickness," a condition characterized by nausea and vomiting, which usually (but not necessarily) occurs in the morning. About 50% of women experience morning sickness during pregnancy. The condition is typically most intense during the first 12 to 13 weeks of gestation LMP, i.e., the rising phase of plasma hCG. The target of hCG is the *area postrema*, the chemosensitive trigger zone of vomiting, which is a circumventricular organ not protected by the blood-brain barrier (BBB).
- regulating masculinization of the genitalia by stimulating fetal testicular androgen secretion (see Intrauterine Sexual Development). This function implies that hCG is also secreted into the fetal circulation, where its concentration is about 10% that of hCG in maternal plasma.

Chorionic gonadotropin increases *luteal hormone production*. In addition to progesterone, the theca lutein cells of the corpus luteum secrete significant quantities of *17-hydroxyprogesterone* in response to LH or hCG (see Fig. 13-4B). Similar to the granulosa lutein cells, the syncytiotrophoblast cells do not express p450c17, and thus do not contribute to circulating 17-hydroxyprogesterone (Fig. 13-24). Plasma levels of 17-hydroxyprogesterone may be used diagnostically as a marker of corpus luteum function in early pregnancy. Whereas plasma progesterone steadily increases toward term, plasma 17-hydroxyprogesterone peaks around the 7th to 8th gestational week LMP (i.e., before the peak levels of hCG are attained) followed by a decline to about two-thirds of peak levels which are maintained during the remainder of pregnancy. The same time-course is followed by another marker of luteal function, plasma concentration of *relaxin*, which is stabilized at 20% of peak levels (Box 13-11). The cause of declining of corpus luteum function is unknown. Maintenance of pregnancy requires an uninterrupted production of progesterone until parturition. A functioning corpus luteum is a mandatory requirement for the maintenance of pregnancy during the first 7 weeks. Starting with about the 7th gestational week (LMP), the placental production of progesterone becomes sufficient to maintain pregnancy in the absence of the corpus luteum. Thus, if an appendicitis involves the right ovary housing the corpus luteum of pregnancy, which necessitates removal of the ovary at appendectomy, pregnancy may normally proceed provided the event occurred after the 7th week of gestation.

The Fetoplacental Unit   The fetoplacental unit refers to the mandatory cooperation between the syncytiotrophoblast and the fetal adrenal gland in the biosynthesis of several steroid hormones. The fetal liver also contributes to the normal steroidogenic process. In terms of estrogen and progesterone production, the fetoplacental unit resembles the cooperation between theca lutein and granulosa lutein cells (see Fig. 13-4B). The steroidogenic pathways of the fetoplacental unit are summarized in Fig. 13-24. The fetoplacental unit is involved in the production of three main hormonal groups: estrogens, progesterone, and corticosteroids.

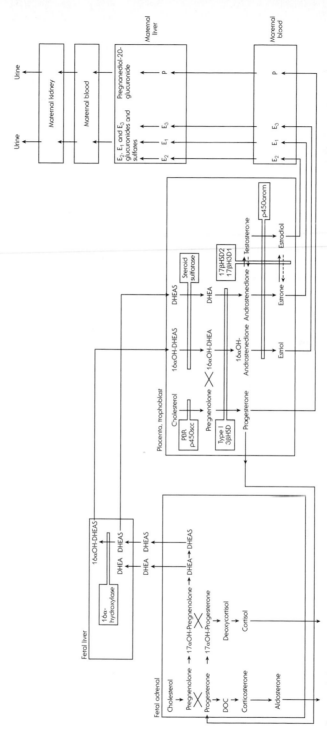

Figure 13-24. Model of the steroidogenesis by the fetoplacental unit. The isoenzyme of 17β-hydroxysteroid dehydrogenase (17βHSD) converting androstenedione to testosterone is uncertain. D-IEA, dehydroepiandrosterone; DHEAS, DHEA sulfate; DOC, 11-deoxycorticosterone; E_1, estrone; E_2, estradiol; E_3, estriol; P, progesterone; PβR, peripheral type benzodiazepine receptor.

555

BOX 13-11   Relaxin

Relaxin is an approximately 6-kDa polypeptide hormone related to insulin and IGFs. Two relaxin genes have been identified (*H1* and *H2*); both are located on the short arm of chromosome 9 and have apparently been derived by gene duplication. The *H2 gene encodes authentic relaxin,* the function of H1 (a relaxin-like peptide expressed in the decidua) is unknown. The primary transcript of the *H2* gene undergoes alternative splicing resulting in two types of mRNAs differing only in their 3' untranslated regions. Similar to insulin, relaxin consists of two polypeptide chains (A and B) linked by two disulfide bonds, and its C-peptide is removed. In males, the prostate secretes relaxin into the seminal fluid. The main source of circulating relaxin in females is the corpus luteum, which produces larger amounts of relaxin during pregnancy than during the menstrual cycle. Relaxin secretion is increased by hCG; the plasma level of relaxin follows the time-course of hCG during pregnancy. Additional sites of expression such as the decidua, heart, and brain may have more importance in local than in systemic actions. The name relaxin reflects the softening of the pubic ligament in guinea pigs, the biologic activity that led to the discovery of this hormone. The main biologic action of relaxin involves the regulation of the gene expression, synthesis, and secretion of matrix metalloproteinases, which are utilized in tissue remodeling during growth of the uterus, the mammary gland, the fetal membranes and the birth canal as a preparation for delivery. Relaxin is essential for cervical ripening and for the preparation of the breast for lactation, including structural changes in the glandular epithelium and the nipple. Relaxin decreases uterin motility- and induces vasodilation in several organs, including the uterus, the mammary gland, lungs and the heart. By inducing matrix metalloproteinases, exogenous relaxin may counteract various factors (such as the anticancer drug busulfan) that induce pulmonary fibrosis. Relaxin inhibits histamine release by mast cells thereby antagonizing experimental asthma. It also depresses aggregation of platelets and their release by megakaryocytes. The relaxin receptor has not yet been cloned but it is presumed to be related to the insulin receptor. The nitric oxide-cyclic GMP pathway is involved in the signal transduction of relaxin, an effect compatible with its vasodilatory action.

• *Production of estrogens* by syncytiotrophoblast from androgenic precursors provided by the fetal zone of the adrenal cortex. The effects of estrogens during pregnancy are listed in Table 13-11; their plasma levels are shown in Fig. 13-23.

   • The placenta is unable to generate 17-hydroxyprogesterone because it does not express the p450c17 enzyme (see page 554). This also means that neither DHEA nor androstenedione can be produced by the placenta. The lack of androgen production by the placenta is important in protecting the female fetus from masculinization. In contrast, the placenta protects the female fetus against masculinization by either maternal or fetal androgens because the placenta has a strong aromatase activity.

- The fetal zone of the adrenal cortex does not express 3β-hydroxysteroid dehydrogenase (3βHSD). Thus, all the pregnenolone generated by the p450scc is processed into DHEA and its sulfate.

- *Progesterone* is synthesized de novo by the syncytiotrophoblast from cholesterol obtained from maternal plasma LDL. (The placenta is unable to synthesize cholesterol.) Placental progesterone secretion (unlike placental estrogen production) does not require the presence of a viable fetus. The syncytiotrophoblast expresses high levels of p450scc, which is also indicated by the tubulovesicular mitochondria. Pregnenolone is converted into progesterone by the type I isoenzyme of 3βHSD. In the absence of p450c17 and p450c21, progesterone is the end product of this pathway. Progesterone as a lipophilic hormone readily enters both the maternal and the fetal circulation. The effects of progesterone during pregnancy are listed in Table 13-11 and their plasma levels are shown in Fig. 13-23. In the fetus, progesterone is an important precursor of adrenocortical hormones produced by the fetal zone of the adrenal cortex.

- *Fetal* production of *glucocorticoids* and *mineralocorticoids*. In general, glucocorticoids are inhibitors of growth, and as such are kept at minimum concentrations throughout much of fetal development. Type II 11βHSD expressed by the placenta protects the fetus against exposure to maternally derived cortisol. Nevertheless the fetus produces corticosteroids. Whereas the fetal zone of the adrenal cortex does not express 3βHSD, the definitive zone expresses type II 3βHSD. During the 13th to 24th gestational weeks, the definitive zone only scarcely expresses p450c21, a mandatory enzyme for the biosynthesis of mineralocorticoids and glucocorticoids. However, the undisturbed human fetus during 16th to 20th gestational weeks actively secretes cortisol, corticosterone, and aldosterone. The apparent conflict is resolved by the processing of placentally produced progesterone by p450c21 followed by p450c11 or p450aldo, which are all expressed at low levels in the fetal zone (see Table 12-6).

- After the 20th gestational week, the trophic action of ACTH is essential for both the fetal and the definitive zones, as indicated by their atrophy in anencephalic fetuses.

- After about the 25th gestational week, the definitive zone grows and matures more rapidly under the influence of increasing plasma ACTH levels, and contributes to the rising levels of corticosteroids. The concomitant increase of ACTH and cortisol implies that the setpoint of the negative feedback is shifting (see also Intrauterine Sexual Development). The rise in cortisol near term promotes maturation of several organ systems such as the lungs (surfactant production) and the gastrointestinal tract (cessation of macromolecular absorption, development of enzyme systems).

Table 13-11   The Main Effects of Estrogens and Progesterone Related
to Pregnancy

Target	Estrogens	Progesterone
Endometrium	—	Decidualization and maintenance of the endometrial lining
Myometrium	Sensitization to OT (promotes contractions)	Decreases uterine contractility
Extrauterine smooth muscle	—	Decreases the contractility of smooth muscles in general; may cause constipation (GI smooth muscle); contributes to the development of venous varicosities by vascular smooth muscle relaxation
Uterine cervix	—	Decreased production of cervical mucus; viscosity of the mucus increases
Vagina	Increased proliferation, thickness, glycogen accumulation, and cornification of the epithelium; increased numbers of surface cells in vaginal smears	Increased contribution of polymorphonuclear leukocytes and parabasal epithelial cells in vaginal smears
Breast	Growth and development of mammary ductal epithelium; inhibition of milk production (both lactogenesis and galactopoiesis); precipitous fall after parturition allows lactation to commence	Growth and development of alveolar epithelium; inhibition of lactogenesis but not galactopoiesis
Bones	Prevention of osteoporosis (see Table 8-7)	?
Brain	—	Increases body temperature by a hypothalamic action; increased ventilatory response to CO_2; precipitous drop at parturition may cause postpartum depression
Liver/ metabolism	Increased production of vitamin K-dependent clotting factors (II, VII, IX, X). Increased glycosylation (and synthesis?) of SHGB, TBG, and CBG leading to increased plasma levels of carrier proteins Increases HDL, decreases LDL, with slight decrease of total cholesterol; slightly increases triglycerides	Glucocorticoid-antagonist and agonistic effects in the development of insulin resistance — —
Electrolytes	—	Compensated state of aldosterone antagonism on the mineralocorticoid receptor

Table 13-11 (*Continued*)

Target	Estrogens	Progesterone
Pituitary/ Hypothalamus	Direct pituitary action: increased PRL gene expression; lactotroph hyperplasia	—
	Via the hypothalamus: increased synthesis and secretion of PRL in part by inhibiting the tuberoinfundibular dopaminergic activity	—
	Suppression of gonadotropin secretion and pituitary GnRH responsiveness	
Skin	Chloasma gravidarum; increased pigmentation of the areola, nipple and the vulva; looser consistency of sebum; decreased formation of acne	—

ABBREVIATIONS: OT, oxytocin; GI, gastrointestinal; SHBG, sex hormone-binding globulin; TBG, thyroxine-binding globulin; CBG, cortisol-binding globulin; PRL, prolactin.

Estriol is the main estrogenic product of the placenta. Its daily production rate is usually assessed by measuring maternal urinary estriol excretion. Subnormal estriol excretion may indicate:

- Placental insufficiency and/or fetal pathologies.
- *Aromatase* deficiency. In this case, plasma androgen levels increase, and lead to virilization symptoms in the pregnant mother as well as severe/ complete masculinization of the female fetus. Virilization in pregnant women is alarming. Normally the estrogen-mediated increase in plasma SHBG decreases free androgen levels in spite of an increase in total plasma testosterone.
- *Steroid sulfatase* (arylsulfatase C) deficiency. As mentioned, the gene encoding steroid sulfatase is located near the Kallmann's syndrome gene on the short arm of the X chromosome. In the case of isolated steroid sulfatase deficiency, the decrease of estriol is not accompanied by increased levels of androgens, and virilization does not occur. The fetus, however, is born with *X-linked ichthyosis* (the name refers to fish-like scales of the skin), which occurs with a frequency of 1 in 2000 to 1 in 6000 and mainly affects hemizygotic males or homozygotic females born usually from consanguinous parents. The skin condition is due to the accumulation of cholesterol sulfate in the epidermis, which usually presents in the 2nd to 3rd month of age. Steroid sulfatase is expressed by leukocytes; the differential diagnosis of ichthyosis vulgaris and X-linked ichthyosis includes the laboratory test of leukocyte-mediated hydrolysis of DHEAS into DHEA. The test is also useful in identifying heterozygotic carrier females.

Decreased placental production of estrogens may cause abnormal patterns of labor because estrogens are important in sensitizing the uterine smooth muscle to oxytocin. Sulfatase deficiency may cause impaired lactation because

- estrogens mediate the gestational hyperplasia and hypertrophy of the pituitary gland by promoting the growth of PRL-producing mammotroph cells; estrogens also stimulate their secretory activity, which contributes to the preparation of the breast for lactation.
- estrogens directly promote the growth of the ductal epithelium of the mammary gland.

The high levels of circulating estrogens are responsible for the development of *chloasma gravidarum* (mask of pregnancy), a cutaneous hyperpigmentation usually occurring after the 16th gestational week, which is accentuated by exposure to sunlight.

Maternal Pituitary Gonadotropin and GH Secretion Are Suppressed During Pregnancy   At the time of implantation, progesterone secreted by the corpus luteum under the influence of hCG prevents menstruation. In addition, the sustained function of the corpus luteum (i.e., estradiol, progesterone, inhibin) exert strong negative feedback suppression of pituitary gonadotropin secretion. This role of the corpus luteum is then replaced by the fetoplacental unit. Plasma LH and FSH are suppressed to nearly nondetectable levels and the pituitary gonadotrophs become unresponsive to a GnRH challenge. The GnRH unresponsiveness continues into the first postpartum week.

The placenta secretes a molecular variant of GH expressed from the *GH-V* gene. During the first trimester, pituitary GH is the only measurable GH in maternal plasma, and its concentrations fluctuate in an episodic manner. From about the 15th to 17th weeks of gestation, pituitary GH is progressively replaced by placental GH-V. GH-V is responsible for the continuously rising plasma levels of IGF-1 during pregnancy. By its negative feedback action on the pituitary and the hypothalamus, IGF-1 suppresses pituitary GH secretion. Concurrently the episodic secretory pattern of GH disappears because GH-V is secreted in a continuous, non-episodic manner. The pituitary GH secretion becomes refractory to secretagogues such as hypoglycemia.

The increased GH-like biologic activity includes chorionic somatomammotropin (hCS). This hormone exerts more GH-like than PRL-like actions in humans. GH-specific antibodies may crossreact with hCS. The increased circulating GH-like biologic activity increases lipolysis thereby decreasing insulin sensitivity. Thus, it is potentially diabetogenic in spite of the direct insulin-stimulating action of hCS.

Similar to hCS, GH-like placental hormones enter the fetal circulation. GH-V and/or hCS may be involved in promoting fetal growth by stimulating fetal production of IGF-1. Chorionic somatomammotropin has been implicated as a trophic factor for the developing pancreatic islets.

During Normal Pregnancy, Free Thyroid Hormones Remain Unchanged but Their Total Plasma Concentrations Are Elevated by Estrogen-Induced Increase of Thyroxine-Binding Globulin Estrogens increase plasma concentration of thyroxine-binding globulin (TBG), which leads to an initial decrease in plasma levels of *free* T_4 and T_3. The normally functioning feedback regulation increases thyroid hormone production. Restoration of normal plasma concentrations of free T_4/T_3 is achieved at an elevated concentration of *total* T_4 and T_3. Thus, in spite of increased total T_4 and T_3, healthy pregnant women remain euthyroid.

During pregnancy, iodine turnover is increased, and the iodine demand of the fetus must be met. This may result in a usually compensated state of iodine deficiency in pregnant women especially toward late gestation. The compensation involves *euthyroidism at elevated TSH levels*, which may result in enlargement of the thyroid gland.

At very high levels (such as seen in trophoblastic diseases), hCG may crossreact with the TSH-receptor and cause true hyperthyroidism. Up to 10% of postpartum women experience lymphocytic thyroiditis, which presents with an initial hyperthyroid phase followed by a prolonged phase of hypothyroidism (see Chap. 11). The condition is usually self-limited.

The Partial Corticosteroid Agonist/Antagonist Effects of High Plasma Progesterone Are Important Determinants of Maternal Adrenocortical Function Progesterone competes with aldosterone on mineralocorticoid receptors, and functions mainly as an antagonist. This is the most likely cause of the activation of the renin-angiotensin system in pregnant women, which leads to a progressive increase of plasma *aldosterone* until reaching plateau levels toward the end of the second trimester (Fig. 13-23). The substantial increase in plasma aldosterone is best interpreted as a *compensatory* feedback mechanism in response to an endogenous receptor antagonist, which explains why neither hypertension nor hypokalemic alkalosis are present.

Maternal ACTH and Cortisol Rise Throughout Pregnancy Due to Placental Production of CRH Plasma total cortisol increases approximately threefold during pregnancy, and the increase in free cortisol is approximately twofold. The circadian rhythm of cortisol secretion is maintained throughout pregnancy, although its relative amplitude (the fluctuation expressed as a percent of the average concentration of cortisol) is blunted. Plasma ACTH also increases throughout pregnancy. The main cause of the concomitant increase in ACTH and cortisol is the physiologic ectopic production of CRH by the placenta. Placental CRH secretion increases during pregnancy (see Parturition). ACTH stimulates adrenal production of both cortisol and androgens.

Cortisol, unlike aldosterone, circulates mainly in association with CBG (cortisol-binding globulin; see Tables 4-1 and 4-2). Plasma CBG levels are elevated by estrogens during pregnancy. This explains why the increase of free cortisol is lower than the increase of total cortisol. The increase in CBG-bound cortisol results in an increased plasma half-life of cortisol. As a C21 steroid, progesterone also binds to CBG. Progesterone competes with cortisol for the glucocorticoid receptor, ameliorates the biologic effect of increased free cortisol, and prevents the development of overt Cushingoid features.

The elevated cortisol nevertheless contributes to

- the development of abdominal striae, which may lead to permanent stretch marks;
  - hyperphagia and weight gain;
  - the development of gestational diabetes in susceptible individuals.

Some of the adrenal androgens may be processed by 17βHSD into testosterone. The increased production of adrenal androgens does not result in virilization for several reasons:

- increased levels of SHBG outpace the increase of androgens and free androgen levels decrease.
- placental aromatase activity rapidly converts androgens into estrogens.

The Calcium and Phosphate Demands of the Fetus Are Primarily Met by an Increase in Plasma Calcitriol of the Pregnant Mother   Calcium transport into the fetus is stimulated mainly by the autocrine action of placental PTHrP (see Chap. 8). This maternal calcium loss can be replenished from two sources:

- mobilization of calcium from maternal skeletal tissues by secondary hyperparathyroidism;
  - increased absorption of dietary calcium and phosphate.

Under physiologic conditions, provided that dietary calcium intake is appropriate (1.2 g/d), no significant secondary hyperparathyroidism occurs. In contrast, circulating calcitriol increases about four- to fivefold during pregnancy. Estrogens, GH, and PRL, which increase during pregnancy, are all inducers of renal 1α-hydroxylase. However, placentally expressed 1α-hydroxylase is the main determinant of increased calcitriol and increased intestinal absorption of calcium. Calcium together with the direct parathyroid action of increased levels of calcitriol prevent the development of secondary hyperparathyroidism.

The Potentially Diabetogenic Changes in Maternal Fuel Homeostasis Support Fetal Nutrition   For their survival, cells depend on the constant supply of fuel present in the extracellular fluid (ECF). Regulatory processes assure that the fuel supply in the ECF is continuously present in spite of the intermittent feeding of the organism. As discussed, an important feature of fuel homeostasis includes adpatational mechanisms to the fasting and the fed states. The fed state promotes fuel conservation (*anabolic state*), whereas the fasting state mobilizes stored fuel (*catabolic state*). Pregnancy complicates this regulatory process because the continuous supply of nutrients to the conceptus must be integrated with the nutritional requirements of the mother. *To prevent fetal growth retardation, amino acids and glucose must be spared for, and preferentially delivered to, the fetus during periods of fasting.* This means that maternal fuel requirements must be primarily satisfied from mobilization of FFA during fasting (Fig. 13-25).

Glucose is transported into the fetus by a concentration gradient-dependent passive transport via GLUT1. In cases of diabetes mellitus (either IDDM or *gestational diabetes mellitus* [GDM]), maternal hyperglycemia results in an increased flux of glucose into the fetus. The fetal pancreas responds to the glucose challenge with insulin secretion starting with the 15th fetal week. The ensuing fetal hyperinsulinemia delivers supranormal amounts of glucose to the intracellular fluid (ICF) for utilization (increased fuel). In addition, high insulin levels exert growth factor-like biologic effects acting on both insulin and IGF-1 receptors. These mechanisms together lead to *fetal macrosomia* (see also in Chap. 10), i.e., a birth weight of >4000 g. Macrosomia may lead to *cephalopelvic disproportion,* which necessitates cesarean section. Infants born from diabetic pregnancies often experience postpartum hypoglycemia because their increased β-cell mass produces insulin that is inappropriately high for the glucose obtained during feedings.

By the third trimester, the increase in cortisol and GH-like biologic activity in maternal plasma results in a significantly altered metabolic state, which is characterized by a *compensated state of insulin resistance.* Therefore, hyperglycemia is prevented at the expense of hyperinsulinemia. During the last trimester, plasma insulin levels are 1.5 to 2.5 times higher than in nonpregnant women. GDM develops when the increase of insulin output does not match the degree of insulin resistance. Compared to nonpregnant women, the oral glucose tolerance test during late *normal* pregnancy displays higher amplitude and prolonged increases of both plasma glucose and insulin. The increase in insulin *secretory rate* is even higher than expected from the increase in plasma levels: the half-life of insulin is shorter during pregnancy due to its placental degradation.

Although the high secretory rate of insulin suppresses glucagon production, the glucagon response to amino acids is retained. This constellation is important in minimizing use of amino acids for gluconeogenesis *during fasting* (which equals accelerated starvation during the third trimester), thereby conserving amino acids for the fetus. During hyperaminoacidemia, the surplus amino acids may be diverted to gluconeogenesis.

In Cushing's disease, hypercortisolemia suppresses the pituitary GH–IGF-1 axis. An unusual feature of late gestation is the concurrent increase

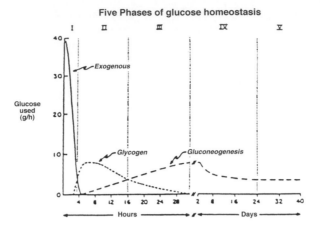

Five Phases of glucose homeostasis

Phase	I	II	III	IV	V
Origin of blood glucose	Exogenous	Glycogen, gluconeogenesis	Gluconeogenesis glycogen	Gluconeogenesis	Gluconeogenesis
Tissues using glucose as fuel	All	All except liver. Muscle, adipose at diminished rates	All except liver, but rate is diminished	Brain/RBC/renal medulla. Small amount by muscle	Brain at lower rates. RBCs, renal medulla.
Major fuel of brain	Glucose	Glucose	Glucose	Glucose, ketone bodies	Ketone bodies, glucose

Figure 13-25. A. The sources of glucose during the feeding/fasting cycle in nonpregnant individuals. Gluconeogenesis becomes the preeminent source of plasma glucose about 16 hours after the last meal. B. Physiologic "accelerated starvation" during late pregnancy. Upon fasting, free fatty acids and ketone bodies more rapidly and more substantially increase in plasma of late pregnant than in nonpregnant women. In nonpregnant women, this coincides with an increase in gluconeogenesis that maintains euglycemia, whereas pregnant women become hypoglycemic. At the same time, plasma alanine in nonpregnant women remains unchanged, which reflects an equilibrium between gluconeogenesis and cortisol-induced mobilization of alanine from muscle tissue. In contrast, plasma alanine decreases in pregnant women because of fetal uptake. The decrease in plasma glucose is the consequence of fetal glucose uptake and subnormal gluconeogenesis. The limited gluconeogenesis in late pregnancy is mainly explained by the elimination of the main substrate (alanine) by fetal uptake. (*Source:* A: from Ruderman NB et al, in Hanson RW, Mehlman MA (eds): *Gluconeogenesis: Its Regulation In Mammalian Species*, New York, Wiley, 1976, p 518; B: Fig. 14-6 in Freinkel N: Metabolic changes in pregnancy, in Wilson JD, Foster DW (eds): *Williams Textbook of Endocrinology*, 8th ed., Philadelphia, Saunders, 1992.)

of cortisol and (placental) GH. The lipolytic effect of GH requires the permissive action of cortisol. Thus, these hormones are synergistic in mobilizing FFA and decreasing insulin sensitivity. The protein catabolic effects of hypercortisolemia, however, are offset by the protein anabolic action of the increased GH–IGF-1 axis and by hyperinsulinemia.

Parturition

The Timing of Parturition Is Determined by the Placental CRH Clock   Natural birth is the physiologic end point of pregnancy, when the

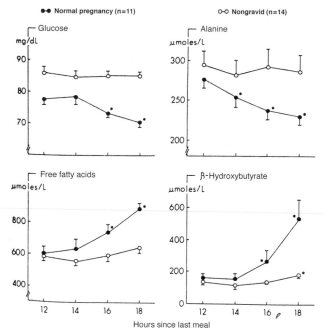

Figure 13-25. (*Continued*)

fetal membranes rupture, the amniotic fluid is lost, and the newborn is expelled from the uterine cavity by active contractions of the myometrium followed by the delivery of the placenta. Recent evidence indicates that the initiating factor of parturition is placental CRH.

CRH and CRH-binding protein (CRH-BP) are synthesized in the placenta and secreted into both the maternal and fetal circulation. Placental CRH is bioactive but causes relatively modest increases in ACTH and cortisol in the pregnant woman because of high levels of CRH-BP. CRH concentrations increase exponentially in maternal plasma as gestation advances. During the last month of pregnancy, there is a significant decrease in CRH-BP resulting in a steep rise in the concentration of free CRH both in the maternal and fetal circulation (Fig. 13-26A). Elevated concentrations of CRH, compared with gestational age-matched controls, occur in patients in preterm labor. In pregnancies complicated by preterm labor, a premature decrease of plasma CRH-BP level occurs. The exponential curve describing the CRH increase is shifted to the left in women who will subsequently deliver preterm and to the right in women who will deliver post-dates, indicating that CRH is linked to a *placental clock* that determines the length of gestation (Fig. 13-26B). Measurement of the maternal plasma CRH concentration as early as 16 to 20 weeks of gestation identifies groups of women who are destined to experience normal term, preterm or postterm delivery.

In the fetus, CRH not only targets the pituitary gland but also exerts a direct action on the fetal zone of the adrenal cortex, and stimulates

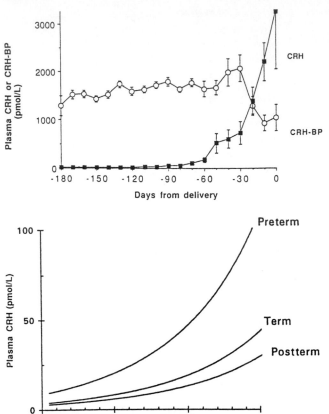

Figure 13-26. A. The concentrations of corticotropin-releasing hormone (CRH) and its binding protein (CRH-BP) in maternal plasma during the last 180 days of gestation in pregnancies ending in spontaneous term labor (37–42 weeks of gestation from the last menstrual period). B. Concentrations of CRH in maternal plasma during midgestation in women whose pregnancies ended in spontaneous preterm labor, spontaneous term labor, or postterm delivery. Premature increase of plasma CRH is a predictor of preterm labor. (*Source:* Fig. 2 and Fig. 1D in McLean M et al: A placental clock controlling the length of human pregnancy. Nature Med 1:460–463, 1995.)

preferential secretion of DHEAS over cortisol. The increased production of DHEAS provides an increased substrate load for the placenta, which results in an increase of estrogen production and an increase in the *estrogen/progesterone ratio* in spite of the sustained plasma progesetrone levels. This, in turn, increases oxytocin-receptor expression in the myometrium.

CRH-R1 is expressed in the myometrial smooth muscle and in fetal membranes; CRH-R2 is expressed at lower levels and only in the myometrium. Toward parturition, CRH-R1 is upregulated in the myometrium of the lower uterine segment, but remains unchanged in the fundus. Stimulation of the CRH-receptors in the myometrium and fetal membranes may be causally linked to parturition by several mechanisms:

- *stimulation of CRH-Rs increases the production of locally acting prostaglandins*, mainly PGE_2 and $PGF_{2\alpha}$;
- stimulation of CRH-Rs potentiates the contractile response of smooth muscle to oxytocin via a prostaglandin-dependent mechanism.

Unlike their inhibitory effect on hypothalamic CRH, glucocorticoids stimulate placental CRH-production. However, glucocorticoids inhibit prostaglandin production.

Androstenedione infusion to pregnant monkeys leads to premature labor and live delivery. Androstenedione-induced preterm labor also increases placental CRH messenger RNA and fetal plasma peptide to concentrations observed at term in pregnant monkeys.

Clinically Observed Labor Gradually Evolves from Prelabor Uterine Activity The coordinated contraction of uterine smooth muscle cells is

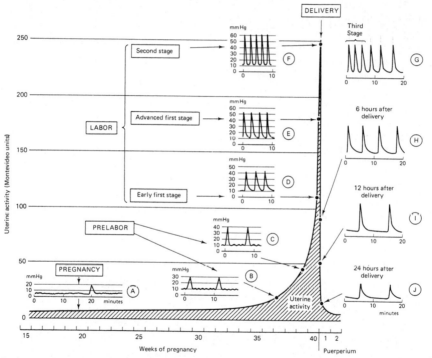

Figure 13-27. Uterine activity after the 15th gestational week. Note the exponential increase uterine activity and compare it with the time-course of CRH (Fig. 13-26). The Montevideo unit is obtained by multiplying the number of contractions/10 min with the average amplitude of the contractions measured in mmHg. Both components of the uterine activity (frequency and amplitude) increase until delivery, followed by an abrupt decrease. The puerperial activity is a functional component of postpartum uterine involution. (*Source:* Fig. 12, p 141 in Elstein M, Chantler EN: Functional anatomy of the cervix and uterus, in Philipp EE, Barnes J, Newton M (eds): *Scientific Foundations of Obstetrics and Gynecology,* 3rd ed., William Heinemann Medical Books publication distributed by Year Book Medical Publishers, Inc., 1986; Figure originally appeared as Fig. 8.12 in Caldeyro-Barcia R: *The Cervix in Pregnancy and Labour,* Churchill Livingstone, 1959.)

assured by gap junctions. During the first trimester, the uterus is relatively quiescent. *Braxton-Hicks contractions* are defined as contractions increasing intrauterine pressure by 10 to 15 mmHg and have a duration of at least 30 seconds. The intensity as well as the frequency of these contractions increases in an exponential manner following the time-course of the exponential increase in plasma CRH (Fig. 13-27). Especially during the last 5 weeks of pregnancy, the myometrial work (often referred to as *prelabor*) results in "taking up" the cervical canal: the internal os of the cervical canal expands, the lumen of the cervical canal unifies with the uterine cavity, but the diameter of the external os of the cervical canal remains narrow. The process continues the ripening of the cervix that was initiated early in pregnancy by luteal relaxin. Before the onset of labor, these changes result in the development of two functionally distinct segments of the uterus:

- The *upper segment* has a thicker and more muscular wall. Its function is the delivery of the fetus by active contractions. Uterine contractions progress from the fundus toward the lower segment.
  - The normal site of implantation and the placenta is in that portion of the endometrium, which belongs to the developing upper segment. This anatomic arrangement assures that the placenta detaches and is delivered only after fetus. Thus, while passing through the birth canal, the fetus continues to be supplied with oxygen by the placenta.
- The *lower segment* becomes progressively thinner and less muscular. If the lower segment were as muscular as the upper segment, its contractions would block the passage of the fetus. Thus, the function of the lower segment is to unify with the vagina during labor and provide a relatively passive fibromuscular birth canal. Unification with the vagina is observed as the dilatation of the external os of the cervix. The dilatation rapidly progresses during labor from about 1 to 2 cm to about 10 cm (the diameter of the head of the fetus).
  - The implantation of the placenta at the lower segment is known as *placenta previa* ("placenta ahead" [of the fetus]). Because detachment and delivery of the placenta would precede the birth of the fetus, this life-threatening condition is a mandatory indication of cesarean section.

The mother is alerted to labor by 2 to 4 relatively intense contractions per 10 minutes and/or by the rupture of the fetal membranes. The latter may present either as a sudden loss of a significant volume, or just a slow leakage of fluid.

Oxytocin Enhances the Uterine Contractions During Labor   As discussed, CRH-stimulated prostaglandins are involved in the onset of labor by directly increasing uterine contractions. The resulting descent of the fetus activates stretch receptors located in the cervix and upper vaginal wall, which in turn results in the release of oxytocin from the posterior pituitary gland (*Ferguson reflex*). More importantly, both the elevated estrogen/progesterone ratio and CRH-induced prostaglandins sensitize uterine smooth muscle to oxytocin: an approximately eightfold increase in responsiveness to oxytocin develops in an exponential manner between the 20th and 39th gestational week. Oxytocin stimulates uterine production of prostaglandins; thus, the relationship between prostaglandins and oxytocin may be viewed as a positive feedback. The positive feedback is terminated by the delivery of the fetus and the placenta: plasma concentrations of CRH (due to the elimination of its source) and oxytocin (due to the lack of stretch receptor activation) precipitously drop thereby decreasing prostaglandin production.

Oxytocin [*oxy,* rapid; *tocos,* parturition] is a nonapeptide hormone (see Fig. 10-5) with a circulating half-life of about 5 to 12 min. Oxytocin is mainly eliminated by the kidney and the liver. In addition to cervicovaginal stretch receptors, oxytocin secretion is stimulated by stimulation of the clitoris or the nipple (see milk ejection reflex, The Structure of the Breast). In lactating women, oxytocin is released by psychosensory input: hearing the baby's cry, seeing the baby, or performing baby care. Similar to ADH, oxytocin secretion is increased by dehydration and stress, and decreased by ethanol. Ethanol was utilized as a *tocolytic* agent to suspend uterine contractions in premature labor.

Oxytocin enhances both the amplitude and the frequency of contractions. The oxytocin receptor, which is encoded by chromosome 3, is a heptahelical receptor coupled by $G\alpha_{q/11}$ with the PLC signaling pathway that leads to liberation of Ca^{2+} from intracellular stores. The initial increase of intracellular calcium opens calcium-activated chloride and cation channels leading to depolarization of the myometrial cells. In turn, depolarization opens voltage-dependent calcium channels and the calcium influx from the ECF results in contraction.

The traditional quantitative measure of oxytocin is the "uterine-stimulating potency" (USP) unit. One USP unit equals about 2 μg synthetic hormone. Synthetic oxytocin is utilized in clinical practice to *induce labor* and/or to *augment contraction* during labor. At low infusion rates (0.5–1 mU/min) the endogenous rhythmic uterine contractions are enhanced. The infusion can be gradually increased until the duration of contractions reaches 40 to 60 seconds occurring at 2.5- to 4-min intervals. Further increase of the dose may lead to *uterine tetany,* when the uterus does not relax between contractions. During contraction, venous efflux of the placenta through the uterine wall becomes severely compromised. The rhythmic contractions allow appropriate oxygenation of fetal blood, but prolonged contractions may result in fetal hypoxia and *cerebral palsy*. Oxytocin continues inducing uterine contractions after delivery (i.e., stage 3 of labor, see Fig. 13-27). These contractions are accompanied by vasoconstriction and vasocompression, which are important in minimizing postpartum bleeding.

When the uterine tone is weak (*uterine atony*), life-threatening bleeding may develop.

When administered at high doses, oxytocin may crossreact with V_2 receptors of ADH in the kidney and cause fluid retention similar to SIADH (syndrome of inappropriate ADH).

Oxytocin is not only a neurohormone but also a neurotransmitter:

- Oxytocin promotes maternal behavior (including acceptance of the newborn).
- In contrast with ADH, which improves memory/retrieval, oxytocin inhibits these cognitive functions by a hippocampal action. This action has been interpreted as the means to prevent recalling the intense pain associated with labor.

Adrenergic Receptor Stimulation Modulates Uterine Contraction
Uterine smooth muscle cells express both α_1- and β_2-adrenergic receptors (see Table 12-4). The ratio of the two receptor types changes during pregnancy. In the nonpregnant uterus and during the last month of gestation, β_2-adrenergic receptors are dominant, and adrenaline causes uterine relaxation by increasing intracellular concentration of cyclic AMP. In clinical practice, this mechanism is utilized for tocolysis by β-adrenergic agonist drugs. In contrast, α_1-adrenergic agonists increase intracellular Ca^{2+} and induce uterine contraction. The ergot alkaloid *ergonovine*, which acts in part by activating α_1-adrenergic receptors, is used especially in cases of uterine atony to induce protracted uterine contraction; the drug must be administered only after the delivery of the fetus and the complete placenta.

The Puerperium

OBJECTIVES

1. Define the timeframe of puerperium. Identify the role of breastfeeding in uterine involution and *afterpains*. Identify the cellular mechanisms of *uterine involution*. Define *lochia*. Describe the regeneration of the uterine cervix.
2. Describe the role of the corpus luteum in the puerperal transition of gonadotropin regulation. Compare and contrast gonadotropin secretion, prolactin secretion and the return of the ovarian cycles in lactating versus nonlactating women. Discuss postpartum depression.

The Puerperium Is a 6-Week Postpartum Period During Which All Reproductive Organs Return to an Approximately Preconceptual State
Immediately after delivery, the uterus weighs close to 1 kg, it has an extensive wound area (the detachment site of the placenta), and the cervix is fully dilated and often torn.

The *uterus* involutes to a weight of <100 g within 6 weeks. The involution mainly involves a decrease of the size of the hypertrophied smooth muscle upon *decreased exposure to estrogens.* However, degradation of the collagenous matrix by activated matrix metalloproteinases and tissue breakdown by infiltrating macrophages also take place. The enlarged uterine cavity shrinks to nearly its original size. Uterine contractions play an active role in this process. These uterine contractions are stimulated by *nursing-induced oxytocin.* Thus, uterine involution proceeds at a faster pace in breastfeeding women, and is accompanied by more intense *afterpains.*

Uterine involution includes regeneration of the *cervix.* Although the originally rounded shape of external os of the cervix changes permanently into a transverse horizontal slit, the regeneration is usually rapid and complete. By the end of the first week, the at least 10-centimeter dilatated cervix narrows to about 1 cm in diameter.

Uterine contractions are important in stopping the *bleeding* from the placental attachment site. One of the reasons for recommending early breastfeeding is to induce oxytocin thereby decreasing blood loss. The *detachment site* is a potential entryway for microorganisms. Before the discovery of antisepsis/asepsis by Semmelweis in the nineteenth century, a dreaded and usually fatal complication of childbirth was *puerperal fever*– sepsis that develops from an iatrogenic infection of the placental detachment site.

Due to the postpartum *decrease of progesterone,* the retained portion of the decidua is shed as *lochia rubra* (red lochia), a blood-tinged discharge containing shreds of tissue. The lochia gradually becomes serous in a few days, then mucoid during the 2nd or 3rd postpartum week. Lochial discharge ceases during the 5th week and the endometrium completely regenerates by the 6th postpartum week. The postpartum regeneration process is much slower than after menstruation, which is in part due to the *very low circulating levels of estrogens.*

After the Postpartum Involution of the Corpus Luteum, the Secretion of Gonadotropins Resumes and Leads to Ovulation About 6 Weeks After Parturition in Nonlactating Women   At the time of delivery, the hormones produced by the placenta sharply decrease in the circulation. Plasma progesterone decreases to *luteal phase levels* within 24 h. As indicated by 17α-hydroxyprogesterone concentration in maternal plasma (see Fig. 13-23), the corpus luteum still functions under the influence of hCG at the time of parturition. After parturition, plasma hCG decreases in an exponential manner to follicular phase levels of LH-like biologic activity by the early 2nd postpartum week, and becomes undetectable between the 11th and 16th day postpartum. Because pituitary LH secretion remains suppressed and hCG decreases, the corpus luteum involutes with a timecourse comparable with that observed during the second half of the luteal phase (Fig. 13-28). During this time, the pituitary gland is unresponsive to exogenous GnRH, which explains low levels of FSH and pituitary LH.

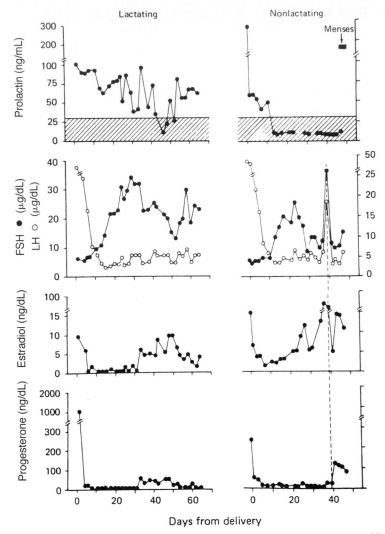

Figure 13-28. Serum concentrations of progesterone, estradiol, prolactin, FSH, and LH-like immunoreactivity during the puerperium in a lactating (left) and a nonlactating woman (right). The LH assay measured both hCG and LH. Note that estradiol fails to follow the rise in plasma FSH in lactating women indicating suppressed follicular development. In nonlactating women, first preovulatory gonadotropin surge occurs about 6 weeks postpartum. (*Source:* From Reyes FI et al: Pituitary-ovarian interrelationships during the puerperium. Am J Obstet Gynecol 114:589–594, 1972.)

- In lactating women, the stimulation of the nipple and hyperprolactinemia inhibit the GnRH pulse generator; the slow pulse frequency and the low levels of circulating inhibin allow increased FSH secretion that is not accompanied either by increased LH or by increased estradiol production. The latter may indicate a direct ovarian action of PRL to inhibit follicular growth and aromatase expression.

• In nonlactating women, the rising FSH stimulates follicular growth and estradiol production, which lead to a positive feedback/preovulatory gonadotropin surge by approximately 6 weeks postpartum. This timing coincides with the complete regeneration of the endometrial lining, including the placental attachment site. If no fertilization occurs, the first menstrual bleeding follows in 14 days.

The sharp decrease of placental steroid hormones often precipitates a usually self-limiting *postpartum depression* ("postpartum blues"). Postpartum depression coincides with the first attempts to breastfeed the infant. Unsuccessful attempts may worsen the depression, and conversely, the depression may hamper the attempts of breastfeeding.

Lactation

OBJECTIVES

1. Identify the main roles of breastfeeding.
2. Discuss the structure and development of the breast. Identify the relationship between mammary epithelium and the underlying mesenchyme, the regulation of morphogenesis, ductal growth, and lobuloalveolar development. Describe the fetal, neonatal, pubertal, pregnant, and lactational phases of mammary development.
3. Discuss the relationship between normal development, growth, and differentiation of the breast and *breast cancer*. Identify hormonal risk factors and potential endocrine markers of breast cancer.
4. Discuss *prolactin* (PRL): its synthesis, secretion, regulation, biologic actions, and signal transduction mechanisms. Identify cellular sources of PRL. Discuss the hypothalamic PRL-inhibiting and -releasing factors. Describe the causes and consequences of hyperprolactinemia in nonlactating individuals. Discuss the physiologic regulators of PRL secretion (such as suckling, stress, and hydration status), and the role of PRL in lactation.
5. Discuss the composition of milk. Define the terms *lactogenesis, galactopoiesis, colostrum, mature milk, foremilk* and *hindmilk*. Identify components of milk responsible for immunologic defense of the infant. Consider the potential physiologic roles of hormones present in milk. Compare and contrast merocrine and apocrine secretory mechanisms. Discuss the regulation of milk protein gene expression, carbohydrate and lipid synthesis.
6. Discuss the relationship between the caloric and fluid requirements of the newborn, and how these relate to the composition of milk. Identify the mechanisms resulting in, and the physiologic need for, milk as an isosmotic but low-sodium fluid. Discuss calcium homeostasis during lactation and the transport of calcium into milk. Identify minerals, iodide and other trace elements in milk and discuss their delivery to the infant.
7. Discuss the regulation of milk yield by PRL, locally acting factors in the breast and the mechanism of *milk ejection*. Consider possible mechanisms of *lactational failure*, measures to improve milk yield in breastfeeding mothers and

to suppress lactation in women who do not elect breastfeeding. Discuss the process of *weaning* and *postlactational involution* of the mammary gland.

The survival of the *fetus* depends on maternal bodily functions tuned to pregnancy by the *fetoplacental unit.* Similarly, the survival of the *newborn* depends on a maternal bodily functions tuned to lactation by signals emanating from the *"neonatomammary unit."* The healthy term newborn is well prepared to adapt to certain aspects of extrauterine life such as breathing through the lungs. Several physiologic systems of the term infant (the infant born between the 37th and 42nd weeks of gestation LMP) are normally immature at birth, such as the digestive system, the kidneys, and all main regulatory systems (nervous, endocrine, and immune systems). Although the placental influences are lost in an abrupt manner, maternal influences over the developing infant are only gradually diminished as the infant gains independence:

- Breast milk is suitable for digestion and absorption by the immature digestive system.
- For its caloric value, breast milk provides the optimal proportion of water and electrolytes. This prevents fluid and electrolyte imbalance that could develop because of the narrow functional reserve of the immature renal system.
- Breast milk provides immunologic protection to the newborn against infections, thereby compensating for the immature immune system.
- Maternal behavior helps to maintain body temperature, and is crucial for the emotional and intellectual development of the infant.
- Breast milk contains hormones which may contribute to the infant's endogenous hormonal regulatory processes.

The natural point of reaching *metabolic independence* is the completion of weaning, when breast milk is replaced by adult-type food.

We now discuss the basic aspects of lactation and its regulation.

The Structure of the Breast   The mammary gland is a modified sweat gland. Each breast contains 15 to 25 lobes, which are in effect separate *compound tubuloalveolar* glands that open independently on the nipple (Fig. 13-29). Before pregnancy, the terminal (lobuloalveolar, secretory) portion of the gland is rudimentary. The secretory product of each lobe is collected into a *lactiferous duct*, which has an expansion near the nipple (*lactiferous sinus*). The secretory alveoli form clusters known as the *lobules*, which are embedded in *loose, cellular, intralobular connective tissue.* The initial segment of the duct system draining the alveoli is the *intralobular duct.* Several intralobular ducts open into each *terminal (inter)lobular duct* which, by definition, drains milk from a whole lobule. Separate lobules, which are drained by distinct terminal (inter)lobular ducts, are demarcated from each other by *dense* interlobular connective tissue.

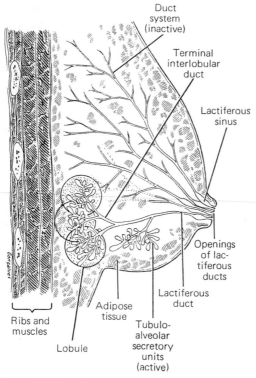

Figure 13-29. Schematic drawing of the female breast. (*Source:* Fig. 23-23 in Junquieira LC et al: *Basic Histology,* 7th ed., Norwalk, CT, Appleton & Lange, 1992.)

The acini and the duct system, until reaching the lactoferous sinus, are lined by an inner *glandular epithelium* and an outer, discontinuous layer of *myoepithelial cells* that rest on a shared basal lamina. The myoepthelial cells are typically absent from breast cancers. The acinar (alveolar) epithelium secretes milk into the lumen. The myoepithelial cells contract in response to oxytocin leading to increased intraluminal pressure and *milk ejection* (milk letdown). The loose intralobular connective tissue of the lactating mammary gland normally contains lymphocytes and plasma cells, which are responsible for producing the immunoglobulins present in milk. The duct system has both secretory and absorptive functions, and actively modifies the composition of milk.

The *nipple* is a multifunctional organ: it is a sensory organ in the milk-ejection reflex, it is the site where the lactiferous ducts open, and it functions together with the areola as *an adaptor that fits the sucking device* formed by the lips, gingiva/hard palate and tongue of the infant. The nipple is a protruding structure that consists of highly innervated modified skin. The nipple and the areola are hairless areas, whose pigmentation depends on race and is promoted by estrogens. Sparse hair may normally grow in the periareolar skin, and may become abundant in hirsutism. The thoracic *spinal nerves* (T4–T6) communicate sensory and sympathetic (mainly vasomotor) nerves to the breast. The sensory nerves are important in signaling oxytocin release by the posterior pituitary gland, PRL release by the anterior pituitary gland via a hypothalamic action, and mediating sexual arousal. Stress-induced vasoconstriction in the breast may decrease milk production and the availability of circulating oxytocin to the myoepithelial cells. Sympathetic fibers activate smooth muscles and cause *erection* of the nipple upon exposure to cold, mechanical and/or erotic stimulation.

Most of the lymphatic drainage of the breast leads into various groups of *axillary lymph nodes*. The *apical group* is also known as *sentinel lymph nodes* because lymph from all other axillary groups is finally conveyed to them making their histologic evaluation especially important in assessing the spread of breast cancer. By the axillary nodes, the lymphatic drainage of the upper limb and the breast have a common final pathway, which explains the *lymphedema* of the upper limb following *radical mastectomy*. Lymph from the medial part of the breast is drained through the chest wall to *parasternal nodes*.

The shape and size of the female breast is due to the combination of its connective tissue fibers and adipose tissue. The connective tissue fibers spread from the interlobular dense connective tissue to the overlying dermis; these fibers together form the *suspensory ligaments of Cooper*. The suspensory ligaments also serve as septa which, together with the dermis, provide enclosed spaces for the subcutaneous adipose tissue. The adipose tissue of the breast (often referred to as the *fat pad*) accumulates under the influence of estrogen and PRL. The fat pad produces locally acting factors and is a highly active metabolic tissue. Invasive breast cancers often cause retraction of the connective tissue fibers, *dimpling* of the skin and asymmetry of the breast, which is especially obvious upon raising the arms. The cancerous infiltration of the fibers may also cause *retraction of the nipple.*

Functional Development of the Breast   Carcinogenesis involves a derangement of the balance between proliferation and differentiation, which implies an intrinsic relationship between these processes during normal development. This relationship is particularly evident in the breast, as exemplified by the existence of endocrine risk factors for breast cancer that are related to the timing of normal developmental events. In the United States, women face a $1:8$ lifetime risk of developing breast cancer. The following discussion focuses on the normal developmental process with references to its relationship with carcinogenesis.

The Development of the Mammary Gland Depends on Epithelial-Mesenchymal Interactions   The development of several organs depends on epithelial-mesenchymal interactions, including the teeth (dental papilla), hair (dermal papilla of the hair follicle), and the sweat and mammary glands (milk lines). *The mammary gland and hair are mammalian-specific features* *shared by all mammals. The developmental regulation of their morphogenesis involves genetic switches adapted from tooth development.*

- *Ulnar-mammary syndrome* is an autosomal dominant disorder characterized by developmental anomalies of posterior elements of forearm, wrist and hand, apocrine/mammary gland hypoplasia and/or dysfunction, diminished to absent axillary hair, abnormal dentition, delayed puberty in males, and genital anomalies. Mutations in *TBX3* (chromosome 12q23-q24.1), a member of the T-box gene family, cause ulnar-mammary syndrome.
- *X-Linked hypohidrotic ectodermal dysplasia* is a congenital disorder resulting in abnormal tooth, hair, and mainly eccrine sweat gland development. The condition is due to the mutations of the *EDA1* gene (the human homolog of the murine *Tabby* gene). Carrier females, who are by definition mosaics for X-linked genes, often present with difficulties with lactation.
- In mice, expression of the *Msx-1* and *Msx-2 homeobox genes* have been shown to be coordinately regulated with the bone morphogenetic protein-2 and -4 (BMP-2 and BMP-4) ligands in the developing mammary gland and teeth.
- The epidermal mesenchymal signaling involves parathyroid hormone-related protein (PTHrP; see Chap. 8). PTHrP secreted by the epithelium targets *PTH/PTHrP receptors* expressed in the underlying mesenchyme. According to experiments with knockout mice, PTHrP is required for epidermal, mammary gland and tooth morphogenesis during embryonic life. PTHrP is probably involved in the branching ductal development of the mammary gland in puberty and pregnancy.

The development of the mammary glands begins during the 4th week of fetal life, when the epidermis forms bilateral *mammary ridges* (milk lines) extending from the axillary to the inguinal regions of the developing limbs. This anatomic arrangement explains both the upper limb and the genital abnormalities in the ulnar-mammary syndrome. By the 6th week, the mammary ridges involute, except in the pectoral area, where normal breast development proceeds. Incomplete involution of the mammary ridges may results in *supranumerous mammary glands and nipples* (*polythelia*) in both sexes.

The Development of the Mammary Gland Occurs in Four Main Stages: Embryonic Morphogenesis, Pubertal Growth, Pregnancy-Induced Growth, and Terminal Differentiation During Lactation During *embryonic/fetal life*, the lobes of each breast are formed by repeated bifurcations of the primary bud. This process leads to the development of the main lactiferous ducts. Although the morphogenesis of the mammary gland proceeds in a manner independent of traditional hormonal influences, the rudimentary mammary gland of the fetus and newborn is responsive to hormones. During pregnancy, the fetal and maternal mammary glands are exposed to essentially identical hormonal environments. When the maternal mammary gland is released from the influence of estrogens and progester-one, which inhibited lactogenesis (the onset of milk production), active secretion may proceed. Palpable mammary tissue and milky discharge ("witch's milk") normally occur in newborns of both sexes during the first few postpartum days.

After the early postpartum days, the mammary gland remains quiescent and rudimentary until puberty. During *puberty*, under the influence of ovarian *estrogens*, pituitary PRL and locally produced EGF, the duct system grows and bifurcates rapidly. GH, which has intrinsic PRL-like activity might contribute to the process. PTHrP produced by the epithelium may be required for the branching pattern of growth. The developmental process is first evident by the protrusion of the areola from its originally flat surface (primary mound, Tanner stage B2). The initiation of breast development (*thelarche*) is usually the first *noticed* sign of puberty in females. During pubertal development, adipose tissue accumulates to form a secondary mound, and finally the primary mound recesses to yield the contour of the mature breast (Fig. 13-30). When *ovulatory* menstrual cycles begin, a *progesterone-mediated* rudimentary lobuloalveolar development accompanies the cyclic growth and regression of the duct system. In the absence of pregnancy, this mechanism results in a slow overall growth of the mature breast until about the age of 30 years.

During *pregnancy*, several systemic hormones acting jointly cause rapid growth and maturation of the mammary gland. These hormones include estrogens, progesterone, PRL, hCS, GH-V, cortisol, insulin, EGF, and probably PTHrP. Under their influence, the epithelial tissue expands and becomes activated, but (mainly because estrogens inhibit terminal differentiation and progesterone inhibits lactogenesis) milk production does not commence. Estrogens and PRL cause deposition of adipose tissue leading to engorgement of the breasts, which is often accompanied by tenderness (*mastodynia*). *Mammary development by the 2nd trimester becomes sufficient to initiate milk production in cases of premature birth.*

The final stage of development is active *lactation*. During lactation estrogen and progesterone levels are low and several factors lead to *amenorrhea* (see below). Lactation is mainly regulated by PRL, but also requires insulin and cortisol. During lactation, further proliferation of the mammary epithelium is arrested, and the epithelium undergoes terminal differentiation leading to *lactogenesis* (the *onset* of milk production). During the first 1 to 3 days of lactation, milk (colostrum) production is minimal. PRL induced by the stimulation of the nipples by the sucking neonate induces further engorgement of the breasts and increased milk production. The term *galactopoiesis* refers to the *maintenance* of ongoing milk production. Progesterone inhibits lactogenesis thereby contributing to the lack of substantial mammary secretion during pregnancy. However, *progesterone does not inhibit galactopoiesis*; thus, progestin-only contraceptive pills are acceptable during lactation.

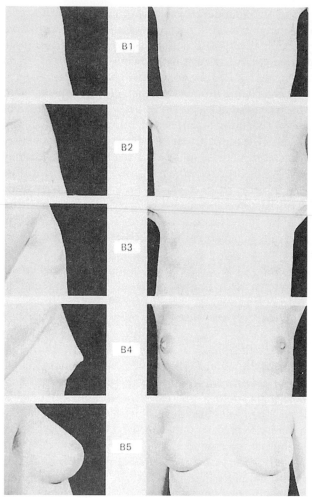

Figure 13-30. Stages of breast development according to Marshall and Tanner. Stage B1: Preadolescent—elevation of the papilla only. Stage B2: Breast bud stage—elevation of the areola as a primary mound and enlargement of the areolar diameter. Stage B3: Further enlargement of the breast and the areola, with no separation of their contours. Stage B4: Development of a secondary mound; the primary mound protrudes from the contour of the secondary mound. Stage B5: Mature stage—the areola no longer protrudes from the contour of the secondary mound. (*Source:* Van Wieringen JC et al: Growth diagrams 1965 Netherlands: Second National Survey on 0–24 Year Olds. Groningen, Netherlands Institute for Preventive Medicine NO Leiden, Wolters-Noordhoff Publishing, 1971. Marshall WA, Tanner JM: Variations in the pattern of pubertal changes in girls. Arch Dis Child 44:291, 1969.)

The CCAAT/Enhancer Binding Protein Family of Transcription Factors Plays a Pivotal Role in the Hormonal Control Determining the Proliferative vs. the Terminally Differentiated Phenotype of Mammary Epithelial Cells The ductal growth and lobuloalveolar development of *CCAAT/enhancer binding protein β* (C/EBPβ) knockout mice is rudimentary even when exposed to the adequate ovarian hormones. In wild-type mice, estrogens promote ductal growth and inhibit terminal differentiation by modulating the expression of C/EBPβ isoforms.

The expression of three C/EBPβ isoforms known as the *liver-enriched activating proteins* (LAPs), and a *dominant-negative isoform* of C/EBPβ known as the *liver-enriched inhibiting protein* (LIP) are elevated throughout pregnancy. LIP can form heterodimers with LAPs and suppress their transcriptional activity, thereby preventing terminal differentiation and facilitating continued proliferation. During pregnancy, LIP expression increases over 100-fold, which exceeds the increase in the expression of LAPs leading to a low LAP/LIP ratio (<5). The drop in circulating estrogens at parturition results in a decrease of LIP to preconceptual levels, and an over 100-fold increase in the LAP/LIP ratio occurs. LAPs are apparently positive regulators of the expression of β-casein, a major milk protein: the promoter region of the β-casein gene contains a C/EBP-binding cis-acting element.

Elevated expression levels of LIP have been detected in various human and experimental breast cancers. Estrogens (provided the estrogen receptor is expressed by the cell) promote growth of breast cancer cells, and antiestrogens such as *tamoxifen* are used in the therapy of breast cancer.

The Extracellular Matrix Plays a Crucial Role in the Attainment of the Terminally Differentiated Phenotype   In the normal mammary gland, *matrix metalloproteinases* are expressed when remodeling of the basement membrane is required for the physiologic processes including ductal growth during puberty/pregnancy, lobulo-alveolar development during pregnancy and involution after weaning. *Relaxin* is required for MMP expression in the mammary gland during pregnancy (see Box 13-11). Relaxin-deficient knockout mice fail to expand their mammary glands during pregnancy and their young die due to lactation failure in spite of the onset of milk secretion from the underdeveloped gland. Dysregulated expression of matrix metalloproteinases, especially *stromelysin-1*, may play a role in *tumorigenesis* by elimination of a differentiation signal normally provided by the basal lamina and in *tumor progression* by facilitating invasion and metastasis of malignant cells through degradation of the basal lamina and the extracellular matrix.

Mammary-Derived Growth Inhibitor Is an Autocrine Factor Inducing Terminal Differentiation and Lactational Phenotype   *Mammary-derived growth inhibitor* (MGDI) is a member of the fatty acid-binding protein (FABP) family (see Chap. 9), and is identical with the heart type FABP. Independent of its fatty acid-binding activity and probably related to its C-terminal 11 amino acids, MGDI functions as an inhibitor of epithelial (but not stromal) cell proliferation. MDGI inhibits ductal growth and induces the formation of fully developed lobulo-alveolar structures. MDGI stimulates its own epithelial-restricted expression and promotes milk protein synthesis. Selective inhibition of endogenous MDGI expression suppresses the appearance of alveolar end buds and lowers the β-casein level in organ cultures. MDGI and EGF are functional antagonists in their effects on cell proliferation.

Proliferating Mammary Epithelial Cells Acquire DNA Damages that Are Repaired by Various Tumor Suppressor Gene Products, Including hRAD51, BRCA1, BRCA2, and ATM   Any proliferating cell is bound to acquire DNA damage. These damages activate DNA repair mechanisms, which may involve *base excision repair* or *nucleotide excision repair* of single-stranded DNA damages, or *recombination-mediated repair* of double-stranded DNA damages. These DNA repair mechanisms are essential for the genetic stability of the cell.

hRAD51 is one of at least five recombination and repair proteins that are involved in ATP-dependent DNA strand exchange reactions, such as recombination-mediated DNA repair, normal meiotic and mitotic recombination (Fig. 13-31). In its absence, the proliferating cells are hypersensitive to ionizing radiation, and develop spontaneous chromosomal abnormalities. The failed repair leads to the presence of the damaged DNA, which is a signal for *checkpoint activation* in the cell cycle and increases the activity of p53 (protein 53), a major tumor suppressor gene. In turn, p53 induces p21$^{wafl/cip1}$ which leads to cell cycle arrest, and Bax which induces apoptosis.

hRAD51 is part of a nuclear multiprotein complex, which includes RNA polymerase II (see transcription, Chap. 3), BRCA1, and BRCA2. The association between hRAD51 and BRCA2 is a direct noncovalent binding involving at least two sites; BRCA1 is only indirectly associated with hRAD51. Both *BRCA* genes were originally identified as "*breast cancer genes*" (hence their name), whose mutation is responsible for a high percentage of *familial breast cancer* cases. They behave as tumor suppressor genes: the mutation of both copies is required for the development of malignancy (Knudson's two-hit model of tumorigenesis; see also Box 10-3). Individuals carrying a germline mutation in a heterozygous form have a fifteen- to twentyfold higher risk for developing breast cancer than the general population. In these cases, the "second hit" is a somatic mutation that inactivates the only normal copy of the gene in a proliferating cell.

hRAD51/BRCA2/BRCA1 dysfunction is expected to cause cell cycle arrest and apoptosis rather than uncontrolled proliferation. However, the unrepaired DNA damage may have inactivated the p53 mechanism, and breast cancer develops. This model suggests that the mutation of *BRCA* genes results in breast cancer by indirect mechanisms.

BRCA genes are expressed in several tissues. Interestingly, their mutations are typically associated with cancers of hormone-sensitive tissues: mutations of *BRCA1* predispose to *ovarian cancer*, those of *BRCA2* to

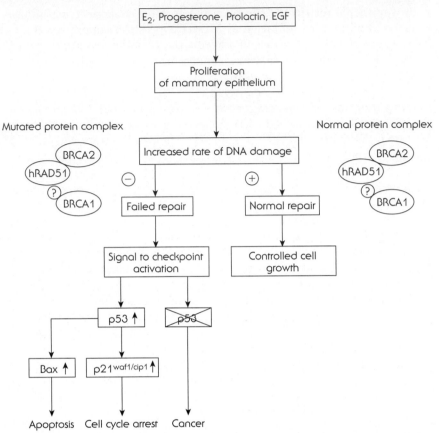

Figure 13-31. A model describing the function of breast cancer genes *BRCA1* and *BRCA2*. Note that the initial damage of the DNA is a normal feature of proliferating cells, and mammary epithelial cells regularly undergo a cycle of limited proliferation and involution as a consequence of exposure to ovarian hormones produced during the menstrual cycle. BRCA proteins are involved in the normal maintenance of genetic integrity by recombination-mediated DNA repair. (*Source:* Modified from Brugarolas J, Jacks T: Double indemnity: p53, BRCA and cancer. Nature Med 3:721–722, 1997.)

prostate cancer. A common feature of the affected tissues is the physiologic hormone-dependent proliferation of cells, and the normal function of the BRCA genes appears to be the recombination-mediated repair of the proliferation-associated DNA damage.

Another gene, whose heterozygous mutation predisposes to breast cancer by similar mechanisms, is the *ATM* gene. The homozygous form of this mutation results in *ataxia telangiectasia*, an ultimately fatal degenerative neurological disease. The ATM gene encodes a PI3-kinase-related enzyme, which is involved in DNA repair and cell cycle checkpoint regulation (see Chap. 9).

The *BRCA* and *ATM* genes are not involved in *sporadic breast cancer*.

The Postlactational Involution of the Breast Is Mainly Due to a Decrease of Circulating PRL   At the time of weaning, the stimulation of the nipple gradually decreases, resulting in a decreased secretion of PRL. As a consequence, the breasts involute: the alveoli atrophy, the duct system undergoes apoptosis, and the adipose tissue regresses until approximately prepregnancy conditions are reinstated. The mechanism might also involve the autocrine inhibition of lactation by a factor accumulating in the lumen of the breasts (see The Composition of Milk and the Regulation of Milk Production).

Some aspects of the maturational changes, however, are apparently irreversible: pregnancy carried to term at an early age (up to the age of 30 years) provides relative protection against breast cancer development. Within this group of women, the risk progressively increases with age. Lactation contributes little, although statistically significant, additional protection against breast cancer. If the first pregnancy occurs after the age of 30 years, the risk for breast cancer seems to be increased. This is probably related to the hormonal stimulation of preexisting cancer. It is estimated that the clinical presentation of the breast cancer occurs only about 8 to 10 years after the development of the cancerous clone of cells.

After menopause, when ovarian hormone production ceases, the mammary epithelium and the connective tissue stroma involute substantially. This may lead to significant changes in the shape, size, and consistency of the breasts. Typically the involution is less severe in obese women, whose adipose tissue aromatase maintains higher levels of estrogens by converting adrenal androgens. It is noteworthy that obesity is associated with an increased risk for breast cancer.

Prolactin   PRL, a member of the lactogenic hormone group of the helix bundle peptide (HBP) family, developed from a GH-like ancestral gene in teleost fish during evolution (see Chap. 10). The main source of plasma PRL is the lactotroph (mammotroph) cell population of the pituitary gland. Pituitary PRL is secreted in an episodic manner with a pulse frequency of about 90 min. Plasma PRL follows a bimodal circadian pattern with a diurnal and a larger nocturnal increase of pulse amplitude but not frequency. The nocturnal PRL surges are usually associated with non-REM sleep.

PRL in the circulation shows molecular heterogeneity: in addition to the monomeric (23-kDa) hormone, disulfide-linked dimers (big PRL), tetramers (big-big PRL), glycosylated, phosphorylated PRL, and PRL cleavage products are present. A 16-kDa N-terminal fragment of PRL (16K PRL) has been demonstrated to exert its effects via a distinct receptor and inhibit angiogenesis in rodents, but the mechanism might not be operational in humans. PRL circulates in plasma with a half-life of about 20 to 30 minutes. PRL is mainly eliminated by hepatic receptor-mediated internalization and proteolysis, and by renal filtration of the intact hormone.

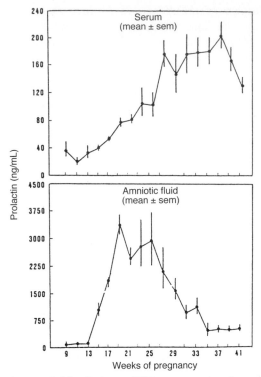

Figure 13-32. Prolactin (PRL) concentrations in maternal serum and amniotic fluid during gestation. About 50% of amniotic fluid PRL is glycosylated; it is mainly synthesized and constitutively secreted by the decidua, which explains the different time course of PRL in the two fluid compartments. The lactotroph cell develops last among anterior pituitary hormones. The fetal pituitary starts secreting significant amounts of PRL only after the 25th week (now shown). (*Source:* Kletzky OA et al: Dynamics of human chorionic gonadotropin prolactin, and growth hormone in serum and amniotic fluid throughout normal human pregnancy. Am J Obstet Gynecol 151:878–884, 1985.)

PRL is widely expressed in tissues including the decidua, normal and tumorous mammary gland, endothelial cells, a specific set of neurons in the CNS, and T lymphocytes. At least the decidual expression is driven by a promoter distinct from that utilized in the pituitary gland. Extrapituitary PRL may be involved in local actions. PRL is present in several biologic fluids, including milk, CSF, and amniotic fluid (Fig. 13-32).

The PRL receptor (PRL-R) is a member of the cytokine receptor family; it is closely related to the GH receptor, and utilizes the Jak–STAT pathway. During evolution PRL acquired its classical target with the appearance of mammals. However, due to the widespread expression of PRL receptors, PRL exerts several biologic actions (Table 13-12).

Similar to GH, PRL is under a dual hypothalamic control (Fig. 13-33). However, PRL is unique among the anterior pituitary hormones in that it is primarily under an inhibitory control: *disruption of the pituitary stalk*

Table 13-12 Selected Biologic Actions of Prolactin

Category of action	Biologic effect(s)
Lactation	Increases milk yield. Promotes gene expression of milk proteins. Stimulates biosynthesis of lactose. Induces lipoprotein lipase in the breast. Stimulates reabsorption of sodium from milk.
Reproduction	Hyperprolactinemia inhibits gonadotropin secretion by hypothalamic actions. In nonlactating individuals: hyperprolactinemia induces galactorrhea amenorrhea syndrome in females, and impotence with or without galactorrhea in males. During lactation: PRL and nipple stimulation per se inhibit gonadotropin secretion; inhibits follicular growth and aromatase expression. In rodents: PRL is luteotrophic (LH-like) in females and synergizes with androgens to stimulate male accessory gland function.
Water and electrolyte homeostasis	Milk production is a regulated loss of fluids and electrolytes. Electrolyte/volume homeostasis provides important feedback to PRL secretion. Stimulates intestinal absorption of sodium. Renal action of PRL on sodium reabsorption is minimal in humans. Stimulates renal 25(OH)vitamin D 1α-hydroxylase, thereby increasing intestinal Ca^{2+} and phosphate absorption (weak action).
Effects on the ectoderm and the skin	Mammary gland (a skin appendage): stimulates proliferation of epithelium during puberty and pregnancy, promotes maturation at the onset of lactation. Growth factor for keratinocytes (in culture). Regulates seasonal change of pelage in sheep.
Metabolism	Trophic factor for pancreatic islets. Stimulation of extrapancreatic PRL receptors may induce insulin resistance. Accumulation of breast adipose tissue especially after priming by estrogens. Modulates steroidogenesis in the adrenal cortex and the gonads.
Growth and morphogenesis	Depending on the signals from the extracellular matrix, stimulates either the growth or the differentiation of mammary epithelium. Inhibits morphogenesis of tadpoles (antagonizes T_4).
Immunoregulation	Promotes lymphocyte proliferation. May be involved in the mechanism of autoimmune arthritis.
Behavior/sleep	Stimulates REM sleep and decreases aggressive behavior.

ABBREVIATIONS: PRL, prolactin; LH, luteinizing hormone.

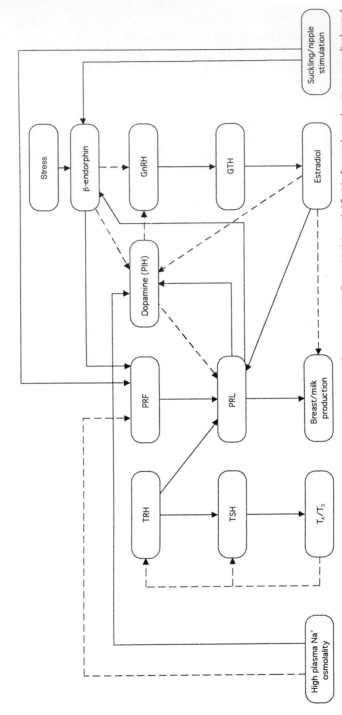

Figure 13-33. A model of the regulation of prolactin (PRL) secretion. Compare with Figs. 11-11 and 13-11. Several mechanisms are displayed which do not necessarily occur simultaneously. TRH, thyrotropin-releasing hormone; TSH, thyroid stimulating hormone; T_4/T_3, thyroid hormones; PRF, PRL-releasing factor(s); PIH, PRL-inhibiting hormone; GnRH, gonadotropin-releasing hormone; GTH, gonadotroph hormone(s). See text for details.

results in hyperprolactinemia. Note that this hyperprolactinemia is moderate, and usually does not reach the plasma PRL levels associated with PRL-secreting tumors of the pituitary gland. As opposed to most hypothalamic neurohormones, which are peptides, the *PRL-inhibiting factor* (PIF) is *dopamine.* Dopamine is produced by the *tuberoinfundibular* (TIDA) and in part by the *tuberohypophyseal* (THDA) dopaminergic neurons; the perikarya are located mainly in the arcuate nucleus of the hypothalamus. Dopamine acts on D_2 dopamine receptors (expressed from chromosome 11q22), which are coupled by $G\alpha_i$ to inhibit adenylyl cyclase activity. In addition, D_2 receptor stimulation activates K^+-channels and decreases intracellular concentration of Ca^{2+}. These effects inhibit both the release and (via the Pit-1 transcription factor) the synthesis of PRL. PRL stimulates dopaminergic activity of the TIDA, which constitutes a *short-loop negative feedback.* No hormone has been identified that would provide a long-loop negative feedback signal to PRL secretion in humans.

During the reproductive ages, PRL levels are higher in women than in men (Table 13-13); the difference is attributed to the difference in circulating estrogens. *Estrogens* stimulate PRL secretion mainly by three mechanisms:

- In concert with the Pit-1 transcription factor, estrogens directly stimulate PRL gene expression in the lactotroph.
- Estrogens inhibit the turnover of dopamine (i.e., inhibit the activity of TIDA) and decrease pituitary D_2 receptors which leads to disinhibition of PRL secretion.
- Estrogens induce lactotroph hyperplasia (chronic exposure to high levels of estrogens). Estrogens are trophic factors for PRL-secreting pituitary adenomas (*prolactinoma*; see Chap. 10). By this mechanism, oral contraceptives may lead to "postpill amenorrhea," usually manifesting as galactorrhea–amenorrhea syndrome. Development of hyperprolactinemia may sometimes present with symptoms while the individual continues her contraceptive pill regimen. In these cases unusually light menstrual flow (hypomenorrhea) may be observed during the days of steroid withdrawal and, in rare cases, mild galactorrhea may be continuously present.

Table 13-13 Normal Values of Serum Prolactin

Physiologic conditions	Concentration (ng/mL)
Adult male, postmenopausal female	3–15
Adult cycling female	5–25
Typical prolactinoma patient	>100
Pregnant female, third trimester	100–250
Newborn (1–7 d)	30–250
Prepubertal child	<10

Whereas *estrogens* are very important in the preparation of the breast for lactation and in inducing lactotroph hyperplasia/hyperprolactinemia during pregnancy, they *are not involved in the regulation of PRL secretion during lactation.*

Ample experimental evidence suggests the involvement of *PRL-releasing factor* (PRF) in the physiologic regulation of PRL secretion, including PRL release induced by nipple stimulation and stress. The chemical nature of the physiologic PRF(s), however, has remained elusive. A number of putative PRFs have been proposed to fulfill this function including the following selected examples:

- TRH is not a physiologic PRF during lactation. In *primary hypothyroidism*, TRH release from the median eminence is increased and stimulates both TSH and PRL secretion. The resulting hyperprolactinemia inhibits GnRH secretion and causes *galactorrhea-amenorrhea syndrome* in women, a condition similar to *lactational amenorrhea*. High levels of estrogens (such as those seen in pregnancy) may sensitize the lactotroph cells to the action of TRH by inhibiting their expression of the TRH-degrading ectoenzyme (see Fig. 11-11).
- VIP, a member of the secretin-GHRH family, produced by parvocellular neurons of the paraventricular nucleus and released into the pituitary portal circulation stimulates PRL secretion in vitro via activating adenylyl cyclase. At least in rodents, the expression of VIP is enhanced during lactation and after adrenalectomy, and bilateral lesion of the paraventricular nucleus inhibits suckling-induced release of PRL. VIP is also produced by the lactotroph cells and stimulates PRL secretion in an autocrine/paracrine manner.
  - In contrast with the vasodilatory VIP, the vasoconstrictor *endothelin-1* (ET-1) acting on endothelin A receptors inhibits PRL secretion both in humans and rodents. It is currently unclear whether the ET-1-mediated inhibition is a physiologic regulator of PRL secretion. At least in rodents, ET-1 is produced by the lactotroph cells suggesting an autocrine function.
- *Oxytocin* is released both in the median eminence and in the posterior pituitary, and may stimulate PRL secretion. However, whereas audiovisual stimuli related to the infant (such as baby cry) stimulate oxytocin secretion and cause milk let-down, plasma PRL does not rise without nipple stimulation.
- *Angiotensin-II* (A-II) stimulates PRL secretion in vitro. A-II is secreted by pituitary gonadotrophs in response to GnRH. This explains why an acute GnRH challenge may increase plasma PRL. PRL is a weak regulator of renal Na^+ reabsorption, intestinal Na^+ absorption, and thus a regulator of plasma volume and osmolality. A-II primarily stimulates renal Na^+ reabsorption via aldosterone, but may cause Na^+ retention in part via PRL.

Various neurotransmitters influence PRL secretion via PRF and/or dopamine. Some of these neurotransmitter systems are targeted by commonly used drugs:

- *Histamine* has a dual role in PRL secretion. Via H_2 receptors, histamine inhibits PRL. Thus, H_2 receptor blockers (used for suppressing gastric acid production) stimulate PRL secretion and may cause gynecomastia in men. In contrast, H_1 receptor blockers (used for alleviating allergic symptoms) inhibit PRL secretion. This indicates a PRL-simulating role of histamine via H_1 receptors.
- *Serotonin* and *adrenaline* (produced by CNS neurons) stimulate PRL secretion. At least in rodents, the serotonin-induced release of PRL is mediated by PRF(s), mainly VIP.
- Morphine and its derivatives are strong stimuli of PRL secretion. These drugs utilize the physiologic mechanism of endogenous opioid peptides that are involved in nursing-induced PRL release.

The preeminent physiologic role of PRL is the regulation of lactation. In the presence of physiologic concentrations of insulin and cortisol, plasma PRL levels and the emptying of the mammary gland are the main determinants of milk yield (see The Composition of Milk and the Regulation of Milk Production). The three most important regulators of PRL secretion are nipple stimulation, hydration status, and stress.

- *Sucking the nipple* is the main regulator of PRL secretion during lactation. During any stage of lactation, the more the daily nipple stimulation, the higher the average plasma PRL level. Nocturnal breastfeeding is an important stimulus in maintaining high daily PRL output. When the mother is not nursing for several hours (a typical setting for working women), plasma PRL levels are very low and pulsatile secretion is suppressed. Upon nursing or using a breast pump, PRL secretion is rapidly stimulated. When spontaneous nursing activity (as dictated by the needs of the infant) is uninterrupted, PRL levels fluctuate in a pulsatile manner and follow a circadian pattern.
- *Hydration status* is an important regulator of PRL secretion, although no direct relationship between plasma osmolality and PRL levels has been demonstrated. *Milk production is a regulated fluid and electrolyte loss*. In concert with stimulation of mineralocorticoid receptors in the lactiferous ducts, PRL promotes sodium reabsorption from milk. Thus, milk secretion represents the loss of hyponatremic fluid, which could lead to hypovolemia and increased plasma osmolality. Under hyperosmotic conditions when ADH is increased to the level to yield a concentrated urine, PRL secretion is suppressed at least in part by an increased dopaminergic tone. Thus, to maintain milk yield, lactating women need to drink enough fluid to achieve *diluting* renal function. In essence, this calls for a physiologic primary polydipsia. Indeed, at a stage of lactation when fluid loss with milk is 500 mL/d (approximately half-maximal milk yield), lactating women drink about 2 L more water than nonlactating women. Angiotensin-II, which is elevated upon hypovolemia, stimulates thirst, and the secretion of ADH and PRL. This mechanism ameliorates the decrease in PRL and maintains milk production in cases of mild dehydration. It is noteworthy that this process is similar to that of salmonids: for spawning, salmonids swim from seawater to freshwater, a hyposmotic environment that induces

PRL secretion. In turn, PRL stimulates sodium reabsorption by acting on the gill and the skin. A role for PRL has been suggested in decreasing the volume of amniotic fluid by stimulating sodium reabsorption in humans.

  • *Stress* has a complex effect on PRL secretion. In general, stress stimulates PRL secretion in both sexes. Unless the blood samples are collected under stress-free conditions, this mechanism may lead to a mistaken conclusion of hyperprolactinemia. On the other hand, stress inhibits nursing-induced PRL secretion in agreement with the everyday observation that stress inhibits lactation. Note, however, that stress-related inhibition of lactation includes additional components.

Increased secretion of PRL is *associated with non-REM sleep* in both sexes. PRL *stimulates REM sleep*. It has been suggested that PRL expressed by CNS neurons is the physiologic source of REM-stimulating PRL, but under conditions of hyperprolactinemia sufficient amount of PRL may cross the choroid plexus by a receptor-mediated transport to exert a somnogenic action.

Most women are amenorrheic during lactation. The mechanism of *lactational amenorrhea* is only partially understood. Immediately after parturition, the corpus luteum renders the pituitary gland unresponsive to GnRH. Hyperprolactinemia and the suckling stimulus per se inhibit GnRH secretion. The decreased pulse frequency of GnRH is a stronger inhibitor of LH than FSH secretion. In spite of the increase in plasma FSH, estrogen secretion remains low because of the ovarian actions of hyperprolactinemia (The Puerperium). Although in theory lactational amenorrhea could be utilized as a method of contraception, it is unreliable probably because todays' lifestyle does not permit sufficiently frequent (13 to 18 times per day) nursing. As a consequence, PRL is insufficiently elevated to antagonize follicular maturation induced by the normally increased FSH (see Fig. 13-28). If pregnancy occurs during the first ovulation, its discovery may be delayed because the continued amenorrhea is assumed to be related to lactation. In spite of breastfeeding at a frequency that leads to amenorrhea in most women (6 to 7 nursings per day), a minority of women experience menstrual periods during lactation. In some of these women, milk production ceases with the onset of the ovarian/endometrial cycle mainly because of the inhibitory action of estrogens on milk secretion. For reasons unknown, other women continue milk production in spite of the endogenous production of estrogens.

Prolactinomas secrete PRL in an autonomous fashion. Although endogenous production of dopamine is insufficient to suppress PRL to the physiologic range, its inhibitory action can be demonstrated by administration of D_2 receptor antagonist drugs, such as *metoclopramide*. The functional evaluation of prolactinomas may also include provocation tests with bolus injections of TRH or VIP. Prolactinomas may be treated by the dopamine agonist *bromocriptine* (see Fig. 10-2). The shrinkage of the tumor during bromocriptine therapy indicates that cyclic AMP mediates important tro-

Table 13-14 Composition of Human Colostrum and Milk in Comparison with Cow's Milk

	Human colostrum	Mature human milk	Mature cow's milk
Caloric content (kcal/L)	671 (588–730)	747 (446–1192)	701 (587–876)
Fat (g/100 g milk)	2.9	4.5	3.8
Cholesterol (mg/L)	280	139	110
Lactose (g/100 mL)	5.3	7.3	4.8
Protein (g/100 mL)	2.7	1.0	3.3
Whey : casein ratio	—	70 : 30	22 : 78
Albumin (g/100 mL)	—	0.4	0.4
Globulin (g/100 mL)	1.5	0.2	0.2
Casein (g/100 mL)	1.2	0.4	2.7
Total ash (g/L)	3.08	2.02	7.15
Selected minerals			
Na (mEq/L)	48	7.8	22
K (mEq/L)	15–19	13–14	36
Ca (mg/100 mL)	30	34	117
P (mg/100 mL)	15	15	92
Fe (mg/L)	0.1	0.3	0.5
I (mg/L)	0.045–0.450	0.044–0.093 (mean, 0.061)	0.036–1.05 (mean, 0.116)
Selected vitamins			
Vitamin D (IU/L)	—	22	14
Vitamin K (μg/L)	—	15.0	60.0
Vitamin C (mg/L)	72	40	11
Carotenes (mg/L)	1.37	0.25	0.37

phic action in these cells. This finding is comparable with the somatotroph hyperplasia caused by the GHRH-cyclic AMP pathway.

The Composition of Milk and the Regulation of Milk Production

Milk Yield and the Composition of Milk Depend on the Stage of Lactation The composition of milk is summarized in Table 13-14. *Colostrum* (early milk) is produced during the first 2 to 4 days postpartum. Colostrum is yellowish due to its high β carotene content, and has a high protein concentration with a high whey : casein ratio. Colostrum is gradually replaced by transitional milk (days 6 to 10) and finally *mature milk*. Milk yield, which is mainly determined by the demand of the infant, rapidly increases during this period: from about 120 mL on the 2nd or 3rd day postpartum to 240 to 300 mL by the end of the 2nd week. The maximum milk yield is approximately 0.8 to 1.2 L/d, which is usually achieved during the 6th to 7th months of lactation, right before supplementation and/or weaning begins.

After an accumulation of milk in the breast during a 2- to 4-h period of nonsuckling, the composition and caloric value of split milk displays marked differences: *foremilk* (milk ejected first) differs from *hindmilk* (milk ejected last). This difference must be taken into consideration when breastfeeding twins.

The Role of Colostrum Is to Provide Defense Factors for the Newborn   The immune system of the newborn is not fully developed, and even if it were, it cannot rely on immunologic memory. Breast milk and in particular, colostrum, represents a significant protective mechanism. Breast-fed infants are less likely to acquire infections than formula-fed babies. Defense factors in human milk include

- *antimicrobial agents*: secretory IgA (antigen-binder), lactoferrin (iron chelator), lysozyme (muramidase, degradation of bacterial wall), mucins and oligosaccharides (antirotavirus activity as a decoy receptor), and digestive products of milk lipids (disruption of viral envelope);
- *bifidus agent*: milk promotes colonization of the intestines by the harmless *lactobacillus bifidus*, thereby preventing colonization by pathogenic bacteria.
- *antiinflammatory factors* (antioxidants, epithelial growth factors, cellular protective agents, and enzymes that degrade mediators of inflammation);
- *immunomodulators*: IL-1 (activator of T cells), IL-6 (enhances IgA production), TNF-α (enhances secretory component production of IgA), TGF-β (induces isotype switching of antibodies in B cells), and antiidiotypic antibodies;
- *leukocytes* (neutrophils, macrophages, and lymphocytes).

Breast Milk Is a Liquid Diet that Simultaneously Satisfies Thirst and Hunger   The *protein composition* of human and cow's milk is different. Casein is the mixture of cheese-generating proteins in milk (*case*, cheese) that precipitate on acidification to pH 4.0. The supernatant of this precipitate is known as *whey*, which contains albumins, immunoglobulins, and *whey acidic protein* in high concentrations. Cow's milk contains more casein than human milk does. Casein is not as rich in essential amino acids as albumin, and is more difficult to digest than albumin. Thus, the nutritional value of human milk proteins is higher.

The promoter region of most milk proteins has multiple cis-acting elements and requires the coordinated function of several *hormone-regulated transcription factors*, including STATs and steroid hormone receptors (see also C/EBPβ in Functional Development of the Breast). Via STAT5, PRL stimulates the expression of several milk proteins, including β-casein, whey acidic protein, UDP-galactosyl transferase, and α-lactalbumin. Stimulation of the glucocorticoid receptor by physiologic levels of cortisol is required for the expression of these proteins. The relatively high type II *11β-hydroxysteroid dehydrogenase* (11βHSD) *activity* in the fat pad and the epithelium of the mammary gland during pregnancy significantly declines after parturition thereby allowing normal glucocorticoid action in lactogenesis and galactopoiesis.

The main *carbohydrate* in milk is lactose, a disaccharide formed by galactose and glucose. About 42% of the caloric value of mature human milk is derived from lactose. Lactose synthesis requires two enzymes in the mammary epithelium: the ubiquitous *UDP-galactosyl transferase* and the mammary specific α*-lactalbumin*, which is a major whey protein. The latter is required for the *lactose synthase* activity; without it, UDP-galactosyl transferase may only glycosylate polypeptides. Immunoreactive α-lactalbumin has been demonstrated in about 70% of various breast cancers and can be used for the detection of micrometastases. Minor quantities of glucose, galactose and fucose are also present in milk; fucose may be part of the "bifidus factor."

On the average, about 50% of the caloric value of mature human milk is derived from lipids. PRL stimulates lipoprotein lipase activity in the breast, which aids synthesis of milk fat by the mammary epithelium. Unlike proteins, which are secreted by exocytosis of secretory vesicles (*merocrine secretion*), lipids enter milk as *fat globules* generated by pinching off the budding apical cytoplasm which contains large lipid droplets (*apocrine secretion*). Some lipid-laden epithelial cells become shed altogether and appear in milk as foam cells. Breast milk contains *fatty acids* that are important for myelinization and the maturation of brain. Infant formulas are deficient in the same fatty acids, which may contribute to a statistically significant difference in IQ test scores observed between 7- to 8-year-old children who were breastfed or formula-fed as infants.

Breastfed infants are less likely to develop *obesity* than formula-fed babies, in spite of the same caloric content of the two diets, and an essentially identical distribution of caloric content among the three main nutrients. The difference may be explained at least in part by the difference in work on behalf of the infant to obtain food. In spite of the oxytocin-mediated milk-ejection reflex, the infant has to suck hard to obtain sufficient volumes of milk. In contrast, sucking from the bottle requires minimal effort, and babies tend to overeat. The appetite-suppressing hormone leptin is present in human breast milk, and is absorbed from the GI tract of the newborn. Milk-derived leptin might be a physiologic regulator of appetite.

The *energy requirement* of the infant during the first year is approximately 100 kcal/kg body weight/24 h. The *fluid requirement* under normal circumstances is about 130 mL/kg/24 h. The caloric content of milk is approximately 70 kcal/100 mL. Thus, 100 kcal/kg energy is delivered by 143 mL breast milk. This means that the breastfed infant does not require fluid supplementation. However, infants may become rapidly dehydrated under conditions such as hot climate, diarrhea, or vomiting. Fluid supplementation with fruit juice (for water loss) or commercial pediatric electrolyte solutions (for electrolyte loss) is important under these circumstances.

Milk Is an Isosmotic Solution Containing Low Concentrations of Sodium Although milk is isosmotic, its *osmotically active constituents* are quantitatively different from those of plasma. Instead of sodium, which is the main determinant of plasma osmolality, lactose accounts for about 70% of the osmolality of milk. The low sodium concentration in milk is due to the actions of PRL and mineralocorticoid receptor stimulation (see below). The latter also increases K^+ concentration in milk, which is needed for the expanding ICF of the growing infant. The low sodium concentration in milk prevents hypernatremia in the infant. In term infants, the osmolality of maximally concentrated urine is 500 to 700 mOsm/kg water, i.e., about half of that in adults (1200 mOsm/kg). Thus, unlike adults who tolerate physiologic (0.15 M) saline as an intravenous fluid *maintenance*, newborns require a mixture of 1 volume physiologic saline: 3 volumes 5% glucose. This isosmotic fluid is designed to be closer to the sodium load infants receive with breast milk. Cow's milk contains enough sodium to induce hypernatremia in the newborn human infant.

The *mineralocorticoid receptors* are preferentially expressed in the duct system of the mammary gland. This arrangement is similar to that observed in salivary glands and eccrine sweat glands (see Chap. 12). As pointed out, 11βHSD is expressed in the nonlactating mammary epithelium. The function of this enzyme in the kidney is to assure that the mineralocorticoid receptor is not stimulated by glucocorticoids. The postpartum decline of 11βHSD suggests that sodium reabsorption and potassium secretion by the lactating mammary gland is regulated by cortisol. This mechanism may coordinate fuel and electrolyte composition of milk.

Lactation and Milk Play a Central Role in the Calcium Homeostasis of the Mother and the Infant Milk contains several essential components of *calcium homeostasis*, including magnesium, calcium, phosphorous and vitamin D. A significant portion of phosphorous is present in milk in the form of casein, a highly phosphorylated protein. The vitamin D content of milk is often insufficient; the supplementation of the infant is influenced by the seasonal changes of exposure to sunlight.

Milk contains several hormones (see second section on page 595), including *PTHrP*, a product of the mammary epithelium. PTHrP is an autocrine factor of the mammary gland that stimulates calcium transport into milk. PTHrP is expressed by breast cancer cells and, depending on the amount secreted, its PTH-like action may either cause *humoral hypercalcemia of malignancy* (systemic effect) or localized osteolytic metastatic bone lesions (see also in Chap. 8).

Maternal calcium homeostasis is different during pregnancy and lactation. Because placental 25(OH)vitamin D 1α-hydroxylase is absent after birth and estrogens are low, renal 1α-hydroxylase activity is maintained by two hormones: PRL and PTH. Because the effect of PRL is weak, *secondary hyperparathyroidism* normally develops during lactation and leads to a significant (6–7%) decrease of bone mineral content by the 6th month of lactation. Dietary calcium supplementation of lactating women is therefore exceedingly important. Maternal vitamin D stores decline during lactation as indicated by the decrease in plasma 25(OH)vitamin D levels. The decrease is due to losses of vitamin D with milk.

Breast Milk Is an Adequate Source of Trace Elements Such as Iron and Iodide   The absorption of *iron* is facilitated from human milk by the presence of lactoferrin. Iron is absorbed together with intact lactoferrin from the GI tract of the newborn. Although the iron concentration of cow's milk is higher, it is less absorbed probably related to the very high concentration of casein, and the generation of ferrous phosphate.

Iodide is actively transported into milk by mechanisms similar to those involved in its transfer into the follicular lumen of the thyroid gland (see Figs. 11-3 and 11-10). Because the transfer of thyroxine with breast milk is minimal, the newborn relies on the iodide content of breast milk to support endogenous synthesis of thyroid hormones.

Milk also contains other trace elements such as *selenium, copper, zinc* and *fluoride*.

Protein and Peptide Hormones Are Present at High Concentrations in Breast Milk   Several *hormones*, mainly peptides/proteins, have been demonstrated in milk, including leptin, PRL, releasing hormones (TRH, GnRH), growth factors (EGF, IGF-1), relaxin, PTHrP, and the lipophilic amino acid derivative melatonin. These hormones often reach concentrations in milk exceeding that in plasma. The GI tract of the newborn and especially the prematurely born infant is not mature; thus, these hormones may escape degradation and may be absorbed as intact, biologically active molecules. Some of these hormones, such as EGF, may act locally on the GI tract and promote the proliferation, maturation or function of the intestines. The impact of certain milk hormones in experimental animals has been demonstrated, but definitive human studies have not yet been reported.

Most of the PRL in breast milk is derived from the circulation by transcytosis. However, PRL is also expressed by the mammary epithelium. Because pituitary PRL is a mandatory requirement for lactation, mammary PRL presumably does not reach the basolateral surface of the epithelium where the PRL receptors are preferentially located. Together with appropriate attachment to the basal lamina, the epithelial polarity is lost in breast cancer. PRL has been suggested to function as an autocrine/paracrine growth factor under these circumstances.

Steroid hormones are also present in milk. Vitamin D is a prohormone steroid, and milk is a physiologic source of vitamin D for the newborn. Estrogens and progesterone are low during lactation. However, steroid compounds produced by the regressing corpus luteum are present in colostrum, and may contribute to the physiologic jaundice of the newborn by competing with bilirubin for the limited glucuronyl transferase activity of the maturing liver.

Milk Production Is Mainly Regulated by Two Types of Humoral Signals: Systemic Hormones and Locally Acting Autocrine Factors Galactopoiesis is stimulated by *systemic hormones*. PRL, cortisol, and insulin stimulate synthesis and secretion of milk, oxytocin induces milk-ejection. The receptors of hydrophilic galactopoietic hormones are located in the basolateral membrane of the alveoli.

Humoral factors acting locally on receptors at the luminal surface of the alveoli inhibit milk secretion. A partially characterized protein hormone appears to mediate the *local autocrine inhibition of milk production*. Its function is to adapt milk production to the demand of the infant. If milk is completely emptied from the breast, the galactopoietic function becomes maximal. Milk retention decreases galactopoiesis even in the presence of appropriate circulating galactopoietic hormones. Preferential feeding from one breast may therefore result in different milk yields of the two breasts.

As mentioned, demand of the infant is the main determinant of milk production. The decreasing sucking activity of the infant during weaning results in the accumulation of the local inhibitor in the breast and the decrease of circulating PRL. Both factors are important components in the *cessation of lactation*. In several species, weaning, tooth eruption, and gastrointestinal function are coordinated during development. It is recommended that until tooth eruption (about 6 months of age), infants should receive no supplementation to breast milk. Supplementation of food may be initiated without weaning if it is given *after* breastfeeding. During the weaning process, supplemented food *precedes* breastfeeding, which satisfies appetite, decreases milk ingestion and nipple stimulation. Weaning in western cultures is usually completed by 1 year of age.

Breastfeeding is the best biologic support for the infant. In spite of advocacy by pediatricians, many healthy women *elect* formula feeding instead of breastfeeding: in the United States in 1993 less than 56% of women attempted breastfeeding, and less than 20% of women nursed their infants beyond 6 months postpartum. When required, *suppression of lactation* can be accomplished by several approaches:

- The chest/breasts are tightly wrapped with a cloth. Stimulation of the nipples is avoided and fluid intake is minimized. The initially accumulating milk inhibits further secretion by a local action. Nonsteroidal antiinflammatory drugs (NSAIDs) such as indomethacin or aspirin can be used to control the pain associated with the engorgement of the breasts. These drugs also inhibit the local synthesis of vasodilatory prostaglandins, and may decrease mammary blood flow and milk yield.
- Pharmacologic suppression of lactation is a controversial issue. The dopamine receptor agonist bromocriptine and (before the availability of bromocriptine) estrogens have been used for this purpose.

Some women experience difficulty with breastfeeding. Total absence of lactation in postpartum women may suggest *Sheehan's syndrome*, a postpartum infarction of the pituitary gland (see Chap. 10). In other cases, insufficient milk production can be overcome by

- Appropriate hydration of the mother and stress-free environment.
- Complete emptying of the breast every 3 hours: after the infant stops sucking, the remaining milk is removed by a breast pump. This method eliminates the locally acting inhibitor of milk secretion, which otherwise accumulates in the lumen of the mammary gland because the initially weak sucking activity of the newborn.
- Pharmacologic approaches: dopamine antagonist drugs (such as metoclopramide) are in use when other attempts have failed. Recombinant human GH may also improve milk-yield; this expensive drug has only been used in limited clinical tests.

ONTOGENY OF THE REPRODUCTIVE SYSTEM

OBJECTIVES

1. Discuss the main checkpoints of sex determination: chromosomal sex, gonadal sex, genital sex, sexual/gender identity, and sexual orientation. Define the terms *hermaphroditism, pseudohermaphroditism,* and *ambiguous genitalia.*
2. Discuss the structure and main genes of the X and Y chromosomes. Describe the process of *lyonization* of the X chromosome, its role and physiologic consequences, particularly in sex determination. Discuss the significance of the *Barr body.*
3. Discuss intrauterine sexual development. Discuss the autosomal and sex chromosomal genes that are involved in the determination of testicular versus ovarian development from the *indifferent gonad.* Define the relationship between the development of the gonads and the adrenal glands. Contrast the timing of events in males versus females. Identify the onset of testicular hormone production (AMH and testosterone), and identify the critical timeframe of androgen exposure of the external genitalia in the process of masculinization. Describe the role of androgens in the development of Wolffian duct structures and the prostate, and identify dihydrotestosterone-dependent processes.
4. Discuss potential mechanisms of deranged intrauterine sexual development. Discuss chromosomal translocation of the *SRY* gene and the consequences of duplication and deletion of the *DSS* locus. Discuss deletions of *SF-1, WT1* and the *SOX9* genes. Discuss *androgen insensitivity syndrome* and enzyme defects (including the various types of *adrenogenital syndrome, type II 5α-reductase deficiency, aromatase deficiency,* and *17βHSD3 deficiency*), which may result in pseudohermaphroditism. Discuss the physiologic basis of the

potential intrauterine treatment of the classic form of 21-hydroxylase deficiency.

5. Discuss the four phases of increased pituitary gonadotropin secretion in females. Compare and contrast these phases with the three corresponding phases in males. Describe the intrauterine, postpartum, and pubertal activation of testosterone secretion. Identify the mechanisms resulting in pubertal development. Describe the physiologic changes associated with puberty. Be familiar with the *Tanner staging* of pubertal development and the timing of developmental milestones.

6. Discuss deranged pubertal development and its potential causes. Discuss delayed puberty, sexual infantilism (absent puberty), and *hypergonadotropic* and *hypogonadotropic hypogonadism*. Discuss *Klinefelter's* and *Turner's* syndromes. Discuss *precocious puberty* leading to either *isosexual* or *contrasexual* development. Compare and contrast *complete* (*true*) and *incomplete precocious puberty*.

7. Define the terms *menopause, andropause,* and *adrenopause*. Discuss the mechanism of perimenopause and the hormonal regulation in postmenopausal women. Distinguish early and late manifestations of menopause. Discuss the physiologic mechanism of *hot flashes* in early menopause, postpartum, and after orchiectomy. Review postmenopausal osteoporosis. Discuss postmenopausal alterations in plasma lipoproteins and the risk for cardiovascular disease. Discuss the benefits and risks associated with hormone replacement therapy in postmenopausal women.

Introduction

During embryonic development, the initially indifferent (bipotential) gonad differentiates into either an ovary or a testis determined by the sex chromosomes present. Human gonadal sex determination is synonymous with testis determination. The presence of the Y chromosome results in the development of a testis, which secretes AMH (the product of Sertoli cells) and *androgens* (the product of Leydig cells) during embryonic life.

- AMH is required for the regression of the Müllerian ducts, the primordia of the female genital tract (Fallopian tubes, uterus, and the upper third of the vagina).
- If the inherently female primordial external genitalia are exposed to sufficient androgen receptor stimulation within the critical period of embryonic development, scrotum and phallus develop. The androgens are also needed for the obliteration of the *urogenital sinus*, the development of the prostate, and the Wolffian duct-derived structures (vas deferens, accessory glands).

In the absence of the Y chromosome, ovaries develop that secrete neither AMH nor androgens during fetal life.

- In the absence of AMH, the female genital tract develops from the Müllerian ducts by default.

- In the absence of androgen exposure, the lower two-thirds of the vagina (from the urogenital sinus) and the vulva develop, also by default.

During the childhood years, psychological sexual identity develops, which is primarily based on the appearance of the external genitalia. During pubertal development, the hypothalamic–pituitary gonad axis is activated, and the gonad secretes the sex steroids appropriate for the sex of the individual, leading to either male or female secondary sexual characteristics, which reaffirm sexual identity, enhance interest in sexuality, and direct sexual orientation toward the opposite sex.

As we shall see, this simplified and seemingly deterministic developmental pattern is not always followed. However, it allows us to consider the main checkpoints of *sex determination*:

- *Chromosomal sex:* The presence of the Y chromosome determines male chromosomal sex.
- *Gonadal sex:* The presence of testis determines male gonadal sex. In cases of *pseudohermaphroditism*, when there is a mismatch between the gonad, the external genitalia, and secondary sexual characteristics, gender is designated by gonadal sex. In the unusual case when both testicular and ovarian tissue are present, the gonadal sex is assigned with the term *true hermaphroditism*.
- *Genital sex:* Genital sex is determined by the anatomy of the external genitalia irrespective of the internal genitalia (such as Wolffian and Müllerian duct structures). The term *ambiguous genitalia* refers to conditions that may reflect *intersex* developmental disorders. These include cryptorchidism, partial labioscrotal fusion, varying degrees of *hypospadias* (urethral opening on the ventral surface of the penis due to incomplete fusion of the urethral folds/labia minora), micropenis, clitoromegaly, a combination of these conditions, and other disorders.
- *Sexual/gender identity* is the psychological self-identification either as a male or a female.
- *Sexual orientation* is attraction/arousal felt toward the opposite sex (*heterosexual* orientation), the same sex (*homosexual* orientation), or both sexes (*bisexual* orientation).

An important feature of the developmental process that the structure and/or function has an *innate bisexual potency*, and these checkpoints decide whether the development proceeds toward male versus female direction. A consequence of this is a wide variety of mismatches between any of the above components of sex determination. These may include mismatches such as those between chromosomal sex and gonadal sex, gonadal sex and genital sex, genital sex and sexual identity, or sexual identity and sexual orientation.

In this section, we discuss the normal regulation of these developmental processes and some of the consequences of deranged development. The subject matter has serious moral and ethical dimensions that are beyond the scope of this text.

Intrauterine Sexual Development

Except for Its Pseudoautosomal Regions, All But One Copy of the X Chromosome Is Permanently Inactivated in Each Cell   Due to the fusion of haploid male and female pronuclei during fertilization, the zygote and all normal human somatic cells contain a diploid set of chromosomes consisting of 22 pairs of autosomes and a pair of sex chromosomes. The oocyte may contribute only an X sex chromosome; the spermatozoon may contribute either an X or a Y sex chromosome. Thus, the normal karyotype is 46,XX in females, and 46,XY in males. (By convention, the number reflects the *total* number of chromosomes, including the sex chromosomes.)

A unique feature of the sex chromosomes is that only one X chromosome may be active in each cell, whereas the other X chromosome is permanently inactivated, a mechanism originally proposed by Mary Lyon in 1961, and now termed *lyonization*. This constitutive heterochromatin appears in the cells as *Barr body* or *sex chromatin* (Box 13-12; see also Chap. 3). During the blastocyst stage of embryonic development, the maternal and

BOX 13-12   Barr Body

Demonstration of the Barr body (sex chromatin) can be used for the diagnosis of *chromosomal sex* by microscopic examination of thionine-stained buccal smear cells. The Barr body appears as a clump of chromatin associated with the nuclear envelope. In normal females, 20 to 80% of the cells are identified as sex chromatin positive. Up to 2% of the cells may be positive for Barr body-like chromatin clump in normal men. Although the buccal smear is not as accurate as karyotyping, it is fast, inexpensive and in case of unambiguous results, may be sufficient. The *drumstick configuration* of the chromatin structure of circulating polymorphonuclear neutrophilic granulocytes has the same significance as the Barr body; 1.5 to 15% of neutrophils display the drumstick configuration in normal females.

The number of Barr bodies equals the total number of X chromosomes minus one. The buccal mucosa of phenotypically female *Turner's syndrome* (45,X) patients is negative for Barr bodies, similar to normal males. Most *Klinefelter's syndrome* (47,XXY) patients are hypogonad males with a Barr body count normally observed in females (i.e., 20 to 80% of the cells displaying a *single* Barr body).

The *Y chromosome* can be detected in buccal smears by quinacrine staining and fluorescence microscopy: the Y chromosome appears as a highly fluorescent clump known as the *F body*.

paternal X chromosomes in the *inner cell mass* are assigned for inactivation in a random manner. However, only paternal X chromosomes are inactivated in the *trophoblast* cells (compare with Box 13-10). All daughter cells of the blastocyst inherit the same assignment of maternal and paternal X chromosomes. As a consequence, the adult female is a mosaic for the active X chromosome: in certain cell populations the paternal X chromosome is active; in others the maternal X chromosome is active. By chance, all cells may carry the same active parental (either maternal or paternal) X chromosome. This condition is known as *extreme lyonization*, which may result in the full manifestation of X-linked recessive genetic diseases typically encountered in males who are normally hemizygous for the X chromosome. The inactivation of an X chromosome in 46,XX females equalizes the active X chromosomal genes present in males and females, a phenomenon known as *gene dosage compensation*.

The telomeric regions of both arms of the X and Y chromosomes contain the same set of genes and are known as the *pseudoautosomal regions* (Figs. 13-34 and 13-35). *The pseudoautosomal region is not inactivated with the rest of the X chromosome, irrespective of the number of the X chromosomes present, and participates in meiotic crossing over between the X and Y chromosomes during spermatogenesis.* The rest of the X and Y chromosomes contain different loci and recombination between them outside the pseudoautosomal regions does not normally occur.

During meiosis, the homologous chromosomes that line up for meiotic crossing over occasionally fail to separate from each other. This phenomenon, known as *meiotic nondysjunction*, results in haploid gametes that either lack or gain a chromosome. Fertilization involving such gametes typically results in *aneuploidia*. As a rule of thumb, the consequences of autosomal meiotic nondysjunction are more severe than those of the sex chromosomes. In the simplest form of nondysjunction, gametes with 24,XX, 22,0 and 24,XY may be formed.

- Fertilization of a 24,XX egg with a 23,Y spermatozoon results in a zygote with a karyotype of 47,XXY (*Klinefelter's syndrome*).
- Fertilization of a 22,0 egg with a 23,X spermatozoon results in a zygote with a karyotype of 45,X (*Turner's syndrome*).
- For viability of the embryo, at least one X chromosome must be present; i.e., 45,Y is lethal.

Klinefelter's and Turner's syndromes are common conditions, which may serve as prototypes of deranged development and will be covered in this chapter.

The chance for meiotic nondysjunction increases with maternal age. Pregnant women above 35 year of age are screened by karyotyping of their fetus by amniocentesis for diseases due to meiotic nondysjunction, including Down's syndrome. Note that this maternal age coincides with the earliest

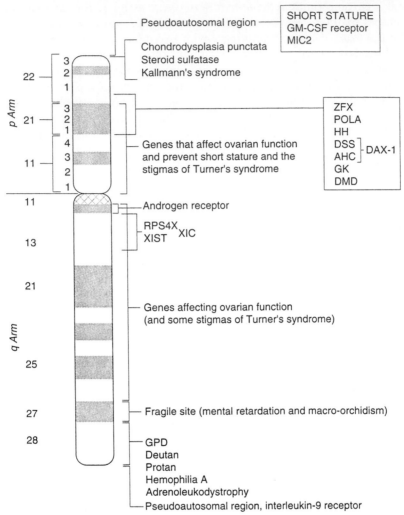

Figure 13-34. Diagrammatic presentation of the Giemsa- (G-) banded X-chromosome. Selected X-linked genes are shown. GM-CSF, granulocyte-macrophage colony-stimulating factor; MIC2, a cell surface antigen; ZFX, zinc finger X; POLA, RNA polymerase; HH, hypogonadotropic hypogonadism; DSS, dosage-sensitive sex reversal locus = AHC (adrenal hypoplasia congenita) = DAX-1 (DSS–AHC-critical region); GK, glycerol kinase; DMD, Duchenne muscular dystrophy; RPS4X, ribosomal protein S4; XIST, inactive X chromosome-specific transcripts; XIC, X inactivation center; GPD, glucose-6-phosphate dehydrogenase; Deutan & Protan, color blindness genes. Note that *XIST* is expressed only from *inactive* X-chromosomes. (*Source:* From Grumbach MM, Conte FA: Disorders of sex differentiation, in Wilson JD, Foster DW (eds): *Williams Textbook of Endocrinology,* 8th ed., Philadelphia, Saunders, 1992.)

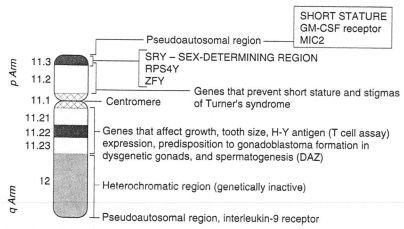

Figure 13-35.   Diagrammatic presentation of the Giemsa- (G-) banded Y-chromosome. Selected Y-linked genes are shown. GM-CSF, granulocyte-macrophage colony-stimulating factor; MIC2, a cell surface antigen; RPS4Y, ribosomal protein S4; ZFY, zinc finger Y; DAZ, deleted in azoospermia. (*Source:* From Grumbach MM, Conte FA: Disorders of sex differentiation, in Wilson JD and Foster DW (eds): *Williams Textbook of Endocrinology,* 8th ed., Philadelphia, Saunders, 1992.)

perimenopausal symptoms and a depletion of ovarian follicles to 25,000, a "critical number" below which the fine-tuning of the hypothalamic–pituitary–ovarian axis deteriorates.

Gonadal Sex Is Determined by the Temporal and Dosage-Dependent Expression of Several Genes Encoded by Autosomes and Sex Chromosomes, Including WT1, SF-1, SRY, DAX-1, and SOX9

The *urogenital ridge* develops by the 5th week of embryonic life adjacent to the developing adrenal gland at the medial aspect of the *mesonephros.* The *indifferent gonad* develops from the urogenital ridge during the 6th embryonic week (Fig. 13-36). The development of the indifferent gonad and the adrenal cortex requires the expression of the *WT-1* gene and the nuclear orphan receptor steroidogenic factor-1 (SF-1; Fig. 13-37).

- The *WT-1* gene, located on chromosome 11p13, encodes a zinc-finger transcription factor. Its loss-of-function mutation in a heterozygous state results in *Denys–Drash syndrome*, which is characterized in XY individuals as gonadal dysgenesis, persistent Müllerian structures, feminization of the external genitalia, nephropathy, and nephroblastoma (Wilms' tumor). Homozygous WT-1 knockout mice fail to develop kidneys and gonads.
- The *SF-1* gene is located on chromosome 9q33. Experiments with knockout mice indicate its role in inducing steroidogenic enzymes and development of the adrenal glands, gonads, and the ventromedial nucleus of the hypothalamus. SF-1 is involved in the development of both the indifferent gonad and in its differentiation into *testis.*

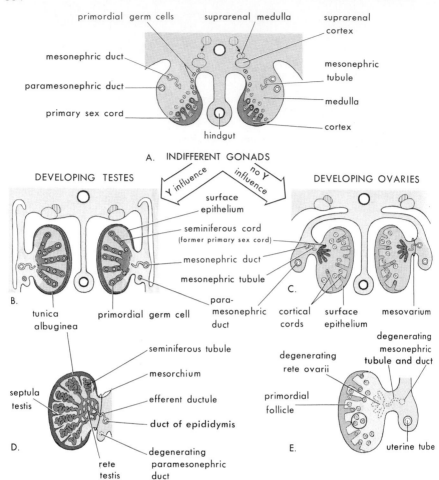

Figure 13-36. Schematic illustration of the morphologic differentiation of the indifferent gonads into testes and ovaries. Compare with regulatory steps shown in Fig. 13-37. Note the different timing of testicular and ovarian development. The primordial germ cells originate from the yolk sac. A. Sixth embryonic week (day 42): indifferent stage (bipotential gonad). B. Seventh embryonic week (days 43 to 50): the primary sex cords develop into seminiferous sex cords which consist of Sertoli cells expressing anti-Müllerian hormone (AMH). AMH acts on ipsilateral structures reaching them by diffusion. Testosterone-producing Leydig cells appear by day 60 (not shown). C. Twelfth embryonic week (days 77 to 84): in the absence of testicular differentiation, ovarian differentiation commences. The cortical cords develop into the follicular epithelium of oogonia. D. Twentieth embryonic week: under the influence of AMH, the paramesonephric (Müllerian) duct degenerated (by the 9th week), and upon androgen exposure the mesonephric (Wolffian) duct developed (by the 12th week). E. Twentieth embryonic week: in the absence of AMH and androgens, the Müllerian duct developed, the Wolffian duct degenerated. (*Source:* Fig. 13-21, p 264 in Moore, KL: *The Developing Human. Clinically Oriented Embryology,* 4th ed, Philadelphia, Saunders, 1988.)

• The common embryologic origin explains the presence of *adrenal rest tissue* in the gonads, particularly in the testis. This ectopic adrenocortical tissue is typically negligible but may present as an ACTH-dependent testicular "tumor" in congenital adrenal hyperplasia, especially in the nonclassic form of p450c21 deficiency.

The development of the testis requires the mandatory expression of the sex determining region Y (*SRY*) gene encoding the *SRY transcription factor* also known as *testis determining factor* (TDF). The most likely function of SRY is the suppression of the developmentally expressed *dosage-sensitive sex reversal* (*DSS*) gene, which is probably identical with DAX-1. DAX-1 is a potent suppressor of SF-1. Thus, the effect of SRY is the disinhibition of SF-1 (see Fig. 13-37). In turn, SF-1 stimulates testicular differentiation via SOX9, which leads to the appearance of Sertoli cells. SF-1 also stimulates the production of AMH by Sertoli cells and the expression of steroidogenic enzymes by the Leydig cells that develop a few days later (see Regulation of the Gonadotropin–Gonad Axis in Postpubertal Males).

• SRY is a transcription factor. Its DNA-binding domain is an *HMG box*, i.e., it is homologous with the DNA-binding domain of the high mobility group (HMG) proteins. The *SRY* gene is closely linked with the pseudo-autosomal region of the *short arm* of the Y chromosome, and may occasionally become *translocated* to the X chromosome during meiosis.
> • The presence of an X chromosome harboring the translocated *SRY* gene leads to the development of *46,XX males*, whose clinical presentation is similar to that of Klinefelter's syndrome patients.
> • The presence of a Y chromosome, whose *SRY* gene was translocated to an X chromosome during meiosis leads to the development of 46,XY females (*complete gonadal dysgenesis*). Note that this condition is distinct from 46,XY females whose condition is due to androgen insensitivity syndrome, or dosage-sensitive sex reversal.

• The SOX genes are related to SRY; they are termed for SRY HMG box. The *SOX9* gene is located on chromosome 17q24.1-25.1. This transcription factor is crucial in the development of cartilage and the testis. Its mutation results in *campomelic dysplasia* and partial male-to-female sex reversal as an autosomal dominant condition indicating that dosage of this factor is critical for its normal function (*haploinsufficiency*).

• DAX-1 has been localized to chromosome Xp21, the same location where the DSS locus had been mapped. Males and females have the same dosage of this gene because of X chromosome inactivation in females. The model shown in Fig. 13-37 explains clinical observations related to this gene:
> • Duplication of Xp21 (i.e., two copies of the gene on the *same* X chromosome) results in the development of 46,XY females because the double dose of DAX-1 cannot be sufficiently suppressed by SRY. This condition is referred to as *dosage-sensitive sex reversal* (DSS). Note that 47,XXY individuals do not express a

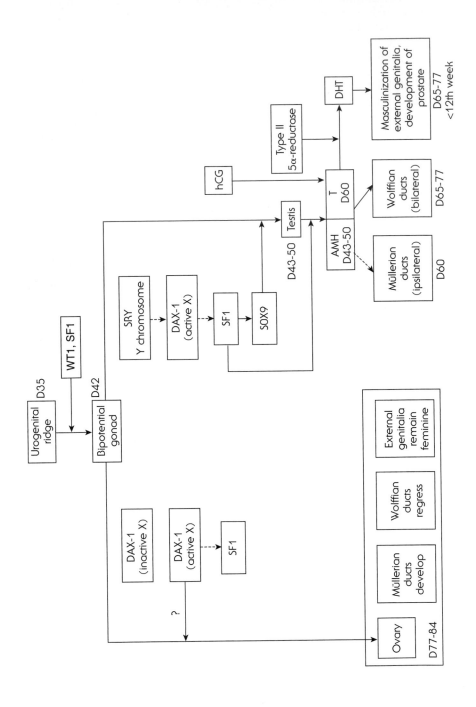

606

double dose of DAX-1 because of the inactivation of the extra X chromosome.

- Deletion of DAX-1 in 46,XY males results in normal sexual differentiation, which indicates that in males DAX-1 must be either suppressed (by SRY) or altogether absent for normal testicular development.

In females, SRY is absent, DAX-1 remains sustained, the SF-1/SOX9 pathway becomes suppressed, and ovaries develop. Note that *none of the classic hormones are required for the development of the ovaries and the testes.*

AMH and Testosterone Secreted by the Testis, Type II 5α-Reductase-Mediated Generation of Dihydrotestosterone by Target Cells, and Tissue Responsiveness to These Hormones Determine the Development of the Genital Tract, Accessory Sex Glands, and External Genitalia The Sertoli cell population is the first to develop in the testis and starts secreting AMH (chromosome 19p13.2-13.3) as early as days 43 to 50 of embryonic life (see Fig. 13-37). AMH, as a typical member of the TGF-β family (see Regulation of the Gonadotropin–Gonad Axis in Postpubertal Males), acts locally and causes the involution of the *ipsilateral* paramesonephric (Müllerian) duct by a paracrine mechanism. The cells of the Müllerian duct express the AMH-specific type II TGF-β receptor (chromosome 12q13). In the absence of AMH or AMH receptor, the Müllerian ducts develop irrespective of the sex steroid hormone environment, and give rise to the Fallopian tubes, uterus, and the upper third of the vagina. In females, this is the physiologic condition. In males, mutations of either AMH or AMH receptor cause *persistent Müllerian duct syndrome*, which is characterized by the coexistence of Müllerian and Wolffian structures, the prostate, and male external genitalia. Similar constellation may be seen in females who were exposed to high levels of androgens during the critical weeks (8th to 12th weeks) of embryonic life either from an exogenous source or by adrenocortical overproduction (see below).

The Leydig cells secrete testosterone from about embryonic day 60 (8th to 9th week). Because the pituitary hormones are first detectable at 12 weeks after conception and pituitary gonadotropins display a peak only during midgestation (see Fig. 13-41), testosterone production at this stage cannot be under the control of the hypothalamo–hypophyseal system. Instead, testosterone is stimulated by hCG, which is still rising to reach peak

Figure 13-37. A model of the regulation of normal sexual differentiation. Solid arrows indicate stimulation, dashed arrows indicate inhibition, the letter D with a number indicates the day of embryonic life. The steps are dosage-sensitive and must occur within specified time windows. Transcription factors: WT1, Wilms' tumor 1; SF1, steroidogenic factor 1; SRY, sex-determining region Y; DAX-1, dosage-sensitive sex reversal/adrenal hypoplasia congenita-critical region of chromosome X; SOX9, SRY high mobility box gene 9. Extracellular signals: AMH, anti-Müllerian hormone; hCG, human chorionic gonadotropin; T, testosterone; DHT, dihydrotestosterone.

levels during the latter part of the first trimester (11th to 12th embryonic week, Fig. 13-23). This peak activity of hCG is crucial in the masculinization of the male fetus. Unlike hCG, which declines after the 12th week, testosterone remains elevated throughout midgestation because of pituitary LH secretion (see Fig. 13-42). The pituitary-stimulated testicular androgen secretion is important in the descent of the testicles into the scrotum, a process completed by the 32nd week. The *absence of functional LH receptors* result in androgen deficiency throughout life: pseudohermaphroditism in newborn males is followed by hypergonadotropic hypogonadism and sexual infantilism (lack of pubertal development). Like the testis, the developing ovary is also exposed to hCG; however, it does not produce steroid hormones.

The testosterone secreted under the influence of hCG has the following roles (see Table 13-4):

- Testosterone stimulates the development of Wolffian duct structures: epididymis, vas deferens, and seminal vesicle.
- Androgens may achieve complete masculinization of the external genitalia only if they are present before the 12th week of embryonic life (Fig. 13-38). After the 12th week, exposure to androgens may only achieve clitoromegaly/phallic enlargement.
- Masculinization of the external genitalia and the proper development of the prostate require conversion of testosterone into dihydrotestosterone (DHT). If the type II 5α-reductase is absent, male pseudohermaphroditism develops (see Box 13-1) in spite of retaining the Wolffian structures. The 5α-reductase deficiency is also known as *"penis at twelve syndrome"* because pubertal testosterone production causes clitoromegaly that usually proceeds to the development of a functional penis. Pubic hair develops without a male escutcheon. Although these individuals are usually raised as females, they change gender identity at the time of phallic development and develop sexual orientation toward women. Their phallus enables them to have intercourse and the seminal vesicle produces a near-normal volume of seminal fluid.

The androgenic action requires the presence of functional androgen receptors. *Androgen insensitivity syndrome* (*Morris syndrome*), a form of male pseudohermaphroditism, is due to the loss of function mutation of the androgen receptors (Fig. 13-39). Because of its psychological impact, it has been recommended to avoid using the term *testicular feminization* when relating this condition to patients. Because the gene of the androgen receptor is located on the X chromosome, *the X chromosome is a determinant of male sexual development.* Mutations of the androgen receptor are without negative consequences in heterozygous females (carriers). If the male infant of a carrier female inherits the X chromosome with the nonfunctional androgen receptor, a phenotypically female cryptorchid XY individual develops.

- *During embryonic development,* androgens are produced by the testis but fail to masculinize the external genitalia, to induce prostate devel-

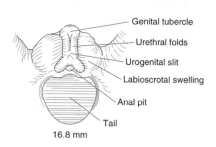

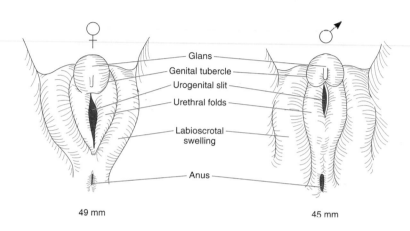

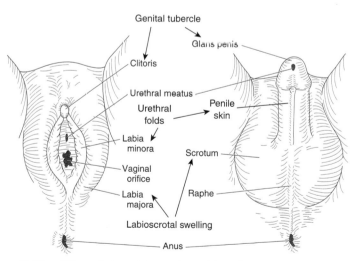

Figure 13-38. Differentiation of the male and female external genitalia from bipotential primordia. (From Fig. 14-9, p 495 in Conte FA, Grumbach MM: Abnormalities of sexual differentiation, Chapter 14 in Greenspan FS, Stewler GJ (eds): *Basic & Clinical Endocrinology*, 5th ed., Stamford, CT, Appleton & Lange, 1997.)

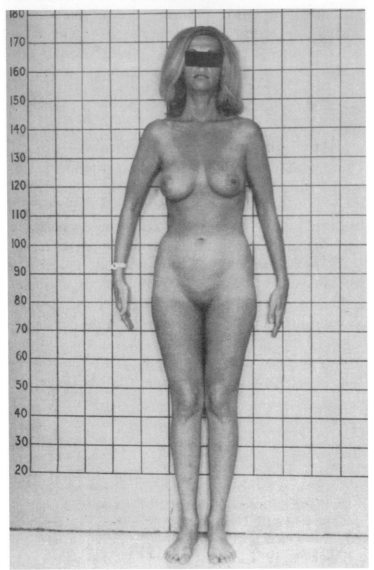

Figure 13-39. Complete androgen insensitivity syndrome (male pseudohermaphroditism). The karyotype is 46,XY. Note the perfectly female phenotype, including the external genitalia, breasts, hips and acne-free complexion. The pubic and underarm hair is absent (or scanty), which is characteristic for the condition. The patients are usually taller than average phenotypic females with somewhat larger than average hands and feet. The condition is usually inherited from the mother, and follows an X-linked recessive pattern because the androgen receptor is encoded by the X chromosome. The vagina ends blindly; Müllerian duct-derived structures are absent due to the intrauterine action of antiMüllerian hormone (AMH) secreted by Sertoli cells. (*Source:* Fig. 5-20, p 121 in Stenchever MA, Jones Jr HW: Genetic disorders and sex chromosome abnormalities, in DeCherney AH, Pernoll ML: *Current Obstetric and Gynecologic Diagnosis and Treatment,* 8th ed., Norwalk, CT, Appleton & Lange, 1994.)

opment and to sustain the Wolffian duct structures. However, AMH action leads to the involution of the Müllerian ducts, including the upper third of the vagina. The lower two-thirds of the vagina develops from the urogenital sinus just as in normal females; thus, the vagina ends blindly. In cases of complete androgen resistance, the male infant is born with female external genitalia and the condition may remain unsuspected until puberty. The condition in the newborn is the *mirror image* of the persistent Müllerian duct syndrome of males and the fetal masculinization of females.

• *Puberty* is delayed for a female, and about normal for a male, which results in a relatively tall stature with normal epiphyseal closure mediated by estrogen receptors. With puberty, testosterone production commences but no androgenic effects are exerted. In the absence of androgenic effects, AMH production by Sertoli cells remains high (see also Regulation of the Gonadotropin–Gonad Axis in Postpubertal Males). The lost *androgenic feedback* to the hypothalamus usually results in an increased LH output, and increased Leydig cell aromatase activity. Testosterone is converted into estradiol mainly within the testis, exerts its actions unopposed by testosterone or progesterone and results in feminization: female contours and breasts develop, but no menstruation occurs (primary amenorrhea). Although the vagina is shorter than average, it is distensible, and is appropriate for normal intercourse. Androgen-dependent hair growth is missing or scanty (this the condition is also known as *"hairless woman syndrome"*), neither male-type balding nor acne develops. The psychosexual development is typically normal female. The phenotypically female individual presents with cryptorchidism, a condition predisposing for testicular malignancy. For this reason, after pubertal development is complete, removal of the testes is recommended. After orchiectomy, *female* hormone substitution is indicated to maintain secondary sexual characteristics and to prevent osteoporosis. Inguinal hernias in preadolescent/adolescent females may direct attention to this condition.

Certain mutations of the androgen receptor result in *incomplete androgen resistance (Reifenstein's syndrome)*. Typical features include the presence of testes, regression of Müllerian ducts, postpubertally elevated estrogen production (compared to normal male levels), and resultant gynecomastia. The development of androgen-dependent features is highly variable.

Dysfunction of the Enzymes of the Steroidogenic Pathway May Interfere with Sexual Development by Altered Gonadal and/or by Altered Adrenocortical Hormone Secretion   Disturbances in the core steroidogenic pathway may have two consequences:

• Defects that result in *decreased production of androgens* result in *male pseudohermaphroditism*, but cause no sexual abnormalities in females.
• Defects that result in *overproduction of androgens* cause varying degree of masculinization/virilization in females (*female pseudohermaphroditism*), and may present as a type of precocious puberty in males.

The defects may involve enzymes specific for either the corticosteroid or the sex steroid synthetic pathway, and the enzymes shared by these two pathways (see Fig. 12-8). The types of congenital adrenal hyperplasia affecting genital development are also referred to as *adrenogenital syndrome*. The common feature of congenital adrenal hyperplasia is the defective production of cortisol, which leads to increased ACTH production (see Box 12-6). Table 13-15 summarizes the various types of congenital adrenal hyperplasia. Note that whereas the effects of these enzyme defects on sexual development may be influenced by gonadal sex, the effects on adrenal function, electrolyte homeostasis, and blood pressure are independent of gonadal sex.

The phenotypes in Table 13-15 can be explained with the aid of Fig. 12-8 as follows:

- *StAR deficiency* precludes steroid hormone biosynthesis in both the adrenals and the gonads. The absence of androgen does not alter

Table 13-15 Enzyme Defects Causing Congenital Adrenal Hyperplasia (Adrenogenital Syndrome)

Enzyme	Gonad	External genitalia	Postnatal sexual development	Salt-loss/ Addisonian crises	Hypertension, hypokalemic alkalosis
StAR	Male	Female	Sexual infantilism	Yes	No
	Female	Female			
3βHSD type II	Male	Ambiguous	Moderately decreased secondary sex characteristics	Variable	No
	Female	Ambiguous	Moderate virilization		
p450c17	Male	Female	Sexual infantilism	No	Yes
	Female	Female			
p450c21	Male	Male	Precocious "puberty" (adrenal virilization)	Variable	No
	Female	Ambiguous/ female	Virilization		
p450c11	Male	Male	Precocious "puberty" (adrenal virilization)	No	Yes
	Female	Ambiguous/ female	Virilization		

the external genital development of females, but prevents the normal masculinization in males. During puberty neither androgens nor estrogens are produced, leading to sexual infantilism. Corticosteroid deficiency presents as Addisonian crises mainly because of the absent mineralocorticoids.

• The deficiency of type II 3βHSD prevents the synthesis of all corticosteroids, the synthesis of potent androgens (androstenedione, testosterone) and their aromatized estrogenic derivatives (estrone, estradiol). However, DHEA (a weak androgen) is overproduced due to the increase in ACTH (absent feedback by cortisol). Thus, in the absence of testosterone the male is insufficiently androgenized by the increased DHEA both in utero and during postnatal development. The female is exposed to unusually high androgenic stimulation both in utero and during postnatal/pubertal development. During puberty, appropriate estrogen production is missing. Depending on the degree of enzyme deficiency, the presentation is variable both in terms of sexual function and in Addisonian crises.

• The deficiency of p450c17 does not affect the zona glomerulosa where its absence is physiologic. Thus, mineralocorticoid production is not prevented and Addisonian crises do not occur. However, the *zona fasciculata* produces overt quantities of DOC, a potent mineralocorticoid, which leads to hypertension. In the absence of the 17,20-lyase activity of p450c17, neither androgens nor estrogens may be produced. Thus, masculinization of the external genitalia does not occur in males, and no sexual development may occur in either sex during puberty. Rare cases have been reported with an isolated defect of the 17,20-lyase activity of p450c17. In these cases neither congenital adrenal hyperplasia nor mineralocorticoid excess occurs, but the impact on sexual development remains.

• The deficiencies of p450c21 (Fig. 12-9) and p450c11 have variable manifestation. The classic forms are associated with severe virilization of the female fetus and severe manifestations of the corticosteroid defect. In terms of the corticosteroid defect, p450c21 and p450c11 deficiencies present with opposite clinical pictures explained by the overproduction of DOC in p450c11-deficiency (see Chap. 12). The nonclassic and cryptic forms manifest only postnatally and the external genitalia of females is normal at birth. The classic forms may be treated by prenatal exposure to glucocorticoids. Dexamethasone administered to the mother crosses the placenta and prevents masculinization and virilization of the external genitalia if the treatment is started in early gestation (preferably before the 7th to 10th week of gestation LMP). The success of this treatment implies that *the fetal pituitary already secretes physiologically relevant amounts of ACTH by the 8th to 12th fetal week, and this ACTH secretion is subject to feedback regulation by glucocorticoids*. Indeed, the corticotroph lineage appears to diverge the earliest during development from the rest of the anterior pituitary hormone-producing cells.

It is noteworthy that the masculinization of the external genitalia is rarely complete in females presenting with any of the virilizing types of congenital adrenal hyperplasia. Although under the influence of ACTH the fetal zone of the adrenal cortex already produces substantial amounts of DHEA and DHEAS during the critical period of external genital development (8th to 12th fetal weeks) as evidenced by placental estriol production (see Fig. 13-23), the androgenic activity of DHEA is insufficient to effect *complete* masculinization even at drastically elevated concentrations. As noted, masculinization depends on the presence of 5α-reductase activity and DHT. In the rare cases of complete masculinization, enhanced peripheral conversion of DHEA by 3βHSD and 17βHSD is assumed to provide testosterone for DHT production in its targets.

The deficiencies of sex steroid specific enzymes (see Fig. 12-8) include *aromatase*, 17βHSD3, and type II 5α-reductase.

- Absence of p450arom (*CYP19*) results in *female pseudohermaphroditism*, which is usually characterized by complete masculinization of the external genitalia, and transient *virilization of the pregnant mother*, which resolves after parturition. This indicates that in the absence of placental aromatase, the fetal adrenal and maternal androgens may reach both the fetus and the mother in high concentrations. Undiagnosed female patients grow up as boys and their Müllerian duct structures persist. During puberty, the ovaries are unable to aromatize androgens. Because the negative feedback to gonadotropin secretion is mainly performed by estrogens, pituitary gonadotropins become elevated. The stimulated ovarian androgen production results in multicystic ovaries and mild virilization. The lack of estrogens explains the absence of breast development, the severely retarded bone age, the delayed epiphyseal closure leading to tall stature, and the early development of osteoporosis. Aromatase deficiency *in males* does not prevent male sexual development. The affected male presents with elevated plasma androgens and *macroorchidism* due to the lost estrogenic feedback suppression of gonadotropins. The delayed epiphyseal closure leads to tall stature with eunuchoid proportions (low upper-to-lower segment ratio), severely retarded bone age, and osteoporosis. The high levels of androgens decrease HDL, and increase plasma LDL, total cholesterol, and triglycerides. The associated hyperinsulinemia is probably the consequence of insulin resistance secondary to increased plasma FFA.

- Type 3 17β-hydroxysteroid dehydrogenase (17βHSD3) is a testis-specific isoenzyme that converts androstenedione into testosterone (see The Biosynthesis, Mechanism of Action and Metabolism of Sexual Steroids). In its congenital absence, male pseudohermaphroditism develops. During puberty, the testes may descend into the labioscrotal folds and produce large amounts of androstenedione, which is converted into testosterone by extratesticular 17βHSD isoenzymes. This leads to phallic development and virilization (Fig. 13-40). When these pubertal changes take place, most affected individuals request sex reassignment to male and develop sexual orientation toward females. This pattern is similar to that observed in cases of 5α-reductase deficiency.

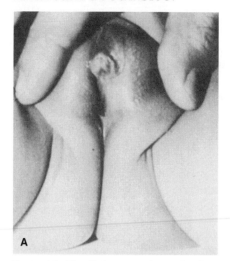 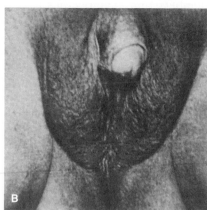

Figure 13-40. Deficiency of type 3 17β-hydroxysteroid dehydrogenase. Affected males are born with almost completely female external genitalia (A) but marked virilization occurs during puberty (B) which typically leads to a change in gender identity. (*Source:* Fig. 109-6, p 1918 in Forest MG: Diagnosis and treatment of disorders of sexual development, Chapter 109 in DeGroot LJ (ed): *Endocrinology,* 3rd ed., Philadelphia, Saunders, 1995.)

Masculinization of the fetus is sometimes caused by exogenous steroids. A potential exogenous source of androgens for the fetus is the mother. In rare cases of *mildly virilizing adrenocortical adenomas of the pregnant mother* which obviously did not cause infertility, the androgen output of the adenoma is increased during pregnancy along with cortisol, and may overwhelm both the SHBG and the capacity of placental aromatase. The consequence on the female fetus is comparable with aromatase deficiency, except that the perfectly masculinized female who is raised as a boy undergoes a quasinormal female puberty. Another exogenous source of steroids are the *synthetic progestins* that possess androgenic activity such as medroxyprogesterone. Before their masculinizing side effect was recognized, these drugs were administered to pregnant women to maintain pregnancy.

Fusions of the labia majora due to the intrauterine masculinizing effect of overt androgen exposure should not be confused with *labial adhesions.* Labial adhesions are characterized by the adherence of labia minora immediately under the clitoris. This condition arises only postpartum on the basis of the hypoestrogenic state of the infant, and may involve an inflammatory mechanism. The condition responds to topically applied estrogen ointments.

Psychosexual Development Is Primarily Determined by the Appearance of the External Genitalia and the Secondary Sex Characteristics Studies in rodents conclusively demonstrated the role of prenatal exposure to sex steroids in the development of sexual behavior on reaching maturity. Such a mechanism does not seem to dominate human psychosexual development. *Gender identity* is usually firmly established by the age of 18 to 30 months. Gender identity is usually based on self-observation of unambiguous external genitalia, comparison of the genitalia with those of the siblings and parents, verbal reinforcement of the gender identity by the family members, and unambiguous rearing. As we have seen, in cases of severe pubertal virilization of male pseudohermaphrodites (17βHSD3 and 5α-reductase deficiency), gender identity may change. It has been suggested that androgens are responsible for the development of *sexual orientation* toward female sexual partners. However, the development of sexual orientation involves complex psychological mechanisms and environmental influences.

Puberty

Pituitary Gonadotropin Secretion Displays Four Phases of Increased Activity Corresponding with Midgestational Fetal Life, the Neonatal Period, the Reproductive Period, and, in Women, the Postmenopausal Years

We have discussed the regulation of the hypothalamic–pituitary–gonad axis in postpubertal males and females. This pattern of regulation is attained by a cascade of events that starts with the intrauterine development of the structures involved. The adult regulation dramatically changes in women with menopause; the decline of testicular function is more subtle. Throughout the lifespan of an individual, four phases of increased *pituitary* gondotroph function can be identified; the first three are present in both sexes (Fig. 13-41):

- Midgestational fetal life.
- Neonatal period.
- Adult reproductive period attained during pubertal development.
- Postmenopausal rise of gonadotropin secretion.

In females, *the ovaries respond to the high levels of gonadotropins with follicular maturation and sex steroid production only during the third phase, i.e., starting with puberty and ending with menopause.* The ovary remains quiescent during fetal and neonatal life, and does not respond to placental hCG or pituitary gonadotropins. In contrast, *the testis responds to each of the three phases of increased gonadotropin exposure with testosterone secretion* (Fig. 13-42).

The *fetal increase* of gonadotropin secretion is attributed to the immaturity of the negative feedback system and, in females, to the absence of gonadal sex steroid production. Some degree of negative feedback function during the midgestational peak is indicated by the higher gonadotropin levels in female than in male fetuses. Gonadotropin levels decrease in both sexes and remain low during the third trimester. This decrease may be explained by the development of the negative feedback regulatory system of

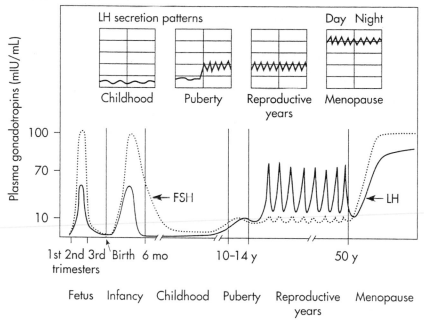

Figure 13-41. The four phases of increased pituitary gonadotropin secretion during the human lifespan. The figure shows the pattern seen in women. Men follow a similar pattern except for (1) the cyclic secretion (seen only in women during their reproductive years), (2) the average age at the onset of puberty, and (3) the absence of menopause. The inset shows the changes in pulsatile secretory pattern and the nyctohemeral rhythm of LH secretion. Note that the ovaries secrete sex steroids in response to gonadotropins only during the reproductive years. (*Source:* Fig. 9-15 in Porterfield SP: *Endocrine Physiology.* St. Louis, Mosby 1997; the figure originally appeared in Braunwald E et al: *Harrison's Principles of Internal Medicine,* 4th ed., New York, McGraw–Hill, 1987.)

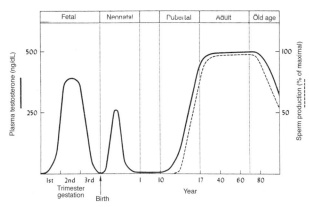

Figure 13-42. The phases of increased testosterone secretion during the lifespan of men. Compare with Fig. 13-41. Note that testosterone increases before the increase in pituitary gonadotropin secretion during fetal life. The early rise of testosterone is in response to hCG. (*Source:* Fig. 10-17, p 271 in Griffin JE, Wilson JD: Disorders of the testes and male reproductive tract, Chapter 10 in Wilson JD, Foster DW (eds): *Williams' Textbook of Endocrinology,* 7th ed., Philadelphia, Saunders, 1985.)

hypothalamic GnRH, and the high concentrations of placentally produced estrogens and progesterone.

The *neonatal increase* of gonadotropins is the consequence of the elimination of placentally provided negative feedback. A curious feature of this period is that gonadotropin secretion remains high for several months even in males, who respond to the increased gonadotropin exposure with up to midpubertal levels of androgen secretion. This androgen output by the neonatal testes is not the cause of the decrease of gonadotropin secretion to childhood levels.

During the *childhood years*, the circulating levels of sex steroids and gonadotropins are low *(juvenile pause of gonadotropin secretion)*. The neuroendocrine mechanisms of this period are still enigmatic. The negative feedback regulation responds to 10 to 25% of the concentration of sex steroids required for comparable suppression of gonadotropins in adults. This exquisite sensitivity is undoubtedly a component of the *low setpoint of the negative feedback regulation* as evidenced by the supranormal gonado-tropin levels of Turner's syndrome patients (Fig. 13-43). Turner's syndrome patients have streak gonads, which are devoid of follicles and do not secrete sex steroids. Although their gonadotropin levels are always higher than those of age-matched controls, they still display a characteristic decrease between the neonatal period and puberty, suggesting that mechanisms other than sex steroid feedback are primarily responsible for the juvenile pause of gonadotropin secretion. There is some evidence that the low levels of gonadotropins are related to the action of a specific group of GABAergic neurons that tonically inhibit GnRH secretion, and that NMDA receptors are also involved in the mechanism. The involvement of pineal melatonin secretion has also been suggested as a mechanism of the juvenile pause of gonadotropin secretion (see Chap. 14).

The *prepubertal/pubertal increase of gonadotropin secretion* is the result of poorly understood maturational changes in the CNS. The tonic inhibition responsible for the juvenile pause is relinquished. Leptin plays a gatekeeper role in this process to assure that adequate energy resources are available to support the energy expenditure required by the reproductive system (see Regulation of the Gonadotropin–Gonad Axis in Postpubertal Males). Both circulating gonadotropins and gonadal hormones increase during pu-berty indicating that the setpoint of negative feedback is gradually elevated to attain a new equilibrium characteristic of adults. The increased plasma concentration of sex steroids brings about the physiologic changes of pu-berty (see below). The onset of puberty is heralded by the reawakening of a partially quiescent GnRH pulse generator.

• Even though plasma gonadotropin levels are very low during the juvenile pause, a low-amplitude pulsatile secretion can be demonstrated. The GnRH/LH *pulse frequency* displays an approximately twofold increase from midchildhood (about 6 years of age) to the clinical onset of puberty,

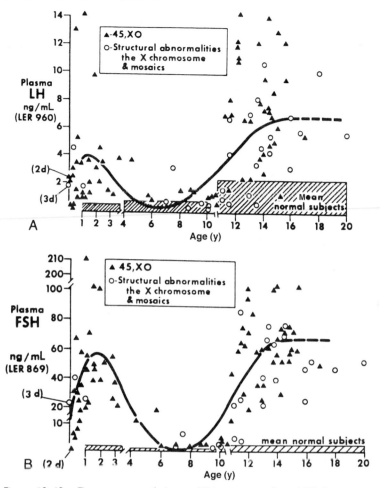

Figure 13-43. The ontogeny of plasma LH (upper panel) and FSH (lower panel) in normal subjects and Turner's syndrome patients. The ontogenetic pattern in the two groups is practically identical, except that it is accentuated in Turner's syndrome patients due to the absence of gonadal feedback-suppression of pituitary gonadotropins. The neonatal peak is followed by a juvenile pause of gonadotropin secretion. Note that Turner's syndrome patients who present with the absence of pubertal development due to gonadal dysgenesis, still display the pubertal onset of gonadotropin secretion. (*Source:* Redrawn from Conte FA et al: A diphasic pattern in gonadotropin secretion in patients with the syndrome of gonadal dysgenesis. J Clin Endocrinol Metab 40:670–675, 1975.)

with no subsequent changes during the continuing development toward adulthood. The twofold increase in GnRH pulse frequency *enhances the GnRH responsiveness of the pituitary* to increase the mass of LH produced to a standardized bolus of exogenous (or a pulse of endogenous) GnRH.

* From midchildhood to sexual maturity, LH production rate increases about fortyfold. Approximately 90% of this increment is accounted for by an increase in the *amplitude* of a preexisting pulsatile secretion. It

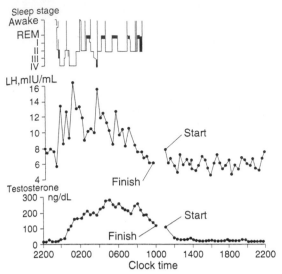

Figure 13-44. Nyctohemeral rhythm and sleep-entrained secretion of LH in a 14-year-old boy in pubertal stage 2. The top panel shows the sleep stages as evaluated by electroencephalogram. Peak LH levels mostly coincide with non-REM sleep. The circadian rhythm of plasma testosterone is shown at the bottom panel. (*Source:* Fig. 15-5 in Styne D: Puberty, Chapter 15 in Greenspan FS, Strewler GJ (eds): *Basic & Clinical Endocrinology,* 5th ed., Stamford, CT, Appleton & Lange, 1997; originally appeared in Boyar RM et al: Simultaneous augmented secretion of luteinizing hormone and testosterone during sleep. J Clin Invest 54:609, 1974.)

has been suggested that the enhanced amplitude of LH is mainly a result of the increased pituitary responsiveness to GnRH.

- GnRH/LH pulses coincide with non-REM sleep. This *sleep-entrained GnRH/LH secretion* is already present in midchildhood, but no circadian changes are seen in the amplitude of the LH pulses or the average plasma concentrations of LH. During the pubertal activation of the GnRH—gonadotropin axis, the appearance of a *nyctohemeral LH rhythm* is the first event (Figs. 13-41 and 13-44). *The amplification of sleep-entrained GnRH/LH secretion occurs about 2 years before the clinical onset of puberty.* The nyctohemeral rhythm of GnRH/LH secretion disappears during young adulthood, when the fairly regular LH pulses occur throughout the entire 24-h day and result in a continuously elevated concentration of plasma LH (see Fig. 13-41). This ontogenetic pattern is useful in the evaluation of pubertal development: low levels of plasma LH in blood samples collected during the daytime are far less informative than those collected during normal sleep.

Adrenarche (the increased production of adrenal androgens; see Chap. 12) normally precedes pubertal development by about 2 years, but there is no clear causal relationship between adrenarche and puberty. Neither Addison's disease nor premature (but otherwise normal) adrenarche has a clear influence on the age of the onset of puberty. In contrast, exposure to high levels of androgens such as in virilizing adrenogenital syndrome may result in *precocious puberty* even if treatment of androgen production is instituted in the meantime. Although adrenarche contributes to physiologic changes at puberty, pubertal maturation is primarily due to the activation of the gonads (*gonadarche*).

The *postmenopausal increase* of gonadotropins reflects the exhaustion of the nonrenewable pool of ovarian follicles: the decline of ovarian hormone production (sex steroids and inhibin) release gonadotropin secretion from the negative feedback suppression. A similar pattern of gonadotropin secretion is seen in cases of testicular failure and after castration (see Figs 13-12 and 13-41).

Pubertal Development Is a Sex Steroid-Regulated Process that Begins Earlier and Does Not Last as Long in Females as in Males Puberty is characterized by the attainment of secondary sexual characteristics and the pubertal growth spurt, which is normally terminated by epiphyseal closure. Pubertal development is assessed by *Tanner staging* of the breasts and pubic hair development in females (Figs 13-30 and 13-45), the genital (penis, testis, scrotum) and pubic hair development in males (Fig. 13-46). The typical time-course of developmental stages is shown in Fig. 13-47.

The *first sign* of puberty in males is the *increase in testicular volume* (from 1 mL to >3 mL). This occurs between the ages of 9 and 14 years, and reflects the combined effects of FSH and LH-driven testosterone on the seminiferous tubules. In contrast, the first sign of puberty in females is related to the effect of increased estrogen production. (As mentioned, the first menstrual cycles are usually anovulatory; thus progesterone is not involved in the first manifestations of female puberty.) Breast development (*thelarche*) is usually noticed first between the ages of 8 to 13 years, although the onset of pubertal growth spurt usually precedes thelarche. Similar to the testis, the ovary grows in size, and follicles appear with diameters of ≥9 mm. These changes in the ovary can be evaluated by ultrasonography.

Underarm and *pubic hair* development (*pubarche*) requires androgenic action. Although the adrenal cortex is a significant source of androgens in females, normal ambisexual hair development also requires ovarian testosterone production. Thus, in Turner's syndrome patients whose streak ovaries do not secrete steroid hormones, pubic hair growth is either absent or markedly decreased as a part of sexual infantilism (Fig. 13-48), in spite of normal adrenarche. A major difference between mature female and male pubic hair distribution is the *escutcheon* (the spreading of pubic hair to the umbilicus), the development of which depends on a normal production rate of testosterone plus local conversion into DHT. Thus, patients with type II 5α-reductase deficiency or Klinefelter's syndrome (a condition with decreased testosterone secretion, Fig. 13-49) present with mature *female* type of pubic hair. In males, the growth of mustache and beard is initiated with some delay after pubarche. The appearance of androgen-dependent hair usually coincides with the activation of other (type I 5α-reductase-

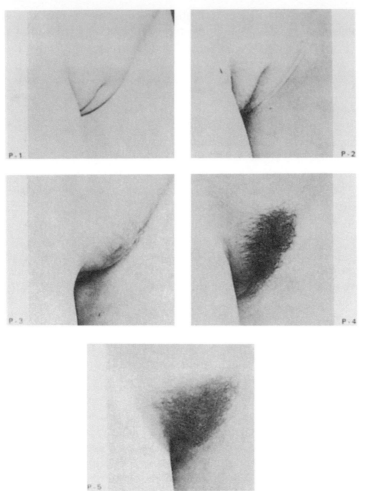

Figure 13-45. Stages of female pubic hair development according to Marshall and Tanner. P-1: Preadolescent; no pubic hair (no difference in the vellous hair over the mons and the abdomen). P-2: Sparse, downy, long, straight, slightly pigmented pubic hair chiefly along the labia majora. P-3: The hair spreads over the superior junction of the labia majora, it is darker, curlier, coarser and grows more densely. P-4: Adult type but covers an area smaller than in the average adult. There is no spread to the medial surface of the thighs. P-5: Adult type and spread. Appears as an inverse triangle (fan), without spreading along the linea alba, but spreading to the medial thighs. (*Source:* Van Wieringen JC et al: Growth diagrams 1965 Netherlands: Second National Survey on 0–24 Year Olds. Groningen, Netherlands Institute for Preventive Medicine NO Leiden, Wolters-Noordhoff Publishing, 1971. Marshall WA, Tanner JM: Variations in the pattern of pubertal changes in girls. Arch Dis Child 44:291, 1969.)

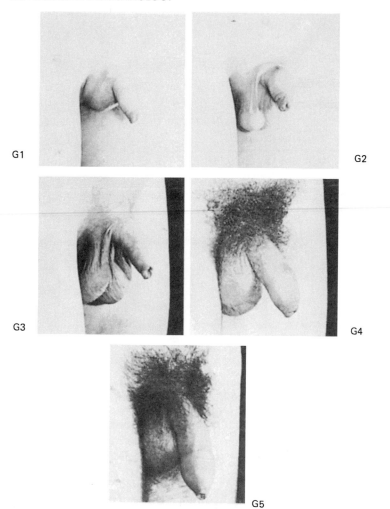

Figure 13-46. Stages of male genital and pubic hair development. Compare with Fig. 13-45. Pubic hair: P-1: Preadolescent; no pubic hair (no difference in the vellous hair over the mons and the abdomen). P-2: Sparse, downy, long, straight, slightly pigmented pubic hair chiefly at the base of the penis on the mons pubis. P-3: The hair spreads laterally on the mons without reaching the medial surface of the thighs; it is darker, curlier, coarser, and grows more densely. P-4: Adult type but covers an area smaller than in the average adult. There is no spread to the medial surface of the thighs or to the umbilicus. P-5: Adult type and spread involving the medial surface of the thighs. The *escutcheon* (spread to the umbilicus) appears with some delay ("P-6"). Genital: G1, Preadolescent. Testes, scrotum and penis about the same size and proportions as in early childhood. G2, Scrotum and testes enlarged, scrotal skin texture and color change commences. G3, Penis is enlarged mainly in length and some increase in diameter. Testicular and scrotal changes are further advanced. G4, Penile growth is marked in both diameter and length, the glans becomes prominent. Testes grow larger, scrotum becomes more wrinkled and pigmented. G5, Adult size and shape are attained. No further growth occurs. (*Source:* Van Wieringen JC et al: Growth diagrams 1965 Netherlands: Second National Survey on 0–24 Year Olds. Groningen, Netherlands Institute for Preventive Medicine NO Leiden, Wolters-Noordhoff Publishing, 1971. Marshall WA, Tanner JM: Variations in the pattern of pubertal changes in boys. Arch Dis Child 45:13, 1970.)

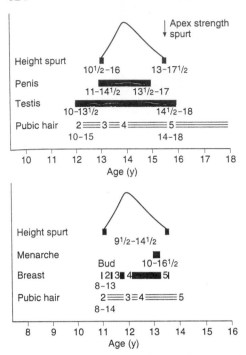

Figure 13-47. Sequence of secondary sexual development in British males (top) and females (bottom). (*Source:* From Marshall WA, Tanner JM: Variations in the pattern of pubertal changes in boys. Arch Dis Child 45:13, 1970.)

dependent) cutaneous structures leading to the development of *body odor* (and pheromonal signaling of sexual maturity) by secretions of *apocrine* sweat glands and *acne* due to overproduction of sebum.

The onset of menses (*menarche*) is an important developmental milestone indicating that estrogen production is sufficient to stimulate endometrial proliferation. In the United States, the average age at menarche is 12.8 years; African American girls experience menarche about 4 months earlier than Caucasians. Menarche is expected to occur within 5 years after thelarche. The absence of menarche beyond 16 years of age is termed *primary amenorrhea*, which may indicate deranged development of the gonadal axis. The first menstrual cycles are usually anovulatory bleedings. The relative number of ovulatory cycles gradually increases to over 80% within 4 to 5 years after menarche. Under the influence of estrogens, the uterus grows to reach adult size. However, this growth can be evaluated only by ultrasonography. Bimanual examination is not only imprecise but is also a traumatic experience during childhood that should be avoided.

In males, the developmental milestone comparable with menarche is termed *spermarche*, which is associated with the appearance of spermatozoa in early morning urine samples, usually in the absence of previous ejacula-

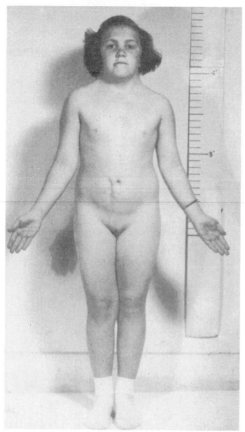

Figure 13-48. A 14-year-old 45,X female with characteristic manifestations of Turner's syndrome. Note the short stature, the absence of pubic hair or breast development, broad chest with widely spaced nipples, webbed neck, increased "carrying angle" of the elbow, and the old-looking face. (*Source:* Photograph by Earl Plunkett; courtesy of G.H. Valentine; Fig. 4, Chapter 8 in Mange AP, Mange EJ: *Genetics, Human Aspects,* 2nd ed., Sinauer Associates, 1990.)

tion. This developmental milestone, however, is not apparent unless urine sediment is microscopically evaluated. The average age at spermarche is 13.4 years at gonadal stage 3 to 4. The ejaculation-independent appearance of spermatozoa subsides later in development. Stage 5 pubertal development is expected within 4.5 years after the first sign of puberty.

The pubertal *growth spurt* is related to an increase in GH pulse *amplitude* and average concentration of IGF-1, which indicates resetting of the negative feedback exerted by IGF-1 on GH at a higher IGF-1 level. This is gradually achieved by the increasing concentrations of testosterone and estradiol. Sexual steroids are unable to effect pubertal growth spurt in Laron dwarves (GH receptor deficiency). In males, the growth spurt starts later, growth velocity is higher, and epiphyseal closure occurs later than in

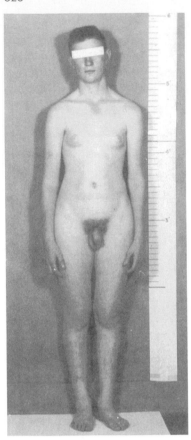

Figure 13-49. A 47,XXY male with Klinefelter's syndrome. The condition is associated with hypogonadism with increased of estrogen: androgen ratio. Note the relatively tall stature with lower than normal upper-to-lower segment ratio (eunuchoid body proportion) and long arms. The breasts are Tanner stage 3 for a female (gynecomastia) and pubic hair displays female distribution. The testes are firm, the testicular volume and the stretched length of the penis are below average. (*Source:* Photograph by Earl Plunkett; courtesy of G.H. Valentine; Fig. 4, Chapter 8 in Mange AP, Mange EJ: *Genetics, Human Aspects,* 2nd ed., Sinauer Associates, 1990.)

females (Fig. 13-50). Thus, males attain a 9-cm taller stature *before* the onset of pubertal growth spurt, and they add 3 cm more to their height *during* the growth spurt (28 cm in men versus 25 cm in women). These two factors together explain that on the average males are about 12 cm taller than females.

The sexual differences in *body contour and composition* develop during puberty. In males, androgen production increases lean body mass: muscle mass increases and fat stores may become decreased. The shoulders become prominent, the hip is narrow. The same presentation in females is a component of virilization. Females are normally under the predominant influence of estrogens (and progesterone), depositing more body fat and less lean muscle mass than males. The hips become more prominent than the shoulders and adipose tissue accumulates in the developing breasts, buttocks, and thighs.

A number of biochemical differences emerge during puberty, including a higher hematocrit, plasma LDL, and lower plasma HDL in males than in females.

The Main Forms of Deranged Pubertal Development Include Delayed Puberty, Sexual Infantilism (Absent Puberty), and Precocious Puberty Leading to Either Isosexual or Contrasexual Development   Deranged pubertal development is often indicated by the abnormal time-course of puberty.

- *Delayed puberty* is considered either in a male ≥14 years or in a female ≥13 years of age if no sign of pubertal of pubertal development is present. Because this definition is based on ±2.5 standard deviations around the mean onset of puberty, in 0.6% of the population the delayed puberty does not indicate a disease but *constitutional delay*. In certain conditions, such as Kallman's syndrome or Turner's syndrome, pubertal development is absent permanently, i.e., does not occur without treatment.
- *Precocious puberty* is defined by the commencement of secondary sexual development either in males <9 years, or in females <8 years of age.
  - *Complete* (true) *precocious puberty* involves the activation of the hypothalamic–pituitary–gonad axis, indicating that the normal mechanism of puberty is activated prematurely. In most males presenting with complete precocious puberty, the underlying cause is a hypothalamic tumor such as that of the pineal gland, which involves the posterior hypothalamus. These tumors destroy the neural structures responsible for the juvenile pause of gonadotropin secretion and involute during puberty in healthy individuals. In most females with complete precocious puberty, no pathology is found and, in the absence of familial predisposition to precocious puberty (which is known as *constitutional precocious puberty*), the diagnosis of *idiopathic complete precocious puberty* is made.
  - *Incomplete precocious* puberty indicates that sex steroid production is not regulated by the hypothalamo–hypophyseal system.

Pubertal development may be isosexual or contrasexual.

- *Isosexual pubertal development* indicates that the secondary sexual characteristics developing during puberty are appropriate for the presumed gonadal sex of the individual.
- *Contrasexual pubertal development* indicates that the secondary sexual characteristics developing during puberty are opposite to the presumed gonadal sex of the individual. Examples of contrasexual pubertal development include
  - conditions leading to virilization/masculinization in *presumed* females, such as certain types of *male* pseudohermaphroditism (type II 5α-hydroxylase deficiency, deficiency in 17β-HSD3) and the nonclassic form of p450c21 deficiency.
  - conditions leading to feminization in *presumed* males, such as certain types of *female* pseudohermaphroditism (fetal masculinization by exogenous androgens).
  - In cases such as androgen insensitivity syndrome, pubertal

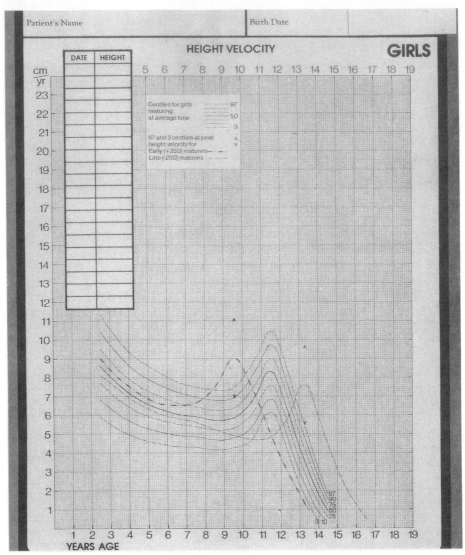

Figure 13-50. Height velocity charts for girls (A) and for boys (B). The three temporally different peaks reflect early, average, and late maturing children. The numbers at the bottom of the curves indicate the percentiles of height velocity for children with the average *timing* of pubertal growth spurt (average height velocity = 50th percentile). Note that the onset of pubertal growth spurt occurs later, but the peak growth velocity is higher in boys than in girls. Epiphyseal closure terminating further gain of height occurs earlier in girls than in boys. (*Source:* From Tanner JM, Davies PW: Clinical longitudinal standards for height, and height velocity for North American children. J Pediatr 107:317–329, 1985. © Castlemead Publications, Distributed by Serono Laboratories, Inc., Randolph, MA.)

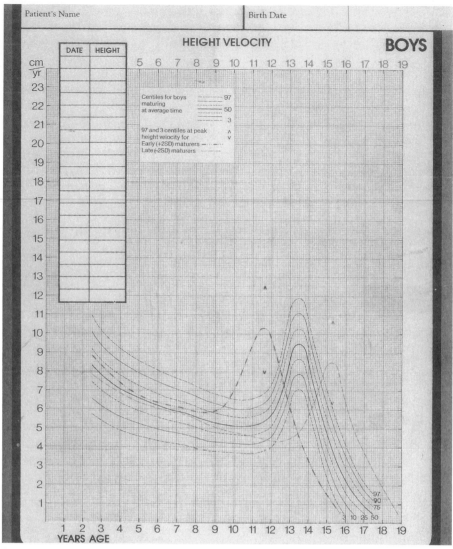

Figure 13-50. (*Continued*)

development results in feminization, which is appropriate for the *presumed* gender, but contrary to the gonadal sex.

Hypogonadism Is Classified into Hypogonadotropic and Hypergona-dotropic Forms In cases of delayed, decreased, or absent pubertal development, the immediate cause is the decreased or absent pubertal rise of sexual steroid production, i.e., *hypogonadism.*

Hypogonadotropic hypogonadism indicates that the gonads do not secrete sexual steroids because of the absence of stimulation by pituitary gonadotropins. This is the case in conditions such as *Kallmann's syndrome* (see Regulation of the Gonadotropin–Gonad Axis in Postpubertal Males), defective GnRH gene, pituitary gonadotropin deficiency (which may either be isolated or part of combined pituitary hormone deficiency or *panhypopituitarism*), CNS tumors disrupting the normal adult-type regulation of the pituitary gland (such as craniopharyngioma), anorexia nervosa, hypothalamic amenorrhea (involving increased opioid-mediated inhibition of the GnRH pulse generator), low body weight (leptin mechanism), and genetic defects (such as Prader-Willi, Laurence-Moon and Bardet-Biedl syndromes).

Hypergonadotropic hypogonadism indicates gonadal failure and the absent negative feedback suppression of gonadotropin secretion. The condition may be due to cryptorchidism and various forms of *gonadal dysgeneses* (see Intrauterine Sexual Development).

Klinefelter's and Turner's Syndromes Are the Most Prevalent Forms of Hypergonadotropic Hypogonadism in Males and Females, Respectively

Klinefelter's syndrome (*seminiferous tubule dysgenesis;* 47,XXY) and its variants (e.g., 48,XXYY) are due to meiotic nondysjunction and are the leading cause of infertility in males (see Fig. 13-49). The gonocytes are present at birth but disappear before the age of 2 years, which results in azoospermia in adults. The timing of puberty is usually normal, but the pubertal development reflects hypogonadism. The impaired Sertoli cell function leads to the *gonadotropin-dependent* hyalinization and fibrosis of the tubules; thus, the testes remain small and become firm to the touch during puberty. The associated destruction of the Sertoli cells leads to a marked decrease in the circulating levels of inhibin B. The primary cause of Leydig cell dysfunction is unknown. Although pseudoadenomatous clusters of Leydig cells give the histologic impression of hyperplasia, the *total number* of Leydig cells is decreased. The *total volume* of Leydig cells is normal, which indicates hypertrophy of the cells. The hypertrophic cells often display abnormal ultrastructure. The subnormal testosterone production increases the pulsatile release of GnRH. The decreased inhibin and androgen feedback to the pituitary together with a longer plasma half-life of FSH result in a disproportionately higher increase in FSH than in LH. The existing Leydig cells are overstimulated by LH and increase their aromatase activity. Because the condition develops in a gonadotropin-dependent manner, the decline in the production of testosterone is progressive. The progressive nature is also indicated by normal fetal masculinization of the genitalia and the typically normal descent of the testes in utero. The progressively subnormal pubertal production of testosterone is associated with normal to supranormal production of estradiol *compared to normal males*. The estrogen production is *subnormal for a female*. The consequences include *hypogonadism* (the *total androgen and estrogen levels are low*) and an elevated *estrogen:androgen ratio,* which leads to varying degrees of *feminization*. The hypogonadism results in delayed epiphyseal closure, which manifests in low upper-to-lower body segment ratio, long upper limbs, and relatively tall stature. The decreased levels of androgens lead to varying degrees of *eunuchoid habitus* including the decrease in the pubertal growth of the penis, female-type pubic hair distribution, decreased facial hair growth, absence of hair line recession, relatively high-pitched voice, decreased libido, and impaired erectile function. The high estrogen:androgen ratio often causes *gynecomastia*; the stimulated ductal growth increases the risk of breast cancer twentyfold over normal males. The condition often remains undiagnosed before puberty. In childhood, behavioral problems and/or mild mental retardation may be present, and the lower limbs may be disproportionately longer than the trunk. The latter indicates a genetic component of the low upper-to-lower body segment ratio independent of delayed epiphyseal closure. Note that in the *Sertoli cell only syndrome* (also known as *germinal cell aplasia;* Spermatogenesis) only the FSH levels are increased (due to impaired inhibin secretion), but testosterone production and secondary sexual characteristics are normal.

Turner's syndrome (45,X), a condition due to meiotic nondysjunction, is the female prototype of gonadal dysgenesis and hypergonadotropic hypogonadism (Fig. 13-48). Similar to Klinefelter's syndrome, the germinal cells rapidly disappear from the gonad. The follicular epithelial cells, the female developmental equivalents of the Sertoli cells, also involute, and in their absence the ovarian stroma is unable to differentiate into a steroidogenic tissue. The result is an inert connective tissue termed *streak gonad*. At the time of puberty, gonadotropin secretion increases to postovariectomy levels (see Fig. 13-43) indicating normal hypothalamic and pituitary mechanisms of both puberty and gonadotropin regulation. As opposed to Klinefelter's syndrome, Turner's syndrome invariably results in *short stature*. The short stature is related to decreased gene dosage involving the pseudoautosomal region of the short arm of chromosome X (see Fig. 13-34). Growth hormone secretion is normal for a prepubertal female. Nevertheless, the affected children fail to show pubertal growth spurt and their growth can be stimulated by exogenous GH. The epiphyseal closure is finally achieved by adrenocortical androgens after their conversion to estrogens. This indicates normal adrenarche and adrenocortical function, which may also cause the appearance of *scanty* pubic hair. The hypogonadism manifests in *primary amenorrhea, absent breast development,* and decreased growth of ambisexual hair. The manifestations of physical stigmata (such as webbing of the neck, short neck with low hairline, broad chest, coarctation of the aorta, cubitus valgus, and [rarely] mild mental retardation) are variable and in their absence the diagnosis may be delayed until puberty.

Most Forms of Incomplete Precocious Puberty Are Associated with Low Levels of Pituitary Gonadotropin Secretion Apart from rare cases of pituitary gonadotroph tumors, the secretion of pituitary gonadotropins is suppressed by feedback mechanisms in the incomplete forms of precocious puberty. In the absence of the appropriate endogenous pulsatile pattern of GnRH, the gonadotropin response to exogenous GnRH is decreased.

In males, due to the absence of increased FSH levels, incomplete precocious puberty is characterized by the absence of an increase in testicular volume. Testosterone production can be stimulated by extrapituitary gonadotropin-secreting tumors, most notably *hCG-producing tumors* of the testis. The hyperstimulation of Leydig cells increases aromatization just like in Klinefelter's syndrome, increases the estrogen:androgen ratio, and often results in gynecomastia. However, unlike Klinefelter's syndrome, the condition is not hypogonadism. Testosterone may be hypersecreted in an autonomous manner in *male-limited familial precocious puberty* (*testotoxicosis*), which is due to an activating mutation of the LH receptor (see Regulation of the Gonadotropin–Gonad Axis in Postpubertal Males). A similar condition may develop if a temperature-sensitive mutation of the $G\alpha_s$ subunit of the trimeric G-protein complex occurs; the mutation functions as a gain-of-function mutation at low temperature (scrotum) but as a loss-of-function mutation at core body temperature (see also Chap. 8). Virilizing forms of *congenital adrenal hyperplasia* (CAH) may present as isosexual incomplete precocious puberty in males. The ACTH-dependent growth of "adrenal rest tissue" usually appears as a bilateral testicular mass rather than the mostly unilaterally presenting testicular tumors. Congenital adrenal hyperplasia may present as contrasexual incomplete precocious puberty in females, who enter pubertal growth spurt, develop muscular male habitus, body odor, pubic, and axillary hair, but these quasipubertal changes are unaccompanied by breast development and menarche (see Fig. 12-9).

McCune-Albright syndrome is an activating somatic mutation of the $G\alpha_s$ subunit of the trimeric G-protein complex that occurs during early embryonic life (Fig. 13-51). Because the mutant protein is used by several hormone receptors, the mutation has variable consequences depending on the contribution of the mutant cell population in the development of hormone target cells (see Chap. 8). The prolonged exposure of the hypothalamus to the sexual steroids may advance pubertal development and the initially incomplete precocious puberty may be converted into the complete form.

Menopause, Andropause, and Adrenopause

Menopause, Andropause, and Adrenopause Are Characterized by the Decreased Production of Sexual Steroids by the Ovaries, Testicles, and Adrenal Cortex, Respectively   *Menopause* is defined as the permanent cessation of the menstrual cycle secondary to the cessation of the ovarian cycle. The diagnosis of menopause is based on the absence of menstrual bleedings for at least 12 months. Thus, the diagnosis of menopause and its

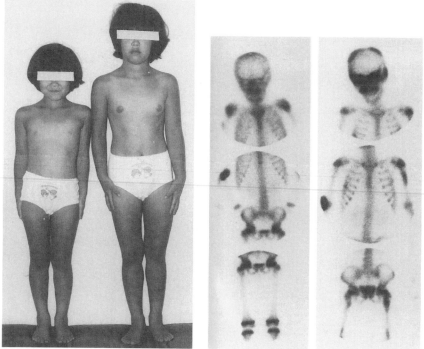

Figure 13-51. McCune–Albright syndrome in 4-year-old monozygotic twins discordant for presenting with precocious puberty and polyostotic fibrous dysplasia. The discordance indicates that a somatic mutation occurred in one of the two sisters only after the separation of the two embryonic cell masses. A. Twin 1 (right) has entered the pubertal growth spurt and has reached Tanner stage 3 breast development. B. ^{99m}Tc-MDP scintigram of the bone indicating bone lesions in twin 1 (right) in the frontal bones, the base of the skull and the left humerus. The high density in the right arm is the site of injection of the radioisotope. (*Source:* Figs. 1 and 2 in Endo M et al: Monozygotic twins discordant for the major signs of McCune–Albright syndrome. Am J Med Gen 41:216–220, 1991.)

timing is always retrospective. On average, last menstrual bleeding occurs at the age of 51.4 years (ranging between 42 and 60 years). Whereas life expectancy has increased over the past 100 years, the timing of menopause has remained the same. Thus, postmenopausal life has increased dramatically, and today's women are postmenopausal for approximately one-third of their entire lifespan. The absence of menstrual bleeding indicates that the endometrium is no longer exposed to sufficient cyclic stimulation by estrogens and progesterone. The average time elapsing between menarche and menopause (i.e., the reproductive phase) is approximately 38 to 39 years. A prolonged reproductive phase due to early menarche and/or late menopause indicates a prolonged exposure of the breasts to estrogens and progesterone, which is associated with an increased risk for breast cancer.

Andropause is defined as the age-dependent decrease of free testosterone in plasma below the low end of the normal range of young (30- to 35-year-old) adult men. The condition is due to a decreased number of Leydig

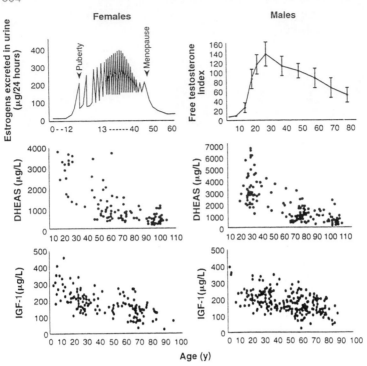

Figure 13-52. Age-related changes in various hormones in females (left) and males (right). Note the modified bell-shaped curves of sexual steroid parameters, the different scales for dehydroepiandrosterone sulfate (DHEAS) for females vs. males, the exponential decrease of DHEAS after the age of 30 years, and the approximately linear decrease of IGF-1 after its pubertal peak. Elderly men, who normally maintain higher production of sexual steroids (including DHEAS) than elderly women, also maintain higher levels of IGF-1. (*Source:* Fig. 3, p 421 in Lamberts SWJ et al: The endocrinology of aging. Science 278:419–424, 1997.)

cells. More than 60% of healthy men over the age of 65 years fulfill the laboratory diagnostic definition of andropause (Fig. 13-52). Nevertheless, significant amounts of testosterone continue to be secreted into old age, and the only unequivocal andropause is castration (*surgical andropause*).

Adrenopause is defined similar to andropause, and it is related to the age-dependent decrease in the production of DHEA and DHEAS by the zonae reticularis and fasciculata of the adrenal cortex.

The Mechanism of the Perimenopausal Process Involves the Decrease of Ovarian Follicles Below a Critical Number and Possibly the Age-Related Derangement of the Hypothalamic Regulation of Circadian Rhythms

Puberty is due to the maturation of the hypothalamus, and menarche is a developmental milestone that signals an underlying process that began years earlier. *Menopause is explained by a combination of the decline/exhaustion of the nonrenewable pool of ovarian follicles and probably the aging of the hypothalamus.* Similar to menarche, menopause is also the result of a process that began years earlier. This process is termed *perimenopause*, which commences at about the age of 35 to 40 years. During perimenopause, fertility is decreased and the rate of meiotic nondysjunction progressively increases.

Perimenopausal symptoms usually begin with irregular menstrual cycles at the age of 35 to 40 years, when the depletion of the ovarian follicles reaches a *critical number*, when the total number of remaining follicles in the two ovaries is <25,000. In age-matched women, who still display regular menstrual cycles, the number of ovarian follicles is higher. Unilateral oophorectomy accelerates the onset of irregular cyclicity by decreasing the total follicular pool.

The exponential decrease of ovarian follicles implies that the number of follicles entering follicular development and becoming available for FSH-mediated rescue also decreases. The decreased follicular numbers translate into decreased granulosa cell mass and weaker inhibition of FSH secretion. As a consequence, the first signs of menopause are the irregular cycles (see below), *increased levels of plasma FSH, and decreased levels of inhibin and estradiol during the early follicular phase in cycling women.* The derangement is progressive (see Fig. 13-52), and is often associated with *hot flashes* and sleep disturbances. At the early stages, no change in the average plasma LH is observed, but the pulse frequency of LH decreases and the pulse duration increases during the follicular phase. In postmenopausal women, both FSH and LH are elevated, similar to those in castrated men (see Figs. 13-12 and 13-41).

The circadian rhythmicity of several hormones and neurotransmitters is regulated by the hypothalamic suprachiasmatic nucleus (see Chap. 14). As a part of the aging process, the biologic clock deteriorates. The consequence is the progressive derangement of the temporal organization of several functions, including the regulation of gonadotropin secretion. It has been proposed that the perimenopausal endocrine changes are at least in part secondary to hypothalamic aging. Although this notion has gained recognition, there is overwhelming experimental evidence supporting the role of the declining ovarian function as the primary cause of menopause.

The *irregularity* of the menstrual cycle (menometrorrhagia) is due to the unpredictable combination of several factors:

- Depending on the FSH responsiveness of the dominant follicle (which was selected from a very limited pool of developing early antral follicles), the follicular phase may either be shortened or prolonged, which leads to varying overall length of the menstrual cycle. A rapidly growing dominant follicle may achieve plasma estradiol *concentration* that results in positive feedback and ovulation earlier, but the total *amount* of estrogen secreted during the follicular phase is diminished.
- The decreased production of estrogens during the follicular phase may result in a diminished proliferation of the endometrium. Luteal progesterone prevents further proliferation as expected. After the involution of

the corpus luteum, the endometrial shedding is decreased: the menstrual bleeding is shorter and lighter.

- Estradiol secretion during the follicular phase may become insufficient to result in positive feedback, ovulation, and formation of the corpus luteum. In the absence of corpus luteum and progesterone, breakthrough bleeding may occur at irregular intervals.

Surgical menopause is the consequence of bilateral oophorectomy. Its manifestations are usually more severe than those due to natural menopause because the gradual perimenopausal endocrine changes are replaced by the abrupt elimination of ovarian hormones. However, even in the absence of hypothalamic aging and in the presence of relatively high adrenal production of androgens, the main manifestations and gonadotropin secretory patterns are essentially identical.

Postmenopausal Physiologic Changes Are Attributed to the Decrease of All Ovarian Steroid Hormones, Including Estrogens, Progesterone, and Androgens Menopausal changes are usually classified as early and late manifestations (Table 13-16). A leading early manifestation of menopause is a thermoregulatory vasomotor imbalance known as "hot flashes" (Fig. 13-53). *Hot flashes develop because of the sudden, transient decrease in the temperature setpoint of the hypothalamic "thermostat."* It appears that the same mechanism that results in pulsatile release of GnRH is also responsible for the phasic resetting of the hypothalamic thermostat (Fig. 13-54). The new setpoint results in the sensation of a hyperthermia, which activates countermeasures by the "cooling center" (see Box 11-3). Hot flashes are defined as recurrent, transient periods of sensation of heat, sweating, and (sometimes) flushing, which are accompanied by increased heart rate, the sensation of palpitations and anxiety, and are followed by chills. The cutaneous vasodilatation and sweating result in an acute heat dissipation which leads to a decrease of core body temperature ranging between 0.1 to 0.9°C. Hot flashes affect 24 to 93% of postmenopausal women in western countries. They occur with the highest frequency during the first 2 years after menopause, followed by gradual dissipation of the symptoms.

Table 13-16   Manifestations of Menopause

Early	Late
Perimenopausal irregularity of the menstrual cycles	Coronary heart disease
Hot flashes	Osteoporosis and periodontal disease
Atrophy of estrogen-dependent tissues: breast, genitourinary system (vaginal atrophy, urinary incontinence)	Cutaneous changes: loss of elastic fibers, decreased dermal water content and turgor, loss of ambisexual hair
Decreased sexual activity	
Depression	

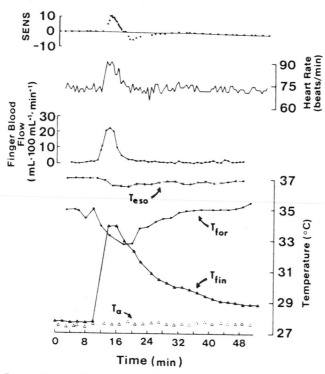

Figure 13-53. Characteristic physiologic changes during a hot flash. SENS, sensation; T, temperature; T_a, ambient, T_{fin}, finger, T_{eso}, esophagus; T_{for}, forehead. The cutaneous/peripheral vasodilatation increases finger temperature, but such an effect is offset by sweating-related heat-loss of the forehead. Note the slight decrease of core body temperature (T_{eso}). (*Source:* Fig. 1 in Kronenberg F, Downey JA: Thermoregulatory physiology of menopausal hot flashes: a review. Can J Physiol Pharmacol 65:1312–24, 1987.)

The ultimate cause of the deranged hypothalamic temperature regulatory mechanism is the decrease of the sex steroids, including progesterone. Thus, hot flashes are not specific for menopause: they occur during the puerperium (postpartum drop of placental steroids), and in men upon orchiectomy. Replacement of these hormones alleviates hot flashes; progesterone appears to be more effective than estrogens administered alone. In women experiencing surgical menopause secondary to salpingoophorectomy combined with hysterectomy, a combined regimen of estrogens and *androgens* instituted immediately after oophorectomy has been found most effective in eliminating or decreasing these symptoms. The sexual steroids have two sites of action:

- feedback regulation to neurotransmitters that directly regulate the GnRH pulse generator and the hypothalamic thermoregulatory centers; and
- direct action on the thermoregulatory centers to decrease their sensitivity to the feedback-regulated neurotransmitters.

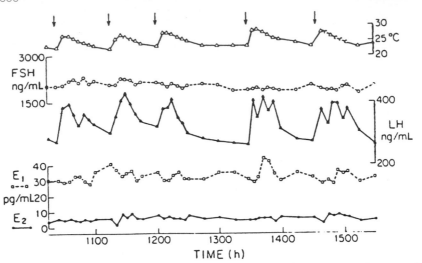

Figure 13-54. Serial measurements of finger temperature and luteinizing hormone (LH) indicate a close association between the pulsatility of gonadotropin releasing hormone (GnRH)/LH and hot flashes. The onset of hot flashes is indicated by the arrows. The association is due to (probably central adrenergic) mechanisms that simultaneously increase GnRH output and decrease the setpoint of temperature regulation. (*Source:* From Meldrum DR et al: Gonadotropins, estrogens, and adrenal steroids during the menopausal hot flash. J Clin Endocrinol Metab 50:685–689, 1980.)

Chronic absence of the steroid hormones results in adaptive changes in the heat center responsiveness, which explains why pulsatile LH secretion continues after hot flashes have disappeared.

Postmenopausal *osteoporosis* is a severe consequence of estrogen deficiency. It is discussed in detail in Chap. 8.

During the reproductive years, women enjoy a decreased risk for *coronary heart disease* and *stroke* in comparison with men. The risk for these cardiovascular diseases increases after menopause and equals that of men of the same age. The main determinant of cardiovascular risk is the plasma lipoprotein profile. Estrogens decrease LDL and increase high density lipoprotein (HDL) levels is plasma. The effect on LDL is related to the estrogen-induced expression of LDL receptors that are crucial for the plasma clearance of LDL by binding its apolipoprotein B-100 (see Box 9-5).

Hormonal Therapy Alleviates the Symptoms of Menopause but Might Increase the Risk for Breast Cancer Various combinations and regimens of hormone therapy are in use, which are adjusted to the risk factors and preferences of the individual. Most postmenopausal complaints can be alleviated by estrogens. The early start of estrogen replacement is crucial for maintaining bone structure because estrogens can only prevent but cannot reverse osteoporosis. Estrogen replacement decreases the risk and severity of Alzheimer's disease, and may be beneficial in the treatment of postmenopausal urinary incontinence. Estrogens increase the risk for endometrial cancer if their action is unopposed by progestins. Thus, in nonhysterectomized women estrogens are never administered without progestins. The estrogen/progesterone regimens may be tailored to yield cyclic bleeding or (by continuous administration) to avoid cyclic bleeding. Progestins, however, attenuate the beneficial effects of estrogens on plasma lipid profile. Prolongation of estrogen exposure of the breast might increase the risk for breast cancer, and this effect may not be antagonized by progestins. Coadministration of low-dose androgens with estrogens (in hysterectomized patients) does not deteriorate the plasma lipid profile compared to treatment with estrogen alone, but is more effective in controlling hot flashes, and in increasing libido and sexual activity.

14

THE PINEAL GLAND AND BIOLOGIC RHYTHMS

OBJECTIVES

1. Define the terms *Zeitgeber, circadian rhythm,* and *entrainment.* Describe the molecular mechanism of the *circadian oscillator* and identify the location of the mammalian *master clock.*
2. Discuss the mechanisms of entrainment of the master clock. Describe the ouput signals of the *suprachiasmatic nucleus,* especially in relationship with melatonin and cortisol rhythms.
3. Discuss the biosynthesis, secretion, plasma transport, and metabolism of melatonin. Discuss the membrane and intracellular receptors mediating the physiologic actions of melatonin.
4. Describe the ontogeny of melatonin production and its potential relationship with reproductive function.
5. Discuss the regulation of circadian melatonin secretion and its relationship with photic cues. Identify melatonin as a *chronobiotic compound* and describe its function in the entrainment of circadian rhythms.
6. Discuss the restorative and anabolic actions of melatonin, including hypothermic, antioxidative and anticancer activities.

INTRODUCTION

The earth's rotation about its axis results in a profound environmental change that requires cyclic adaptation by living organisms. Evolutionary pressure led to the early development of an internal pacemaker (*Zeitgeber* [German: timegiver]) or clock: an endogenous oscillator mechanism with a period length of approximately (but not exactly) 24 h, which generates a free-running *circadian rhythm* in the absence of environmental cues (Latin: *circa diem* = approximately 1 day). Because the earth's axis is not perpendicular to the plane of its orbit around the sun, the proportion of daylight and darkness within the 24-h day varies with the season and latitude. Thus, for appropriate adaptation to these cyclic circadian and circannual changes the organism requires

- a circadian clock/oscillator;
- an entrainment pathway to the oscillator, which resets the clock to sunrise ("Zeitgeber-time 0 hr") or sunset;
- ouput signal(s) from the clock to effect physiologic changes in a temporal manner.

Circadian clocks are genetically determined and their basic principle is conserved as evidenced by their mechanism in *Neurospora, Drosophila,* and mammals. The clock's core consists of intracellular negative feedback loops, in which nuclear proteins inhibit the transcription of their own mRNAs *after a lag,* thereby yielding oscillating levels of both their mRNA and protein.

In vertebrates, the clock mechanism that governs the rest of the organism is expressed at three distinctive sites: the retina, the hypothalamic *suprachiasmatic nucleus* (SCN) and the pineal gland. The pineal gland in lower vertebrates functions as a "third eye" and has photoreceptors, which are rudimentary in the mammalian pineal. The involution of the photoreceptive function was associated with the loss of independent clock function of the pineal gland. However, *melatonin* production (the hormonal output signal of the pineal gland) has been retained and is regulated by the SCN, which functions as the *masterclock* in mammals.

The *entrainment* of the endogenous clock within the SCN is achieved by a direct neuronal input from the retina. The targets of circulating melatonin include the SCN, where it reinforces and/or effects the entrainment of the Zeitgeber. In addition to pineal gland function, the SCN regulates several circadian rhythms by neural connections.

In this chapter, we discuss the molecular mechanism of the circadian oscillator, the function of the SCN as a masterclock, the pineal gland, and the physiology of melatonin.

THE MOLECULAR MECHANISM OF THE CIRCADIAN CLOCK

A model of the molecular pacemaker located in the neurons of the SCN is shown in Fig. 14-1. The proteins involved in the pacemaker machinery contain the *PAS dimerization domain*. The PAS acronym refers to the first three proteins discovered which share this domain: Period (a *Drosophila* pacemaker protein), Arnt (aryl hydrocarbon receptor nuclear translocator, see Chaps. 5 and 12) and Sim (the *Drosophila* "single-minded" protein). PAS is homologous with the bacterial protein *photoactive yellow*, which can convert light signals into biochemical reactions. The main mammalian pacemaker proteins identified thus far include CLOCK, BMAL1, PERs, and TIM.

CLOCK is a member of the basic helix-loop-helix DNA-binding domain (bHLH-PAS) transcription factors. It also contains a glutamine-rich

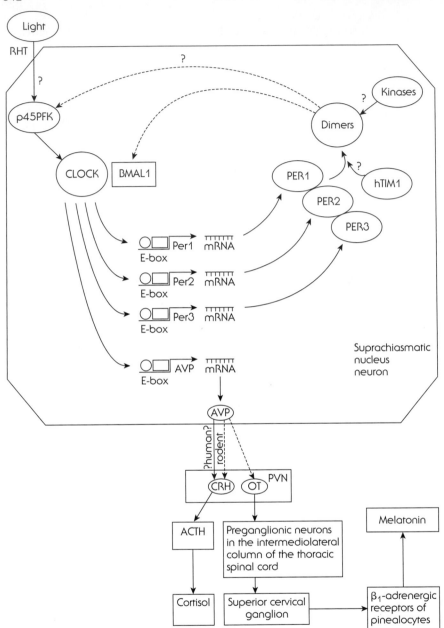

Figure 14-1. Model of the molecular pacemaker located in the neurons of the suprachiasmatic nucleus. Solid arrows indicate stimulation/increase; dashed arrows show inhibition/decrease. The PER-PER and perhaps the PER-hTIM1 protein dimers inhibit the function of the CLOCK–BMAL1 heterodimeric transcription factor after a lag, so that the completion of cycle depicted requires about 24 hours. The entrainment of the cycle by light involves the retinohypothalamic tract (RHT) and glutamate as a neurotransmitter. A potential target of the glutamatergic mechanism is a set of histone H1 kinases termed *periodically fluctuating*

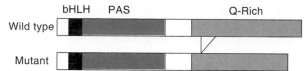

Figure 14-2. The modular structure of the wild type and the mutant murine Clock transcription factor. The DNA-binding domain is a basic helix-loop-helix (bHLH) module. The PAS (Period/ARNT/Single minded) domain is required for dimerization. The glutamine- (Q-) rich domain functions as a transcriptional transactivator. An A–T nucleotide transversion at the splice donor site results in exon skipping and a deletion of 51 amino acids. In a heterozygous state, the mutation results in an endogenous rhythm 1 h (equaling 6 standard deviations) too long. In a homozygous state, the endogenous rhythm is initially 3 to 4 h too long, then becomes abolished in the absence of photic cues. (*Source*: From Fig. 1 in Reppert SM, Weaver DR: Forward genetic approach strikes gold: Cloning of a mammalian *Clock* gene. Cell 89:487–490, 1997.)

(Q-rich) region towards its C-terminus (transcriptional transactivation domain). The human *CLOCK* gene is localized on chromosome 4q12, its coding sequence extends over 20 exons with an intron/exon organization that is identical with that of the mouse *Clock* gene. The coding sequence of human *CLOCK* is 89% identical to its mouse ortholog; its amino acid sequence consists of 846 residues and is 96% identical with the murine Clock protein. Surprisingly, the mammalian Clock mRNA is expressed constitutively without a circadian oscillation. Nevertheless an inactivating mutation of *Clock* ("circadian locomotor output cycles kaput") in mice affects circadian rhythmicity (Fig. 14-2). Mice homozygous for the *Clock* mutation, display very long (27- to 28-h) periods upon initial exposure to constant darkness, and lose rhythmicity upon prolonged (duration of weeks) constant darkness. Conversely, overexpression of the normal clock gene in transgenic mice shortens the length of the endogenous circadian rhythm. Thus, *Clock regulates two fundamental properties of circadian clocks: the length of the circadian period (cycle time) and the persistence of rhythmicity.* *Clock* is highly expressed in the SCN and the retina; however, it is also expressed in other brain regions and peripheral tissues such as the gonads, liver, gut, kidney, lung and heart, where it may be involved in cellular regulation not necessarily related to circadian rhythms.

Brain/muscle Arnt-like protein 1 (BMAL1) is a bHLH-PAS domain transcription factor that forms heterodimers with CLOCK. Unlike the Clock mRNA, BMAL1 mRNA displays a robust circadian rhythm in the SCN reaching peak levels at the dark-light transition.

Figure 14-1. (*Continued*) *protein kinases* (PFKs), especially p45PFK. A major output signal is arginine vasopressin (AVP), which serves as a neurotransmitter connecting the SCN to other areas of the brain including subsets of corticotropin releasing hormone (CRH) and *autonomic* oxytocin (OT) neurons in the paraventricular nucleus (PVN). Vasoactive intestinal peptide (VIP) is another circadian output signal of the SCN-pineal pathway, which is in antiphase with AVP (not shown). The output signal in the model is based on rodent experiments and may be applicable in humans only with modifications. (*Source*: Modified from Dunlap J: Circadian rhythms: An end in the beginning. Science 280:1548–1549, 1998.)

The mammalian PER proteins (Per1, Per2, and Per3) are homologous with the *Drosophila* "period" protein. The promoter region of the *PER* genes contains the CLOCK/BMAL1 response element known as the *E-box*. The PER mRNA levels follow circadian rhythm with peak levels at early night, which is an expression pattern antiphase to that of BMAL1 mRNA. PERs are expressed in several tissues. The expression of rat Per2 mRNA follows a circadian pattern in peripheral mononuclear leukocytes, which is synchronous with that in the SCN and in other peripheral tissues. The peripheral circadian expression of Per2 mRNA is abolished in SCN-lesioned rats. These findings suggest that the circadian pattern of peripheral Per2 is not generated by a complete peripheral clock mechanism, but is driven by some SCN-regulated humoral signal.

The human *TIM* gene (*hTIM*; located on chromosome 12q12-13) is homologous with the *timeless* gene of *Drosophila*."Timeless" and "period" are dimerization partners in *Drosophila*. The significance of the TIM transcription factor in mammals is uncertain; it is expressed relatively weakly in the SCN and shows no circadian rhythm. In the retina of mice, Tim mRNA displays a circadian rhythm, which is particularly robust in the presence of entrainment by light/dark cycles. Reports on the dimerization ability of mammalian TIM with PER have been inconsistent. It has been suggested that in the mammalian SCN, PER–PER interactions have replaced the function of PER–TIM heterodimers.

The neurons of the SCN contain *histone H1 kinase* activity that periodically fluctuates with a circadian rhythm, reaching a maximum at the midpoint of the light phase and a minimum at the midpoint of the dark phase. Three histone H1 kinases termed *periodically fluctuating protein kinases* (PFKs) have been found in the SCN: p45PFK, p100PFK, and p200PFK. The highest circadian fluctuation is exhibited by p45PFK activity. This enzyme phosphorylates the Ser-Pro-rich region of the Clock protein thereby increasing its transcriptional activity. Thus, whereas the expression of CLOCK does not change with the time of day, its phosphorylation state and activity fluctuate.

The model in Fig. 14-1 shows that the CLOCK–BMAL1 heterodimer transcription factor activates the transcription of genes containing the E-box. These genes include

- the PER transcription factors and
- the *arginine vasopresssin* (AVP) gene.

The PER and AVP mRNA rhythms are abolished in the SCN of mice homozygous for the *Clock* mutation, indicating that the transcriptional machinery of the core clockwork directly regulates a clock-controlled output rhythm.

The PER transcription factors form dimers which, after a lag, suppress their own expression by decreasing the activity of the CLOCK–BMAL1 heterodimer. This cycle results in oscillating transcriptional activation of *PER* genes by CLOCK–BMAL1 with an inherent period of time of about 24 h. The mechanism of decreasing CLOCK–BMAL1 activity by PER proteins is unclear. PERs might interact via their PAS domains with the CLOCK–BMAL1, regulate the kinase(s) acting on CLOCK, and/or regulate BMAL1 expression (which shows a clear circadian rhythm). Such an action would be indirect because PERs lack a DNA-binding domain.

THE FUNCTION OF THE SUPRACHIASMATIC NUCLEUS

The suprachiasmatic nucleus (SCN) is the masterclock of mammals. Its neurons contain the circadian molecular oscillator; the single-cell oscillators function in a coordinated manner and are entrained by photic cues, and the neurons regulate circadian functions by their neurotransmitters. Isolated lesion of the SCN abolishes circadian rhythms, including those of hormones, sleep and locomotor behavior.

The appropriate *coordination* of SCN single-cell oscillators requires the highly *polysialated* form of the *neural cell adhesion molecule* (PSA–NCAM). Mice deficient in the PSA–NCAM display the same pattern of deficit in their circadian rhythms as those having a mutant *Clock* gene.

Photic entrainment of circadian rhythms occurs as a consequence of daily, light-induced adjustments. Photic information is transmitted by a unique population of retinal photoreceptors, processed by a distinct subset of retinal ganglion cells, and conveyed to the SCN directly through the *retinohypothalamic tract* (RHT) and indirectly by the *geniculohypothalamic tract* (GHT). The transmitter of the retinohypothalamic tract is *glutamate*, whereas the geniculohypothalamic tract utilizes γ *aminobutyric acid* (GABA) and *neuropeptide Y* (NPY). The excitatory amino acid glutamate utilized by the retinohypothalamic tract activates both NMDA and metabotropic glutamate receptors, thereby inducing the expression of *immediate early genes*, and the synthesis and release of nitric oxide (NO). Out-of-phase exposure to light during the nocturnal period activates the glutamate mechanism and activates the NO signaling. These mechanisms lead to CREB phosphorylation, which ultimately effects phase resetting of the biologic clock by unknown downstream mechanisms.

Serotonergic innervation from the median raphe nucleus of the pons and melatonin from the pineal gland provide nonphotic information to the SCN, which may regulate the response of the SCN circadian clock to light. Other *nonphotic entrainment* signals include environmental factors such as delayed food intake or the onset of sleep.

The main neurotransmitters serving as *circadian output signals* from the SCN are AVP and vasoactive intestinal peptide (VIP), which are apparently produced by the SCN in an antiphase manner. As mentioned above,

CLOCK–BMAL1 induces the expression of AVP. AVP as a neurotransmitter, by direct and indirect means, inhibits

- corticotropin-releasing hormone (CRH) neurons located in the paraventricular nucleus (PVN).
- a group of oxytocin-containing autonomic neurons which project to the upper thoracic intermediolateral column of the spinal cord.

These neurons play central roles in the stimulation of adrenocorticotroph hormone (ACTH) and in the stimulation of sympathetic outflow from the spinal cord to the *superior cervical ganglion,* respectively. VIP fibers emerging from the SCN also communicate signals to the autonomic neurons of the PVN. The postganglionic sympathetic fibers of the superior cervical ganglion stimulate melatonin production by the pineal gland (see details below). The AVP output signal displays the following important features:

- The inhibition of CRH/oxytocin neurons follows the induction of AVP gene expression with a significant lag. This is due to the time requirements of translation and axonal transport to nerve terminals. In addition, AVP release from the terminals requires action potential.
- *The inhibition of the sympathetic–pineal gland pathway occurs during the light phase of the 24-h day* both in rodents (nocturnal species) and in humans (diurnal species) leading to low plasma melatonin levels during the day and high levels at night. In contrast with the similarity in melatonin rhythms, the timing of the ACTH-glucocorticoid rhythm is opposite in rodents and humans. Thus, the SCN/AVP inhibition of the PVN/CRH-ACTH axis demonstrated in rodents may be applicable in humans only with modifications. In depression (a condition probably caused by an increased CRH activity), the ACTH-cortisol axis is inappropriately activated, which is characteristically associated with melatonin level, sleep, and appetite disturbances.

THE PINEAL GLAND AND THE PHYSIOLOGY OF MELATONIN

Melatonin Is a Lipophilic Derivative of Serotonin Synthesized upon β_1-Adrenergic Receptor Stimulation of Pinealocytes

The *pineal gland* (*epiphysis cerebri*) is the pine cone-shaped posterior protrusion of the third cerebral ventricle just above the opening of the aquaeductus cerebri (see Fig. 10-1B). With age, the pineal gland progressively accumulates concretions called brainsand (*acervuli cerebri* or *corpora aranacea*). These concretions display a layered structure, and are predominantly composed of calcium and magnesium phosphate in a glycoprotein matrix.

There is a correlation between the age of the subject and the number of layers in the largest acervuli suggesting that the layers develop due to circannual changes in mineral deposition in the organ. The formation and growth of acervuli is inhibited by normal parathyroid function, and becomes enhanced after parathyroidectomy. Due to their mineral content, acervuli are conspicuous with radiological imaging techniques, and provide a useful landmark in the diagnosis of intracranial diseases.

Unlike the other circumventrical organs of humans or the pineal gland of other mammals, the human pineal is supplied by continuous capillaries and is protected by the blood-brain barrier (BBB). Postganglionic *noradrenergic* fibers arising from the superior cervical ganglion reach the pineal gland by joining the course of blood vessels in the pia mater (see Fig. 14-1). Note that these fibers are on the *abluminal* side of blood vessels; thus noradrenaline gains access to its target cells without a need to penetrate the BBB. The parenchyma of the pineal gland mainly consists of modified neurons termed *pinealocytes,* which synthesize and secrete melatonin upon stimulation by noradrenaline. Melatonin readily crosses the BBB in both directions, which is essential for its secretion into blood and targeting specific brain areas by the circulating hormone.

Melatonin is highly lipophilic. Thus, it is not stored within the pinealocytes but released into the circulation immediately on synthesis. Melatonin (5-methoxy-N-acetyltryptamine) is synthesized from L-tryptophan through serotonin (Fig. 14-3). The synthesis of serotonin is similar to that of dopamine:

- The first reaction is a hydroxylation by *tryptophan hydroxylase* for serotonin and by tyrosine hydroxylase for dopamine synthesis.
- The second reaction is identical in the two biosynthetic pathways and is performed by the same enzyme, *aromatic L-amino acid decarboxylase.*

The next reaction in melatonin biosynthesis is *the rate-limiting step, which dictates the circadian rhythm of melatonin: the N-acetylation of serotonin by arylalkylamine N-acetyltransferase* (AA–NAT).

The final step of melatonin synthesis is reminiscent of that of adrenaline synthesis: a methyltransferase reaction utlizing S-adenosyl-L-methionine (SAM). However, unlike the N-methylation in adrenaline synthesis by PNMT, the reaction is an O-methylation targeting the hydroxyl group of N-acetylserotonin, which is catalyzed by *hydroxyindole-O-methyltransferase* (HIOMT).

Melatonin synthesis is regulated by the SCN via noradrenergic sympathetic nerves. The activated β_1-*adrenergic receptors* stimulate AA–NAT activity via *cyclic AMP*. This action is potentiated by the stimulation of α_1-*adrenergic receptors*. Depending on the species, the activity of AA–NAT varies 7- to 150-fold between daytime minimum and nighttime peak levels, and its regulation may involve transcriptional and/or translational mechanisms. The human AA–NAT gene is located on chromosome 17q25. The

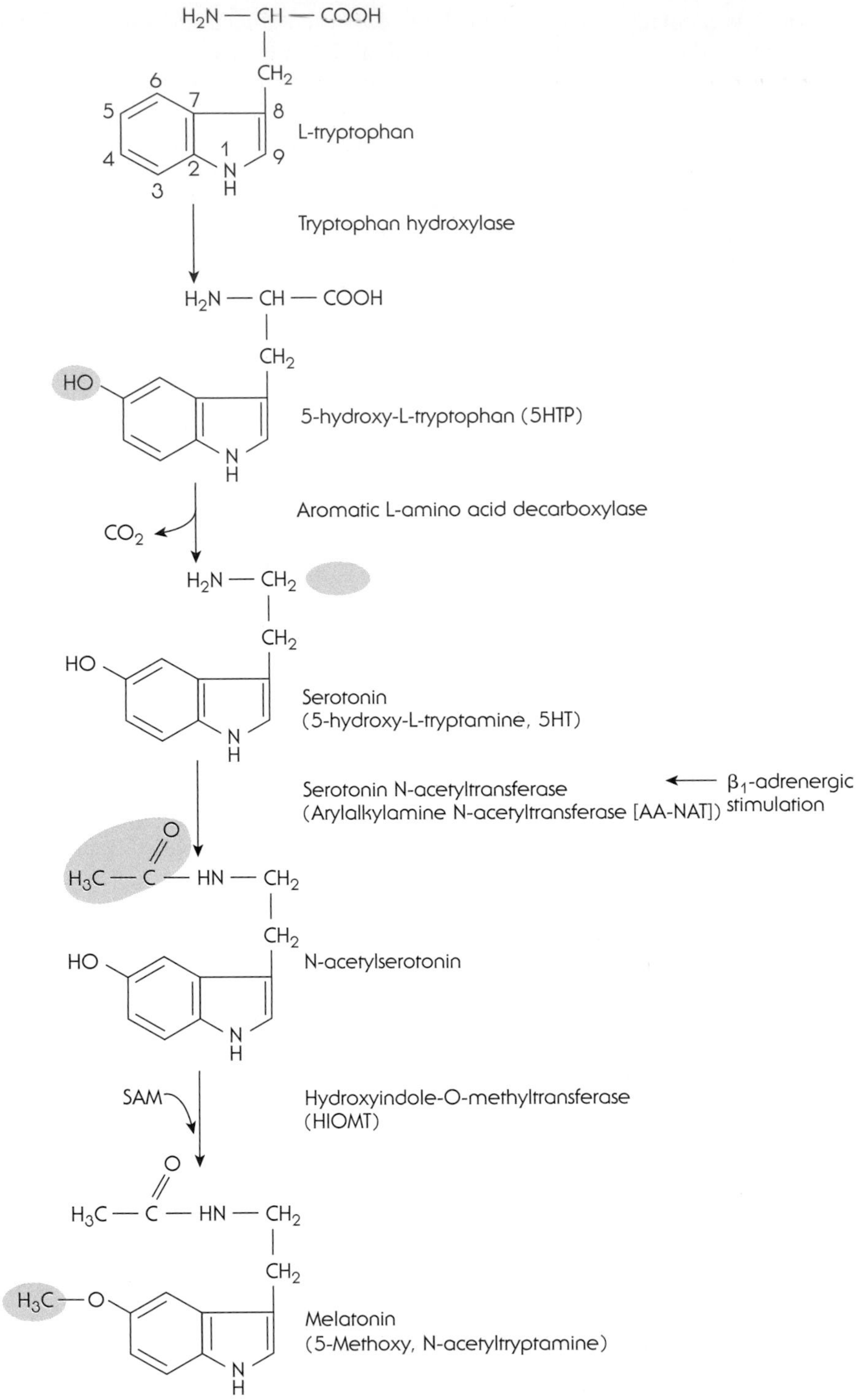

H₂N — CH — COOH

L-tryptophan

Tryptophan hydroxylase

H₂N — CH — COOH

5-hydroxy-L-tryptophan (5HTP)

Aromatic L-amino acid decarboxylase

CO_2

Serotonin
(5-hydroxy-L-tryptamine, 5HT)

Serotonin N-acetyltransferase   ← β₁-adrenergic
(Arylalkylamine N-acetyltransferase [AA-NAT])   stimulation

N-acetylserotonin

SAM   Hydroxyindole-O-methyltransferase
               (HIOMT)

Melatonin
(5-Methoxy, N-acetyltryptamine)

daily fluctuation in AA–NAT *protein levels* and *activity* in monkey pineals is about thirtyfold, but only threefold in AA–NAT mRNA levels. Thus, *the primate AA–NAT/melatonin rhythm is primarily due to the regulated translation of preexisting mRNA*. The AA–NAT gene is also expressed in the retina, where its mRNA levels are approximately 25% of those in the pineal. The function of retinal AA–NAT is unknown; nevertheless the retina does not produce significant amounts of melatonin because of the extremely low levels of HIOMT.

Melatonin Circulates in Plasma as Protein-Bound and Free Hormone with a Half-Life of About 20 to 47 Minutes

As a lipophilic hormone, melatonin circulates in plasma bound to α_1-acid glycoprotein (AGP, also known as orosomucoid; see Chap. 4) and albumin. The protein-bound melatonin is in equilibrium with the free hormone.

In spite of this protein binding, melatonin is rapidly cleared from the circulation by the liver with a significant first passage phenomenon. The first passage phenomenon, however, is not as significant as with sexual steroids, and melatonin can be effectively administered orally. The half-life of melatonin in the circulation has been reported between 15 and 60 min with average values ranging between 20 and 47 min. It appears that the half-life of melatonin is longer in prepubertal individuals than in adults.

In the liver, melatonin is converted into 6-hydroxymelatonin by a microsomal cytochrome P450 followed by sulfoconjugation. The resulting 6-sulfatoxymelatonin is more water-soluble, does not bind with plasma proteins and is rapidly excreted with urine and, to a lesser extent, with bile and feces. A small proportion of intact melatonin is excreted by the kidney.

The Cellular Action of Melatonin Is Mediated by G-Protein-Coupled Membrane Receptors and Intracellular Receptors Related to Retinoid/Rexinoid Receptors

In spite of being a lipophilic hormone, melatonin acts at least in part on membrane receptors. Two mammalian melatonin membrane receptor subtypes have been identified:

- The *Mel1a* melatonin receptor is expressed at most sites displaying ^{125}I-Mel binding, including the SCN and the pars tuberalis of the adenohypophysis (the latter is weak in humans).
- The *Mel1b* melatonin receptor is expressed in the retina and brain.

Figure 14-3. The biosynthetic pathway of melatonin in the pineal gland. The stimulation of β_1-adrenergic receptors is potentiated by α_1-adrenergic receptors, and mainly involves cyclic AMP-mediated upregulation of the translation of preexisting AA–NAT mRNA. SAM, S-adenosyl-L-methionine. Compare with Fig. 12-4.

Both membrane receptors are coupled with a pertussis toxin-sensitive $G\alpha_i$ protein, and inhibit the activity of adenylyl cyclase. By incompletely understood mechanisms, melatonin inhibits the activity of nitric oxide synthase. In addition, as a "free radical scavanger" antioxidant, melatonin may antagonize the action of nitric oxide (NO).

The intracellular/nuclear receptors of melatonin belong to the *ROR/RZR family* (ROR = retinoic acid-related orphan receptor; RZR = retinoid Z receptor), a group of the steroid hormone receptor superfamily. Melatonin is a specific ligand for the brain-specific nuclear receptor RZRβ. RZRα and its splicing variant RORα_1 also serve as nuclear receptors for melatonin with binding affinities in the low nanomolar range. In contrast to RZRβ, RZRα/RORα are expressed in many tissues and cells outside the brain. The thiazolidinedione CGP 52608 is a synthetic RZR ligand that acts as a functional agonist of melatonin at its nuclear receptor, but does not bind to the high-affinity melatonin membrane receptors. Note that the prototypes of thiazolidinediones are troglitazone, rosiglitazone, and pioglitazone, which are PPARγ (peroxisome proloferator-activated receptor γ) agonists that form heterodimers with the RXR (rexinoid) receptor (see Chaps. 5, 9, and 15).

The RZRs may bind as monomers to half-sites of the natural retinoid response elements. RZRs can bind as homodimers to specific response elements formed either by palindromes or by direct repeats of two TAGG-TCA half-sites. These RZR-specific response elements display dramatically decreased affinity for RAR–RXR heterodimers.

The intracellular receptors of melatonin might be involved in the interactions between melatonin and estrogens, and in the anticancer actions of melatonin.

- Melatonin (but not other indole derivatives) at nanomolar concentrations antagonizes estrogen action via a nuclear receptor which, upon melatonin binding, destabilizes the binding of the estradiol-estrogen receptor complex to the estrogen response element. The inhibitory effect caused by melatonin is saturable and does not appear to be mediated by RZR nuclear receptors.
- Melatonin inhibits the cellular uptake of linoleic acid and its metabolism to 13-hydroxyoctadecadienoic acid (13-HODE) by 5-lipoxygenase. 13-HODE is growth-signaling molecule which stimulates epidermal growth factor (EGF)-dependent mitogenesis. RZRα and RORα_1 receptors mediate the melatonin-induced repression of 5-lipoxygenase.

The Physiologic Functions of Melatonin Include Temporal Organization, Restorative/Anabolic, and Reproductive Actions

Melatonin was discovered as a hormone that induced perinuclear aggregation of melanin granules within the dermal melanophore cells of frogs (hence the name), thereby lightening their skin color. This function of melatonin is characteristic in amphibians but absent in mammals. In general, melatonin is a timing signal to which each species has adapted the timing of physiologic processes. The physiologic role of melatonin in humans falls into three categories:

- Self-regulation of circadian timing by the suprachiasmatic nucleus-pineal complex.
- Promotion of restorative or anabolic physiologic processes. These include
  - hypothermic action (decrease of core temperature),
  - promotion of sleep/decrease of alertness,
  - decreased cardiovascular output,
  - antioxidant function,
  - anticancer activities.
- Interaction with reproductive function.

In the following section, we discuss these actions in relation with the ontogeny and daily secretory profile of melatonin.

Melatonin Secretion Commences Postpartum, Peaks in Early Childhood, and Becomes Diminished in Old Age

Melatonin crosses the placental barrier and enters the circulation of the fetus. It has been suggested that maternal plasma melatonin levels are reflected in the fetus and provide the first entrainment signal for the developing fetal circadian rhythms. Such a function might be taken over by breast milk, which contains melatonin derived from maternal plasma. Nevertheless, plasma melatonin levels are very low in the newborn, and melatonin rhythm in term infants is first detectable at the age of 9 to 12 weeks (Fig. 14-4).

Nighttime peak melatonin levels reach their maximum in 1- to 5-year-old children, then rapidly decrease to adult levels by the late teenage years. The transition from Tanner stage 1 to Tanner stage 5 of sexual maturation is associated with a significant decrease in nocturnal melatonin levels. It has been suggested that the prepubertally high levels of melatonin are responsible for the juvenile pause of gonadotropin secretion and the decline of melatonin is causative in the onset of pubertal gonadotropin secretion. This theory is still unsettled. In certain mammals such as the hamster, melatonin possesses a gonadostatic function, but such a role in humans is uncertain. As noted, melatonin may antagonize the *action* of estrogens, and thus might inhibit both negative and positive estrogenic feedback to gonadotropin secretion. Estrogens have been demonstrated to suppress supranormal melatonin secretion in amenorrheic patients. Thus, it is unclear whether the high melatonin inhibits the production of sexual steroids or melatonin is high because of the low levels of circulating sex steroids.

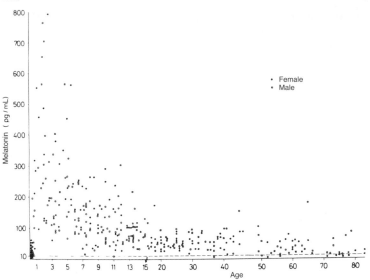

Figure 14-4. The ontogeny of melatonin secretion. The figure shows the age-dependent nighttime (i.e., circadian peak) serum concentrations of melatonin in 367 subjects (210 males, 157 females). Note that between the ages of late teens and forties, peak melatonin levels are relatively steady, usually ranging between 60 and 100 pg/mL. (*Source*: From Waldhauser F et al: Alterations in nocturnal serum melatonin levels in humans with growth and aging. Clin Endocrinol Metab 66:618, 1988.)

    Menopause is associated with a decrease in circulating melatonin. In males of the same age, melatonin levels also drop with no significant alteration in reproductive physiology. Old age is often associated with severely diminished melatonin secretion. The absence of reinforcement of the circadian clock entrainment by melatonin results in irregularities of circadian rhythms, such as the sleep-wake cycle.

The SCN-Driven Free-Running Circadian Melatonin Rhythm of Blind Subjects Is Overridden by Light-Entrainment in Nonblind Individuals

Under physiologic circumstances, melatonin is best viewed as a "*darkness hormone*" in all species studied: during daylight and/or sufficiently bright artificial light, plasma melatonin levels are low, and the onset of melatonin secretion is strongly correlated ($r > 0.90$) with dusk and/or the onset of darkness (Fig. 14-5). In normal human subjects on a typical daily rest-activity schedule, peak levels of plasma melatonin are usually attained between 2:00 and 4:00 A.M. Melatonin starts decreasing in plasma well before the onset of light/waking up, indicating that an inherent circadian rhythm driven by the SCN "anticipates" sunrise. Staying awake *in darkness* does not influence this rhythm. In contrast, *exposure to bright light during the rising phase of plasma melatonin promptly inhibits further melatonin secretion.* Exposure to 2500 lux is required for the complete suppression of nighttime melatonin secretion in humans (domestic light is approximately 300 to 500 lux). The most effective light is in the green band (= 540 nm), which corresponds with the maximum sensitivity of rods.

Under natural lighting conditions (in the absence of artificial light), the seasonal changes in the length of light and dark periods of the day are reflected in melatonin secretion. Irrespective of the length of darkness (within the normal range of seasonal variations), dusk coincides with the onset of melatonin secretion, and plasma melatonin starts decreasing about 4 hours before sunrise. Thus, the longer the darkness, the more prolonged the melatonin secretion. Exposure to average household artificial light during the evening hours is sufficient to delay the onset of melatonin secretion in most individuals. Thus, in today's society, humans experience summer-like long daylight hours all year round. For individuals suffering from *seasonal affecting disorder* (SAD), exposure to bright (melatonin-suppressing) light is often beneficial.

In blind human subjects, whose retina is unable to sense and/or transmit light signals, and in laboratory animals kept in constant darkness, melatonin

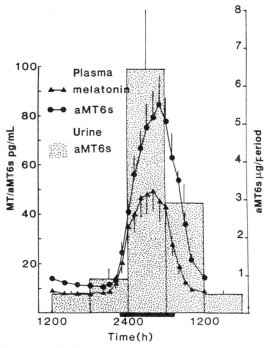

Figure 14-5. Plasma concentrations of melatonin (MT) and 6-sufatoxymelatonin (aMT6s), and urinary excretion of aMT6s during the 24-h day. The thick horizontal bar indicates the time spent in darkness. Note the close association between the onset of darkness and the onset of melatonin secretion. The decrease of plasma melatonin precedes the onset of light reflecting the action of the Zeitgeber in the suprachiasmatic nucleus. (*Source:* From Arendt J: Melatonin. Clin Endocrinol 29:205–229, 1988.)

secretion follows a free-running, endogenous rhythm. The term "free-running" reflects the absence of entrainment by photic or other cues. Although the circadian rhythm is in fact "circa" (around) 24 h for the population, it has a remarkably fixed timing in each individual. As a consequence, exposure to constant darkness leads to the desynchronization of melatonin rhythm in the population, and a progressive shift of melatonin rhythm from the standard clock time in each individual. Thus, *in blind subjects melatonin rhythm is unrelated to the time of day. Bouts of drowsiness typically coincide with rising levels of plasma melatonin, explaining the irregular sleep pattern* observed by most blind subjects.

Due to Its Function as an Entrainer of the Zeitgeber, Exogenous Melatonin May Be Used for the Treatment of Circadian Rhythm Disturbances Such as Jet Lag

Circadian rhythm disturbances are attributed to the discrepancy between the Zeitgeber's setting and the environmentally enforced nyctohemeral (night-day) rhythm. This discrepancy results in sleep disturbances, inappropriately decreased daytime alertness, fatigue, out-of-phase cortisol rhythm, and decreased ability in adapting to stressful conditions. Circadian rhythm disturbances are associated with

- transmeridian travel (jet lag),
- shift work,
- blindness (free-running rhythm),
- age-related decrease of melatonin production.

In the cases of transmeridian travel and shift work, the circadian rhythm disturbance is resolved by photic entrainment, which may take several days. In cases of blindness and age-related pineal involution, photic entrainment is either absent or severely decreased.

Melatonin is a chronobiotic compound that can be administered to enhance, reinforce, or replace the photic entrainment of the Zeitgeber. As discussed above, photic entrainment which signals "light" activates a nitric oxide (NO) mechanism. Conversely, melatonin which signals "darkness" inhibits NO production or antagonizes its action. The endogenous decrease of melatonin precedes the exposure to light. Thus, during photic entrainment, NO production is simultaneously disinhibited and actively stimulated.

Exogenous melatonin may normalize sleep patterns in blind and elderly subjects, and result in a more rapid resetting of the Zeitgeber in shift-workers and after transmeridian flight. The effects include a more rapid resetting of the rhythm in plasma cortisol, core body temperature, sleep, and other physiologic functions. The beneficial effect requires that the timing of melatonin administration is not in conflict with the novel photic entrainment signal. Melatonin preparations that provide prolonged absorption and sustained plasma levels ("time release" capsules) are not suitable for resetting the circadian clock.

The Circadian Rhythm of Melatonin Displays a Strict Inverse Association with That of Core Body Temperature

The nocturnal decrease of core body temperature is temporally associated with the rising levels of plasma melatonin (Fig. 14-6).

- Administration of melatonin during the day, when its levels are normally low, decreases core body temperature by about 0.3 to 0.4°C.
- Suppression of melatonin at night (either by exposure to bright light or by administration of β-adrenergic receptor antagonists) increases core body temperature to approximately the same degree.

The hypothermic effect of melatonin is exerted mainly on the hypothalamic thermoregulatory centers, but the details of its mechanism of action are unclear. Melatonin certainly enhances heat loss, but it might also decrease heat production. When plasma progesterone concentrations are high (such as the luteal phase of the menstrual cycle and pregnancy), melatonin does not exert its hypothermic effects. This might represent a mechanism of keeping core body temperature higher at night to promote better embryo implantation and survival.

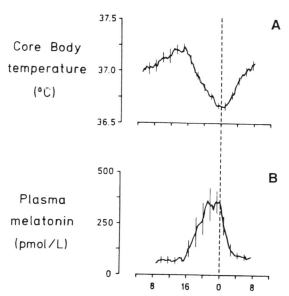

Figure 14-6. Circadian rhythms of core body temperature and plasma melatonin. (*Source:* From Shanahan TL, Czeisler CA: Light exposure induces equivalent phase shifts of the endogenous circadian rhythms of circulating plasma melatonin and core body temperature in men. J Clin Endocrinol Metab 73:227, 1993.)

Melatonin Is a Free Radical Scavenger and Antioxidant, Which Is Delivered in High Concentrations to Inflammatory Sites by Its Binding Protein

Melatonin markedly protects both membrane lipids and nuclear DNA from free radical damage by several mechanisms:

- It has been demonstrated to detoxify a variety of free radicals and reactive oxygen intermediates including the *hydroxyl radical, peroxynitrite anion, singlet oxygen,* and *nitric oxide.*
- It stimulates antioxidative enzymes such as *glutathione peroxidase, glutathione reductase, glucose-6-phosphate dehydrogenase,* and *superoxide dismutase.*
- It inhibits the prooxidative enzyme, *nitric oxide synthase.*

Free radicals are produced in large quantities during inflammation. Whereas these free radicals are important in killing invading microorganisms, they may also inflict damage on host tissues. Free radicals produced by chronic inflammation have been implicated in carcinogenesis. The capillary bed of inflammatory sites has an increased permeability, which allows the delivery of protein-bound melatonin. This mechanism is also involved in the delivery of CBG-associated cortisol, a potent antiinflammatory agent (see Chap. 12). AGP, the binding protein of melatonin, is an acute phase protein that is synthesized by the liver and by activated macrophages. It is a natural antiinflammatory agent displaying antineutrophil, immuosuppressive and anticomplement activities. AGP maintains high melatonin concentration at the site of inflammation; during the local degradation of AGP, melatonin is liberated from binding.

Melatonin inhibits leukotriene production in B lymphocytes. 5-Lipoxygenase is a key enzyme in the biosynthesis of leukotrienes (see Fig. 12-14), which are known to be allergic and inflammatory mediators. 5-Lipoxygenase is repressed by melatonin via its action on RZRα and RORα_1. In contrast, 5-lipoxygenase mRNA levels are not affected by melatonin in differentiated monocytic and granulocytic cell lines, which do not express RZRα.

15

THE ADIPOSE ORGAN: APPETITE, LEPTIN, AND OBESITY

OBJECTIVES

1. Define *obesity*; identify its major causes and consequences. Distinguish hyperplasia and hypertrophy of adipose tissue as causes of obesity.
2. Discuss the regulation of *adipogenesis*, including the regulation of *preadipocyte* differentiation into *mature adipocyte*. Identify adipose tissue as an endocrine secretory "organ."
3. Discuss the principle of the *lipostat* mechanism. Identify the role of *leptin* in the lipostat, and describe the main mechanisms of leptin dysfunction, which may result in obesity. Discuss obesity as a "regulation of body weight at an elevated setpoint."
4. Discuss the regulation of leptin secretion, including its ontogeny and secretory pattern. Discuss leptin receptor isotypes, and the potential mechanisms of leptin resistance.
5. Identify the hypothalamic targets of leptin, and their role in the regulation of the equilibrium between caloric intake and energy expenditure. Discuss the relationship between appetite, energy expenditure, corticotropin-releasing hormone (CRH), leptin, and Cushing's disease.
6. Discuss the mechanism of the termination of food intake during a meal and its integration with energy homeostasis.

ADIPOGENESIS

Clinical Obesity Is Defined by a Level of Adiposity that Is Associated with Increased Morbidity and Decreased Life Expectancy

Obesity is defined by the presence of excessive amount of adipose tissue. However, there are various ways of defining what is considered to be excessive.

- In a cosmetic sense, the "ideal body image" and degree of adiposity are culture-dependent: by today's standard, the beauties pictured in renaissance European paintings are overweight individuals.
- In a clinical sense, obesity is the level of adiposity that is associated with increased morbidity and decreased life expectancy. This occurs at body weights exceeding the "ideal body weight" by 20% or more. The ideal body weight for most individuals is between the *body mass index* (BMI) values of 20 and 26; the variability is mainly accounted for by muscle and bone masses, which influence the BMI (see Box 10-4). *A BMI of ≥28 indicates clinical obesity.* The main long-term adverse effects of obesity include increased risk for diabetes mellitus, syndrome X (see Chap. 9), coronary heart disease, osteoarthritis, and certain types of cancer (prostate and colon cancers in men; breast, endometrial, and biliary cancers in women). Note that obesity is not defined as adiposity exceeding the population average. In fact, such a definition would hide the increasing prevalence of obesity.

Human obesity is due to a combination of environmental and genetic factors. The genetic factors are considered stable, yet the prevalence of obesity has been increasing at an alarming rate in the industrialized world, indicating the impact of changing environmental factors. These environmental factors include sedentary lifestyle (insufficient physical activity, lack of exercise), consumption of highly processed (low fiber/high energy) foods, increasing consumption of refined sugars (including those present in drinks), simultaneous consumption of fat and carbohydrates that promotes lipid storage in white adipose tissue, and increasing overall caloric intake. High-fat diet has also been implicated and highly publicized. The resultant decrease in fat consumption, however, has failed to exert any impact on the increasing prevalence of obesity in the United States.

Adipogenesis Involves Proliferation of Mesenchymal Stem Cells, Their Differentiation into Committed Preadipocytes, and the Clonal Expansion of Preadipocytes Followed by Terminal Differentiation into Mature Adipocytes

The degree of *adiposity* is the relative contribution of *white adipose tissue* to the whole body mass. The degree of adiposity is the main determinant of body weight changes in adults, which varies with the long-term nutritional and metabolic status of the individual. The regulation of body weight and adiposity involves *adipogenesis* (i.e., proliferative and differentiation processes that lead to the generation of adipose tissue). The adipose tissue in turn can be utilized for storing and retrieving lipids. Adipose tissue generation commences in utero, but may also occur any time during postpartum life. In general, generation (expansion) of adipose tissue occurs during *long-term* positive caloric balance.

Adipose tissue growth involves

  • the formation of new adipocytes (*hyperplasia*) from *mesenchymal stem cells* by
          • proliferation and differentiation into *committed preadipo-cytes,* which undergo *clonal expansion*;
          • growth arrest of the preadipocytes associated with terminal differentiation into *mature adipocytes*; and
  • an increase in adipocyte size by the accumulation of lipids (*hypertrophy*).

Whereas lipid stores in the adipocytes increase and decrease depending on the *short-term* balance between caloric intake and energy expenditure (i.e., the hypertrophy is reversible), the hyperplasia of adipose tissue has been regarded as an irreversible process. This serves as the rationale of surgical procedures such as *liposuction,* which are aimed at diminishing the numbers of adipocytes. However, in vitro experiments suggest that decreases in adipocyte number may occur via *apoptosis* of preadipocytes and mature adipocytes (such as following growth factor deprivation or mild heat injury), and possibly via adipocyte *dedifferentiation* of mature adipocytes (such as upon exposure to TNF-α, see below).

Adipogenesis Is Controlled by a Hormonally Regulated Cascade of Transcription Factors, Including the Retinoic Acid Receptor, Members of the C/EBP Family, and Peroxisome Proliferator-Activated Receptor γ

The *mesenchymal stem cell* is pluripotent and may differentiate into any component of blood vessels (including the endothelium), fibroblasts, myoblasts, chondroblasts, osteoblasts, and *preadipocytes (lipoblasts).* Myoblast differentiations is determined by the *MyoD* family of regulatory genes. Bone morphogenetic proteins (BMPs, members of the TGF-β family, see Box 8-1) prompt differentiation toward osteoblasts. The factor inducing differentiation towards the adipocyte lineage is unknown. In vitro experiments suggest that embryonic stem cells may be directed toward preadipocyte differentiation by exposure to *physiologic concentrations* of retinoic acid for a precise period of time via activating retinoic acid receptor (RARα). *Committed preadipocytes* express *preadipocyte factor-1 (*Pref-1), and may undergo a final round (or rounds) of mitosis referred to as the *clonal expansion.*

The *maturation of committed preadipocytes* has been partially characterized, and a current model of the crucial events is presented in Fig. 15-1. The main stimulators and inhibitors of adipocyte differentiation are summarized in Table 15-1. The cascade includes the following main steps:

  • Preadipocytes express *Pref-1* (see below), a transmembrane protein which inhibits differentiation probably by suppressing the expression of peroxisome proliferator activated receptor γ (PPARγ; see Chaps. 5 and

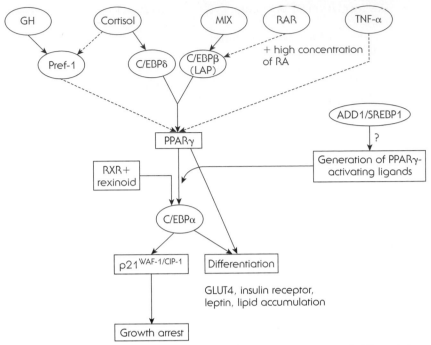

Figure 15-1. A model of the regulatory cascade leading to terminal differentiation of preadipocytes into mature adipocytes. GH, growth hormone; MIX, methylisobutylxanthine; RAR, retinoic acid receptor; Pref-1, preadipocyte factor-1; TNF-α, tumor necrosis factor-α; C/EBPs, CCAAT-enhancer binding proteins; LAP, liver-enriched activating protein; PPARγ, peroxisome proliferator activated receptor γ; RXR, retinoid X receptor; ADD1, adipocyte determination and differentiation factor-1 (also known as SREBP-1c, sterol regulatory element binding protein-1c); GLUT4, glucose transporter 4.

9). Whereas growth hormone (GH) sustains, cortisol inhibits the expression of Pref-1.

• The CCAAT-enhancer binding proteins (C/EBPs) are transcription factors containing a leucin zipper domain, which promotes their dimerization. They are often involved in switching from an undifferentiated proliferative to a differentiated nonproliferative phenotype as we have seen in the development of the mammary epithelium (see Chap. 13). *C/EBPδ* and *C/EBPβ* (also known as *liver-enriched activating protein* [LAP]), probably by forming heterodimers, increase the expression of PPARγ. Their action on the expression of PPARγ is antagonized by Pref-1 and tumor necrosis factor-α (TNF-α). C/EBPδ and C/EBPβ are expressed only in a transient manner during differentiation until they are permanently replaced by C/EBPα.

• The expression of C/EBPδ is induced by *cortisol*. As discussed below, glucocorticoids play such a key role in adipogenesis that their severe decrease is essentially incompatible with obesity.

• The expression of C/EBPβ is induced by *methylisobutylxanthine* (MIX), a drug related to caffeine. MIX is used together with cortisol as a standard experimental agent for inducing differentia-

Table 15-1   Stimulators and Inhibitors of Adipocyte Differentiation

Stimulators	Inhibitors
Glucocorticoids	Pref-1
Experimental drugs in vitro: MIX, phorbol esters (by activating PKC)	EGF, TGF-α
IGF-1, insulin	GH
Physiologic levels of retinoic acid and rexinoids	Supranormal levels of retinoic acid
Activators of PPARγ (such as troglitazone, pioglitazone, and rosiglitazone)	Inhibitors/partial agonists of PPARγ (such as GW0072)
Type IV collagen, laminin	Type I and type III collagen
Angiotensin II (on AT$_2$ receptors)	Cytokines: TNF-α, IL-1β, IL-11, IFNγ
PGI$_2$	PGF$_{2\alpha}$

ABBREVIATIONS: Pref-1, preadipocyte factor 1; MIX, methylisobutylxanthine; PKC, protein kinase C; EGF, epidermal growth factor; TGF, transforming growth factor; IGF, insulin-like growth factor; GH, growth hormone; PPAR-γ, peroxisome proliferator-activated receptor-γ; TNF, tumor necrosis factor; IL, interleukin; IFN, interferon; PGI$_2$, prostacyclin; PGF$_{2\alpha}$, prostaglandin F$_{2\alpha}$.

tion of preadipocyes into mature nonmitotic adipocytes in vitro. Its mechanism of action, however, is uncertain because it has multiple activities, such as inhibition of phosphodiesterase (thereby increasing cyclic AMP) and antagonism on adenosine 1 receptors.

- The expression of C/EBPβ is inhibited by *supraphysiologic* doses of retinoic acid acting via RAR.

- PPARγ is a convergence point of the regulatory pathways. It is a transcription factor that functions as a heterodimer formed with the retinoid X receptor (RXR). PPARγ is potently activated by thiazolidinedione drugs (such as troglitazone, pioglitazone and rosiglitazone), 15-deoxy-ΔPGJ$_2$, and prostacyclin (PGI$_2$). Its physiologic ligand in the adipocyte is still uncertain. It has been proposed that *adipocyte determination and differentiation factor-1* (ADD1, also known as *sterol regulatory element binding protein-1c* [SREBP-1c]) induces adipocyte differentiation by generating the activating ligand for PPARγ. The RXR:PPARγ heterodimer has two functions: it directly induces several adipocyte-specific genes and induces C/EBPα expression.

- *The expression of C/EBPα heralds the terminal differentiation of adipocytes.* C/EBPα induces the expression of several adipocyte-specific genes and the expression of p21[WAF-1/CIP-1] (see Chap. 13) thereby causing growth arrest. The crucial role of C/EBPα has been demonstrated in C/EBPα knockout mice, which fail to develop mature white adipose tissue. Cotransfection experiments indicate that the *synergistic action between PPARγ and C/EBPα is required for full differentiation and expression of the mature adipocyte phenotype.*

Preadipocyte Factor-1 Is a Regulator of Proliferation and Differentiation in Adipocytes, Pancreatic β Cells, and the Adrenal Cortex

Preadipocyte factor-1 (Pref-1) is a transmembrane protein containing several repeats of an epidermal growth factor (EGF)-like sequence in its extracellular domain. Pref-1 is highly expressed in preadipocytes, but is undetectable in mature adipocytes. Constitutive expression of Pref-1 or the addition of its ectodomain inhibits adipocyte differentiation. The cleavage of the Pref-1 *ectodomain* from the transmembrane segment generates a 50-kDa biologically active *soluble* form. There are four major isoforms of *membrane-anchored* Pref-1 that are generated by alternative splicing. Two of these Pref-1 isoforms do not produce biologically active *soluble* ectodomain; the noncleaved ectodomain may be involved in cell–cell contact signaling. *Suppression of Pref-1 gene expression is required for adipocyte differentiation*. Glucocorticoids such as dexamethasone attenuate the transcription of Pref-1 and promote adipogenesis.

Interaction of the *EGF repeats* of Pref-1 with an as yet unidentified receptor may mediate the inhibitory effects of Pref-1 in adipocyte differentiation. It is therefore not surprising that several growth factors, especially *EGF* and the related transforming growth factor-α (TGF-α) are potent inhibitors of adipogenesis. Several *extracellular matrix proteins* contain an EGF domain, which may explain the adipocyte differentiation-inhibiting action of type I and type III collagens and fibronectin. In contrast, type IV collagen and laminin present in basal/external laminae promote adipogenesis.

In addition to preadipocytes, *Pref-1* regulates the differentiation of several tissues.

- Expression of Pref-1 is stimulated by GH and/or prolactin in rat pancreatic islet cells and may play a role both in embryonic pancreas differentiation and in postnatal β cell growth and function.
- Pref-1 has been identified as being identical with the *zona glomerulosa* (ZOG) *protein* in the adrenal cortex, which may be responsible for zonal differentiation. Pref-1 is expressed in the fetal zone of the adrenal cortex and in the zona glomerulosa of the definitive cortex, but is absent from the zonae fasciculata and reticularis.

Although IGF-1 Promotes Adipocyte Differentiation, the Antiadipogenic Action of Growth Hormone Prevails in vivo

GH is an important lipolytic hormone that depletes mature adipocytes of their accumulated triglycerides (Chap. 10). The involvement of the *GH/insulin-like growth factor-1 (IGF-1) axis* in *adipogenesis* involves multiple actions.

- Although GH induces adipocyte differentiation in certain preadipocyte cell lines, experiments with primary cultures of preadipocytres indicate that *GH inhibits the differentiation of preadipocytes by maintaining the expression of Pref-1*.
- GH induces IGF-1 production by preadipocytes, which may act in a paracrine/autocrine manner. Preadipocytes secrete IGF-binding proteins

(IGFBPs) in a differentiation-dependent manner, which probably modulate the biologic action of IGF-1.

- IGF-1 stimulates the proliferation of preadipocytes ("clonal expansion").
- Physiologic doses of IGF-1, or supraphysiologic doses of *insulin*, are required for the differentiation of preadipocytes into mature adipocytes.
  - The main signal transduction pathway of IGF-1-induced differentiation involves Ras (see Fig. 9-13). The downstream signaling of Ras is *in part* mediated by Raf-1, which, however, induces adipocyte differentiation independent of the mitogen-activated protein kinase (MAPK) pathway. Overexpression of Raf-1 induces only partial differentiation indicating that Ras activates Raf-1-independent mechanisms.
    - Activation of protein kinase B (PKB/Akt) contributes to the differentiaton of adipocytes, which may involve upregulation/mobilization of the GLUT4 glucose transporter.

It is uncertain where IGF-1 fits into the differentiation pathway depicted in Fig. 15-1, but might act via C/EBPβ thereby complementing the action of cortisol in a manner similar to the action of MIX. The net in vivo effect of the GH–IGF-1 axis is a decrease in adiposity and, due to action on muscle, an increase in lean body mass. It is of interest that in contrast with IGF-1 and insulin, most growth factors (and the activation of PKC) *inhibit* the differentiation of adipocytes.

TNF-α (Cachectin) Inhibits and Reverses Adipocyte Differentiation

During TNF-α-mediated inhibition of adipocyte differentiation, PPARγ expression stays at low levels. In contrast, TNF-α treatment has no effect on the adipogenesis-related decrease of Pref-1 gene expression. Pref-1 functions as a nonreversible molecular checkpoint whose expression is insensitive to TNF-α-generated signals, whereas PPARγ expression remains sensitive to TNF-α at all stages of the adipogenesis program. Although *dedifferentiated adipocytes* and preadipocytes display similar morphologic features and express mostly the same set of genes, the absence of Pref-1 expression in dedifferentiated adipocytes versus Pref-1 expression in preadipocytes indicates that they represent different states of differentiation.

Adipose Tissue Is a Major Endocrine Secretory Organ

Adipose tissue is not a simple lipid storage depot, but an active component in the regulatory mechanisms that integrate the function of adipocytes with other bodily functions. The integration is in part achieved by using metabolites for signaling, such as free fatty acids (FFA) liberated from mature adipocytes by catecholamines, GH, or glucagon (see Chap. 9).

However, the adipocyte is not only a target but also a source of hormones. Some of these hormones act in an endocrine manner via the circulation (estrone, leptin), whereas others act mainly in a paracrine/autocrine fashion (TNF-α, angiotensin II, prostaglandins). Note that estrogens are *converted* from circulating androgens by aromatase mainly expressed by preadipocytes, whereas the other adipocyte hormones are synthesized de novo.

THE REGULATION OF BODY WEIGHT

The Basic Concepts of the Lipostat Mechanism

The Relatively Constant Degree of Adiposity Is Sustained by Negative Feedback Mechanisms, Which Maintain an Equilibrium Between Caloric Intake and Energy Expenditure   In contrast with continuous energy utilization, the uptake of energy with meals is intermittent, leading to a requirement of storing energy during the *postprandial state*. The stored energy is then mobilized by catabolic mechanisms during the *postabsorptive state*. The highest caloric reserve is in the form of triglycerides present in white adipose tissue.

- *Weight gain* occurs when the caloric intake exceeds the energy expenditure.
- *Weight loss* occurs when the energy expenditure exceeds the caloric intake.

In adults, body weight is relatively constant over prolonged periods of time. This implies a relatively constant degree of adiposity, and a *long-term equilibrium between caloric intake and energy expenditure*. For example, to maintain a weight change of <10 kg over a 10 year period, an average 70-kg adult must have >98% congruency between caloric intake and energy expenditure.

- *Caloric intake* is determined by appetite (the sensation of hunger leading to seeking and ingestion of food) and the availability, composition, and taste of food.
  - *Orexigenic* agents increase, whereas *anorexic* agents decrease, appetite.
- *Energy expenditure* has multiple determinants related to metabolic regulation and is coordinated by the central nervous system (CNS), mainly by the hypothalamus:
  - *Sympathetic activity*: noradrenaline released from postganglionic fibers in white adipose tissue and circulating adrenaline

stimulate lipolysis by activating mainly β_3-adrenergic receptors (see Chap. 12).

- *Insulin* decreases β_3-adrenergic receptor expression in adipose tissue, thereby decreasing the lipolytic effect of noradrenergic mechanisms. In addition, insulin inhibits the hormone-sensitive lipase in adipocytes (see Chap. 9).
- *Thyroid hormones* promote lipolysis and energy expenditure. This involves upregulation of β-adrenergic receptors in several tissues, increased basal metabolic rate (including increased Na^+/K^+-ATPase activity), and upregulation of uncoupling proteins (UCPs), mainly UCP-3 in muscle (see Chap. 11).
- Additional hormonal regulation of metabolism includes the GH–IGF-1 axis (Chap. 10), the CRH–ACTH–cortisol axis (Chap. 12), glucagon (Chap. 9), and sexual steroids (Chap. 13).
- *Physical activity*: a sedentary lifestyle is associated with decreased energy expenditure. The increased energy expenditure induced by exercise exceeds the actual caloric need and the acute duration of the exercise. Exercise increases muscle mass (i.e., the mass of calorie-burning tissue), and converts skeletal muscles from anaerobic to aerobic types of fiber (see Chap. 11), thereby increasing the utilization of FFA. Exercise mobilizes FFA from adipose tissue by activating the sympathoadrenal system and GH secretion. This mechanism is especially effective in decreasing adiposity when the main source of circulating glucose is gluconeogenesis, i.e., after an overnight fasting.

The feedback regulation of caloric intake and energy expenditure that results in constant body weight (degree of adiposity) is known as the *lipostat mechanism* (Fig. 15-2). The main feedback signal emanating from adipose tissue has been identified as a 16-kDa helix-bundle peptide hormone termed *leptin* (Greek: *leptos* = thin). As will be discussed in more detail, leptin secretion is proportionate with adiposity and, by acting on multiple targets, leptin decreases appetite and increases energy expenditure. During starvation, adiposity and plasma leptin levels are decreased, which leads to decreased energy expenditure thereby conserving stored energy. Conversely, increased food intake may result in an initial increase of adiposity and plasma leptin, but the leptin-stimulated suppression of appetite and leptin-induced energy expenditure prevents a long-term weight gain. In an evolutionary sense, individuals have always been more often challenged by starvation than by the possibility of overfeeding. Accordingly, the leptin-based lipostat mechanism is more effective in antagonizing weight loss ("starvation shield" function) than in preventing obesity.

Obesity is defined by the presence of excessive amount of adipose tissue, and is usually quantified by the BMI (see above). It is important to realize that *the body weight is relatively constant in both lean and obese individuals.* Thus, obesity does not indicate perpetual weight gain, but *represents an equilibrium between caloric intake and energy expenditure that*

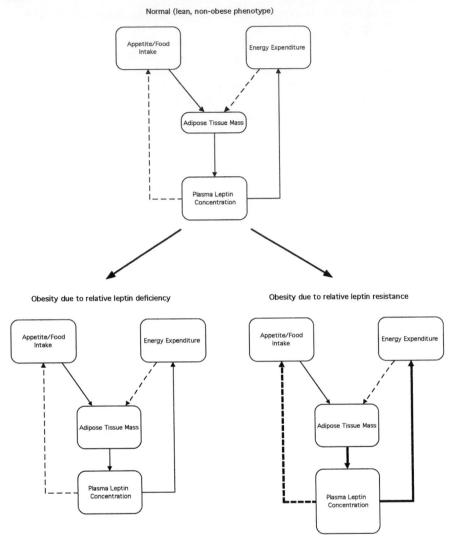

Figure 15-2. Overall model of the lipostat mechanism that maintains the degree of adiposity relatively constant. The solid arrows indicate stimulation/increase, the dashed lines indicate inhibition/decrease. The thickness of the lines and the size of the symbols reflect differences in concentration, mass or activity. In all three cases displayed, there is no net wet gain or weight loss, i.e., the caloric intake equals the energy expenditure. In lean individuals, appropriate feedback by leptin is achieved at low adipose tissue mass. In most cases of human obesity, appropriate feedback is achieved at increased adipose tissue mass. This may compensate for a decreased leptin-production capacity of individual adipocytes (normal plasma leptin at the expense of obesity; left), or (in the vast majority of cases) adiposity via hyperleptinemia compensates for a relative leptin resistance (right).

is achieved at an increased degree of adiposity. Obesity therefore may involve two main mechanisms (see Fig. 15-2):

- The adipocytes produce subnormal amounts of leptin.
    - *Absolute leptin deficiency* is the cause of the obese phenotype of *ob/ob* homozygous mutant mice. The *ob* (*obese*) gene encodes leptin. The human *OB* gene is located on chromosome 7q31.3-32. Although a few mutations of the *OB* gene have been found in morbidly obese humans, *OB* gene mutation is a rare cause of human obesity.
    - *Relative leptin deficiency* means that the plasma leptin levels are *lower than expected for the degree of obesity.* Thus, as a first approximation, normal leptin levels (plasma concentration of nonobese individuals) are achieved at the expense of an increased adipose tissue mass. The situation is somewhat comparable with the nonclassic form of p450c21 deficiency leading to congenital adrenal hyperplasia, in which plasma cortisol is normalized at an increased adrenocortical mass. Relative leptin deficiency may account for 10 to 15% of obesity in the general human population.
- Leptin resistance of the target tissues prevents normal feedback mechanisms.
    - *Absolute leptin resistance* is the consequence of inactivating mutations of the leptin receptor. This has been identified in certain genetic models of obesity, such as the *db/db* (non-insulin-dependent diabetic) mouse and the diabetic fatty Zucker rat. Other than plasma leptin levels, the phenotypes of absolute leptin deficiency and absolute leptin resistance are essentially identical. Similar to absolute leptin deficiency, absolute leptin resistance is a rare cause of human obesity, which has been identified only in a few cases of morbid obesity.
    - *Relative leptin resistance* (as a first approximation) means that the normal appetite suppressing and energy expenditure-increasing effects of leptin are achieved at supranormal plasma concentrations of leptin. This condition is comparable with insulin resistance, in which normoglycemia is maintained by supranormal secretion of insulin. It is estimated that the vast majority of human obesity is the consequence of relative leptin resistance. Note, however, that the apparent leptin resistance may indicate a defect in any downstream mechanism of leptin action, including CNS mechanisms and peripheral sites such as β_3-adrenergic receptors or UPCs.

In Obesity, the Equilibrium Between Caloric Intake and Energy Expenditure is Achieved at an Elevated Setpoint The concept discussed above in a simplified form becomes more meaningful if we take into consideration that the new equilibrium between caloric intake and energy expenditure in obese subjects is achieved *at an elevated setpoint.* The elevated setpoint implies that

  • leptin, which coordinates the components of the equilibrium, is also regulated at an elevated setpoint;
  • the caloric intake of obese individuals is actually higher than that of lean subjects. The increased caloric intake is usually balanced by a proportionately increased energy expenditure. The *basal metabolic rate* (BMR) is about 45 kcal/h/m^2 body surface area, and at any given height an increase of body weight results in an increase of body surface area (see Chap. 11). The increased energy expenditure is in part mediated by the sympathoadrenal system. Indeed, daily norepinephrine production (an indicator of sympathetic activity) is higher in obese subjects, which promotes lipolysis. It must be noted, however, that leptin-induced sympathetic activity is not a mandatory requirement for elevated plasma free fatty acid levels and decreased insulin sensitivity (see autocrine TNF-α mechanism below). Both absolute leptin deficiency and absolute leptin resistance are associated with insulin-resistant diabetes mellitus as seen in mutant rodent models of obesity (see also in Chap. 9).

Leptin

Daytime Plasma Leptin Levels in the Fed State Increase with Adiposity   The *OB* gene is expressed almost exclusively in *white adipose tissue*. In nonpregnant adults, circulating leptin is derived from white adipose tissue. The main source of leptin is the *subcutaneous* adipose tissue; *visceral* (retroperitoneal, omental, mesenteric) fat expresses lower levels of OB mRNA and is not a significant independent determinant of plasma leptin. *In the fed state*, leptin expression and *daytime* plasma leptin levels increase with adiposity in an almost linear manner. For this reason, plasma leptin measurement has been suggested as "the poor man's way to measure body fat." To be precise, the relationship between adiposity and plasma leptin is curvilinear (shallow exponential). In general, leptin gene expression is correlated with the process of fat accumulation and thus the size of adipocytes. During fasting, leptin secretion is acutely inhibited; thus, fasting lipid levels are not reliable estimates of adiposity. The fasting-related decrease of plasma leptin can be avoided by increasing the frequency of meals. This is the basis of the recommendation of frequent meals in several weight-loss programs.

The *placenta* is the other major site of expression. Placental leptin (and a soluble leptin receptor) may contribute to the regulation of maternal fuel homeostasis and might signal satiety to the fetal hypothalamus. During lactation, leptin enters breast milk and is absorbed from the gastrointestinal tract of the newborn. Thus, the placenta and breast milk may serve as exogenous sources of circulating leptin for the fetus and neonate respectively.

The Ratio of Free to Protein-Bound Leptin Increases with Total Plasma Leptin and Body Mass Index   The average *half-life* of leptin in the circulation is 20 to 30 min; it is primarily degraded by the proximal tubules of the kidney. Leptin circulates in plasma as a 16-kDa free hormone, and also as a presumably biologically inactive protein-bound compound. Several *leptin-binding proteins* have been demonstrated in human plasma, some of which are related to the soluble isoform of the leptin receptor. *Total leptin and the relative proportion of free leptin increase with BMI.* During pregnancy, total leptin levels rise between the 20th and 30th weeks of gestation; this rise is caused by the increase in the bound leptin with no significant change in free leptin levels. There is a significant postpartum fall in free leptin levels that may increase appetite in support of lactation.

Plasma Leptin Concentrations Display a Pulsatile Pattern Organized into a Circadian Rhythm Approximately 3 to 4 leptin pulses occur during the 24-h day, mostly 2 to 3 h after meals. Pulse *frequency* correlates negatively with adiposity.

The *temporal organization* of the circadian leptin rhythm is unaltered by varying degree of adiposity. The highest plasma leptin levels occur between midnight and early morning hours, and the lowest levels occur between noon and midafternoon. The nocturnal rise in leptin resembles those reported for melatonin, prolactin, thyroid-stimulating hormone (TSH), and FFA. The nocturnal rise in leptin might be responsible for suppressing appetite during sleep-related fasting.

Although compared to lean subjects most obese individuals are hyperleptinemic at any time point, *the relative amplitude of the circadian rhythm of leptin is attenuated in obesity* (Fig. 15-3). The *relative* increase in the nocturnal leptin concentration is inversely related to the relative gain in total body fat. If the blunted nocturnal rise in serum leptin persists over a prolonged period of time, it may contribute to the development of obesity, either by inadequate suppression of nighttime appetite or by attenuated nocturnal increase of energy expenditure.

The Sexual Difference in Plasma Leptin Concentration Emerges During Puberty Plasma leptin levels and the ontogeny of leptin secretion are similar in both sexes until puberty. Leptin levels are high in the newborn, then decrease to relatively low levels during childhood. As puberty approaches, plasma leptin increases in both sexes. Leptin is not a cause but a permissive "metabolic gate" of puberty and reproductive function (see Chap. 13).

- The pubertal increase of androgens results in an increase of lean body mass and a depletion of fat stores in males. Thus, in males the prepubertal/early pubertal rise of leptin is followed by a decline.
- In contrast, in females, estrogens increase deposition of subcutaneous fat (female contours develop), and leptin levels either remain elevated or increase further. Severe weight loss in postpubertal females results in

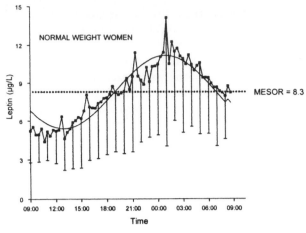

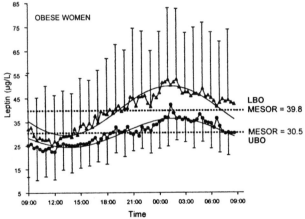

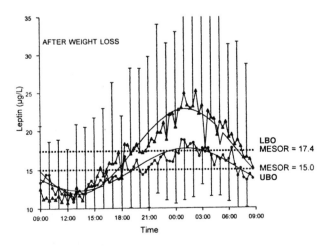

secondary amenorrhea, which involves mechanisms regulated by the *decrease* in leptin. Although plasma leptin decreases after menopause, it remains higher in women than in men of the same age.

Women have a higher percentage of adipose tissue than men, which in part explains the higher *postpubertal* plasma leptin levels of females. However, even after correction for adiposity, females have higher plasma leptin levels than males. This may be related to the sexually dimorphic *regional distribution of adipose tissue*: *android* (central, upper body) fat distribution is mainly abdominal and visceral, *gynoid* (peripheral, lower body) fat distribution predominantly involves the buttocks, thighs, upper arm and the breast. Note that the "android" distribution does not reflect the effect of androgens, which increase lean body mass, but the combined effect of cortisol and insulin.

The fat distribution in obesity may be estimated by the *waist to hip ratio* (WHR): *upper body obesity* in women and men is defined as WHR >0.86 and >0.95, respectively. Visceral adiposity is more precisely assessed by magnetic resonance imaging (MRI). As noted, visceral fat produces less leptin than subcutaneous adipose tissue. In contrast, visceral fat is more correlated with insulin resistance.

Leptin Secretion is Inhibited by Cyclic AMP, Caloric Restriction, and Activators of PPARγ, and Stimulated by Glucocorticoids, Insulin, TNF-α and IL-1β As mentioned, daytime plasma leptin levels in the fed state are primarily determined by the degree of adiposity or, more precisely, the lipid content and corresponding size of individual adipocytes. Thus, hypertrophy of the adipose tissue provides a better negative feedback to appetite than hyperplasia.

In line with its primarily starvation shield function, *fasting acutely* decreases leptin concentrations, prompting hunger. The decrease in leptin occurs in the absence of appreciable depletion of adipocyte triglyceride stores. This mechanism explains the difficulty of losing weight. The mecha-

---

Figure 15-3. Circadian rhythm of plasma leptin in normal weight (body mass index [BMI]: 22.4 ± 2.1 kg/m²) and obese women. Each data point represents the mean leptin concentration at 20-minute intervals and hourly standard deviations calculated from 8 subjects. Obese subjects were divided into lower body obesity (LBO; BMI: 33.2 ± 4.4) and upper body obesity (UBO; BMI: 33.9) subgroups. The waist to hip ratio (WHR) in each subgroup was 0.77 (normal weight), 0.77 (LBO), and 0.96 (UBO). Note that the timing of the circadian rhythm was not influenced by obesity. The average plasma concentration of leptin (dotted line) was higher in obese than in normal weight individuals, but the *relative* amplitude of the rhythm was attenuated. Upon weight loss (bottom panel; LBO BMI: 27.5 ± 3.0; UBO BMI: 28.4), the average plasma concentration of leptin decreased and the relative amplitude of the rhythm increased. The UBO group tended to have lower plasma leptin levels indicating that the abdominal visceral fat does not secrete leptin as well as subcutaneous adipose tissue. (*Source*: Fig. 1 in Langendonk JG et al: Circadian rhythm of plasma leptin levels in upper and lower body obese women: Influence of body fat distribution and weight loss. J Clin Endocrinol Metab 83:1706–1712, 1998.)

nism of decreased leptin secretion may involve an increase in intracellular *cyclic AMP* concentration; a cyclic AMP-response element has been identified in the promoter region of the *OB* gene, which serves as a silencer. During fasting, plasma glucose and insulin levels decrease, which results in upregulation of β_3-adrenergic receptor in adipocytes. Severe hypoglycemia may activate the sympathoadrenal system, which may activate lipolysis directly by acting on the adipocyte β_3-adrenergic receptor, or indirectly via mobilizing glucagon. At a fixed caloric intake, circulating levels of leptin are positively associated with the *dietary fat* content. This observation, in part, provides the rationale for weight-loss programs based on a high fat/low-carbohydrate diet. Note that this diet keeps plasma insulin levels low, thereby enhancing lipolysis and decreasing hepatic cholesterol synthesis.

Cortisol increases leptin expression via a glucocorticoid response element in the *OB* gene. In addition, cortisol promotes obesity when acting in conjunction with insulin, and the resultant lipid accumulation (adipocyte hypertrophy) stimulates leptin secretion. *Insulin* increases leptin gene expression in vitro, and appears to increase long-term (but not short-term) leptin secretion in vivo.

The *OB* gene promoter is positively regulated by C/EBPα. In most cases, C/EBPα and PPARγ act synergistically to induce adipocyte-specific gene expression. The *OB* gene is a surprising exception. Stimulation of *PPARγ* by thiazolidinediones acutely suppresses leptin gene expression and leptin secretion by adipocytes in vitro. In contrast, thiazolidinediones do not alter plasma leptin levels in vivo. This may be due to the insulin-sensitizing action of thiazolidinediones which, in the presence of insulin, results in decreased lipolysis and cytoplasmic cyclic AMP. Such a change might compensate the direct *OB* gene-suppressing action of the activated PPARγ, and explain why troglitazone treatment of NIDDM does not consistently cause weight gain.

TNF-α is probably the agent responsible for cachexia seen in malignancies. It is a potent anorexic cytokine, which decreases appetite by a direct CNS action and also indirectly by *increasing* plasma leptin levels. TNF-α is produced by activated macrophages and also by adipocytes. Thus, its action on adipocytes is at least in part an autocrine/paracrine mechanism. TNF-α is a potent lipolytic agent that induces dedifferentiation of the mature adipocyte (see Adipogenesis). TNF-α production by adipocytes increases with obesity, thereby contributing to elevated FFA and leptin levels in plasma. The increase in plasma FFA may at least in part explain the action of TNF-α to induce insulin resistance (see Chap. 9). Exposure to high levels of macrophage-derived TNF-α (such as seen in cancer), the adipocyte lipid stores become severely depleted and one would expect that TNF-α would decrease *OB* gene expression. In contrast, TNF-α induces leptin mRNA and protein synthesis, which in part might be related to its action to induce cachexia. Thalidomide, a drug that became infamous for causing birth defects, has been demonstrated to inhibit TNF-α synthesis. Promising results have been reported with thalidomide to improve appetite in cancer and HIV-infected patients.

Interleukin 1 (IL-1) increases plasma leptin levels by two mechanisms: a direct action on adipose tissue similar to that of TNF-α, and an indirect action via cortisol by stimulating CRH release from the median eminence.

GH has a complex relationship with leptin. As discussed, GH inhibits adipogenesis and is a potent lipolytic hormone. It does not, however, act via cyclic AMP but via the Jak–STAT pathway. Obesity develops in GH deficiency and GH resistance, and this obesity is associated with increased plasma leptin. Conversely, spontaneous GH and IGF-1 secretion, and the GH response to provocative tests become attenuated in obese individuals whose GH axis was functioning normally before their obesity developed. This has been largely attributed to the hypothalamic action of increased plasma FFA. However, leptin resistance may also be involved; exogenously administered leptin in non-obese (leptin-responsive) individuals stimulates GH secretion.

The Leptin Receptor is a Member of the Cytokine Receptor Family and has Multiple Isoforms Leptin is a helix-bundle peptide (see Table 10-7). Its 3-dimensional structure is therefore similar to those of GH, leukemia inhibitory factor (LIF), IL-6, or ciliary neurotrophic factor (CNTF), and the *leptin receptor* (encoded by chromosome 1p) is a member of the cytokine receptor family. Accordingly, the main signal transduction system of the leptin receptor is the Jak–STAT pathway. The cellular effects of leptin include induction of *suppressor of cytokine signaling 3* (SOCS-3), which may be involved in the development of leptin resistance by inhibiting the Jak-mediated phosphorylation of STAT (intracellular negative feedback).

The mRNA of the leptin receptor undergoes alternative splicing, which yields several leptin receptor isoforms. Only the *long isoform* has the full potency in activating the Jak–STAT pathway, which occurs upon ligand-induced homodimerization. The long isoform is expressed in specific areas within the CNS (see below) and also in peripheral tissues, such as the hematopoietic stem cells, steroidogenic tissues (ovary, adrenal cortex), liver, pancreas, skeletal muscle, lung, and kidney.

- The other (*short*) *isoforms* are truncated at their C-terminus (cytoplasmic domain). The function of the short forms may include
    - *Transport of leptin through the BBB.* A short isoform is predominant in *brain capillary endothelium* and also in the *choroid plexus*. It has been demonstrated that the receptor-mediated leptin transport is less efficient in hyperleptinemic (obese) human subjects. Above the total plasma leptin concentration of 25 to 30 ng/mL, an

increase in plasma leptin does not yield a proportionate increase in cerebrospinal fluid (CSF)/brain extracellular fluid (ECF) levels of leptin. This is probably explained by saturation and receptor downregulation at the transport sites. The transport of leptin into the CNS may be a rate-limiting step of leptin action, and its impairment has been suggested as a primary cause of the relative leptin resistance observed in obese subjects.

- Inhibition of ligand-induced Jak–STAT activation. By forming heterodimers with the long receptor isoform, the pairing/activation (cross-phosphorylation) of the intracellular domain is eliminated.

- The *soluble receptor* isoform is truncated between the N-terminus and the transmembrane domain and functions as a leptin-binding protein in plasma.

The Neuroendocrine Regulation of Body Weight and the Targets of Leptin

Leptin Targets Multiple Neurotransmitter Systems in the Hypothalamus, Including CRH, Neuropeptide Y, Agouti-Related Transcript, and α-Melanocyte-Stimulating Hormone   Lesions of the ventromedial hypothalamus result in hyperphagia leading to "hypothalamic obesity" similar to that seen in *ob/ob* or *db/db* mice. Conversely, lesions of the lateral hypothalamus result in loss of appetite, and the animals starve even when they have access to food (Fig. 15-4). In situ hybridization has revealed mRNA encoding of the *long isoform* of the leptin receptor in neuronal perikarya of several hypothalamic areas, including the arcuate (ARC), paraventricular (PVN), ventromedial (VMN), dorsomedial (DMN) nuclei and, to a lesser degree, the lateral hypothalamus.

The hypothalamus contains several neurotransmitter systems that form a redundant regulation of food/caloric intake (Table 15-2) and energy expenditure. Leptin apparently provides the integrative signal to these neurotransmitters. Figure 15-5 displays a simplified model of body weight regulation by leptin.

A Major Determinant of the Elevated Setpoint of the Equilibrium Between Caloric Intake and Energy Expenditure in Obesity is the Hypothalamic CRH   CRH serves as a main indirect and probably direct feedback target of leptin. There are two functional subsets of parvocellular paraventricular CRH neurons: those that use CRH as a *neurotransmitter*, and those that use CRH as a *neurohormone* for regulating pituitary ACTH secretion. It appears that these neuronal groups are influenced by the suprachiasmatic Zeitgeber (Chap. 14) and are regulated by leptin in a subset-specific fashion.

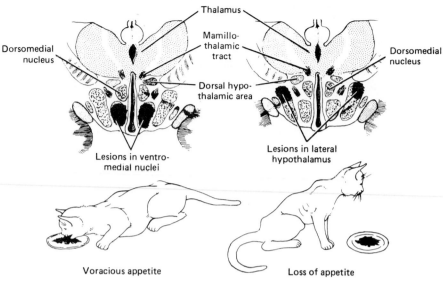

Figure 15-4. The effects of hypothalamic lesions on feeding. The experiment suggests the existence of a satiety center in the ventromedial hypothalamus and a hunger center in the lateral hypothalamus. Compare with Fig. 16-5. (*Source*: Fig. 14-5, p 216 in Ganong WF: *Review of Medical Physiology*, 17th ed., Stamford, CT, Appleton & Lange 1995; redrawn from Netter FH in Ciba Clinical Symposia. Ciba Pharmaceuticals Co., 1956.)

Table 15-2 Hypothalamic Stimulators and Inhibitors of Appetite

Stimulators of appetite (orexigenic agents)	Inhibitors of appetite (anorexic agents)
NPY[a]	α-MSH[b]
ART (AGRP)[a]	CART[b]
MCH	CRH,[b] urocortin
Orexin A and B (hypocretins)	Oxytocin
Galanin	GLP-1[b]
Noradrenaline (on α_2-adrenergic receptors)	Serotonin
GHRH	
	CNTF
	CCK
	Bombesin
	Neurotensin

[a] Experimentally identified *direct* targets of leptin are indicated by [a] (inhibition by leptin) and [b] (stimulation by leptin). Note that NPY is coexpressed with ART, and α-MSH is coexpressed with CART by neurons in the arcuate nucleus.

ABBREVIATIONS: NPY, neuropeptide Y; α-MSH, α-melanocyte-stimulating hormone; ART, agouti-related transcript; AGRP, agouti-related peptide; CART, cocaine and amphetamine regulated transcript; MCH, melanin-concentrating hormone; CRH, corticotropin-releasing hormone; GLP-1, glucagon-like peptide-1; GHRH, growth hormone-releasing hormone; CNTF, ciliary neurotrophic factor; CCK, cholecystokinin.

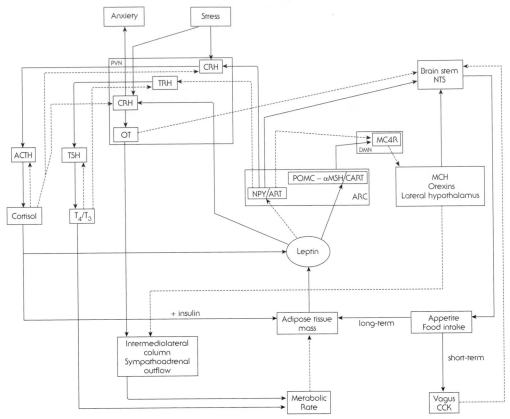

Figure 15-5. Model displaying the hypothalamic actions of leptin and the neuroendocrine regulation of body weight. Note that the figure neglects regulation of appetite by plasma glucose and the action of insulin on glucose uptake in neurons of the ventromedial nucleus. Compare with Fig. 15-4. Solid arrows indicate stimulation/increase; dashed arrows indicate inhibition/decrease. PVN, paraventricular nucleus; ARC, arcuate nucleus; NTS, nucleus tractus solitarii; CRH, corticotropin-releasing hormone; OT, oxytocin; ACTH, andrenocorticotroph hormone; TRH, thyrotropin-releasing hormone; TSH, thyroid-stimulating hormone; T_4/T_3, thyroxine/triiodothyronine; NPY, neuropeptide Y; ART, agouti related transcript; POMC, proopiomelanocortin; α-MSH, α-melanocyte-stimulating hormone; CART, cocaine and amphetamine regulated transcript; MC4R, melanocortin 4 receptor; MCH, melanin-concentrating hormone; CCK, cholecystokinin. (*Source:* Modified from Fig. 1 in Flier JS, Maratos-Flier E: Obesity and the hypothalamus: Novel peptides for new pathways. Cell 92:437–440, 1998.)

CRH acting as a *neurotransmitter*

- suppresses appetite;
- increases anxiety;
- increases sympathetic outflow at least in part via oxytocin-producing parvocellular PVN neurons that project to the intermediolateral column

of the spinal cord. The increased sympathetic activity increases lipolysis and energy expenditure in part via the increased expression of uncoupling proteins.

The activity of these neurons is *stimulated* by leptin and appears to be suppressed by exogenously administered glucocorticoids. Central administration of a CRH *antagonist* attenuates the anorexic effect of leptin. Cushing's disease (pituitary adenoma) and Cushing's syndrome (ectopic ACTH, exogenous glucocorticoids) are associated with hyperphagia, which is attributed to the suppression of CRH tone.

CRH acting as a *neurohormone* increases the activity of the ACTH-adrenocortical axis. Leptin lowers the elevated glucocorticoid levels of *ob/ob* mice by suppressing CRH probably through a mechanism involving *neuropeptide Y* (NPY). NPY is a stimulator of the CRH–ACTH–cortisol axis. *Leptin inhibits NPY, thereby indirectly decreasing neurohormonal CRH activity.*

- In starvation, leptin decreases and allows increased output of cortisol by altering the setpoint of feedback. Cortisol is essential for the adaptation to starvation because it supports gluconeogenesis.
- In obesity (either due to leptin deficiency or leptin resistance), the tone of these CRH neurons is increased, and the negative feedback by cortisol to CRH is operating at an elevated setpoint ("perceived starvation amidst of abundance"). The increased tone of CRH explains that obesity is a mild *pseudocushing state*, with mildly elevated daily production of glucocorticoids. This condition is distinct from Cushing's disease (pituitary corticotroph adenoma), as indicated by the suppressibility of the ACTH–cortisol axis in obese subjects by the *low-dose dexamethasone test* (see Chap. 12). The peripheral action of endogenously overproduced cortisol contributes to the maintenance of obesity.

More severe pseudocushing states include *major depression* and *anorexia nervosa*. As indicated by increased concentrations of CRH in the CSF, the activity of neurohormonal and neurotransmitter-type CRH neurons is augmented in both conditions, which results in significantly increased daily cortisol production and elevated urinary free cortisol. In *major depression,* hypercortisolemia is associated with anxiety and weight loss. Depression may also be associated with weight gain that might be related to an altered circadian pattern of CRH activity. *Anorexia nervosa* patients have very low BMI and thus low circulating levels of leptin. It appears that these patients upregulate leptin receptors, and normalize leptin levels *in the CSF* before their BMI returns to normal.

Although Central Administration of NPY Evokes Virtually all Features of Leptin Deficiency, the Anorexic Effect of Leptin is Enhanced in NPY Knockout Mice NPY neurons in the ARC were the first recognized targets of leptin. NPY is the most potent centrally acting orexigenic agent known to date. Leptin tonically suppresses NPY. In leptin deficiency and leptin resistance, the tone of NPY increases. Central administration of NPY mimics almost every aspect of leptin deficiency, including hyperphagia, increased glucocorticoid secretion, and decreased activity of the TRH–TSH–thyroid axis. NPY knockout mice generated on an *ob/ob* leptin-deficient background display an attenuated degree of obesity, which indicates the physiologic role of the leptin–NPY pathway in the regulation of body weight.

Surprisingly, the anorexic action of exogenous leptin is uniquely amplified in NPY knockout mice. In NPY knockout mice, the response to anorexic agents such as CRH and MC4R agonists is unaltered. These results suggest that NPY may tonically antagonize the anorexic action mediated by other physiologic targets of leptin.

α-MSH and Agouti-Related Transcript are Leptin-Regulated Peptides Which Function as Competitive Antagonists on Melanocortin 4 Receptors

Whereas α-MSH activates both melanocyte MC1 and hypothalamic melanocortin 4 (MC4) receptors, the *agouti* protein (normally expressed only in the skin) functions as its competitive receptor antagonist (see Table 12-10). A mutation in normally lean black mice that results in the *widespread overexpression* of the agouti protein causes yellow (agouti) coat color by MC1R inhibition, and delayed onset obesity by MC4R inhibition (see Box 12-10).

The agouti protein and the *agouti-related transcript* (ART, also known as *agouti-related protein* [AGRP], encoded by chromosome 16q22) share the same molecular mechanism of action. However, in contrast with the agouti protein, ART is normally expressed in the hypothalamus and is a *physiologic* regulator of body weight and adiposity. Whereas NPY is coexpressed with ART, α-MSH (a derivative of proopiomelanocortin [POMC]) is coexpressed with *cocaine and amphetamine regulated transcript* (CART, encoded by chromosome 5). Note that the terms ART and CART refer not only to the mRNA (the transcript per se) but also to the peptide, which directly exerts the biologic effect. α-MSH/CART and NPY/ART are found in two distinct sets of neurons in the arcuate nucleus. Both sets of neurons express the long isoform of leptin receptor. Leptin stimulates α-MSH/CART and inhibits NPY/ART expression and neuronal activity. The peptides expressed by each set of neuron not only respond to leptin in a similar manner, but also exert a similar effect on food intake (Table 15-2).

The action of ART on the MC4R (and agouti on MC1R) requires a cofactor, known as *mahogany*, whose function may be the presentation of ART and agouti as the ligands for their respective melanocortin receptors. Mutations of the mahogany gene in agouti mice prevent the action of agouti, thereby reverting the yellow coat color to mahogany and preventing the development of obesity. Mahogany is a single-transmembrane domain protein that is expressed in many tissues, including pigment cells and the hypothalamus. The extracellular domain of the mahogany protein is the orthologue of human *attractin*, a circulating molecule produced by activated T cells that has been implicated in immune cell interactions.

Stimulation of MC4R exerts an anorexic action. Thus, α-MSH is anorexic, whereas its antagonist, ART, is orexigenic. It is likely that in addition to NPY, these peptides may modulate paraventricular CRH activity. Indeed, the main targets of α-MSH and ART are neurons in the PVN and the DMN. The DMN may provide connection to several areas of the brain, including the lateral hypothalamus, PVN, the reticular formation, and the *nucleus tractus solitarii* (NTS), which have been implicated in the regulation of feeding behavior and/or energy expenditure. Leptin resistance of obese MC4R knockout mice does not prevent the orexigenic actions of exogenous NPY or anorexic actions of exogenous CRF. Thus, CRH and (in part) NPY act downstream of the MC4R signaling (see Fig. 15-5).

Melanin Concentrating Hormone and Orexins are Orexigenic Peptides Produced by Neurons in the Lateral Hypothalamus It appears that the α-MSH/ART competition for the MC4R modulates the activity of orexigenic peptides, such as *orexin A and B* (also termed *hypocretins*) and *melanin concentrating hormone* (MCH). These peptides are produced by neurons found in the *lateral hypothalamus*, which, however, is not a major direct target of α-MSH, ART or leptin. Thus, α-MSH and ART might exert their action on MC4R-expressing neurons in the DMN, which project to the lateral hypothalamus, and inhibit MCH and orexins. Leptin may primarily modulate MCH and orexins via its action on the α-MSH-ART balance.

Hypocretins are *hypothalamic* peptides that have a structure similar to the gut hormone *secretin* (hence their name). Both orexin A and B are generated by the proteolytic cleavage of their common precursor (*preprohypocretin*). The peptides act on two distinct G-protein-linked receptors (*Hcrtr1* and *Hcrtr2*). Insulin-induced hypoglycemia increases the expression of preprohypocretin that eventually effects the hypoglycemia-associated sensation of hunger. In addition to their orexigenic action, hypocretins acting on Hcrtr2 have been implicated in the normal activation of the *motor excitatory* and the *arousal systems*. Dogs homozygous for spontaneous loss-of-function mutations of Hcrtr2 and preprohypocretin knockout mice suffer from *narcolepsy*, a disease characterized by sudden bouts of *cataplexy* (loss of muscle tone) and sleepiness ("sleep attacks").

MCH is a 19-amino-acid peptide originally identified in the intermediate lobe of teleost fish pituitary glands. MCH in the chum salmon causes the aggregation of melanophors (hence its name), thereby lightening skin color. MCH should not be confused with either melatonin or α-MSH. MCH is found in mammals only in the lateral hypothalamus and in the zona incerta.

It is of interest that ancestral pigment-regulating peptides are extensively involved in the mammalian regulation of energy homeostasis. MCH and α-MSH are antagonistic in both systems:

- Whereas α-MSH darkens, MCH lightens skin color in teleost fish.
- Whereas α-MSH decreases, MCH increases appetite in mammals.

In addition, the functions of agouti/ART and mahogany underscore the functional coupling of the regulation of pigment cells and feeding during evolution.

The Leptin-Mediated Long-Term Regulation of Body Weight is Coordinated with Short-Term Satiety Signals Emanating from the Gastrointestinal Tract During Ingestion of Food   Food intake is terminated by the feeling of *satiety*. As mentioned, plasma leptin displays episodic fluctuations which usually reach peak levels 2 to 3 hours after meals. Food intake therefore does not acutely stimulate leptin secretion and leptin is not the cause of the termination of food intake.

The *enterochromaffin cells* are members of the amine precursor uptake and decarboxylation (APUD) system. The enterochromaffin cells are scattered in the simple columnar epithelial lining of the gut, and respond to changes in the luminal fluid composition. These cells are also known as enteroendocrine cells because they secrete hormones into the abluminal ECF. An example of this mechanism is the secretion of glucagon-like peptide-1[7-37] (GLP-1[7-37]), the main incretin that modulates insulin secretion in response to increased luminal concentration of glucose in the gut (carbohydrate-rich meal; see Chap. 9).

Several peptide hormones produced by the enteroendocrine cells have been implicated in mediating the acute satiety during meals and the termination of food intake. The most important of these satiety hormones is *cholecystokinin* (CCK). The main source of circulating CCK is the small intestine, especially the duodenum and jejunum. The amounts of CCK produced by the ileum gradually decrease in an aboral direction. CCK is released upon protein- and lipid-rich ("filling") meals, and to a certain extent in response to acidification of the duodenum. Carbohydrates do not induce CCK secretion. CCK promotes satiety by several mechanisms:

- CCK inhibits gastric emptying. This effect allows proper processing of the duodenal content before the next bout of acidic gastric content reaches the small intestine. Continued feeding in combination with inhibited gastric emptying results in gastric distension. This is sensed by gastric stretch receptors, and the signal is conveyed by afferent vagal nerve fibers to the nucleus tractus solitarii (see Fig. 15-5).
- CCK stimulates CCK receptors expressed on these vagal sensory nerves. Systemically administered exogenous CCK induces satiety in the absence of gastric distension, but this effect still requires intact vagal afferent nerves.

The nucleus tractus solitarii integrates multiple signals that regulate feeding behavior. The effect of CCK and other satiety-inducing intestinal peptide hormones is to decrease *meal size*. However, if the leptin-mediated regulatory mechanisms continue to indicate insufficient lipid stores, *meal frequency* increases. This is well illustrated by an experiment, in which *free-feeding* rats received intraperitoneal CCK injections before each meal they initiated. CCK decreased meal size by 50%, but the animals initiated feeding twice as often, thereby eventually consuming the same amount of food and maintaining the same body weight. Thus, the mechanisms of long-term energy homeostasis supercede the short-term satiety-based regulation of food intake.

During ontogeny, the regulation of thirst and hunger develop in an interrelated manner. The newborn is on a liquid diet (breast milk) that simultaneously satisfies thirst and hunger. It is therefore not surprising that dehydration induces the sensation of hunger even in adults. Weight-loss diets invariably call for proper hydration as an integral part of the program.

RECOMMENDED LITERATURE

Adashi EY, Rock JA, Rosenwaks Z: *Reproductive Endocrinology, Surgery, and Technology.* Lippincott-Raven, 1996.

Bazer FW: *The Endocrinology of Pregnancy.* Clifton, NJ, Humana Press, 1998.

Braverman LE: *Diseases of the Thyroid.* Clifton, NJ, Humana Press, 1997.

Clark OH, Duh Q-Y D: *Textbook of Endocrine Surgery.* Philadelphia, Saunders, 1997.

Conn PM, Melmed S: *Endocrinology. Basic and Clinical Principles.* Clifton, NJ, Humana Press, 1997.

DeGroot LJ: *Endocrinology.* 3d ed, Philadelphia, Saunders, 1995.

Greenspan FS, Strewler GJ: *Basic and Clinical Endocrinology.* 5th ed, Stamford, Appleton & Lange, 1997.

Handwerger S: *Molecular and Cellular Basis of Pediatric Endocrinology.* Clifton, Humana Press, 1998.

Hershman JM: *Endocrine Pathophysiology. A Patient-oriented Approach.* 3d ed, Philadelphia, Lea & Febiger, 1988.

Kettyle WM, Arky RA: *Endocrine Pathophysiology.* Lippincott-Raven, 1998.

Manni A: *Endocrinology of Breast Cancer.* Clifton, NJ, Humana Press, 1998.

McDermott MT: *Endocrine Secrets.* 2d ed, Philadelphia, Hanley & Belfus, Inc., 1998.

Melmed S: *The Pituitary.* Oxford, Blackwell Science, 1995.

Moore WT, Eastman RC: *Diagnostic Endocrinology.* 2d ed, St. Louis, Mosby, 1996.

Norman AW, Litwack G: *Hormones.* 2d ed, San Diego, Academic Press, 1997,

Rosen CJ: Osteoporosis. *Diagnostic and Therapeutic Principles.* Clifton, NJ, Humana Press, 1996.

Sperling MA: *Pediatric Endocrinology.* Philadelphia, Saunders, 1996.

Tietz NW: *Clinical Guide To Laboratory Tests.* 3d ed, Philadelphia, Saunders, 1995.

Weintraub BD: *Molecular Endocrinology. Basic Concepts and Clinical Correlations.* New York, Raven Press, 1995.

Wenig BM, Heffess CS, Adair CF: *Atlas of Endocrine Pathology.* Philadelphia, Saunders, 1997.

Wilson JD, Foster DW, Kronenberg HM, Larsen PR: *Williams Textbook of Endocrinology.* 9th ed, Saunders, 1998.

Yen SSC, Jaffe RB, Barbieri: *Reproductive Endocrinology.* 4th ed, Philadelphia, Saunders, 1999.

ACCESSING MEDICAL INFORMATION ON THE WEB

Biomedical sciences develop at a rapid pace. To obtain up-to-date information, one cannot rely on textbooks alone. An important function of textbooks is to provide the conceptual framework into which one may fit new pieces of information. Quite often, however, medical students are overwhelmed with textbook material, and find little or no time to search for novel information that will not appear on their exams. For those who nevertheless have the time and the inclination for online search, the following web site is of major interest: ⟨http://www.ncbi.nlm.nih.gov⟩. At this web site, Pubmed (Medline) and the Entrez Browser are the most useful.

The Entrez Browser contains information about nucleotide and protein sequences. Most journals require that the authors provide the accession number of the sequence submitted for publication. Thus, the Entrez Browser usually contains information before it appears in Medline. In certain cases, the sequence is deposited but remains unpublished as a scientific paper. To find out whether a gene/cDNA of interest has been cloned, one may enter the name (such as *growth hormone receptor*) and the species (*human*). If chromosomal location is desired, the key word *chromosome* is also entered. A list is generated by the computer, from which one can choose the promising titles. When accessed, these titles display sequences, references, Medline link, and several other features.

Pubmed provides current information published by most biomedical journals. The information can be accessed by key words which appear in the medical subject headings, in the title, or in the abstract. Searches may be conducted by author names. It may be useful to combine the scientific term with the key word *review*. The abstract of most papers published after the late 1970's may be accessed via Medline; however, many review articles do not have an abstract. Review papers usually lag behind original research reports, but are more up to date than textbooks.

When entering key words, some experimentation may be needed. Greek characters should be spelled out (for example, *alpha*). In certain publications, an acronym may be separated from a numeral by a hyphen, in other publications the hyphen may be absent (such as GLUT-4 and GLUT4). There are inconsistencies in the use of terminology. For example, TRH is more frequently used than TRF, yet CRF is more frequently used than CRH. Some texts use the term *-liberin* for hypothalamic releasing hormones, such as *thyroliberin* for TRH. Acronyms can be misleading because the same acronym may be used with different meanings (such as ER for estrogen receptor and endoplasmic reticulum).

INDEX

Note: Boldface numbers indicate illustrations, page numbers followed by the letter *t* indicate tables.

ISBN 0-07-034432-9

90000

9 780070 344327